Recollections of Trauma
Scientific Evidence and Clinical Practice

NATO ASI Series

Advanced Science Institutes Series

A series presenting the results of activities sponsored by the NATO Science Committee, which aims at the dissemination of advanced scientific and technological knowledge, with a view to strengthening links between scientific communities.

The series is published by an international board of publishers in conjunction with the NATO Scientific Affairs Division

A	Life Sciences	Plenum Publishing Corporation
B	Physics	New York and London
C	Mathematical and Physical Sciences	Kluwer Academic Publishers Dordrecht, Boston, and London
D	Behavioral and Social Sciences	
E	Applied Sciences	
F	Computer and Systems Sciences	Springer-Verlag
G	Ecological Sciences	Berlin, Heidelberg, New York, London,
H	Cell Biology	Paris, Tokyo, Hong Kong, and Barcelona
I	Global Environmental Change	

PARTNERSHIP SUB-SERIES

1. Disarmament Technologies	Kluwer Academic Publishers
2. Environment	Springer-Verlag
3. High Technology	Kluwer Academic Publishers
4. Science and Technology Policy	Kluwer Academic Publishers
5. Computer Networking	Kluwer Academic Publishers

The Partnership Sub-Series incorporates activities undertaken in collaboration with NATO's Cooperation Partners, the countries of the CIS and Central and Eastern Europe, in Priority Areas of concern to those countries.

Recent Volumes in this Series:

Series A: Life Sciences

Recollections of Trauma
Scientific Evidence and Clinical Practice

Edited by
J. Don Read
The University of Lethbridge
Lethbridge, Alberta, Canada

and

D. Stephen Lindsay
University of Wales
Bangor, United Kingdom, and
University of Victoria
Victoria, British Columbia, Canada

Plenum Press
New York and London
Published in cooperation with NATO Scientific Affairs Division

Proceedings of a NATO Advanced Study Institute on
Recollections of Trauma: Scientific Evidence and Clinical Practice,
held June 1996,
in Port de Bourgenay, France

NATO-PCO-DATA BASE

The electronic index to the NATO ASI Series provides full bibliographical references (with
keywords and/or abstracts) to about 50,000 contributions from international scientists
published in all sections of the NATO ASI Series. Access to the NATO-PCO-DATA BASE is
possible in two ways:

—via online FILE 128 (NATO-PCO-DATA BASE) hosted by ESRIN, Via Galileo Galilei, I-00044
Frascati, Italy

—via CD-ROM "NATO Science and Technology Disk" with user-friendly retrieval software in
English, French, and German (©WTV GmbH and DATAWARE Technologies, Inc. 1989). The
CD-ROM also contains the AGARD Aerospace Database.

The CD-ROM can be ordered through any member of the Board of Publishers or through
NATO-PCO, Overijse, Belgium.

Library of Congress Cataloging in Publication Data

Recollections of trauma: scientific evidence and clinical practice / edited by J. Don Read
and D. Stephen Lindsay.
    p.   cm.—(NATO ASI series. Series A, Life sciences; v. 291)
    Includes bibliographical references and index.
    ISBN 0-306-45618-4
    1. Adult child sexual abuse victims—Congresses. 2. Recovered memory—Congresses. 3.
Autobiographical memory—Congresses. 4. Psychic trauma—Congresses. I. Read J. Don. II.
Lindsay, D. Stephen. III. Series.
RC569.5.A28R53 1997
616.85'8369—dc21   97-17155
                                                                                   CIP

ISBN 0-306-45618-4

© 1997 Plenum Press, New York
A Division of Plenum Publishing Corporation
233 Spring Street, New York, N. Y. 10013

http://www.plenum.com

10 9 8 7 6 5 4 3 2 1

Printed in the United States of America

PREFACE

The controversy regarding cases in which people report "recovered memories" of childhood sexual abuse may well prove to be the most important issue in professional psychology in the 1990s. Some have argued that such reports often reflect illusory beliefs inadvertently created by suggestive forms of "memory work" in psychotherapy. This claim amounts to a charge of widespread malpractice, and publicity about it threatens the reputation of clinical psychology. From a cultural/historical point of view, this controversy constitutes a crisis point in Western society's belated and still incomplete efforts to acknowledge and respond effectively to the shocking prevalence of child sexual abuse. "Responding effectively" entails both protecting children from abuse and avoiding false accusations. Some professionals who emphasise prevention of false accusations have described the popularisation of therapeutic searches for suspected hidden memories of childhood sexual abuse as a modern "witch hunt" in which suggestive therapies lead to false accusations (e.g., Ofshe & Watters, 1994). In turn, some who emphasise support of abuse victims have dismissed such arguments as anti-feminist "backlash" (e.g., Bloom, 1994). This political polarisation, which has been avidly fanned by the media, overlays the long-standing tension between experimental and clinical psychology. The mixture of a taboo subject, deep politicisation, and a historic rift within psychology creates an explosive cocktail, and it is not surprising that professional discussions of this topic have often generated more heat than light.

The aim of the NATO Advanced Studies Institute (ASI) on which this book is based was to create a situation that would facilitate productive and probing dialogue among an international group of experts with a variety of perspectives on memory for trauma. Most of the 95 participants were psychologists (including practitioners and clinical, cognitive, and neuroscience researchers), but the group also included anthropologists, legal scholars, and experts from other relevant fields. The remote and pleasant setting of the conference (which was held at Les Jardins de l'Atlantique, a lovely resort hotel on the French Atlantic) ensured that participants worked, ate, and socialised together throughout the 11-day meeting. Although gruelling, this situation fostered a convivial atmosphere, which in turn created opportunities for in-depth and probing discussions of difficult and controversial issues as professionals with diverse perspectives struggled to understand one anothers' views. To paraphrase remarks made by several participants, it is difficult to dehumanise someone you've just had breakfast with. The ASI did not, of course, eliminate differences in perspective, but it did succeed in enhancing mutual understanding and respect, promoting serious dialogue, and fostering future collaborative research efforts between researchers and clinicians who often held very different perspectives on the issue.

This book attempts to capture the content, as well as some of the process, of the ASI of the same name as this volume. During the meeting, each of the major lectures (Section I) was followed by a 30-minute commentary, which in turn was followed by a tape-recorded 30-minute discussion period. The book includes the text of thirteen lectures along with a written version of the accompanying peer commentary and selected excerpts from the discussion period. The lectures are presented in the same order in which they occurred during the ASI. There were also fifteen 30-minute papers (Section II), each of which is included (again, in the order in which the papers were given). The same brief format was also used in a single integrated symposium of six paper presentations on the legal issues surrounding recovered memories (Section III) organized and moderated by Daniel Shuman. Subgroups of 10–15 attendees also met over the course of the ASI to discuss particular focal issues (Section IV). These working groups provided opportunities for participants to engage in extended discussions of a particular issue, and the book includes reports on the fruits of these discussions authored by the facilitators: Agenda for Clinical Research (facilitated by Lucy Berliner and Judith McDougall), Agenda for Cognitive/Neuroscience Research (facilitated by Ira E. Hyman, Jr., and Jonathan W. Schooler), Issues Related to Guidelines for Clinical Practice (facilitated by Tara Ney and Fran Grunberg), and Concepts of Sexual Trauma in France (facilitated by Marie-Christine Simon de Bergen). The last chapter in this section represents an ongoing data-collection project completed by a much smaller workgroup of Steve Lindsay and Jonathan Schooler and presents a brief overview of the results of a questionnaire distributed to participants at the beginning of the ASI. The questionnaire asked participants about a range of issues relevant to the controversy regarding recovered memories of childhood trauma. Lindsay and Schooler note that the questionnaire suffered from numerous shortcomings, but contend that its most striking finding may well reflect the current state of knowledge in this area: opinions on many issues varied extremely widely, both between and within subgroups of participants, and rarely if ever did opinions divide neatly between practitioners and researchers. Finally, the ASI also included three evening poster sessions, and abstracts of the 58 posters are presented in the penultimate section (V) of the book. Preceding a subject index (SectionVI) are presented the names, affiliations, mail and e-mail (where available) addresses of all of the participants. Readers are encouraged to contact these individuals for discussion and provision of additional relevant reading materials.

Thus this book is a somewhat polished representation of an 11-day effort by a substantial number of highly regarded experts with a wide range of perspectives to communicate with one another on the topic of the relationship between trauma, memory, and remembering. We owe a tremendous debt to each of the participants in the scientific programme for their thoughtful and stimulating contributions and to all of the attendees for their vigorous participation in the discussions throughout the ASI conference and we record here our gratitude to all of them. We also express our profound appreciation to Sherrill Mulhern for her wonderfully successful efforts in selecting the site for the meeting and working tirelessly with the excellent hotel staff to coordinate the many details of our accommodations. It is no exaggeration to say that the meeting would not have been as successful without Sherrill's efforts. The NATO Scientific Affairs Board is thanked for providing the funding that made both the ASI and this book possible. As well, we would like to thank Elaine Hunter, who worked with the technical staff at the hotel to record all of the discussion sessions following the presentations, for her great success in deciphering and transcribing those comments into written form. Two skillful people at the University of Lethbridge provided tremendous support and assistance during the conference organisational and book preparation stages, Lisa Bjorn and Karen Larsen, respectively, and we also owe them a debt of gratitude. Finally, we thank Robert Wheeler, Eileen Bermingham and, in particular, Meri Zeltser at Plenum for assistance in the speedy production of this book.

J. Don Read
D. Stephen Lindsay

REFERENCES

Bloom, S. L. (1994). Hearing the survivor's voice: Sundering the wall of denial. *Journal of Psychohistory, 21,* 461–477.
Ofshe, R., & Watters, E. (1994). Making monsters: *False memories, psychotherapy, and sexual hysteria.* New York: Scribner.

CONTENTS

I. PRIMARY LECTURES

II. BRIEF PAPERS

III. LEGAL PANEL

IV. REPORTS OF THE WORKING GROUPS

POSTER ABSTRACTS

INCREASING SENSITIVITY

D. Stephen Lindsay

School of Psychology
University of Wales—Bangor
and
Department of Psychology
University of Victoria
Victoria, B.C. V8W 3P5 Canada

The title of this lecture is intended to have two meanings, one having to do with our sensitivity as participants in this Advanced Studies Institute (ASI) and the other having to do with the concept of sensitivity in signal detection theory and its application to the issue of memory work and recovered memories. I shall start with some comments on the former and finish up with the latter, with a discussion of research on memory suggestibility in between.

1. CULTIVATING SENSITIVITY AS PARTICIPANTS IN THE ASI

With regard to the first meaning of my title—our sensitivity as participants in this ASI—I am in danger of preaching. But perhaps that is not entirely inappropriate. Whatever our areas of specialisation, and whatever our perspectives on the controversy surrounding the topic of adulthood recollections of childhood trauma, we are all of us human beings, and the pitfalls that beset our discussions of trauma and memory have as much to do with basic human foibles of the sort often addressed in sermons (e.g., pride, greed, obstreperousness) as they have to do with the scientific evidence. Moreover, this particular topic is fraught with difficult moral issues. Thus a bit of preaching may not be out of order. My hope is that my sermon, in this first lecture of the ASI, will be of some practical use in setting the tone for a genuine and searching exploration of what we do and do not yet know about the relationship between childhood trauma and adulthood recollections.

Social psychological research confirms the commonplace that when people publicly aver a position on an issue—especially an extreme position—they sometimes become overly committed to that position and defend it dogmatically, rejecting out of hand evidence that conflicts with that belief and interpreting questionable evidence (or the absence of evidence) as support for that belief (e.g., Fiske & Taylor, 1991). Scientists seem, to my eye, to be as vulnerable to this "entrenchment effect" as most other people; indeed, a fair

Recollections of Trauma, edited by Read and Lindsay
Plenum Press, New York, 1997

amount of scientific research is driven by scientists who stake out an extreme position and defend it against contrary evidence.

Although there is a place for stubborn defense of one's own beliefs, I hope that most will agree that this ASI is not such a place. Rather than entrenching ourselves in our established positions, I hope we will be open to entertaining new and sometimes qualitatively different kinds of evidence and arguments. I do not mean to suggest that we relinquish our moral principles, or even worse that we abandon critical thinking. On the contrary, we will rely on our keenest critical skills to make progress toward understanding. But I hope that we will be sensitive in the sense of being open to thinking carefully about the arguments and evidence presented. It is true that science—all science, not just psychology—is informed by intuition and carried out with conviction, rather than being conducted in vacuous objectivity, but it is also true that genuine progress in science requires openness to observation and willingness to change.

I also hope that we will be sensitive in the sense of being aware and respectful of one anothers' feelings. In North America and some other areas, this topic has given rise to vitriolic attacks in which individuals on one "side" have vilified individuals on the other. Some individuals have been publicly described as reckless, money-grubbing quacks, others as patriarchal perpetrator protectors. I'm not sure which of these slurs is worse, but I am confident that no one here believes that either sort of epithet can justly be applied to his or her own work, and I am also confident that this sort of name calling is not helpful. To emphasise yet another meaning of my pet term, such attacks have overly sensitised some participants in the debate, such that it is difficult for them not to over-react to certain kinds of stimuli. There may well be people on both sides of this controversy who are unethical opportunists, but the vast majority of participants in this debate do not fit that description. On the contrary, most are people with a deeply felt commitment to responding to a serious problem. Some of us have worked personally with parents whose adult offspring underwent outlandishly suggestive therapies and ultimately came to believe that they had been subjected to years of extremely bizarre and frankly implausible forms of sexual abuse. Some of us have worked personally with clients who were sexually abused by loved ones, and who struggle greatly in trying to come to terms with their histories. Both kinds of cases are heartrending, and it is not surprising that working with them gives rise to strong feelings.

We have a long road ahead of us, both in the immediate future—11 days of working and socialising together cheek and jowl—and in the long term, as psychology and the broader culture come to terms with the various implications and ramifications of this issue. Progress will be swifter and more sure if all parties involved in the discussion maintain a reasoned openness to evidence and argument and a degree of civility and human kindness.

As one means of fostering this kind of sensitivity, I suggest that we all do our best to avoid extremist positions. Doing so will not only enhance our interactions, but will also move us closer to science. For example, surely no one could argue that it is impossible for people to remember long-forgotten childhood traumas. Quite the contrary, the evidence we have on this issue suggests that people can indeed remember previously forgotten childhood traumas (e.g., chapters in this volume by Andrews; Carlson, Armstrong, & Loewenstein; Dalenberg; Schooler, Ambadar, & Bendiksen; and Williams & Banyard). Similarly, surely no one would argue that it is impossible for people to come to believe that they suffered childhood traumas that did not actually occur (e.g., commentary and chapter in this volume by Mulhern and Loftus). Here again, the evidence, to which I will turn shortly, argues against such an assertion. Thus, it is not a simple, dichotomous question of whether or not long-forgotten experiences can later be remembered, nor of whether or not illusory memories can be experienced. We can state with some certainty that both of these happen. Instead, we must grapple with a host of questions regarding how and why and when such phenomena occur, what they mean, and how we should respond to them. These are questions that clinical psychologists and some memory researchers, neuroscientists, and other scholars have studied in their separate and different ways for years, well before the current controversy erupted. I hope the ASI lectures, papers, working groups, and discussions will delve into the intricate subtleties raised by the controversy regarding recovered memories, and that by joining forces we can make substantial progress toward understanding these difficult issues.

In pursuing that objective, it may be helpful to acknowledge that we are, each of us, susceptible to biases that can distort judgment. Classic research by Tversky and Kahneman (e.g., 1974) and others reveals that human reasoners often rely on heuristics, or mental shortcuts, when making judgments. For example, when estimating how common or probable a particular kind of event is, people typically rely on the "availability" heuristic: The more quickly and easily examples of a particular kind of event can be brought to mind, the greater the perceived commonness or probability of events of that kind. To illustrate this with a trivial example, if you ask people which is more common, English words that begin with R or English words that have R as the third letter, most people confidently assert that there are more words that begin with R. In fact, however, there are approximately three times more words that have R as the third letter. The error occurs because it is easier to retrieve words cued by first letter than by third letter. The point is that many factors other than the objective frequency or probability of a particular kind of event contribute to the ease with which examples come to mind, such as the vividness of the examples one has happened to encounter, and these factors can greatly distort judgments about the commonness or probability of events.

Such heuristics are of more than academic interest, because they have direct relevance to clinical work. For example, I recently came across a 1965 study by Oskamp (republished in 1982), in which experienced clinicians and psychology students were given four incremental blocks of information about an actual patient's background, starting with a block of demographic information and progressively providing more and more detailed information about the patient's past. After each block of information, participants answered the same set of questions abut the patient's current attitudes, beliefs, etc. (which they were to answer based on the information about the patient's background) and rated their confidence in their answers. Participants were invited to change their answers to the questions after each successive block of background information, but they rarely did so, and the rate of changing answers decreased sharply across blocks. That is, respondents seemed to lock into answers fairly early on, and stick with them regardless of additional information. Even after all four blocks of information, accuracy was not significantly above chance. Most importantly, even at the outset most respondents were slightly more confident than they should have been given their chance-level accuracy, and over blocks confidence grew dramatically, such that by the end of the task respondents were often very confident in answers—right or wrong. Interestingly, the experienced clinicians in this study were no more accurate, and no less confident in their inaccurate judgments, than the students. Oskamp speculated that participants started out by making their best guesses and thereafter interpreted new information as support for those guesses, eventually becoming quite confident in erroneous conclusions. This is an example of "confirmatory bias"—that is, the human tendency to look for and focus on evidence that appears to support their beliefs.

A related phenomenon is termed "illusory correlation." People often perceive correlations that do not actually exist. For example, in a classic study by Smedslund, nurses studied 100 "case histories," each of which indicated whether or not a patient had a particular symptom and whether or not the patient had a particular disease (see Shweder, 1977). Nurses were asked if the symptom and disease were correlated, and 85% indicated that they were. In fact, however, although there were many cases in which the disease and the symptom co-occurred, there were also many cases in which the symptom occurred without the disease, and there was no correlation between the two. Similarly, Chapman and Chapman (1967) found that psychology students often reported correlations between features of patients' drawings and the patients' psychiatric diagnoses (e.g., students reported that paranoid patients tended to draw faces with large eyes) even though the drawings and diagnoses had been randomly paired and there were no such relationships. One explanation of this phenomenon is that human reasoners tend to focus on the positive cases—that is, they go about assessing a relationship by thinking of cases in which X was positive and Y was also positive; if many positive-positive cases come to mind, they think that the two are correlated. A slightly more careful reasoner might also consider the frequency of cases in which X was positive and Y negative, but this too is insufficient: One cannot assess correlation without considering all four cells.

Don Read and I and others have previously cited evidence of reliance on heuristics and biases in human judgment in the context of arguments regarding the fallibility of clinical judgment (e.g., Lindsay & Read, 1994). I stand by those arguments, but it is important that we keep in mind that researchers too are susceptible to such heuristics and biases. Heuristics and biases can influence scientists' interpretation of findings, summaries of the research literature, and generalisations from studies to other situations. There are countless cases in the history of science—all sciences, not just psychology—in which researchers believed passionately in a particular interpretation of data that ultimately proved to be wrong. I am not saying that scientific psychology is just as vulnerable to distortions and biases as non-scientific approaches. What I am saying is that good scientists must be aware of the role of subjective judgment in their work, and should regard their own beliefs, interpretations, and generalisations with some of the same scepticism with which they view the subjective beliefs of other people.

Another way of putting what I am trying to drive at here is that people on all sides of this issue should try to tolerate uncertainty. Clinician Phil Mollon (1996) recently made some quite elegant arguments in this regard. He pointed out that people seem quite keen on being certain about things, even when there is not sufficient foundation to justify certainty, and even when certainty stands in the way of progress and development. So let's balance our convictions with an acknowledgment of the many uncertainties.

It is not easy to be open to alternative arguments and evidence regarding an issue about which one feels very strongly. In their text on social cognition, Fiske and Taylor (1991) reviewed a body of evidence that shows that when people feel stressed and under pressure they tend to simplify their attitudes and beliefs—that is, tend to view things in black and white terms. Fiske and Taylor noted that, in the heat of controversy, "Research on one's own side of the issue seems flawless and extraordinarily relevant by comparison to evidence for the other side...An impartial observer, who describes both sides as having strong and weak points, will be perceived as biased and hostile by both sides" (Fiske & Taylor, 1991, p. 150). I think it may be useful to acknowledge this human tendency, and to try to avoid it.

I will not pretend to be an "impartial observer." On the contrary, I likely have fairly strong biases, because I do have an agenda. In the interest of communication, let me state that agenda explicitly: I believe that highly suggestive approaches to "memory work" have been widely popularised, that such approaches can lead people to develop illusory memories or false beliefs regarding childhood sexual abuse, and that such approaches have inadvertently harmed substantially numbers of clients and families. My aim is to convince practitioners that they should avoid suggestive approaches to memory work. I seek to pursue this agenda in ways that do not undermine support for survivors of childhood sexual abuse.

It may be helpful, in pursuing that agenda, to clear up some misunderstandings that sometimes get in the way of constructive dialogue on this topic. From my admittedly biased point of view, one of the most important of these is the erroneous belief that anyone who expresses concerns about suggestive approaches to memory wok in therapy is thereby denying the reality of childhood sexual abuse. This is like saying that criticising use of electroconvulsive shock therapy (ECT) as a treatment for schizophrenia amounts to denying the reality of schizophrenia. No doubt there are people who both criticise suggestive memory work and deny the reality of childhood sexual abuse as an important social problem, just as there likely are people who both criticise ECT and deny the reality of schizophrenia as a serious disorder, but such views are thankfully rare exceptions. For my part, although I think that some writers have exaggerated the societal importance of childhood sexual abuse as a psychopathogen (relative to child neglect, child poverty, and other nonsexual forms of child physical and emotional abuse), I do not doubt that harmful sexual abuse of children occurs at rates many times higher than once was thought, and that this is an important social problem that demands continued efforts to protect children, support survivors, and prosecute and treat perpetrators. The vast majority of critics of memory work share these views. Consider the following quotations:

"Sex abuse is a frequent and frightful experience with potentially disastrous consequences..." (Lief, 1992)

"Child sex abuse is a widespread and ancient phenomenon." (Gardner, 1992).

"There is little doubt that actual childhood sexual abuse is tragically common. Child abuse constitutes a serious social problem. I do not question the commonness of childhood sexual abuse . . . . The appearance of abuse statistics is one battle in the war waged against an earlier tendency . . . to disbelieve the abuse reports of women and children—a tendency that we should all deplore." (Loftus, 1993)

"We know that sexual abuse of children exists. There is empirical evidence to substantiate that the sexual abuse of children exists to a much greater extent than we previously recognised. It is a reprehensible crime. Every effort should be made to help victims of sexual abuse and to create a social climate in which abuse does not continue to take place. (FMS Scientific and Professional Advisory Board, 1994)

Similar statements appear in writings by many other critics of memory work, including those by Don Read and myself (e.g., Lindsay & Read, 1994, 1995; Read & Lindsay, 1994). I believe that productive dialogue will be enhanced if clinicians acknowledge that criticisms of memory work do not entail denial of child sexual abuse. Similarly, discussion may be facilitated if critics of memory work acknowledge that concern about the psychological well-being of survivors of abuse does not entail denial of the risks of suggestive memory work.

Productive dialogue regarding memory work and recovered memories has also been stymied by a tendency to simplify complex issues by turning continua into dichotomies: Abused versus not abused; remembered versus forgotten; recovered versus always known. I have been guilty of such dichotomisation at times myself, but I think it gets in the way of understanding, and that we must work on improving both our language and our measures. For example, although psychologists often speak as though individuals either always fully remembered or never remembered a traumatic event, in fact there are many shades of grey here (e.g., remembering in some ways and not in others) (see Schooler et al., this volume).

Having made this point, it is nonetheless worth emphasising that the focus of critics of memory work has been on cases in which people who presented for common psychological problems and appeared initially to believe that they had no history of abuse underwent a prolonged, multifaceted, socially influenced search for hidden memories whose possible existence was suggested by a therapist or self-help guide and who subsequently experienced memory recovery. Conversely, most practitioners whose work includes treatment of sexual abuse focus on clients who report abuse histories without undergoing such suggestive searches. Thus we sometimes talk at cross purposes, because people with different backgrounds use the same words but with quite different concepts in mind.

Another misunderstanding that has sometimes obstructed constructive dialogue has to do with the question of how easy it is to lead people to develop illusory memories or false beliefs about traumatic childhood events. Some sources claim that many practitioners are now afraid even to broach the issue of childhood sexual abuse for fear of being accused of leading their clients to develop false memories. This, in my view, reflects a misunderstanding of the criticisms and of the relevant scientific evidence. I will turn now to a brief review of that literature.

2. RESEARCH ON SUGGESTIBILITY

Researches have learned quite a bit about suggestibility over the course of the last two decades, inspired by the pioneering work of Beth Loftus (e.g., Loftus, 1979, 1991). In my view, that literature indicates that people are unlikely to develop illusory memories or false beliefs regarding traumatic childhood events in response to direct and straightforward questions about their trauma histories. The situation is complicated in this regard by the prevalence of self-help books, newspaper and magazine articles, radio and television shows, novels, and movies that have widely popularised the idea that people with psychological problems often have repressed histories of childhood sexual abuse, and I think it would be good practice to assess the extent to which a client has been exposed to such ideas if one is going to ask about childhood sexual abuse (cf. Courtois, this volume). It may also be that people with certain disorders are extraordinarily susceptible to suggestion. But research does not support the notion that people are likely to develop illusory memories of traumatic events in response to a few straightforward questions (for more detailed and complete reviews of the evidence for this argument, see Lindsay & Read, 1994, 1995).

In my view, scientific research on eyewitness suggestibility tells an impressively consistent and coherent story. Taking that literature as a whole, comparisons across and within studies indicate that, all else being equal, it is much easier to create false memories of trivial details than it is to create false memories of dramatic real-life experiences. For example, a single passing suggestion about a trivial detail in a video tape can lead many people falsely to report that they remember seeing the suggested detail in the video, but a single passing suggestion about childhood sexual abuse would be extremely unlikely to lead people falsely to report remembering non-experienced abuse. On the other hand, research indicates that prolonged, multifaceted suggestive influences can indeed lead people to develop illusory memories and/or false beliefs of traumatic childhood events that never really happened.

It is sometimes claimed that research on suggestibility should not be generalised to memory work. For example, it has been argued that because the participants in research are not all trauma survivors research on memory suggestibility cannot be generalised to trauma survivors. This argument entirely misses the point: Concern about suggestive memory work focuses on its potential ill-effects for clients who are not trauma survivors. (In any case, there is little reason to believe that trauma survivors are less suggestible than other people.) Another argument that has been advanced against generalising from studies of memory suggestibility is that the studies do not involve psychotherapy clients in situations that directly mirror therapy. I see little reason to assume that therapy clients are less suggestible than other people, and the suggestive power of some therapy situations, which I will describe shortly, dwarf those of research studies.

A third argument against generalisation is that the false memories created in research studies are not false memories of childhood sexual abuse. This argument will never be directly refuted by experimental research, because ethics bar researchers from testing the hypothesis that suggestions can lead people falsely to believe that they were sexually abused by their parents. But the argument is not so strong as it might appear. For one thing, there are documented real-world cases in which people recovered memories that are demonstrably false or extremely implausible. Examples include reported memories of bizarre and murderous satanic rituals; memories of abusive events during the first days of life, or even in the womb or during past lives; UFO abductions; and memories of events that would have left unambiguous physical evidence in the absence of such evidence (see Lindsay & Read, 1995, for references). The point of citing such examples is not to imply that all experiences of memory recovery should be attributed to the same mechanisms that give rise to illusory memories and false beliefs such as these; rather, the point is merely that such cases demonstrate that people can experience illusory memories of traumatic childhood events.

This anecdotal evidence is supported by recent studies that provide relatively close analogies to false memories of childhood sexual abuse. Several participants at this ASI have undertaken such research, and I will not steal their thunder by describing their dramatic findings. Instead, I will restrict my report to a brief description of a study that Colleen Kelley, David Amodio, and I recently completed. Our procedure more closely mirrors memory work in therapy than the procedures used in most studies of suggestibility, in that we did not suggest the occurrence of a particular event but rather of a general class of events. In our procedure, right-handed undergraduates performed a series of tests that, we told them, might be able to detect right-handed adults who were born with a left-hand preference. After performing the tests, 15 participants were told that the results indicated that they were probably born with a right-hand preference. Another 30 participants were told that the results indicate that they may have been born with a left-hand preference. We told all participants that our test was new and tentative, and that we were not sure if it worked, and asked each of them to spend an hour doing some take-home exercises to see if they could remember any early childhood experiences that might have encouraged them to switch from a left-hand preference to a right-hand preference. Of the 30 people who were told that the test results indicated a possible congenital left-handedness, 15 were also given instructions, modelled after exercises in *The Courage to Heal* (Bass &

Davis, 1988), that asked them to suspend critical judgment about any thoughts and images that came to mind when trying to remember handedness-shaping experiences. Later, participants completed a questionnaire about their memories and were then debriefed.

Of the 15 people in the right-handed diagnosis condition, 2 (13%) reported memories of early childhood experiences of being discouraged from using their left hand. In contrast, 6 of 15 (40%) in the left-handed diagnosis condition, and 7 of 15 (47%) in the left-handed plus lax memory monitoring condition, reported such memories. Here are some examples:

> I remember my mother saying, "We don't eat with our left hands" . . . I remember my siblings making fun of me and would call me names of left-handed people whenever they saw me doing anything with my left hand, so that I would stop doing it . . . A very faint image of my left hand reaching for something but not being allowed to take it until I reached with my right.

It is possible, of course, that these are accurate memories. It is important to note, however, that all participants worked on remembering such experiences, so the effect of "diagnosis," which tripled reports of memories of handedness-shaping, remains striking and informative; at minimum these results show that diagnoses can have dramatic effects on the likelihood that people will report memories consistent with the diagnosis.

Moreover, diagnosis also affected people's subsequent reports about their beliefs. We asked people to rate the likelihood that they were born left-handed. As shown in Table 1, only 1 of the 15 subjects in the right-handed condition gave a response at the mid-point of the scale, but 9 of those in the left-handed condition, and 12 of those in the left-handed/lax condition, responded at or above the mid-point of the scale. Four of the 30 subjects in the left-hand conditions (13%) indicated that "It is probable that I was born with a left-hand preference." Thus a single suggestive session, followed by a single hour of memory work, had a dramatic effect on both reported memories and reported beliefs about childhood events. (Although there were non-significant trends in the predicted direction, the "lax" instructions did not reliably increase the effects of diagnosis.)

Sceptics can always argue that the analogy from research studies such as this to the clinical situation is imperfect, but the onus shifts to explaining why one should not generalise in the interest of parsimony. Moreover, I would argue that, when in doubt, therapists have a moral responsibility to minimise the risk of harming their clients. By analogy, if small doses of a drug were shown to cause blindness in rats, one would not continue prescribing the drug to humans on the grounds that the studies differed too much from the clinical situation; rather, one would be very cautious in using the drug until it was shown

Table 1. Number of participants selecting each of the response options regarding the likelihood that they were born with a left-hand preference, as a function of condition

Response option	Condition		
	Right	Left	Left+Lax
Almost sure not	6	1	0
Improbable	8	5	3
Possible	1	7	10
Probable	0	2	2
Almost sure	0	0	0

Note. There was a reliable effect of condition, Chi square = 20.23, p < .003.

to be safe. Note that this doesn't mean that one would stop treating people, but simply that one would be cautious in using the controversial intervention.

3. FACTORS THAT DETERMINE THE LIKELIHOOD OF ILLUSORY MEMORIES/FALSE BELIEFS

The procedures used in the Kelley et al. study described above, and in related studies by Loftus and her colleagues (e.g., Loftus & Pickrell, 1995) and Hyman and his colleagues (e.g., Hyman, Husband, & Billings, 1995), create quite powerful suggestive influences. For example, the Kelley et al. study drew on the mystique of science and had people spend an hour working on conjuring up memories. These are powerful suggestive influences, but they are trivially weak compared to some forms of memory work, described in more detail below.

The likelihood that suggestions will lead to false memories depends on several factors (see Lindsay & Read, 1994, for references). These can be divided into three major categories: First, all else being equal, people are more susceptible to suggestions about things that they do not remember very well. For example, a long delay after witnessing or experiencing the event in question generally increases susceptibility to suggestions. Similarly, people may be more susceptible to suggestions regarding childhood events than to suggestions regarding adulthood events. Second, people are more likely to be influenced by "strong" suggestions than weak ones. Many factors determine the overall strength of suggestions, including the perceived authority of the source of the suggestions, perceived plausibility of the suggestions, repetition of suggestions, factors that enhance imagery of suggestions, and factors that lower individuals' criteria for accepting thoughts and images as memories. Third, there is mounting evidence that some people are more susceptible to suggestions than others, perhaps because of individual differences in some of the factors I've just mentioned (i.e., clarity of autobiographical memory, responsiveness to authority, imagery skills, etc.).

The approaches to memory work that most alarm me combine many and sometimes all of the factors that have been shown to increase the likelihood that people will develop illusory memories or false beliefs. In some cases, the therapist, a trusted authority, communicates a rationale for the plausibility of hidden memories of long-ago childhood trauma by telling the client that many people with his or her symptoms have hidden memories, that the client's physical symptoms and dreams evidence them, that doubt is sometimes a sign of "denial," and that healing may depend on recovering hidden memories of childhood trauma. Clients receiving memory work are often repeatedly exposed to suggestive information from multiple sources, such as anecdotes in popular books, other survivors' stories, comments and interpretations offered by a therapist, etc. Such information may provide a "script" for recovering memories and self-identifying as a survivor, as well as suggestions of particular details. Such information may also create biases in the way clients interpret ambiguous events (e.g., dreams, physical symptoms, and emotions may come to be interpreted as evidence of hidden memories of childhood trauma). Memory work may also involve techniques such as hypnosis, guided imagery, sodium amytal, etc., which enhance imagery and lower response criterion such that people are more likely than they would normally be to interpret thoughts, feelings, and images as memories. The therapist may also endorse the client's abuse-related reports as accurate memories, and counter the client's expressions of doubt. These converging suggestive influences often unfold gradually over a period of months of therapy sessions, sometimes supplemented with homework exercises, self-help books, and survivors' meetings. Such approaches need not be overtly coercive—that is, the therapist may neither intend to be nor be perceived as coercive, but rather as a caring guide through uncharted territory.

It is these sorts of long-term, multifaceted approaches to memory work, which combine many of the factors that contribute to the formation of false beliefs and illusory memories, that most alarm me. We know that some therapists have used such approaches (see Lindsay & Read, 1995). Some have published descriptions of such approaches in books and articles in the professional and popular press, and others have released therapy notes in court cases that attest to the use of extraordinarily suggestive searches for suspected hidden memories. Former clients have provided yet other accounts. Of course, most therapists who use memory work do not employ all of the suggestive practices I've enumerated. Approaches to memory work range along a continuum, from those that pose little or no risk to those that pose substantial risk of leading clients to develop illusory memories. My concern focuses on use of particularly risky techniques to help clients search for suspected hidden memories.

4. PREVALENCE OF SUGGESTIVE MEMORY WORK

How prevalent are such approaches? We really do not know, but recent surveys suggest that potentially risky approaches to memory work are not the exclusive domain of a tiny fringe of unqualified therapists. For example, Yapko (1994) surveyed hundreds of U.S. practitioners attending workshops and conventions related to hypnotherapy, and found a truly frightening prevalence of erroneous beliefs concerning the reliability of hypnosis as a tool for helping people remember early childhood events. The results of Poole, Lindsay, Memon, and Bull's (1995) national survey of 145 U.S. doctoral therapists who work with women clients, randomly sampled from the National Register of Health Service Providers in Psychology, was reassuring in some ways but alarming in others. On the one hand, most respondents indicated that searching for hidden memories of childhood trauma is not a central focus of their therapy. On the other hand, 75% indicated that they had made at least some use of special techniques, such as hypnosis and guided imagery, with the specific aim of helping clients remember childhood sexual abuse. There was virtually no agreement about which techniques should and should not be used for this purpose. Collectively, the respondents listed a huge range of symptoms (e.g., sexual dysfunction, relationship problems, low self-esteem, depression, anxiety, sleep disorders, eating disorders, born-again Christianity, etc.) as "indicators" of childhood sexual abuse, and there was very little agreement across respondents about which symptoms are indicators. Furthermore, 25% reported a constellation of beliefs and practices that, in my view, justify concern. This minority indicated that they (a) believe that it is important for survivors to remember the abuse for therapy to be effective, (b) are sometimes "fairly certain" after the first session with a client who reports no abuse that s/he had in fact been abused, and (c) use two or more special techniques to help clients remember childhood sexual abuse. These criteria are too lax to limit this subgroup to those who use the most extreme and suggestive approaches, but they are sufficient to warrant concern. This subgroup, who reported working with a collective total of 3,542 women in the previous 2 years, claimed high rates of memory recovery among their clients. In view of our relatively small sample size (145) and relatively low return rate (40%), these findings may overestimate the prevalence of memory work among U.S. doctoral psychotherapists, but even if the sample is assumed to be maximally non-representative (i.e., even if 100% of those who did not return the survey did not meet criteria for "memory focused" respondents), the results are still alarming. Our results for a small sample of British psychologists indicated less use of hypnosis as a means of fomenting memory recovery but few other differences were found between U.S. and British therapists.

Bottoms, Beety, Goodman, Tyda, and Shaver (1995) reported survey findings from 358 APA clinicians. Of these, 73% reported at least one case in which an adult client had recovered memories of a traumatic event. The more revealing finding, I think, is that a small percentage of respondents reported very large numbers of such cases (e.g., 9 therapists reported more than 100 such cases, including one psychologist who reported 260 clients who had recovered trauma memories). Bottoms et al. reported detailed analyses of 425 reports of cases of recovered memories. Interesting highlights of their findings include the facts that 90% of the recovered traumatic events were of childhood sexual abuse and 90% of the cases involved recovered memories of alleged repeated abuse. Therapy was the most frequently reported trigger of recovered memories.

The BPS survey of 810 Chartered Registered practitioners, published last year, might seem at first glance to present a much more reassuring picture, primarily because it emphasises findings indicating that people often experience memory recovery outside of therapy (Andrews, Morton, Bekerian, Brewin, Davies, & Mollon, 1995). In fact, however, all of the studies to date paint a quite consistent picture: The majority of highly trained psychotherapists do not go on highly suggestive hunts for suspected hidden memories, yet a small but non-trivial percentage do, and a sizable percentage sometimes use potentially risky techniques more selectively.

5. LOWERING RISK WITHOUT LOWERING SENSITIVITY

It has sometimes been claimed that if trauma-oriented therapists avoided use of potentially suggestive approaches to explore the possibility that clients have non-remembered abuse histories, they would inevitably be less likely to detect real survivors. The person who has most clearly articulated the view is cognitive psychologist Kathy Pezdek (1994). Pezdek drew on signal detection theory (SDT) to make her point. SDT is a method that yields separate estimates of "sensitivity," the extent to which a perceiver can discriminate between positive and negative cases, and "response bias," the extent to which the perceiver tends to be liberal or conservative in assessing the evidence for a positive case. SDT was initially developed in the context of perceptual judgment tasks. Imagine, for example, a radar operator trying to discriminate between blips and flashes of light that represent aircraft (referred to as "signal") versus blips and flashes of light that occur on a radar screen due to various uninteresting events such as static or birds (referred to as "noise"). The blips of light vary in their strength. On average, blips that are due to noise are weaker than blips that are due to aircraft, but some noise blips are quite strong—stronger than some of those caused by aircraft. Thus frequency distributions of the signal strengths of many occurrences of the two types of events would overlap (Figure 1, Panel A). Sensitivity is represented by the separation of the two distributions. If the noise and signal distributions overlap a lot, then there is very little sensitivity—that is, the perceiver is not sensitive to differences between noise and signal. If the two distributions overlap very little, then there is high sensitivity—that is, the perceiver is very sensitive to differences between noise and signal.

Sensitivity alone does not determine when the radar operator will hit the alarm button and when he or she won't. Response criterion, also called bias, refers to the signal strength above which the radar operator will identify a blip as a signal. If the operator believes that aircraft are likely to attack, and that it is important that the base be alerted to any possibility of aircraft, then the operator will use a liberal criterion, hitting the alarm button even when the blips are quite weak. This means the operator will rarely miss an aircraft, but it also means that s/he will have many false alarms. Conversely, if the operator believes that aircraft are unlikely, and that false alarms should be avoided, he or she will use a conservative response criterion, only pressing the button if the blips are very strong.

Panel A:

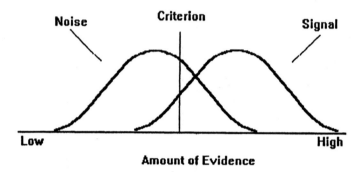

Panel B:

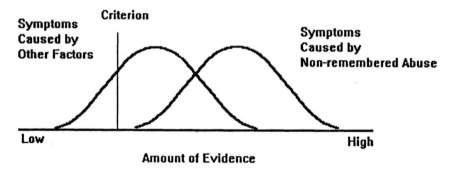

Panel C:

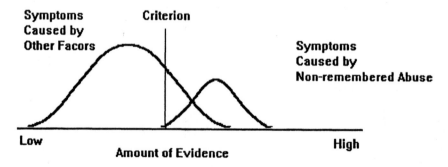

Figure 1. Signal detection theory distributions and response criteria.

This means that the operator will rarely have false alarms but will quite often fail to identify aircraft. Figure 1, Panel A illustrates a somewhat liberal response criterion.

At first blush, the analogy seems quite direct: The therapist is akin to a radar operator, peering into the screen of the client and trying to discriminate between symptoms that evidence childhood sexual abuse versus symptoms that might appear to suggest abuse but that really have other causes. Pezdek argued that to decrease the false alarm rate—that is, avoid falsely identifying non-abused clients as survivors—therapists would have to use a conservative response criterion (i.e., require a lot of evidence before deciding that a client has a CSA history), which would necessarily simultaneously decrease the hit rate—that is, would lead therapists to often fail to detect clients who really are survivors.

There are so many things wrong with this argument that I hardly know where to begin. Let me start by playing along with the SDT analogy, although I will later explain why I think the analogy itself is a poor one. What would happen if we assumed that the extant response criterion—the one that alarms critics—is far to the left of the dimension (i.e., that some therapists identify clients as survivors even when there is very little evidence to support that judgment, as illustrated in Panel B)? If so, such therapists could increase their response criterion a substantial amount before their hit rates were aversely affected. Or what if the base rate of symptoms caused by hidden memories is actually quite low, such that the frequency of hidden memory cases is low compared to that of other causes of such symptoms? I've not discussed this point in my talk, but there are many reasons to believe that only a small percentage of clients in general practice have symptoms caused by non-remembered abuse histories, but a large percentage have symptoms that may be viewed as "indicators" of hidden memories but which in fact are caused by other factors (see Lindsay & Read, 1994, 1995). If this is true, then increasing response criterion would lower false alarms but have little effect on the rate of correct identifications (as illustrated in Panel C).

A more fundamental criticism—although even now I will continue to play along with the SDT analogy—is that response criterion is not the only or even primary factor addressed by critics of memory work. Critics have been at least as concerned that the techniques used by some trauma-oriented practitioners to help clients "explore the possibility" that they were sexually abused as children can lead clients who were not abused to come to experience thoughts and feelings and images that look an awful lot like memories of real abuse. To put this in terms of the SDT metaphor, suggestive memory work can increase the signal strength of the noise distribution, thereby reducing sensitivity. In plain language, suggestive memory work can make it difficult to differentiate between veridical and illusory memories.

As I have hinted, these criticisms, couched as they are within the SDT metaphor, are largely moot because the metaphor itself is a poor one. SDT assumes a single underlying strength dimension, ranging from weak to strong, with a single decision threshold. In reality, the situation is both more complex and more dynamic than this. Moreover, there are many reasons to believe that we can reduce iatrogenesis to trivial levels without lowering detection of survivors of actual abuse. This can be done not by simply tightening response criterion but rather by qualitatively changing the decision processes used to identify survivors.

Consider, for example, work by Rod Lindsay and Gary Wells on eyewitness suspect identification (e.g., R. C. L. Lindsay & Wells, 1985). Most studies of eyewitness suspect identification use the same sort of procedure used by most police officers: People first view a simulated crime and are later shown a set of mug shots or a live line-up and asked if the culprit is among them. Depending on various parameters of the situation, varying percentages of witnesses identify the culprit, others identify an innocent person as the culprit, and yet others say the culprit is not present. What we would like, of course, is a procedure that would lower the likelihood of false identifications of innocent people without lowering the likelihood of correct identifications of culprits. Lindsay and Wells developed a simple procedure that does just that—it virtually eliminates false identifications without lowering correct identifications. The procedure works because it doesn't simply make people more cautious but rather qualitatively changes the way they go about making their identification judgments.

Conversely, Fisher and Geiselman (1988) have been working for more than a decade on an approach to interviewing witnesses to crimes that they term the "cognitive interview." The cognitive interview is designed to increase the amount of accurate information that witnesses report to police without increasing the amount of inaccurate information. There is some controversy about the technique, and it might best be described as in a continuing state of development, but there is no question that it can greatly increase correct reports while having a much smaller, if any, tendency to increase inaccurate reports.

The point is that psychologists can be open, sensitive, and responsive to their clients' histories without using suggestive memory recovery techniques, and hence that the risk of iatrogenesis can be virtually eliminated without reducing support for survivors of actual abuse. Indeed, I think it is only when one has an exclusive focus on detecting abuse survivors, or an exclusive focus on avoiding false memories, that undesirable trade-offs become inevitable. What we need to do is simultaneously maximise both sensitivity to survivors and awareness of the vulnerabilities of memory.

6. CONCLUSION

Some critics of memory work may wish to convince practitioners that therapy should not focus on childhood trauma at all, partly on the grounds that focusing on childhood trauma moves one toward using potentially risky techniques and partly on the grounds that there is little evidence of the differential efficacy of such approaches compared to more present-focused interventions. I lean a bit in that direction myself, but I am not an expert in psychotherapy and I would not feel comfortable telling psychotherapists that focusing on childhood trauma is inappropriate. In any case, the traumagenic model is so deeply rooted in our culture that it would be a Herculean task to root it out. Therefore, I am content with the more modest goal of building a broad consensus about the safety of approaches to memory work at either end of the risk continuum. If experts can agree that certain approaches pose little or no risk, and that reports of abuse that arise via those approaches should not be viewed as suspect, and if experts can agree that certain other approaches pose substantial risk and that reports of abuse that arise via those approaches do justify scepticism, then we will have moved from an unworkable, polarised situation to a workable middle ground.

I suspect that some critics of memory work may hesitate to agree that some approaches to addressing childhood trauma in therapy with adults pose little or no risk. This may partly be because they have committed to a position. And it may partly be because one can always imagine cases in which even the most innocuous questions set in motion a chain of events that ultimately bring powerful suggestive influences to bear on a vulnerable client. Conversely, some trauma-oriented practitioners may hesitate to agree that some approaches to memory work put clients at risk of developing illusory memories or false beliefs. Here again, this may partly be because they have committed to a position, and it may partly be because they can well imagine situations in which essentially accurate accounts of abuse are thrown into doubt on the grounds that suggestive techniques may have given rise to them.

The fears on both sides are understandable, because acknowledging that both essentially accurate and essentially inaccurate recovered memories occur puts one on a slippery slope. But in my view we should be on a slippery slope, or at least in a grey and uncertain topography between the two extremes. That is where the interesting and important questions arise, and where answers can be formulated. Our long-term applied goal is clear enough: to maximise good and minimise harm. More concretely, to maximise the efficacy with which we respond to the very real and important problem of childhood sexual abuse while simultaneously minimising the risk of inadvertently harming non-abused clients and their families.

The real abuse of children is a more important problem than iatrogenic illusory memories or false beliefs. Child sexual abuse has been going on for much longer, has harmed many more people, and is a much more difficult problem to overcome. Iatrogenic false beliefs and illusory memories are nonetheless an important problem: They harm clients and families, they undermine support for survivors of abuse, and they weaken the reputation of psychology. Thus we need to work on both problems. By working together, cognitive and neuroscience memory researchers, psychological practitioners, and clinical researchers can make progress toward answers to important questions such as "Is it helpful to encourage clients with certain symptoms to search for suspected hidden abuse histories?" "If so, can we discriminate between clients who are more versus less likely to be helped by such treatments, and between those who are more versus less likely to be harmed by them?" "If searches for suspected hidden memories are to be undertaken in therapy, how can the risks of such searches by reduced?" It is my devout hope that this ASI will make a substantial contribution toward developing answers to these and related questions. Amen.

REFERENCES

Andrews, B., Morton, J., Bekerian, D. A., Brewin, C. R., Davies, G. M., & Mollon, P. (1995, May). The recovery of memories in clinical practice: Experiences and beliefs of British Psychological Society practitioners. *The Psychologist*, 209–214.

Bass, E., & Davis, L. (1988). *The courage to heal: A guide for women survivors of child sexual abuse*. New York: Harper & Row.

Bottoms, B. L., Beety, K. R., Goodman, G. S., Tyda, K. S., & Shaver, P. R. (1995, June). *Clinical cases involving allegations of repressed memory: Therapists' experiences and attitudes*. Paper presented at the meeting of the American Psychological Society, New York.

Chapman, L. M., & Chapman, J. P. (1967). Genesis of popular but erroneous psychodiagnostic observations. *Journal of Abnormal Psychology, 72*, 193–204.

Fisher, R. P., & Geiselman, R. E. (1988). Enhancing eyewitness memory with the cognitive interview. In M. M. Gruneberg, P. E. Morris, & R. N. Sykes (Eds.), *Practical aspects of memory: Current research and issues* (pp. 34–39). New York: John Wiley.

Fiske, S. T., & Taylor, S. E. (1991). *Social cognition* (2nd ed.). New York: McGraw-Hill.

FMSF Scientific and Professional Advisory Board. (1994). *Frequently asked questions about the False Memory Syndrome Foundation*. Philadelphia, PA.

Gardner, R. A. (1992). Belated realisation of child sex abuse by an adult. *Issues in Child Abuse Accusations , 4*, 177–195.

Hyman, I. E., Jr., Husband, T. H., & Billings, F. J. (1995). False memories of childhood experiences. *Applied Cognitive Psychology, 9*, 181–197.

Lief, H. I. Psychiatry's challenge: Defining an appropriate therapeutic role when child abuse is suspected. *Psychiatric News, August 12, 27(16)*, 14.

Lindsay, D. S., & Read, J. D. (1994). Psychotherapy and memories of childhood sexual abuse: A cognitive perspective. *Applied Cognitive Psychology, 8*, 281- 338.

Lindsay, D. S., & Read, J. D. (1995). "Memory work" and recovered memories of childhood sexual abuse: Scientific evidence and public, professional, and personal issues. *Psychology, Public Policy, and Law, 1,* 846–908.

Lindsay, R. C. L., & Wells, G. L. (1985). Improving eyewitness identifications from lineups: Simultaneous versus sequential lineup presentations. *Journal of Applied Psychology, 70,* 556–564.

Loftus, E. F. (1979). *Eyewitness testimony.* Cambridge, MA: Harvard University Press.

Loftus, E. F. (1991). Made in memory: Distortions in recollection after misleading information. In G. H. Bower (Ed.), *The psychology of learning and motivation: Advances in research and theory,* (Vol. 27, pp. 187–215). San Diego: Academic Press.

Loftus, E. F., & Pickrell, J. E. (1995). The formation of false memories. *Psychiatric Annal, 25,* 720–724.

Mollon, P. (1996, April). *Clinical complexities in the memory debate.* Paper presented at the annual meeting of the British Psychological Society, Brighton, England.

Oskamp, S. (1982). Overconfidence in case-study judgments. In Kahneman, D., Slovic, P., & Tversky, A. (Eds.), *Judgment under uncertainty: Heuristics and biases* (pp. 287–293). Cambridge: Cambridge University Press. (Original work published 1965.)

Pezdek, K. (1994). The illusion of illusory memory. *Applied Cognitive Psychology, 8,* 339–350.

Poole, D. A., Lindsay, D. S., Memon, A., & Bull, R. (1995). Psychotherapy and the recovery of memories of childhood sexual abuse: U.S. and British practitioners' beliefs, practices, and experiences. *Journal of Consulting and Clinical Psychology, 63,* 426–437.

Read, J. D., & Lindsay, D. S. (1994). Moving toward a middle ground on the "false memory debate:" Reply to commentaries on Lindsay and Read. *Applied Cognitive Psychology, 8,* 407–435.

Shweder, R. A. (1977). Likeness and likelihood in everyday thought: Magical thinking in judgments about personality. *Current Anthropology, 18,* 637–658.

Tversky, A., & Kahneman, D. (1974). Judgments under uncertainty: Heuristics and biases. *Science, 185,* 1124–1131.

Yapko, M. (1994). *Suggestions of abuse: Real and imagined memories.* New York: Simon & Schuster.

COMMENTARY ON INCREASING SENSITIVITY

John Briere, University of Southern California School of Medicine

I am pleased to have the opportunity to respond to Dr. Lindsay's chapter, since he and I often find ourselves sharing separate corners of a weakly defined "middle position" in the recovered memory debate. His discussion in the preceding chapter is a good example of the balance and respect for competing perspectives that we should strive for in this area. Of course, because this is a debate in which reasonable people frequently disagree, I do have a few comments. Some merely reinforce Lindsay's points, and some take a different position. Most importantly, however, the central assertion remains: The time for black-and-white thinking in this area has passed. Although extreme positions are often important in social debates, in the sense of raising points that otherwise might be obscured or avoided, they can impede later progress if they stifle discussion or distract from important issues. In this regard, a major theme of Lindsay's chapter is unavoidable: there is little doubt that both accurate recovered memories and inaccurate or "false" memories can occur for childhood sexual abuse. If we accept this as a given, we are afforded the opportunity to explore and understand rather than battle and waste yet more time.

1. SENSITIVITY AND THE RECOVERED MEMORY DEBATE

Beyond issues associated with the understandable need to avoid ambiguity in a contentious area, those of us drawn into the debate have struggled with the affect that inevitably arises in this area. Those who work with victims of abuse and violence can become angry or hurt when others seem to dismiss or discount the effects of such maltreatment, characterize therapy as unduly "soft" or ill conceived, or provide advice to therapists on specific clinical matters without the benefit of clinical training. Similar feeling arise in some of those who have worked with falsely accused individuals, have themselves been affected by false accusations, or do research on memory distortion, especially when they are characterized by others as necessarily part of the "backlash" against child abuse awareness.

Unfortunately, strong feelings have been an especially prominent part of this debate. Both the attacks that many of us have experienced, as well as our defensive responses to them, reflect processes that, at minimum, obscure clear vision. Further, they reveal aspects of this issue that are less scientific or clinical than personal. The intrusion of personal issues into theoretically objective discourse is not new to scientific or clinical affairs, of course, nor does it necessarily signal that either side of the discussion is "wrong." But it does mean that not all expressed opinions on the recovered memory - false memory issues reflect solely their intellectual components. There can be, as well, intrusion of personal history, territoriality, even competitiveness and meanness. That these responses are human is understandable, but they are not acceptable at a public level because they can affect others. For example, psychotherapy clients with incomplete memories of childhood sexual abuse can be hurt by sarcastic or glib commentaries on false memories and those assumed to have them. Similarly, those falsely accused of abuse can suffer when experts state that all abuse disclosures are inherently truthful or that all those accused are guilty. Although there are trials and tribulations inherent in what we, as professionals do, we must not lose track of the fact that others are listening—including those of whom we are speaking.

From this perspective, sensitivity refers to our awareness of how and why we take the positions we take on this issue and whether we are able to change our analyses in response to new information, as well as recognition of the impacts of what we say on others. Too many people are too personally involved for vitriol to be a responsible option in this debate. I, personally, am trying to heed Lindsay's and my own advice in this regard, both in terms of not rising to the emotional bait in discussions with those who harshly reject the viability of recovered memory as a concept, and by working to characterize both sides of the debate in respectful terms when writing or speaking publicly. I know that I have further to go in this process, and I invite others to join me in this effort.

2. THE CONCEPT OF "MEMORY WORK"

One of the phrases often used by Lindsay in his chapter and elsewhere is that of "memory work." The implication is that this phrase refers to the use of especially suggestive psychotherapy techniques to recover memory of events that may or may not have transpired. Unfortunately, at first glance the term seems to describe a process that occurs in many therapeutic approaches. As I note in Chapter 2 of this volume, because adverse childhood events are carried and express themselves in memory, almost any attempt to address such trauma could be characterized as memory work. For example, some of the most efficacious interventions for victims of rape, uncomplicated sexual abuse, war trauma, and other adverse events appears to be the cognitive-behavioral techniques of systematic desensitization and cognitive restructuring (e.g., Frank & Stewart, 1983; Foa, Rothbaum, Riggs, & Murdock, 1991; Jehu, 1989; Keane, Fairbank, Caddell, & Zimering, 1989; Smucker, Dancu, Foa, & Niederee, 1995). In these approaches, the client is asked to recollect and desensitize memories of traumatic events, and is invited to explore objectively the negative assumptions, meanings, and attributions he or she made at the time of the trauma and thereafter. Clearly, such interventions are memory work: they rely on exposure to and processing of traumatic memories in order for a positive treatment outcome to occur. Because almost any therapeutic intervention that requires the client to discuss (and therefore recall) upsetting events can be considered memory work, further information is required when this term is used.

In order for the term *memory work* to be useful, let alone before it can be discounted, it must include information on whether memory is being elicited or merely processed, and whether the memories in question are those currently available or those hypothesized to be "repressed" or dissociated from awareness. Even when the process involves the elicitation of unavailable memories, it must be characterizable as potentially suggestive before it can be reasonably criticized. Unfortunately, despite the work of Lindsay and Read (1994) and others, we have yet to determine empirically just how suggestive most of these techniques actually are. Hypnosis for memory recovery purposes, definitive statements regarding the presence of repression, drug assisted interviews, and pressure to remember supposed past events seem like good candidates for a blacklist in this regard (Briere, 1995a,b); Yet, the data are not yet there. I agree with Lindsay's contention that a reasonable possibility of risk should be sufficient to proscribe a given technique. But, in the absence of definitive data, who defines the level of risk, especially for techniques less dramatic than those listed above? Is guided imagery suggestive? If so, under what conditions? How about invitations to repeatedly visit and revisit childhood events? Is talking to one's family about one's childhood a suggestive process? The danger here, of course, is that those especially critical of "memory work" may include techniques in this list that do not belong there, and may characterize therapists as potentially harmful when, in fact, they are not. Sans data, conjecture may substitute for fact, potentially impeding progress in understanding the impacts of therapy in the alleged recollection of previously unremembered abuse.

In this regard, Lindsay and his colleagues suggest here and elsewhere (e.g., Poole, Lindsay, Memon, and Bull, 1995) that, based on certain criteria, approximately 25% of therapists are likely to be engaging in risky therapy with regard to memory recovery. Among the additional information needed before such conclusions could be made, however, would be (a) whether, as they note, the proportions they report are generalizable to larger samples and greater questionnaire return rates, (b) whether each of the "risky" techniques included as criteria are, in fact, specifically associated with an unacceptable level of suggestibility (i.e., at a level that might lead to confabulation of nonexistent abuse experiences), and (c) whether the respondents in their study understood that they were being asked to list techniques they used specifically for memory recovery (as opposed to methods used to trigger or process readily available memory material). Although not included in their criteria for risky therapy, it would also be helpful to know whether therapists' willingness to list "indicators" of sexual abuse in the Poole *et al.* (1995) study (most of which have been empirically associated with childhood sexual abuse in various studies) means that therapists generally believe that the presence of these indicators necessarily discriminates specific sexual abuse survivors from others. In the absence of such information, Lindsay and colleagues' oft-quoted 25% estimate may be premature.

Despite my concerns about attaching a specific prevalence rate to risky or dangerous therapeutic activities, at least based on currently available data, I agree with Lindsay's contention that some clinicians are uninformed as to the vagaries of memory, especially as they relate to psychotherapeutic practice. Such knowledge gaps may lead to misdiagnosis of the client's difficulties and errors in therapeutic practice. As well, I have no quarrel with the notion that hypnosis (when used for "memory recovery"), drug assisted interviewing, and almost any therapist pressure to recollect unavailable material is contraindicated in good psychotherapy. Finally, there is little doubt that there are therapists working with abuse survivors and others who engage in inappropriate therapeutic practice. Confronting such individuals should not be the sole province of recovered memory critics. In fact, it is ethically incumbent on therapists to monitor our colleagues in this regard, and, in the absence of appropriate response to corrective feedback, to take steps (e.g., through professional organizations or boards) to proscribe their practice in this area.

3. THE HANDEDNESS STUDY AS A RELEVANT PARADIGM

Lindsay describes a study in which he and his colleagues attempted to cause right-handed individuals to believe that they were actually left-handed at birth, through the use of a supposed diagnostic test and exercises modelled after *The Courage to Heal*. Although, interestingly, the addition of Courage to Heal exercises did not seem to increase suggestibility much beyond the effect of "diagnosis" alone, being told that they may have been left-handed at birth substantially increased subjects' self-reported recollections of childhood left-handedness. Lindsay notes that "In some ways, our procedure more closely mirrors memory work in therapy than the procedures used in most studies of suggestibility, in that we did not suggest the occurrence of a particular event but rather of a general class of events" (p. 7).

As noted above, I would take issue with Lindsay's implication that most "memory work" involves significant suggestion of any type. Beyond that concern, however, these data support other studies indicating that being told that one may have experienced one of several things in childhood tends to increase the likelihood that one will, in fact, "remember" such events. As Lindsay notes, however, such studies have been criticized for their limited ecological or external validity vis a vis the actual subject in question: false memories of sexual abuse as a result of therapist activities. In this regard, leading someone to believe they were actually left-handed as a child, or lost in a mall, and so on may be considerably easier that convincing them that a loved or trusted adult had sexual intercourse with them. This does not mean that such convincing cannot occur, only that the handedness study (among others) cited in Lindsay's chapter may not be an especially useful analogue for that more serious scenario. Nevertheless, in my opinion, a therapist who approximated the Lindsay et al study (i.e., telling a client that testing indicates he or she may have been sexually abused as a child) would not be meeting modern standards of practice. In fact, as I have noted elsewhere (e.g., Briere, 1996), there is no good evidence that any psychometric instrument can serve as a litmus test for a history of sexual abuse.

4. SIGNAL DETECTION AND RECOVERED MEMORIES

Lindsay devoted a fair amount of time to criticisms of Pezdek's (1994) discussion of signal detection theory as it might relate to procedures for accessing unavailable abuse memories. Lacking equivalent space here, I will limit my comments in this area. I would merely note that to the extent that Pezdek was supporting a loosening of criteria for determining the presence of sexual abuse (an interpretation I'm not sure she'd agree with), the risk of false positives (viewing the nonabused as abused) might easily be untenable. Further, as Lindsay and others (e.g., Courtois, in this volume) note, it is rarely appropriate for therapists to attempt to uncover a "repressed" sexual abuse history in the first place. As outlined in Chapter ???, the clinician is usually in the best position when he or she works with what is available at any given moment, without ruling in or ruling out a nondisclosed history of childhood trauma.

5. SHOULD CLINICIANS AVOID FOCUSSING ON CHILDHOOD TRAUMA?

Lindsay notes on page 14 that he "leans toward" convincing practitioners that treatment should not focus on childhood trauma at all, but that, as a nonclinician, he may be less qualified on this point and therefore does not assert it. As someone who has been exposed frequently to the results of bad therapy in this area, it is understandable that Lindsay would be tempted to pursue this position. Yet, he is correct when he notes that nonclinicians must be careful to stay within their fields of expertise when discussing such notions. Further, given data suggesting that childhood sexual abuse is a major risk factor for posttraumatic stress disorder in adulthood (e.g., Kessler, Sonnega, Bromet, Hughes, & Nelson, 1995), and the likelihood that other trauma-related symptoms such as dissociative disorders, sexual dysfunctions, conditioned fears, and depression may persist in sexual abuse and assault victims for many years (e.g., American Psychiatric Association, 1994; Frank & Stewart, 1983; Kilpatrick & Resnick, 1993; Neumann, Houskamp, Pollock, & Briere, 1996), discouraging therapists from directly addressing these traumas with desensitization or cognitive techniques would be ill-advised, if not unethical—especially since such techniques have been shown to assist specifically in these areas (e.g., Jehu, 1989; Linehan, 1993; Smucker, Dancu, Foa, & Niederee, 1995).

6. CONCLUSIONS

In summary, although certain specific elements of Lindsay's chapter are subject to dispute, his general points are congruent with good clinical practice. Further, his attention to the implications of his position for people beyond the "false memory" community is a model for those of us who paricipate in this debate, regardless of position. Like other chapters in this volume, Lindsay's contribution is likely to presage the future, especially in terms of the development of overbridging perspectives that allow for respectful dialogue and integrative thinking.

REFERENCES

American Psychiatric Association. (1994). *Diagnostic and Statistical Manual of Mental Disorders (4th ed.)*. Washington, D.C.: Author.

Briere, J. (1995a). Science versus politics in the delayed memory debate: A commentary. *The Counseling Psychologist, 23*, 290–293.

Briere, J. (1995b). Child abuse, memory, and recall: A commentary. *Consciousness and Cognition, 4*, 83–87.

Briere, J. (1996). Psychological assessment of child abuse effects in adults. In J.P. Wilson & T.M. Keane (Eds.), *Assessing psychological trauma and PTSD: A handbook for practitioners* (pp. 43–68). NY: Guilford.

Frank, E., & Stewart, B.D. (1983). Depressive symptoms in rape victims: A revisit. *Journal of Affective Disorders, 7*, 77–85.

Foa, E.B., Rothbaum, B.O., Riggs, D.S., & Murdock, T.B. (1991). Treatment of posttraumatic disorder in rape victims: A comparison between cognitive-behavioral procedures and counseling. *Journal of Consulting and Clinical Psychology, 59*, 715–723.

Jehu, D. (1989). *Beyond sexual abuse: Therapy with women who were childhood victims.* Chichester, UK: John Wiley.

Keane, T.M., Fairbank, J.A., Caddell, J.M., & Zimering, R.T. (1989). Implosive (flooding) therapy reduces symptoms of PTSD in Vietnam combat veterans. *Behavior Therapy, 20*, 245–260.

Kessler, R.C., Sonnega, A., Bromet, E., Hughes, M., & Nelson, C.B. (1995). Posttraumatic stress disorder in the national comorbidity survey. *Archives of General Psychiatry, 52*, 1048–1060.

Kilpatrick, D., G., & Resnick, H.S. (1993). Posttraumatic stress disorder associated with exposure to criminal victimization in clinical and community populations. In J.R.T. Davidson and E.B. Foa (Eds), *Posttraumatic Stress Disorder: DSM-IV and beyond* (113–143). Washington, D.C: American Psychiatric Press.

Lindsay, D. S., & Read, J. D. (1994). Psychotherapy and memories of childhood sexual abuse: A cognitive perspective. *Applied Cognitive Psychology, 8*, 281–338.

Linehan, M. M. (1993). *Cognitive-behavioral treatment of borderline personality disorder.* New York: Guilford

Neumann, D.A., Houskamp, B.M., Pollock, V.E., & Briere, J. (1996). The long-term sequelae of childhood sexual abuse in women: A meta-analytic review. *Child Maltreatment, 1*, 6–16.

Pezdek, K. (1994). The illusion of illusory memory. *Applied Cognitive Psychology, 8*, 339–350.

Poole, D. A., Lindsay, D. S., Memon, A., & Bull, R. (1995). Psychotherapy and the recovery of memories of childhood sexual abuse: U.S. and British practitioners' beliefs, practices, and experiences. *Journal of Consulting and Clinical Psychology, 63*, 426–437.

Smucker, M.R., Dancu, C., Foa, E.B., & Niederee, J.L. (1995). Imagery rescripting: A new treatment for survivors of childhood sexual abuse suffering from posttraumatic stress. *Journal of Cognitive Psychotherapy, 9*, 3–17.

QUESTION AND ANSWER SESSION

Yehuda. I actually want to get back to the data you presented, because I think that one of the interesting things we can work on is how to take an experimental paradigm that is on one end of the spectrum and make it more clinically relevant. It's too easy for clinicians to dismiss what you've done, and say this isn't really relevant to what I need to deal with in a clinical context, but there's a way to make it so. I think clinicians really do struggle with how much or how little to say because on the one hand you really want to give the patient an opportunity to search for traumatic incidents that are not immediately available and that sometimes take a very long time to come forward and at the same time you want to avoid what your data so eloquently shows—that people can be highly suggestible. So the question isn't an either/or, it's a dose response. So how can you take your experimental paradigm and determine at what point people can be convinced they are left-handed? Because the real issue is not that a therapist can convince a patient of anything—unfortunately we know that is true—the question is how little does a therapist actually have to say, before a very sensitive probe that gives permission for the patient to explore something that he or she never considered that's relevant turns into a manipulation?

Lindsay. That's the question, because now we've agreed that we're not going to play the game of "Oh it's impossible that people could have these false memories" or "It's impossible that people could have accurate reports of events." So given that we're not going to do that stupid stuff, which is great, then how can you be open to patients or clients reporting abuse without being suggestively leading of them? We can only sort of speculate at this point because there are so many variables and they all interact with one another. As I said in my talk, my opinion is that from the existing literature we can say with some confidence that people aren't going to go developing false memories of childhood traumas, at least not most people—there may be some psychiatric conditions, but most people aren't going to in respond to some straightforward questions such as "I want you to know this is something we can talk about," that would be included in the other forms of information that you get in your ongoing learning about each other. But the fact is that's a hunch and there could well be people on quote my side of the issue who could disagree with me on that and say no you shouldn't broach the subject unless the person spontaneously brings it up, so we don't know for sure. I'm not completely confident that we'd quickly get experimental evidence that would say boom that amount of suggested probing around is OK. My personal feeling is that beyond communicating to patients or clients that we're interested in trauma histories along with other facts about them and that you're open to talking about it, my personal bias is that you shouldn't do any more encouraging in a particular direction, you should instead be open to what directions are important for the person you're working with.

Yehuda. Yes but can we do better research so that we can have a dose-response effect? See, we talk about how dichotomies are bad and we design our studies so the answer is a dichotomy. So what our challenge is, is to come up with a data set that doesn't look like a dichotomy. The clinicians will handle how they should behave, experimental people don't have to use their data to tell clinicians what to do in their office, what they do have to provide is data that goes away from a dichotomy so people can actually be thoughtful about it. I'm sort of asking you how you would redesign your study so that instead of the question "Can I convince right-handed people that they may have been left-handed and someone messed around with that," that I could ask the question in a different way so that my data would be if I do this then I have this much of a percent chance of versus if I went in with this intervention then I could increase or decrease that.

Lindsay. It was in that spirit that we had our two levels so that some people had this left-handed thing and some people left plus lax instructions. It turned out that our standard instructions for the guided imagery and journaling were just too similar to our standard plus the lax thing. I think it's interesting and important to look at multiple levels of your independent variable. On the other hand, I think it would probably be inappropriate to say that, because in this study there was a 20% increase in the likelihood of false memories when you added this component, therefore in some other situation there would also be a 20% increase. There might be good grounds to argue for a generalisation but not in terms of magnitude of effect. So it's very difficult to, given that we can't do experiments that will lead people to believe they were traumatised in extreme ways—that's going to always limit our ability to generalise from the study in terms of absolute magnitude. Again, my feeling is that we can get so close to zero iatrogenesis without reducing sensitivity to real survivors that we ought to just do it, especially once we clear the air and we don't have a population of people who saw that highly suggestive TV shows etc.

Spencer Eth. My concern is less about the research and more about the treatment, and I would want to raise an issue about a comment that Dr. Briere made which, if I understood it correctly, was in a sense that it's not so important whether it did or didn't happen—just use the material, you work with the patient and hopefully in the process the patients get better. I would argue that it is important whether the patient has had a traumatic history or not and it is not so easy to elicit that in the course of a therapy and where it really becomes problematic is in patients in whom you have the suggestion of traumatic histories because of diagnoses such as depression, anxiety, substance abuse, axis II conditions, which are most of the patients we treat, where there's a suspicion that there's a traumatic history but that information is not forthcoming in the course of therapy and there is a sense that the patient might be resisting, that there might be difficulty recollecting these events, or reluctant to talk about it and in that instance, therapists such as myself, and good therapists who don't use hypnosis or sodium amytal who are trying to treat patients, do make efforts to encourage patients to talk about material that's difficult to talk about. If we have a clinical suspicion that material includes traumatic histories then I think it's incumbent upon ourselves to elicit that information and it's not at all clear to me that research with an undergraduate population is really particularly helpful in that clinical situation where the dilemma is that the more you try to elicit that information the more liable you are to be suggestive, but on the other hand one cannot disprove that clinical intuition without making a focussed effort to elicit information of that sort and I'm hoping this conference will assist clinicians in developing methods to be better able to elicit traumatic history without falling into the trap of suggesting that history and encouraging false reports by patients.

Briere. We probably don't disagree, Spencer, which isn't a surprise, but I think that what we're superficially disagreeing on is, you may know I've developed instruments that ask about history, but if someone in therapy with me, especially someone who has complex PTSD where there are multiple things going on with them at the same time, it's entirely within possibility that I might come to the conclusion that I'm not going to get the information I need to form a definite assessment of their criterion A experience but what I have to do is make it easier for them to do whatever they have to do in terms of talking about things so I would be more towards decreasing the need of the survivor to use avoidance strategies which look like denial and work with them so they can come up with the material, so I do have some concerns that if we press the individual too hard for information that they don't have or don't want to share with us then we end up being part of an adversarial dynamic which I don't want to support in therapy, I want to support the increased likelihood that they will come up with this material on their own. But what you're talking about and what the people in the room who work with extreme trauma know very well is that all this speculation doesn't do you a wit of good when you're in there and there's someone like a torture survivor who's been very badly traumatised. You need to know the information, you need to make the intervention. It's a continuum, but my position is more that I will hold in abeyance an integrated final picture of what's going on with the patient as long as possible, and in the process of treatment assessment may occur. But part of what I would do which other people maybe wouldn't do is my treatment is not going to be trauma specific it's going to be good general psychotherapy which will facilitate the development of material which may then cause us to be more specific later but if we front-end it with specifics you run into problems. I doubt if we're really disagreeing on that too much.

Lindsay. What I'm hearing from both Dr. Briere and Dr. Eth is this belief that someone who's presenting with depression or something like that gives one a basis for believing that there's a trauma history. Dr Eth can you clarify that when you said there was a variety of symptoms such as anxiety or depression?

Eth. I said there were many patients with conditions that we know to be associated with PTSD, such as depression, substance abuse, anxiety disorders, axis II disorders, where given other information you have you develop the clinical suspicion that they have a trauma history, including work with children where you have a strong suspicion that there is an abuse history and the patient doesn't talk about it and you can't confirm that suspicion.

Lindsay. Right that's what I understood you to say. That's of course where we get into our strongest concern. You've obviously asked an open question, you've made it clear that you're open to talking about an abuse history, and the person doesn't, but you have the clinical intuition from their symptoms that they have an abuse history, you may then think, I'm not going to be suggestive, I'm not going to lead the client, I'm not going to push the client, I'm just going to try to set up conditions that will allow the person to discover and talk about these events. My feeling is that that's a risky situation to be in because although it's true that we have data showing that reported histories of abuse are associated with a variety of symptoms, we also know that those symptoms are associated with other etiological factors. I think it would be just as risky to say that based on these things I've formed an intuition that the person has some other kind of background and I'm now going to set the conditions that will allow them to talk about that.

Briere. Although I thought we were coming from the same place, the longer you talked the less I was sure about that. One of the problems about people from outside the area coming into the area is that you just brief yourself on one little area. For instance Spencer could talk for a long time about the Vietnam veteran re-adjustment data which is thousands of Vietnam vets, we know the co-morbidity of PTSD and depression in quite high, we know that anxiety disorders overlap with post traumatic and acute stress disorders, not from a few survivor reports but from a few people who just left Da Nang. The issue is, you can't just say well forget it then. The problem is, when you have co-morbidity, when you have sequelae, clinicians are in the situation where we feel we want to make people better—that's our job. If we just ignore the data, and it's very robust, the co-morbidity for PTSD is extremely high, which means that someone who has an identified traumatic stress is very likely to have at least one other axis I diagnosis, we can't completely ignore that. What I would hope is that we don't mischaracterise though is that if someone comes in with depression, we're going to treat her for abuse history. It's just a question of using all the data that's available to us, in as smart a way as possible to come up with a clinical hypothesis, which the process of the work will help.

2

AN INTEGRATED APPROACH TO TREATING ADULTS ABUSED AS CHILDREN, WITH SPECIFIC REFERENCE TO SELF-REPORTED RECOVERED MEMORIES

John Briere

University of Southern California School of Medicine
1937 Hospital Pl.
Los Angeles, California 90003-1071

1. INTRODUCTION

Research conducted over the last two decades suggests that sexual abuse is both common in North American society and associated with a variety of subsequent psychological difficulties. Although not all child abuse appears to confer significant long-term effects, sequelae of childhood sexual abuse often documented in the literature include anxiety and depression (e.g., Bagley & Ramsay, 1986; Stein, Golding, Seigel, Burnham, & Sorenson, 1989), posttraumatic stress (e.g., Rowan, Foy, Rodriguez, & Ryan, 1994; Saunders, Villeponteaux, Lipovsky, Kilpatrick, & Veronen, 1992), dissociative symptoms (e.g., Briere, Elliott, Harris, & Cotman 1995; Chu & Dill, 1990), cognitive disturbance such as low self-esteem and helplessness (e.g., Gold, 1986; Jehu, Gazan, & Klassen, 1984–85), suicidality (e.g., Briere & Runtz, 1986; de Wilde, Klienhorst, Diekstra, & Wolters, 1992), substance abuse (e.g., Swett, Cohen, Surrey, Compaine, & Chavez, 1991; Rohsenow, Corbett, & Devine, 1988), sexual dysfunction (e.g., Becker, Skinner, Abel, & Treacy, 1982; Wyatt, Newcombe, & Riederle, 1993), interpersonal problems (e.g., Elliott, 1994; Herman, 1981) and personality disorders (Briere & Zaidi, 1989; Ogata, Silk, Goodrich, Lohr, Westen, & Hill, 1990).

A definitive causal relationship between such difficulties and sexual abuse cannot be established, however, given the research methodologies most often used in this area (i.e., retrospective, cross-sectional studies), and the possibility that other coexisting "third" variables such as family dysfunction or low socioeconomic status may confound the relationship between abuse and hypothesized effects (Briere, 1992a). Nevertheless, the aggregate of consistent findings in this literature, as well as the existence of a small handful of longitudinal studies on abuse effects (e.g., Egeland, Sroufe, & Erickson, 1983), has led many researchers and clinicians to conclude that childhood sexual abuse is, in fact, a risk

Recollections of Trauma, edited by Read and Lindsay
Plenum Press, New York, 1997

factor for a variety of psychological problems (see, for example, a meta-analysis by Neumann, Houskamp, Pollock, & Briere, 1996).

Given the various clinical correlates of childhood sexual victimization, as well as the likelihood that such distress and disorder represents at least some actual effects of sexual abuse, there has been growing clinical interest in the specific psychotherapeutic treatment of sexual abuse survivors. Early interventions in this area typically were not grounded in sophisticated psychological theory or explicit standards of practice, partially because little information was available on how such abuse-related trauma might be addressed. More recently, however, cognitive, behavioral, and self psychological perspectives have been combined with the insights of those working with victims of more acute traumas (e.g., war veterans and rape victims). The result has been a growing convergence in the field regarding an integrated approach to treating adults sexually abused as children.

In this chapter I outline one view of this evolving perspective. In doing so, however, I intentionally focus on a specific scenario: the treatment of individuals with significant abuse-related symptomatology. I do not address the issue of inappropriate treatment of non-abuse-survivors for nonexistent abuse-related problems, as sometimes may occur in badly conducted treatment or in those seemingly rare instances when the client presents with factitious symptoms or history that is not detected by the therapist. As well, this discussion is limited to those whose abuse has produced long-term effects; Because not all child abuse experiences are associated with lasting psychological difficulties, an abuse history, alone, is insufficient reason for involvement in therapy. Instead, the focus here is on how to treat effectively those who have been abused and who suffer from that abuse, while, at the same time, not complicating the issue by producing adverse treatment effects.

Unfortunately, the development of modern clinical theory and standards of practice in this area have been far from linear nor has it been free from controversy or error. Most significantly, the treatment of sexual abuse survivors has become inextricably entangled in the "recovered memory" versus "false memory" debate. Briefly stated, individuals sometimes report that they have (or had) incomplete or no knowledge of abuse experiences they now recall having occurred in childhood, as described later in this chapter. This self-reported lack of memory for abuse often has been referred to as "repressed" memory, although most modern clinicians and clinical researchers prefer the term *dissociative amnesia*, as per the current Diagnostic and Statistical Manual (DSM-IV) of the American Psychiatric Association (American Psychiatric Association, 1994).

Reports of amnesia and later recall of sexual abuse are controversial for several reasons. First, on a legal or forensic level, accusations of abuse based on events thought to have occurred many years ago are hard to support or defend against, since the evidence surrounding the accusation is likely to have gone "stale" and to lack current corroboration. As a result, the courts generally have been reluctant to consider uncorroborated recovered memory reports as sufficient evidence of a crime or malfeasance. Second, many people have difficulty accepting the entire notion that especially negative events can be forgotten—it seems counterintuitive to some that they would not be, in fact, more vividly remembered. Third, a minority of recovered memories appear to be fantastical or are for events that occurred so early in life that they could not have been encoded without further brain and cognitive development. These reports are referred to as *false memories* by some. Such reports may arise from a variety of processes, but critics of the concept of recovered memory especially point to badly conducted therapy as an etiologic factor (e.g., Lindsay, 1994; Loftus, 1993). In this regard, there is little question that a minority of therapists have used questionable "memory recovery" techniques, have told their therapy clients that their problems were due to repressed memories of abuse despite the client's statements that no abuse occurred, or, perhaps more typically, did not question clearly impossible "memory" content or work to inhibit ongoing confabulatory processes (Briere, 1995a,b). Such errors can create victims both of clients who have come to believe nonexistent abuse histories and those who have been falsely accused based on such pseudomemories (Lindsay, 1995). On the other hand, recent research by Elliott (Elliott & Briere, 1995a; Elliott, 1995) suggests that recovered memory reports in the general population does not arise solely (or even primarily) during psychotherapy.

Although some undetermined number of recovered memory reports may be distorted or confabulated, it is likely that many others represent actual instances of temporarily inaccessible memories of childhood trauma that, for some reason, return to conscious awareness. In fact, the notion of psychogenic amnesia for trauma is not at all new to psychiatry or psychology. For example, articles published around World Wars I and II suggest that nonorganic (often referred to as "hysterical") amnesia was an accepted concept among combat physicians and was often documented in reports of war effects (e.g., Henderson & Moore, 1944; Parfit & Gall, 1944; Sargant & Slater, 1941; Thom & Fenton, 1920; Torrie, 1944)—phenomena unlikely to be the results of errant psychotherapy. For example, in a study of war stress in 1,000 admissions to a neurological hospital unit, Sargant and Slater (1941) reported that "severe" war stress ("prolonged marching and fighting under heavy enemy action") produced amnesia for war events in 35% of patients, whereas "moderate" stress (e.g. "experiences like periodical dive-bombing at home bases and aerodromes") resulted in amnesia for 13% of patients (p. 758). Other traumatic events, such as torture, concentration camps, physical assaults, and rape also have been linked to dissociative amnesia (Loewenstein, 1993). Tromp, Koss, Figueredo, and Tharan (1995), for example, found that, as compared to other unpleasant memories, women's recollections of adult rape experiences were significantly "less clear and vivid, contained a less meaningful order, were less remembered, and were less thought and talked about" (p. 607). In Elliott's (1995) study of trauma and memory in a large sample of the general population, subjects reported having had periods of incomplete or absent memories for a wide variety of traumatic experiences, ranging from war to accidents to instances of sexual or physical assault.

Apropos of this significant literature, DSM-IV identifies five forms of memory disturbance that may occur as dissociative amnesia: *localized amnesia*, wherein "the individual fails to recall events that occurred during a circumscribed period of time ... (e.g., the uninjured survivor of a car accident in which a family member has been killed may not be able to recall anything that happened from the time of the accident until two days later)" (p. 478), *selective amnesia*, in which "the person can recall some, but not all, of the events during a circumscribed period of time (e.g., a combat veteran can recall only some parts of a series of violent combat experiences)" (p. 478), *generalized amnesia*, involving rare circumstances wherein there is no memory for the person's entire life, *continuous amnesia*, in which there is "the inability to recall events subsequent to a specific time up to and including the present" (p. 478); and *systematized amnesia*, involving a "loss of memory for certain categories of information, such as all memories relating to one's family or to a particular person" (p. 478).

Most modern research on amnesia, however, has been concerned with amnesia specifically for severe childhood abuse experiences. A number of studies of clinical and nonclinical subjects have found either (a) that a substantial proportion of those who report childhood trauma experiences (especially sexual abuse) also describe periods of partial or complete memory loss for said traumas (Briere & Conte, 1993; Elliott & Briere, 1995a; Feldman-Summers & Pope, 1994; Herman & Schatzow, 1987; Loftus, et al., 1994; Williams, 1995), or (b) that some subjects with independently established histories of childhood sexual abuse will, upon follow-up as adults, fail to report any recollection of these experiences (Williams, 1994).

Although all of these studies suffer from methodological limitations of one sort or another, their reliable replication across samples and research methods suggests that some real phenomenon is in operation. These data appear to demonstrate that amnesia for sexual abuse can occur, and that these memories sometimes can be recovered at a later point in time. In this regard, for example, a recent publication of the American Psychological Association (1996) notes that

> The APA Working Group on Investigation of Memories of Child Abuse Final Report (1996), APA's release of Questions and Answers About Memories of Childhood Abuse (1995), and the APA Presidential Task Force on Violence and the Family Final Report (1996) have reported that experiences of early child abuse that have been forgotten can be remembered later. Even though this may not happen often, and most people who were abused during childhood remember part or all of the abusive experiences, adults can forget and then later remember childhood abuse. This has been demonstrated in a variety of research and clinical reports, but additional studies are needed to determine the precise processes and mechanisms that occur during this situation. (p. 3)

However, given the false memory reports described earlier, it is not reasonable to assume that all recovered memory reports represent real childhood occurrences. Instead, it appears that any given report must be evaluated in the same ways as should be any other allegation of past events.

An important issue for abuse-focused therapy in this debate is therefore whether a given intervention increases access to previously dissociated memories, or, instead, iatrogenically produces pseudomemories of nonexistent events. If, as will be suggested, verbal processing of traumatic memory is helpful in recovering from trauma, it will not be enough to counsel clinicians to avoid any attention to (or encouragement of) recollections of previous events. As well, clinicians report that some clients spontaneously recover memories of painful childhood events, including abuse, during the process of generic psychotherapy. Thus, any modern approach to abuse-related trauma must take memory into account, both in terms of its role in therapy and its vulnerability to distortion, confabulation, or restimulation. The remainder of this presentation will therefore address memory issues while outlining the process of abuse-focussed therapy.

2. THE GOALS OF TREATMENT

The first issue to be considered in the treatment of abuse survivors is the goals of therapy. Briefly stated, these fall into three areas: (1) Continued or improved stability, (2) symptom and/or distress reduction, and (3) improved response to future stressors. Stability refers to the client's general level of psychological and social functioning. Although treatment of any sort of traumatic state may involve temporary periods of decreased stability, the ultimate goal of treatment should include psychosocial functioning at the highest level possible.

Similarly, an important result of abuse-focused psychotherapy is the reduction of symptomatology and psychological distress. Clinical experience suggests that affective symptoms (e.g., anxiety and depression) may respond somewhat faster to treatment than, for example, chronic posttraumatic stress or enduring symptoms of personality disorder (e.g., Briere, 1996b). As well, some individuals' childhood trauma and current cognitive or defensive style (e.g., avoidance, substance abuse) may be of sufficient severity that not all abuse-related difficulties can be resolved. Nevertheless, good psychotherapy can reduce posttraumatic symptomatology (Linehan, 1993; Rothblum & Foa, 1992), and the client has a right to expect that symptom reduction be a primary goal of treatment.

A final goal of abuse-focused therapy is improved resilience for future stressors. A well-known phenomenon is for those severely abused as children to have a lower threshold for the development of symptoms when confronted with later traumatic or detrimental events (e.g., Zaidi & Foy, 1993). By desensitizing abuse-related trauma and increasing tolerance for (and modulation of) negative affective states, successful therapy may allow the client to withstand moderate level stressors and have less extreme reactions to major stressors.

Note that none of these goals require a specific technical outcome, such as total (or, in fact, any) memory recovery or therapeutic "abreaction" of abuse-related material. As noted by Riviere (1996), the goal of treatment is greater psychological health, not exorcism of specific traumatic memories. Because memories are our record of the past, can intrude as symptoms, and can carry with them painful affects and cognitions, they must be addressed at some level during treatment. In this regard, however, and contrary to the assumptions of some (e.g., Fredrickson, 1992), memory recovery, itself, is not an explicit goal of abuse-focused therapy.

3. ETHICS OF TREATMENT

Beyond the intended effects of abuse-focused psychotherapy, the clinician must be aware of (and adhere to) certain ethical standards with regard to the conduct of treatment. The ethical issues involved in the treatment of abuse survivors are similar to those for any other client population. Even greater vigilance and technical skill is required in work with abuse survivors, however, because sexual abuse can produce interpersonal difficulties, self-other boundary confusion, and significant transferential dynamics in the therapy session. These phenomena, in turn, may activate therapist countertransference and thereby potentially decrease therapeutic effectiveness (Pearlman & Saakvitne, 1995).

Perhaps most important to abuse-focused therapy, the client should be made aware of (a) therapeutic confidentiality and, significantly, its limits (e.g., in cases of danger to self or others, or the therapist's duty to report child abuse), (b) potential negative side effects (both psychological and forensic) of certain therapeutic interventions, such as hypnosis or medication, and (c) the potential for treatment to temporarily activate or intensify certain symptoms (e.g., posttraumatic stress or dysphoria) (Briere, 1996c). As well, the therapist should be aware of the limits of his or her expertise in treating abuse survivors, seeking out consultation, supervision, and/or additional training when indicated. For example, therapists should not hold themselves out to the public as experts or specialists in treating abuse survivors without, in fact, additional specialized training or experience in this area. Similarly, clinicians without training or experience in treating child abuse survivors should exercise special caution when making determinations regarding the presence or absence of (a) an abuse history, (b) false memories, or (c) the specific impacts of child abuse on an individual client. Finally, those clinical interventions used by the therapist should be among those generally accepted by specialists in the field, and should be appropriate to the survivor's specific difficulties.

It is also especially important that the clinician be sufficiently self aware, psychologically healthy, and under sufficient self-control that he or she does not act out counter-transferential issues or social biases on the client (Elliott & Briere, 1995b). Such issues obviously include inappropriate anger, sexual expression or behavior, and physical or psychological boundary violation, as well as instances of sexism or especially sex-role stereotyped expectations.

4. ASSESSMENT ISSUES

Because sexual abuse appears to produce a variety of symptoms and disorders, assessment is an especially important part of treating abuse survivors. Not only should treatment begin with a psychosocial evaluation and, when appropriate, psychological testing, some form of assessment should be an ongoing component of the treatment process. Abuse-related symptoms frequently wax and wane across treatment, and can be masked or distorted by initial avoidance responses that decrease as treatment continues—processes that may not be detected if assessment only occurs at the outset of therapy. When psychological testing is indicated, the instruments used should have adequate sensitivity and specificity in terms of detecting abuse-relevant symptomatology (Briere, 1996b, in press).

If or when the client is able to tolerate discussion of his or her childhood history, assessment should include taking a detailed history regarding the abuse and its characteristics (e.g., age at onset and offset, number of incidents, use of threats or force, presence of penetration, number of perpetrators and their relationship to the victim). The presence of other childhood and adult traumas also should be evaluated, since many sexual abuse survivors have also experienced psychological abuse, emotional neglect, and physical maltreatment, and may have been revictimized as adults. It should not be assumed that any given symptom is the result of sexual abuse, per se, as opposed to the many other potentially harmful events that the survivor may have encountered (Courtois, 1995). As well, the individual may have had psychological, neurological, or neurochemical difficulties that preceded child abuse—problems that should not be confused with child abuse effects, per se.

As per this NATO conference, the clinician must be attuned to the complexity of long-term recall as it related to abuse reports, especially in terms of potential memory distortion effects, and the increased suggestibility of some survivors (e.g., those with significant dissociative symptoms or reduced self capacities). In this regard, it is suggested that (a) assessment of abuse memories be as nondirective as is reasonably possible, such that the client is neither pressured to recall unavailable material nor unduly discouraged from describing what is possible to remember, (b) drug-assisted interviews and assessment-focused hypnosis be avoided whenever possible, and (c) amnesia neither be assumed nor prematurely ruled-out. For further discussion in this area, there are several thoughtful statements on "recovered memory" and therapy by the American Psychological Association, American Psychiatric Association, American Society of Clinical Hypnosis, British Psychological Society, and other professional organizations, as well as an excellent set of guidelines by Christine Courtois, the most recent version of which can be found in this volume.

Attention to potential therapeutic influence over recall should not inhibit reasonable exploration of the client's self-reported history, however, nor should the subject of abuse memories be avoided during treatment. As Lindsay (1995) notes,

> Criticisms of memory work in psychotherapy are not directed at survivors of CSA [child sexual abuse] who have always remembered their abuse or at those who spontaneously remember

previously forgotten abuse. Furthermore, most critics of memory work in psychotherapy do not claim that all memories of CSA recovered in therapy are false. Finally, most critics do not suggest that practitioners should never broach the subject of CSA, nor do they claim that a few probing questions about CSA are likely to lead clients to create illusory memories." (p. 281)

5. THE PROCESS OF PSYCHOTHERAPY

Many clinically presenting survivors of severe childhood abuse appear to spend considerable time and energy balancing trauma-related distress and intrusion with self-protective avoidance mechanisms such as dissociation, externalization, or substance abuse (Briere, 1996a; McCann & Pearlman, 1990). Such avoidance, although reinforced by its immediate effectiveness in reducing the felt impacts of posttraumatic symptoms and associated dysphoria, may prevent adequate exposure to and processing of traumatic material (Resick & Schnicke, 1993), thereby leaving posttraumatic symptoms relatively undiminished.

Because the survivor tends to counter abuse-related distress with avoidance, it is important that psychotherapy proceed slowly and carefully so as not to motivate over-use of this response. A primary goal is to keep from overwhelming the client—either by exposing him or her to unacceptable levels of posttraumatic distress during treatment, or by inappropriately discouraging access to needed avoidance activities such as denial, intellectualization, or dissociation. At the same time, however, the clinician seeks to facilitate exposure to traumatic material so that it can be desensitized and integrated. As a result, effective abuse-focused interventions are neither so nondemanding as to be useless, nor so evocative or powerful that the client is retraumatized. Such interventions allow emotional and cognitive processing, but do not activate internal protective systems that produce excessive avoidance and neutralize treatment.

In addition to balancing challenge with stability, the clinician must work to provide a safe therapeutic environment. In the absence of continual and reliable safety and support during treatment, the survivor is unlikely to reduce his or her reliance on avoidance defenses nor attempt to form an open relationship with the psychotherapist.

Effective therapeutic responses tend to occur on a continuum, with one end anchored in interventions devoted to greater exposure to potentially threatening but therapeutically important memories (exploration), and the other involving interventions that support and solidify previous progress, or that provide a more secure base from which the survivor can operate without fear (consolidation). Exploratory interventions typically invite the client to examine and process material related to his or her traumatic history. For example, exploration might involve asking the client to describe a specific abuse incident in detail, or to use slightly less intellectualization when discussing a painful aspect of his or her childhood. Consolidation, on the other hand, is less concerned with exposure or processing than with safety and foundation. Such interventions involve activities that reduce arousal, keep the client focused on the "here and now," interrupt escalating internal states, and increase internal stability. The decision to explore or consolidate at any given moment reflects the therapist's assessment of which direction the client's balance between stresses and resources is leaning. The overwhelmed client, for example, will require less exploration and more consolidation, whereas the stable client may gain most from the opposite.

5.1. Increasing Self Capacities

Implicit in modern abuse-focused therapy is the importance of "internal" or "self" capacities during trauma processing. In the absence of sufficient internal resources, for example, even very small amounts of distress or dysphoria will be experienced as overwhelming by the client. So important are self resources to effective therapeutic intervention that some clients may require extensive work in this area before any significant trauma-focused interventions can occur (Courtois, 1991; McCann & Pearlman, 1990).

Although a number of self capacities and functions have been hypothesized (e.g., McCann & Pearlman, 1990), perhaps most important to the successful processing of traumatic material are the related concepts of affect tolerance and affect modulation. Affect tolerance refers to the relative ability of the client to feel painful feelings without needing to avoid them through activities such as dissociation, externalization, substance abuse, etc. For example, people with good affect tolerance may be able to experience considerable frustration, anxiety, or anger without engaging in tension-reduction behaviors such as aggression, self-mutilatory activities, sexual "acting out," or self-destructiveness. Affect modulation refers to the ability to alter or reduce painful affects, also without major reliance on avoidance. Activities thought to assist in affect modulation include self-soothing, positive self-talk, placing upsetting events in perspective, and self-distraction. As noted above, in the absence of such skills, traumatic reexperiencing and dysphoria can easily overwhelm the client.

A cognitive-behavioral approach to affect regulation training is outlined by Linehan (1993). She notes that distress tolerance and affect modulation are both internal behaviors that can be learned during therapy. Among the specific skills taught by Linehan's treatment model are distraction, self-soothing, and self-relaxation. The survivor also learns to, for example, identify and label feelings, reduce vulnerability to hyper-emotionality (i.e., through decreased stress), and develop the ability to experience emotions without judging or rejecting them.

Affect tolerance and modulation is also learned implicitly during effective abuse-focused therapy. Because, as outlined in the next section, trauma-focused interventions involve the repeated evocation and processing of distressing but non-overwhelming memories, such treatment slowly teaches the survivor to become more "at home" with some level of distress, and to develop whatever skills are necessary to de-escalate moderate levels of emotional arousal. This growing ability to move in and out of strong emotional states, in turn, fosters an increased sense of emotional control and reduced fear of negative affect, per se.

5.2. Processing Traumatic Memories

Assuming that the client either has sufficient affect regulation skills or that these functions have been strengthened in therapy, the treatment of trauma symptoms is relatively straightforward. There are at least three major steps in this process, although they may recur in different orders at various points in treatment: (1) identification of traumatic (i.e., abuse-related) events; (2) gradual re-exposure to the affect and cognitions associated with a memory of the abuse, while keeping avoidance responses minimal; and (3) emotional and cognitive processing.

5.2.1. Identification of Traumatic Events. In order for traumatic material to be processed in treatment, it must be identified as such. Although this seems an obvious step, it is more difficult to accomplish in some cases than might be expected. The survivor's avoidance of abuse-related material may lead either to conscious reluctance to think about or speak of upsetting abuse incidents, or to less conscious dissociation of such events. In the former case, the survivor may believe that a detailed description of the abuse would be more painful than he or she is willing to endure, or that exploration of the abuse would overwhelm his or her self resources. Dissociation of abuse material, on the other hand, may present as incomplete or absent recall of the events in question.

Whether denial or dissociation, avoidance of abuse-related material by an abuse survivor should be respected, since it indicates his or her judgement that exploration in that area would exceed his or her capacities to handle the associated negative affect. The role of the therapist at such junctures is not to overpower the client's defenses, push him or her to discuss painful things, or in any way to convince him or her that abuse occurred. Rather, the clinician should work to provide the conditions (e.g., safety, support, and a trustworthy environment) whereby avoidance is less necessary. Because this can require significant time and skill, the specific enumeration and description of abusive events is far from a simple matter. Further, it is likely that in some cases recollection of painful childhood experiences may not occur at all. For example, the abuse may have transpired prior to the offset of infantile amnesia (Reviere, 1996), it may have been sufficiently overwhelming or disruptive that accurate memory encoding may not have occurred (Briere, 1992b), excessive stress-related neurohormone production (e.g., of cortisol) may have irrevocably altered the functions of memory-specific brain structures, perhaps especially the hippocampus (Bremner, Davis, Southwick, Krystal, & Charney, 1993), or the memory material may be sufficiently distressing that it is continually dissociated despite therapeutic intervention (Briere, 1996b). Obviously, in any of these instances, recall of abuse-related material will not occur, regardless of the therapist's clinical activities. The potential for permanently nonavailable memories in any given instance further reinforces the inadvisability of pushing for "repressed" abuse memories, per se, as opposed to interventions that focus on support and the processing of already available abuse-related material.

5.2.2. Gradual Exposure to Abuse-Related Material. If, at some point, there is sufficient abuse material available to the treatment process, the next step in the treatment of abuse-related trauma is that of careful, graduated exposure to various aspects of the abuse memory. Exposure treatment can be defined as "repeated or extended exposure, either in vivo or in imagination, to objectively harmless but feared stimuli for the purpose of reducing anxiety" (Abueg & Fairbank, 1992, p. 127). In the current context, the memory of abuse is harmless (in the sense that the abuse, itself, is not occurring) but is feared (produces distress) because of its prior association with actual harm or danger. The goal of exposure techniques for abuse trauma is not just the eradication of irrational anxiety, however. The intended outcome also includes the reduction of intrusive (and secondarily, avoidant) symptomatology associated with unresolved traumatic events.

Support for the ameliorative effects of exploring painful memories in a safe environment can be found in the experimental work of Pennebaker and colleagues (e.g., Murray & Segal, 1994; Pennebaker, Kiecolt-Glaser, & Glaser, 1988; Petrie, Booth, Pennebaker, Davison, & Thomas, 1995). They have found in various studies, for example, that merely asking university students in the laboratory to repeatedly write about a previous upsetting experience appears to reduce psychological and physical indices of distress and improve immune functioning (known to be negatively affected by posttraumatic stress). Although Pennebaker does not suggest this in his research papers, the fact that merely writing about a traumatic event during an experiment measurably reduces psychophysiological indicators of distress appears to validate the potential benefits of expressing and processing abuse-related memories during therapy.

The exposure approach suggested here for abuse trauma is a form of systematic desensitization (Wolpe, 1958), wherein the survivor is asked to recall non-overwhelming, but somewhat painful abuse-specific experiences in the context of a safe therapeutic environment. The exposure is graduated according to the intensity of the recalled abuse, with less upsetting memories being recalled, verbalized, and desensitized before more upsetting ones are considered. It should be noted that this form of exposure is self-administered: the client is asked to recall painful material, as opposed to a fear hierarchy approach in which the client is presented with a series of gradually more upsetting or frightening stimuli. The use of exposure or desensitization procedures appears to be effective in the treatment of various types of trauma survivors, including sexual abuse survivors (Smucker, Dancu, Foa, & Niederee, 1995), rape victims (e.g., Frank & Stewart, 1983; Foa, Rothbaum, Riggs, & Murdock, 1991) and war veterans (e.g., Bowen & Lambert, 1986; Keane, Fairbank, Caddell, & Zimering, 1989).

In contrast to more strictly behavioral interventions, however, the current approach does not adhere to a strict, pre-planned series of exposure activities. This is because the survivor's ability to tolerate exposure may be quite compromised, and may vary considerably from session to session as a function of outside life stressors, level of support from friends, relatives, and others, and the extent to which internal resources are available. Regarding the last point, the client may be sufficiently stressed by previous therapeutic events or aspects of the therapeutic relationship (e.g., restimulated attachment dynamics; Elliott & Briere, 1995a) that his or her ability to handle any further distressing material is limited. Further exposure at such times usually leads to avoidance responses, or even to some level of cognitive disorganization. Instead of further exposure, the focus of therapy at this point should become consolidation, arousal reduction, and the shoring up of self resources as indicated earlier. In addition, if previous exposure has led to enduring feelings of revulsion, self-hatred, or helplessness, the client may require cognitive-behavioral interventions that interrupt or contradict cognitive distortions before he or she can move on to more exposure (e.g., Jehu, 1988).

Exposure to abuse memories is complicated by the fact that there may be a number of different memory encoding-retrieval systems to address including, minimally, those involving verbal versus nonverbal material. The former is thought to be more narrative and cognitive, whereas the latter may involve the encoding and recovery of emotion-laden or sensory material (Metcalfe & Jacobs, 1996; van der Kolk, 1994). McCann and Pearlman (1990) note that both cognitive and emotional material should be processed—the first by repeatedly exploring the factual aspects of the event (e.g., who, what, where, and when), and the second by recollection/reexperiencing and recounting of the physical environment and bodily sensations associated with the abuse.

The need to address nonverbal material may be especially relevant because, as indicated by van der Kolk and Fisler (1995) and others, it is likely that some components of posttraumatic memory are intrinsically sensory or sensorimotor. As a result, good trauma work is both cognitive and affective, addressing not only distorted cognitions and the acquisition of insight, but also the need for emotional expression, processing, and desensitization.

As indicated earlier, for abuse-focused therapy to work well, there should be as little avoidance as possible during the session. Specifically, the client should be encouraged to stay as "present" as he or she can during the detailed recall of abuse memories, so that desensitization is maximized. The extremely dissociated survivor may have little true exposure to abuse material during treatment, despite what may be detailed verbal renditions of a given memory. On the other hand, the therapist must keep the client's overall emotional resources in mind and not interrupt survivor dissociation that is, in fact, appropriate in the face of potential overstimulation. This might occur, for example, when the client accesses memories whose affective characteristics exceed his or her internal capacities. It is not uncommon, however, for avoidance responses such as dissociation to become so overlearned that they automatically (but unnecessarily) emerge during exploration of stressful material. In this case, some level of encouragement of the client to reduce his or her dissociation during treatment is not only safe but frequently imperative for significant desensitization to occur.

5.2.3. Emotional and Cognitive Processing. The last component of abuse-focused desensitization of traumatic memories involves the emotional and cognitive activity that must occur during self-exposure to traumatic memories. This is an important step because, without such processing, exposure may result only in re-experienced pain, not resolution. In other words, therapeutic interventions that focus solely on the narration of abuse-related memories will not necessarily produce symptom relief.

Although past approaches to trauma resolution have included some version of cognitive processing, as outlined below, the concept of *emotional* processing is newer to the trauma field. This growing attention to affect, as opposed to solely cognitive or psychodynamic issues, no doubt arises in part from the effectiveness of behavioral interventions that desensitize conditioned emotional responses during treatment. Behavioral writers such as Rachman (1980) view emotional processing as a normal part of human functioning that, when effective, reduce emotional distress. According to Rachman

> Emotional processing is regarded as a process whereby emotional disturbances are absorbed, and decline to the extent that other experiences and behavior can proceed without disruption... If an emotional disturbance is *not* absorbed satisfactorily, some signs become evident. These signs are likely to recur intermittently... The central, indispensable index of unsatisfactory emotional processing is the persistence or return of intrusive signs of emotional activity (such as obsessions, nightmares, pressure of talk, phobias, [and] inappropriate expressions of emotion... (p. 51).

I have suggested (e.g., Briere, 1996a) that such processing is a central component of effective therapy for trauma, especially in instances when, as Rachman notes, this process has been blocked by other factors. In this regard, there appear to be two aspects of abuse-related emotional processing immediately relevant to abuse-focused treatment: facilitation of emotional discharge and titration of level of affect.

Interestingly, although emotional processing appears to be an important activity in recovery from trauma, classical behavioral exposure therapists have not been especially concerned with emotional expression or release during therapy. Instead, traditional behavior therapy tends to involve one of two approaches. In the first approach, *exposure alone*, the client is repeatedly exposed to a stimulus (e.g., a tape recording or detailed description of an assault) that triggers conditioned emotional responses (e.g., fear) until the emotional response fades away (habituates) for lack of reinforcement (i.e., because there is, in fact, no current danger). In the second approach, *exposure and relaxation* (i.e., the classic systematic desensitization paradigm), the traumatic stimulus also becomes associated with an anxiety-incompatible state (relaxation) that, by virtue of its presence during exposure to traumatic memory, disrupt the linkage between recollection and current distress (see Marmar, Foy, Kagan, & Pynoos, 1993; Rothblum & Foa, 1992 for descriptions of these approaches).

Although repeated client descriptions of abuse memories during therapy, alone, often result in some habituation and counterconditioning of painful emotional responses (i.e., via the experienced safety of the therapy office), abuse-focused therapy also capitalizes on the positive effects of emotional release. Specifically, crying or other emotional discharge often engenders a relatively positive emotional experience, affect that can then countercondition the fear and related affects initially associated with the trauma. In other words, the lay suggestion that someone "have a good cry" or "get it off of your chest" may reflect support for emotional activities that naturally desensitize posttraumatic distress. From this perspective, just as traditional systematic desensitization pairs a formerly distressing stimulus to a relaxed (anxiety-incompatible) state, and thereby neutralizes the original anxious response over time, repeated emotional release during nondissociated exposure to painful memories both disrupts the previous connection between memory and distress and pairs traumatic stimuli to the relatively positive internal states associated with emotional release.

Although appropriate emotional expression may facilitate the counterconditioning of abuse-related trauma, such activity should not be forced. Most importantly, appropriate emotional expression is not equivalent to the recently rediscovered notion of "abreaction" of chronic abuse trauma. These more dramatic procedures often involve pressure on the client to engage in extreme emotional discharge, often in the context of an hypnotic state. Unfortunately, such techniques run the risk of greatly exceeding the client's internal capacities, with resultant flooding of painful affects. In addition, by their very nature, such interventions encourage dissociated emotional release — a phenomenon that, while easily accomplished by many survivors, is unlikely to be therapeutically helpful. As noted by Cornell and Olio (1991), "[abreactive] techniques may appear to deepen affect and produce dramatic results in the session, but they may not result in the client's sustained understanding of, or connection to, their experience of abuse" (p. 62).

At the same time that the client is encouraged to remember and to feel, he or she is also asked to think. For example, the client might explore the circumstances of the abuse, the basis for his or her reactions, and the dynamics operating in the abuser. This process is likely to alter the survivor's internal schema so that the abuse experience can be cognitively integrated, as described by Horowitz (1976). In the absence of such activities, the client may experience a reduction in painful affect but not improve in the cognitive domains of self-blame, helplessness, hopelessness, or low self-esteem (Resick & Schnicke, 1993).

Cognitive processing also allows the survivor to rework abuse-related cognitive distortions and negative self-perceptions (Jehu, 1988). These distortions typically involve harsh self-judgments of having caused, encouraged, or deserved the abuse (Jehu, Gazan, & Klassen, 1984/1985), as well as those broader self-esteem problems typically associated with child maltreatment (Briere, 1992b). By exploring with the survivor the inadequate information and logical errors associated with such beliefs and self-perceptions, the therapist can assist in the development of more positive cognitive schemas regarding self and others.

Together, emotional and cognitive processing change considerably the original associations to traumatic abuse; the first by counterconditioning distress, and the second by providing insight and altering the cognitive matrix in which the abuse was imbedded. In this way, the survivor who remembers his or her abuse (both narratively and through intrusive re-experiencing), who expresses emotions related to it, and who repetitively talks and ruminates about it is engaging in a natural healing response. This process may occur best during therapy, where the clinician can provide a safe and organized structure for the unfolding of each component and can be counted on to keep the exposure process well within the client's capacities. As noted earlier, the survivor's existing self resources will determine how much exposure and processing can occur without overwhelming the survivor and stimulating avoidance responses.

5.3. Access to Previously Unavailable Material

Taken together, the approach outlined in this chapter allows the therapist to address the impaired self functioning, cognitive distortions, affective disturbance, and posttraumatic stress found in some adults who were severely abused as children. The serial desensitization of painful memories is likely to slowly reduce the survivor's overall level of posttraumatic stress — a condition that eventually lessens the general level of avoidance (e.g., dissociation) required by the survivor for internal stability. This process also increases self resources; As noted earlier, progressive exposure to nonoverwhelming distress is likely to increase the client's repertoire of affect regulation and affect tolerance skills (Linehan, 1993). As a result, successful ongoing treatment allows the survivor to confront increasingly more painful memories without exceeding the survivor's (now greater) emotional capacities.

In combination, decreasing stress levels and increasing self resources can lead to a relatively self-sustaining process: As the need to avoid painful material lessens with treatment, memories previously too overwhelming to address may become more available for processing. As this new material is, in turn, desensitized and cognitively accommodated, self capacity is further improved and the overall stress level is further reduced —thereby permitting access to (and processing of) even more previously avoided material. Ultimately, treatment ends when traumatic material is sufficiently desensitized and integrated, and self resources are sufficiently learned and strengthened, that the survivor no longer experiences significant intrusive, avoidant, or dysphoric symptoms.

This progressive function of abuse-focused therapy removes the need for any so-called "memory recovery" techniques. Instead of relying on hypnosis or drug-assisted interviews, for example, to somehow facilitate recollection of previously unavailable material, this approach allows increased access to these memories as a natural function of the survivor's reduced need for avoidance. Whereas authoritarian memory recovery techniques might easily exceed the client's self capacities and flood him or her with destabilizing memories and affects, careful abuse-focused therapy only allows access to dissociated memory when, by definition, the client is able to handle such material.

In addition to their potential problematic nature as clinical interventions, some memory recovery techniques are associated with a greater risk of suggestion. Although the actual suggestibility potential for hypnosis, drug-assisted interviews, or continued probing for memories is less known than some critics claim, there is little doubt that such techniques can increase the likelihood that at least some of what is "uncovered" is inaccurate or confabulated. Because psychology has yet to develop definitive methods of separating the wheat (true memories) from the chaff (pseudomemories or grossly distorted ones), the use of aggressive memory recovery techniques may further confuse, rather than clarify, the psychotherapy process.

Finally, it is possible that extreme pressure for clients to recall that which is unavailable or unreal can lead to the development of pseudomemories as an avoidance or distraction device. This may occur either because the client believes that he or she must come up with *some* memories in order to discontinue the memory recovery process, or the client may attempt to develop fantastical memories as a way to avoid accessing less bizarre but actually more painful ones (e.g., abuse by a previously beloved father figure).

. It should be noted that it is not memory exploration, per se, that is at fault here, but rather the use of techniques that either place undue pressure on the client or that unduly capitalize on suggestibility. In this regard, the type of treatment advocated in this chapter supports the processing of recollected trauma when possible, but does not support methodologies that coerce or exceed the survivor's existing capacities. In fact, modern abuse-focused therapy reverses an assumption held by those who advocate aggressive memory retrieval: It suggests that clients do not get better when they remember more, but rather, that they may remember more (i.e., avoid less) as they get better.

6. CONCLUSIONS

This chapter outlines a model of abuse-focused psychotherapy that can facilitate both the desensitization of traumatic memory and the strengthening of internal resources. Its primary focus is on the client's internal state—the intent is to provide sufficient processing without overwhelming the client with excessive traumatic material. This model does not require "memory recovery," per se, although improved access to traumatic memory may occur during the process. In fact, it suggests that memory recovery techniques may do harm in some instances, either by overwhelming the client or by producing material of questionable accuracy. On the other hand, available abuse memories must be addressed in treatment, since desensitization can only occur upon exposure to (and processing of) such recollections. Ultimately, then, the issue may not be whether "memory work," per se, is inappropriate. Instead, clinicians must determine the most optimal ways in which such work can be accomplished, such that posttraumatic distress is reduced, but unwanted iatrogenic effects do not occur.

REFERENCES

Abueg, F.R. & Fairbank, J.A. (1992). Behavioral treatment of posttraumatic stress disorder and co-occurring substance abuse. In P.A. Saigh (Ed.), *Posttraumatic stress disorder: A behavioral approach to assessment and treatment* (pp.111–146). Needham Heights, MA: Allyn & Bacon.

American Psychiatric Association (1994). *Diagnostic and statistical manual of mental disorders (4th ed.)*. Washington, D.C.: Author.

American Psychological Association (1995). *Questions and answers about memories of child abuse*. Washington, D.C: Author.

American Psychological Association (1996). *APA Presidential Task Force on Violence and the Family final report*. Washington, D.C.: Author.

American Psychological Association (1996). *Working Group on Investigation of Memories of Childhood Abuse final report*. Washington, D.C.: Author.

Bagley, C., & Ramsay, R. (1986). Disrupted childhood and vulnerability to sexual assault: Long-term sequels with implications for counseling. *Social Work and Human Sexuality, 4*, 33–48.

Becker, J., Skinner, L., Abel, G., & Treacy, E. (1982). Incidence and types of sexual dysfunctions in rape and incest victims. *Journal of Sex and Marital Therapy, 8*, 65–74.

Bowen, G.R., & Lambert, J.A. (1986). Systematic desensitization therapy with post-traumatic stress disorder cases. In C. R. Figley (Ed.), *Trauma and its wake*, Vol. II. New York: Brunner/Mazel.

Bremner, J.D., Krystal, J.H., Southwick, S.M., & Charney, D.S. (1996). Functional neuroanatomical correlates of the effects of stress on memory. *Journal of Traumatic Stress, 8*, 527–553.

Briere, J. (1992a) Methodological issues in the study of sexual abuse effects. *Journal of Consulting and Clinical Psychology, 60*, 196–203.

Briere, J. (1992b). *Child abuse trauma: Theory and treatment of the lasting effects*. Newbury Park, CA: Sage.

Briere, J. (1995a). Science versus politics in the delayed memory debate: A commentary. *The Counseling Psychologist, 23*, 290–293.

Briere, J. (1995b). Child abuse, memory, and recall: A commentary. *Consciousness and Cognition*, *4*, 83–87.

Briere, J. (1996a). A self-trauma model for treating adult survivors of severe child abuse. In J. Briere, L. Berliner, J. Bulkley, C. Jenny, & T. Reid, (Eds.). *The APSAC handbook on child maltreatment* (pp. 140–157). Newbury Park, CA: Sage Publications.

Briere, J. (1996b). *Therapy for adults molested as children, Second edition.* New York: Springer Publishing Co.

Briere, J. (1996c). Treating adults who were sexually abused as children: Central principles. *National Center for PTSD Clinical Quarterly*, *6*, 29–33.

Briere, J. (in press). *Psychological assessment of adult posttraumatic states.* Washington, D.C.: American Psychological Association.

Briere, J., & Conte, J. (1993). Self-reported amnesia for abuse in adults molested as children. *Journal of Traumatic Stress 6*, 21–31.

Briere, J., Elliott, D.M., Harris, K., & Cotman, A. (1995). Trauma Symptom Inventory: Psychometrics and association with childhood and adult trauma in clinical samples. *Journal of Interpersonal Violence*, *10*, 387–401.

Briere, J., & Runtz, M. (1986). Suicidal thoughts and behaviours in former sexual abuse victims. Special issue on family violence, *Canadian Journal of Behavioural Science*, *18*, 413–423.

Briere, J., & Zaidi, L.Y. (1989). Sexual abuse histories and sequelae in female psychiatric emergency room patients. *American Journal of Psychiatry*, *146*, 1602–1606.

Chu, J.A., & Dill, D.L. (1990). Dissociative symptoms in relation to childhood physical and sexual abuse. *American Journal of Psychiatry*, *147*, 887–892.

Cornell, W.F., & Olio, K.A. (1991). Integrating affect in treatment with adult survivors of physical and sexual abuse. *American Journal of Orthopsychiatry*, *61*, 59–69.

Courtois, C.A. (1991). Theory, sequencing, and strategy in treating adult survivors. In J. Briere (Ed.), *Treating victims of child sexual abuse* (pp. 47–60). San Francisco: Jossey-Bass.

Courtois, C. (1995). Assessment and diagnosis. In C. Classen (Ed.), *Treating women molested in childhood* (pp. 1–34). San Francisco: Jossey-Bass.

de Wilde, E.J., Kienhorst, I.C., Diekstra, R.F., & Wolters, W.H. (1992). The relationship between adolescent suicidal behavior and life events in childhood and adolescence. *American Journal of Psychiatry*, *149*, 45–51.

Egeland, B., Sroufe, L.A., & Erickson, M. (1983). The developmental consequences of different patterns of maltreatment. *Child Abuse & Neglect*, *7*, 459–469.

Elliott, D.M. (1994). Impaired object relationships in professional women molested as children. *Psychotherapy*, *31*, 79–86.

Elliott, D.M. (1995, August). *Trauma, memory loss, and subsequent recall: Prevalence and triggers to memory recall.* Paper presented at the annual meeting of the American Psychological Association, New York.

Elliott, D.M., & Briere, J. (1995a). Posttraumatic stress associated with delayed recall of sexual abuse: A general population study. *Journal of Traumatic Stress*, *8*, 629–647.

Elliott, D.M., & Briere, J. (1995b). Transference and countertransference. In C. Classen (Ed.), *Treating women molested in childhood* (pp. 187–226). San Francisco: Jossey Bass.

Feldman-Summers, S., & Pope, K.S. (1994). The experience of "forgetting" childhood abuse: A national survey of psychologists. *Journal of Consulting and Clinical Psychology*, *62*, 636–639.

Foa, E.B., Rothbaum, B.O., Riggs, D.S., & Murdock, T.B. (1991). Treatment of posttraumatic disorder in rape victims: A comparison between cognitive-behavioral procedures and counseling. *Journal of Consulting and Clinical Psychology*, *59*, 715–723.

Frank, E., & Stewart, B.D. (1983). Depressive symptoms in rape victims: A revisit. *Journal of Affective Disorders*, *7*, 77–85.

Fredrickson, R. (1992). *Repressed memories: A journey to recovery from sexual abuse.* New York: Simon and Schuster.

Gold, E.R., (1986). Long-term effects of sexual victimization in childhood: An attributional approach. *Journal of Consulting and Clinical Psychology*, *54*, 471–475.

Henderson, J.L., & Moore, M. (1944). The psychoneuroses of war. *The New England Journal of Medicine*, *230*, 273–279.

Herman, J.L. (1981). *Father-daughter incest.* Cambridge: Harvard University press.

Herman, J.L., & Schatzow, E. (1987). Recovery and verification of memories of childhood sexual trauma. *Psychoanalytic Psychology*, *4*, 1–14.

Horowitz, M.J. (1976). *Stress response syndromes.* New York: Jason Aronson.

Jehu (1988). *Beyond sexual abuse: Therapy with women who were childhood victims.* Chichester, UK: John Wiley.

Jehu, D., Gazan, M., & Klassen, C. (1984/85). Common therapeutic targets among women who were sexually abused in childhood. *Journal of Social Work and Human Sexuality*, *3*, 25–45.

Keane, T.M., Fairbank, J.A., Caddell, J.M., & Zimering, R.T. (1989). Implosive (flooding) therapy reduces symptoms of PTSD in Vietnam combat veterans. *Behavior Therapy, 20*, 245–260.

Lindsay, D.S., (1994). Contextualizing and clarifying criticisms of memory work. Special Issue: The recovered memory/false memory debate. *Consciousness & Cognition: An International Journal, 3*, 426–437.

Lindsay, D.S., (1995). Beyond backlash: Comments on Enns, McNeilly, Corkery, and Gilbert. *The Counseling Psychologist, 23*, 280–289.

Linehan, M. M. (1993). *Cognitive-behavioral treatment of borderline personality disorder.* New York: Guilford.

Loftus, E.F. (1993). The reality of repressed memories. *American Psychologist, 48*, 518–537.

Loftus, E.F., Polonsky, S., & Fullilove, M.T. (1994). Memories of childhood sexual abuse: Remembering and repressing. *Psychology of Women Quarterly, 18*, 67–84.

Marmar, C.R., Foy, D., Kagan, B., & Pynoos, R.S. (1993). An integrated approach for treating posttraumatic stress. In R.S. Pynoos (Ed.), *Posttraumatic stress disorder: A clinical review* (99–132). Lutherville, MD: Sidran.

Metcalfe, J., & Jacobs, W.J. (1996). A "hot-system/cool-system" view of memory under stress. *PTSD Research Quarterly, 7*, 1–6.

McCann, I.L., & Pearlman,L.A. (1990). *Psychological trauma and the adult survivor: Theory, therapy, and transformation.* New York: Brunner/Mazel.

Murray, E.J., & Segal, D.L. (1994). Emotional processing in vocal and written expression of feelings about traumatic experiences. *Journal of Traumatic Stress, 7*, 391–405.

Neumann, D.A., Houskamp, B.M., Pollock, V.E., & Briere, J. (1996). The long-term sequelae of childhood sexual abuse in women: A meta-analytic review. *Child Maltreatment, 1*, 6–16.

Ogata, S.N., Silk, K.R., Goodrich, S., Lohr, N.E., Westen, D., & Hill, E.M. (1990). Childhood sexual and physical abuse in adult patients with borderline personality disorder. *American Journal of Psychiatry, 147*, 1008–1013.

Parfit, D.N., & Gall, C.M.C. (1944). Psychogenic amnesia: The refusal to remember. *The Journal of Mental Science, 379*, 519–531.

Pearlman, L.A., & Saakvitne, K.W. (1995). *Trauma and the therapist: Countertransference and vicarious traumatization in psychotherapy with incest survivors.* New York: W.W. Norton.

Pennebaker, J.W., Kiecolt-Glasser, J.K., & Glaser, R. (1988). Disclosure of trauma and immune function: Health implications for psychotherapy. *Journal of Consulting and Clinical Psychology, 56*, 239–245.

Petrie, K.J., Booth, R.J., Pennebaker, J.W., Davison, K.P., & Thomas, M.G. (1995). Disclosure of trauma and immune response to a Hepatitis B vaccination program. *Journal of Consulting and Clinical Psychology, 63*, 787–792.

Rachman, S. (1980). Emotional processing. *Behavior, Research, and Therapy, 18*, 51–60.

Resick, P.A. & Schnicke, M.K. (1993). *Cognitive processing therapy for rape victims: A treatment manual.* Newbury Park: Sage.

Reviere, S.L. (1996). *Memory of childhood trauma: A clinician's guide to the literature.* New York: Guilford.

Rohsenow, D.J., Corbett, R., & Devine, D. (1988). Molested as children: A hidden contribution to substance abuse? *Journal of Substance Abuse, 5*, 13–18.

Rothblum, B.O. & Foa, E.B. (1992). Cognitive-behavioral treatment of posttraumatic stress disorder. In P.A. Saigh (Ed.), *Posttraumatic stress disorder: A behavioral approach to assessment and treatment* (pp. 85–110). Needham Heights, MA: Allyn & Bacon.

Rowan, A.B., Foy, D.W., Rodriguez, N., & Ryan, S. (1994). Posttraumatic stress disorder in a clinical sample of adults sexually abused as children. *Child Abuse & Neglect, 18*, 51–61.

Sargant, W., & Slater, E. (1941). Amnestic syndromes of war. *Proceedings of the Royal Society of Medicine, 34*, 757–764.

Saunders, B.E., Villeponteaux, L.A., Lipovsky, J.A., Kilpatrick, D.G., & Veronen, L.J. (1992). Child sexual assault as a risk factor for mental disorders among women: A community survey. *Journal of Interpersonal Violence, 7*, 189–204.

Smucker, M.R., Dancu, C., Foa, E.B., & Niederee, J.L. (1995). Imagery rescripting: A new treatment for survivors of childhood sexual abuse suffering from posttraumatic stress. *Journal of Cognitive Psychotherapy, 9*, 3–17.

Stein,, J.A., Golding, J.M., Siegel, J.M., Burnam, M.A., & Sorenson, S.B. (1988). Long-term psychological sequelae of child sexual abuse: The Los Angeles Epidemiological Catchment Area Study. In G.E. Wyatt, & G. Powell, (Eds.), *The lasting effects of child sexual abuse* (Newbury Park, CA: Sage.

Swett, C., Cohen, C., Surrey, J., Compaine, & Chavez, R. (1991). High rates of alcohol use and history of physical and sexual abuse among women outpatients. *American Journal of Drug & Alcohol Abuse, 17*, 49–60.

Sargant, W., & Slater, E. (1941). Amnestic syndromes of war. *Proceedings of the Royal Society of Medicine, 34*, 757–764.

Thom, D.A, & Fenton, N. (1920). Amnesia in war cases. *American Journal of Insanity*, 76, 437–448.

Torrie, A. (1944). Psychosomatic casualties in the Middle East. *Lancet*, 1, 139–143.

Tromp, S., Koss, M.P., Figueredo, A.J., & Tharan, M. (1995). Are rape memories different? A comparison of rape, other unpleasant, and pleasant memories among employed women. *Journal of Traumatic Stress*, 8, 607–627.

Williams, L.M. (1994). Recall of childhood trauma: A prospective study of women's memories of child sexual abuse. *Journal of Consulting and Clinical Psychology*, 62, 1167–1176.

Williams, L.M. (1995). Recovered memories of abuse in women with documented child sexual victimization histories. *Journal of Traumatic Stress*, 8, 649–673.

van der Kolk, B.A. (1994). The body keeps the score: Memory and the evolving psychobiology of posttraumatic stress. *Harvard Review of Psychiatry*, 1, 253–265.

van der Kolk, B.A., & Fisler, R. (1995). Dissociation and the fragmentary nature of traumatic memories: Overview and and exploratory study. *Journal of Traumatic Stress*, 8, 505–525.

Wolpe, J. (1958). *Psychotherapy by reciprocal inhibition*. Stanford: Stanford University Press.

Wyatt, G.E., Newcombe, M.D., & Riederle, M.H. (1993). *Sexual abuse and consensual sex: Women's developmental patterns and outcomes*. Newbury Park, CA: Sage.

Zaidi, L.Y., & Foy, D.W. (1993). Childhood abuse experiences and combat-related PTSD. *Journal of Traumatic Stress*, 7, 33–42.

COMMENTARY ON AN INTEGRATED APPROACH TO TREATING ADULTS ABUSED AS CHILDREN WITH SPECIFIC REFERENCE TO SELF-REPORTED RECOVERED MEMORIES

J. Don Read, University of Lethbridge, 4401 University Dr., Lethbridge, AB, T1K 3M4, Canada

1. GENERAL COMMENTS

I very much appreciated hearing Dr. Briere's presentation in which he described a therapeutic approach for abuse survivors with strong theoretical and empirical foundations, an approach that is so well formulated that I wonder whether there is anything, beyond praise and admiration, at all useful for me to say here. On the other hand, I do want to be sure that I understood his position correctly and in that spirit my comments have been formulated and have been cast in the form of questions that I had about what the presentation did or did not tell me. None of my comments however is intended to take away from Briere's thoughtful presentation and my enthusiastic response to it. My focus here will be upon the overlap between cognitive psychology and clinical psychology with a specific emphasis on the implications of Briere's comments for our understanding about trauma memory and relevant research.

For me, Briere's clinical orientation to clients who have suffered childhood trauma properly assigns much control to the client within a positive humanistic or "self" framework that also seems remarkably sensitive to the potential for distortion of clients' verbal reports following the lapse of time since childhood and the inevitable reconstructive memory processes. As well, the approach taken in his presentation explicitly reflects a recognition of the dangerous potential of suggestive influences by therapists and the multiple bases to any presenting symptom or verbal report made by a client. As the professed goals of the self-trauma model are not "archaeological" with respect to memory but do reflect the central role of memory seen in most psychotherapy, I would anticipate there would be much less likelihood of clients distorting memories within this kind of approach than within what have been called "memory-recovery therapies", which Briere characterises as inappropriately focused on memory work.

Second, had this particular orientation and obvious caution been widely evident in much of the clinical and popular literature that Steve Lindsay and I reviewed in recent papers on "memory recovery" techniques and therapy over the last 3 years, our concerns about the potential for the production of false memories (on the basis of research within cognitive psychology) would have been substantially reduced (e.g., Lindsay & Read, 1994, 1995). Third, as a general comment, I also found Briere's summary statement very appealing in which he argues it is not that the recovery of memories facilitates mental health but that the recovery of memories is a marker of improved mental health.

However, I also find myself pondering a potential caveat to my enthusiastic response. The caveat embraces the question of whether clients understand (or need to understand) the distinction Briere has made between the emergence of memories as the prelude to therapy (followed by anticipation of improved psychological health) and the emergence of memories as evidence of having attained the goal of improved psychological health. This distinction might be better cast in the question: Should traumatic memories be exorcised so the client can get started on the road to better mental health (as in the memory-recovery approaches he cautions against) or should the presentation of traumatic memories be taken as evidence of psychological improvement (as in Briere's self-trauma model)? Perhaps there is no need for clients to understand this distinction because Briere's description of the model in this chapter includes no discussion of what the client might be told about the potential emergence of memories at the outset of therapy. Perhaps nothing need be said about memories of trauma such that what happens in therapy just happens. My assumption however, based on Briere's general approach and his other written materials (e.g., Briere, 1996), is that he would recommend that the matter be raised with clients early on and its absent discussion here is simply an oversight. However, with or without such discussion, I believe that a misinterpretation by clients of the role and importance of memories could arise for at least two reasons. First, a national sample of clinical psychologists recently reported to Polusny and Follette (1996) that more and more frequently they have seen clients enter therapy with an expectation of a process of memory recovery. If true, clinicians may already have the problem of countering clients' expectations and beliefs about the importance of memory recovery. Second, if the potential emergence of trauma memories as markers of good therapeutic outcome is discussed, some clients might be encouraged to present their trauma memories as the desired demonstrations of the therapeutic success they and the therapist seek. Many clinicians (including Briere, Courtois, and Lynn, this volume) have regularly reminded us of the subtle influences exerted by even the most intentionally neutral therapists. However, there is no way, nor would we wish a way, around the interactive process between client and therapist. My question then, asks whether memories might nonetheless be eagerly sought by clients in the self-trauma approach and, if so, are there hazards for them in doing so?

2. INITIAL ASSESSMENT OF CLIENTS

In listening to and reading the core of Briere's presentation (see also Briere, 1996), I find that there also remains for me the nagging question as to the basis for the initial assessment of a client as an abuse survivor. On the one hand, Briere indicates that the self-trauma model is presented for discussion here in the context of "the treatment of individuals with significant abuse-related symptomatology," and is "limited to those whose abuse has produced long-term effects" and those "who have been abused and who suffer from that abuse". Thus, although apart from the title of Briere's presentation, because he never actually said so, I think we must assume that he refers *only* to clients for whom an abuse history is known and, presumably, reported by the client. I did find this issue somewhat ambiguous because at later points in his presentation Briere refers to those who either deny or have absent recall of abuse (as a result of dissociative processes or one of four possible encoding problems) and describes the way in which the self-trauma model would encourage the emergence and later desensitisation of those memories that are not "permanently unavailable", although he indicates that for some clients such recall apparently will never occur. In the end, I had to assume that in every case Briere was referring to clients who at least initially reported some knowledge of abuse and, as a result, could not be clients for whom complete amnesia about the abuse exists. Otherwise, we are left with the logical conundrum as to how the therapist knows there is an abuse history that produced the long-term effects inferred from the clients' presentation.

From his remarks I also understand however that some survivors will not disclose abuse at the outset or, apparently, even after extensive therapy within the most facilitative environment for doing so *because* their self resources are not yet strong enough to provide the support to allow them to do so. Admittedly, I don't know an easy way around the problem of the inherent circularity of this kind of argument but it is possible, of course, that whenever clients do not recall traumatic events in question (known or hypothesised), we can always say that the memories exist but the clients just do not yet have the internal self resources to deal with them. And, of course, if they did recall the events of interest, then it follows that they must have had sufficient self resources to do so. Distinguishing between those clients who don't have any (or additional) traumatic experiences to recall from those who do have such experiences but lack the resources to recall them would be difficult, to say the least.

In this same connection, Briere indicates that in his clinical experience the "dissociation of or disconnection from abuse-related material may present as incomplete or *absent* recall of the events in question". This I find also takes us back to the same thorny issue and to much of the basis of a conference like this. That is, how do we know what the "events in question" are or whether there even are *any* events in question? Further, Briere states that such absent recall can also reflect denial. And, he indicates that traumatic events can be so upsetting that even therapeutic intervention cannot get through. I think that much of the debate surrounding the issue of recovered memories could be enlightened if we had knowledge of the relative proportions of clients who present with one versus another kind of behaviour or complaint. For example, to satisfy the criteria for post-traumatic stress disorder as per the DSM-IV, a client must present symptoms that involve, among other things, intrusive recollections of the trauma and evidence of avoidance of thoughts about the trauma, such as psychogenic amnesia. It is argued often (see Yehuda, this volume, for example) that these two symptoms frequently co-present within the same client. Because the simultaneous experience of both intrusive recollection and dissociative amnesia in the same client is a logical mind twister (and on the surface, at least, would seem to rule out the possibility of diagnosing them as having "complete amnesia"), empirical data that speak to such reportedly commonly observed, joint appearances would be rather important. In this vein I would similarly ask, what proportion of clients do therapists anticipate for whom dissociation appears to present as absent recall? For that matter, what is the proportion of clients considered to be absent the recall of abuse at the termination of therapy? Because I would like to understand what kinds of clients are being referred to, my question asks which clients are included in Briere's discussion: those who have some knowledge of traumatic experiences, or those with none, or both?

Some work on this issue has been completed recently by Polusny and Follette (1996) and, from their sample of clinical psychologists, it appears that clients who have no memory of sexual abuse trauma (among those who have been determined to have been abused) are very infrequent (i.e., less than 15% of clinical psychologists reported having *ever* seen a single client who initially reported no memory followed by the recollection of sexual abuse during the course of therapy.

3. THERAPEUTIC GOALS AND PROCESS

What I assume is being recommended throughout Briere's presentation is that the therapist must be cognizant of the possibility of abuse or past trauma and proceed on that basis. What I hear is that as the client becomes healthier he or she will recall memories that reflect that progress toward health. My assumption is that even when no additional memories are recalled, there will be a point reached during therapy at which the therapist engaged in self-trauma work no longer anticipates recovery of further memories. My question here is, given the goals of this self-trauma model and the assumption that memories may be recovered as products and demonstrations of successful therapy, can the therapeutic goals be considered to have nevertheless been met and therapy judged successful when no additional memories are brought forward? On this point Briere argues that for such clients there simply is no need to provide a relentless search for memories. One hopes for equivalent restraint from other therapists.

However, does this perspective not put the therapist in conflict if the success of therapeutic intervention is, mistakenly I think, indexed by the amount of traumatic material recalled? If no memories can mean a lack of success in returning the client to mental health would there not be an ethical obligation to continue with therapy when no memories have emerged? Obviously, this approach has more inherent accountability than those therapies which suggest no perceptible indicator of success within the client's reach. Hence there may be both a positive and negative side to this approach: on the one hand, more accountability for the client, but, on the other hand, a larger investment in observable success by the therapist. It seems to me that in other forms of trauma therapy (including so-called memory-recovery therapies) a therapist's success is not as directly observable as in Briere's self-trauma model.

Given Briere's emphasis upon various models of trauma theory, there is an explicit belief that desensitisation of trauma experiences must occur in order for the client to make the most effective use of his or her own resources. Because I am not a clinician, I will accept on faith Briere's statements regarding the clinical rationales that underlie some of the intervention techniques he described. However, Briere describes four reasons for the failure of trauma-related material to be recalled and, as a result, not be available for desensitisation and subsequent cognitive processing: (1) childhood amnesia; (2) inadequate encoding at time of trauma; (3) hypothetically excessive neurohormone activity (it is not clear to me how or why this is not simply a subset of (2)); and (4) events were so distressing (solidly repressed, disconnected, or dissociated) that not even therapeutic intervention could break through. With clients who have not provided any recollection of any trauma, it seems to me that there should be a fifth alternative: there was no traumatic event to recall. As I mentioned at the outset, this was a point about which I could not be certain: on what bases did the therapist reach the conclusion that the client had indeed been abused but, because of one of the four reasons described, does not remember the abuse?

4. RETROSPECTIVE ASSESSMENTS OF TRAUMA MEMORY

The terms "complete amnesia", "partial amnesia" and "dissociative amnesia" all made appearances within Briere's presentation. I have some difficulty with his use of these terms because I'm not convinced that the clients' psychological states necessarily match the pathology suggested by the terms. Complete or total amnesia for some events is clearly evident for some people and there are many abnormalities of memory functioning, some organic, some functional, many of which Michael Kopelman (this volume) has documented particularly well. However, from a cognitive psychologist's perspective, I do question the wisdom of referring to the incomplete remembering or recollection of an event or set of events as evidence of "partial amnesia" And, I particularly question the wisdom of categorising clients and survey respondents as partial amnesics who, perhaps on the basis of a single question by therapist or survey researcher, have reported that there has been a period of time during which they now think they did not well remember the events they are now describing.

More specifically, the belief that traumatic events are often not recalled or are not recallable is based upon clinical observation as well as many empirical studies and surveys. The retrospective reports from participants in the various research studies of Briere and Conte (1993) and Elliott and Briere (1995), Williams (1994a, 1994b, 1995), and Loftus, Polonsky and Fullilove (1994), as well as others, frequently asserted that they previously remembered less about the abuse than they did at the time of being asked the question. From these multiple reports, Briere suggests that "some real phenomenon is in operation". I would not disagree but suspect that Briere does not intend this statement to be as ambiguous as I take it to be. I believe that he means to imply that there is something special about the experience of trauma that can have unusual consequences for memory, notably a reduction in access to or retrieval of relevant events from memory. I also think there may be some real phenomenon here but I am not convinced that it is either a single phenomenon or that the possibly multiple phenomena are necessarily related to trauma.

Other researchers, including several at this meeting (i.e., Brewin, Andrews, Schooler, Williams, Loftus) as well as John Briere, have critiqued the various methodological difficulties of the kinds of retrospective questions used in these studies (see, for example, Williams, this volume). The only point I wish to make here is that Briere's presentation neglects detailing such critiques and we are left with the impression that he believes such reports of perceived improvements in recall to reflect the amnestic characteristics of trauma. From a cognitive psychological perspective however, I would emphasise the likely influence of cognitive heuristics upon these kinds of metamemorial judgments.

For example, I can say now with considerable certainty that there has been a period of many years in my past wherein I had much less recall of the French language than I do today. But the reason for my judgment has neither anything to do trauma nor with any attempt at relearning French prior to getting on a Paris-bound plane. Instead, in my role as a meeting organiser I was intermittently, and frequently cued and reminded of French for several months prior to this meeting. In other words, my judgment that there was a period of time in which I remembered French less than I do now was based entirely upon my experiences over recent months during which I surprised myself as to how much French I remembered. Had I also been asked at some point whether there was a period during which I had forgotten French, I likely would have said yes.

The important point is that I would not, however, have referred to this perception of a prior impoverished recollection period as a demonstration of partial or complete amnesia for French. I raise this, of course, not because I believe that memories of a language studied in high school and memories of trauma have much in common but because I think we have to remain alert to the possibility of other interpretations and other bases for the kinds of retrospective metamemorial judgments being made in the work described by Briere. When a client has been in therapy and childhood abuse has been a focus of treatment and discussion, should we really be surprised to learn that such clients reach a point when they believe they formerly had less recall of the abuse than they do now? Unless they had been similarly focused for several years on the abuse prior to therapy, how could it be otherwise? It should be noted that questions about the reliability of these latter judgments are very different from questions about the reliability and accuracy of recall of specific life events, a topic addressed by Brewin, Andrews, and Gotlib (1993).

5. SUGGESTIONS FOR FUTURE RESEARCH

From a researcher's perspective several intriguing research ideas present themselves as a result of Dr. Briere's stimulating presentation. First, if his position on memories as consequences of successful therapy (rather than as anticipatory stage-setting) has validity, one should be able to trace with a sample of clients the extent of disclosure of sexual abuse in therapy and relate it to their improvements in mental health. A second goal of research could be to compare, if possible, whether false recollections, as anticipated, are much less likely within the Briere self-trauma model than within the aggressive memory-recovery therapies that he argues may have done clients a disservice. Finally, in this model we can ask whether and how the treatment programs and progress of two potential clients would differ, one suspected of a history of trauma and the other a documented victim of similar abuse but who both present with absent recall of the events? There is the possibility that at least some of these research suggestions could be studied within laboratory experimental paradigms in the manner of Pennebaker and colleagues, as described in Dr. Briere's presentation. I look forward with optimism to the scientific testing of some of the model's recommendations.

REFERENCES

Brewin, C., Andrews, B.,& Gotlib (1993). Psychopathology and early experience: A reappraisal of retrospective reports. *Psychological Bulletin, 113,* 82–98.

Briere, J. (1996). A self-trauma model for treating adult survivors of severe child abuse. In J. Briere, L. Berliner, J. Bulkley, G. Jenny, & T. Reid (Eds.). *The APSAC handbook on child maltreatment* (pp. 140–157). Newbury Park, CA: Sage Publications.

Briere, J., & Conte, J. (1993). Self-reported amnesia for abuse in adults molested as children. *Journal of Traumatic Stress, 6,* 21–31.

Elliott, D. M., & Briere, J. (1995). Posttraumatic stress associated with delayed recall of sexual abuse: A general population study. *Journal of Traumatic Stress, 8,* 629–647.

Lindsay, D. S., & Read, J. D. (1994). Psychotherapy and memories of childhood sexual abuse: A cognitive perspective. *Applied Cognitive Psychology, 8,* 281–338.

Lindsay, D. S., & Read, J. D. (1995). Memory work and recovered memories of childhood sexual abuse: Scientific evidence and public, professional, and personal issues. *Psychology, Public Policy, and Law, 1,* 846–908.

Loftus, E. F., Polonsky, S., & Fullilove, M. T. (1994). Memories of childhood sexual abuse: Remembering and repressing. *Psychology of Women Quarterly, 18,* 67–84.

Polusny, M. A., & Follonette, V. M. (1996). Remembering childhood sexual abuse: A national survey of psychologists' clinical practices, beliefs, and personal experiences. *Professional Psychology: Research and Practice, 27,* 41–52.

Williams, L. M. (1994a). Recall of childhood trauma: A prospective study of women's memories of child sexual abuse. *Journal of Consulting and Clinical Psychology, 62,* 1167–1172.

Williams, L. M. (1994b). What does it mean to forget child sexual abuse? A reply to Loftus, Garry, and Feldman (1994). *Journal of Consulting and Clinical Psychology, 62,* 1182–1186.

Williams, L. M. (1995). Recovered memories of abuse in women with documented child sexual victimization histories. *Journal of Traumatic Stress, 8,* 649–673.

QUESTION AND ANSWER SESSION

Lynn. I was curious about what I sensed was a sense to demonize hypnosis as a vile technique, so I find myself in the position of defending hypnosis. One of the things you talked about was the resource-building process as very important. Then you mentioned things like self-development, self-soothing, ego strengthening, relaxation. These are the kind of techniques I associate with hypnotic techniques. I fully agree that we don't use hypnosis with very dissociative clients, or in the middle of a dissociative episode, but it seems to me there are appropriate uses in this phase of treatment. I was concerned because it seemed you were saying there was some altered state of hypnosis that people get zonked into, and personally, I don't think the research supports an identifiable altered state. In fact, I think that people now are essentially agreeing that we don't really agree that there is an altered state that is very measurable. So, could you comment on that?

Briere. Yes. What you are saying is what some other people have said on this issue, in terms of using hypnosis to build internal resources. I think that may be a good use of hypnosis. My concern is that I'm not sure of its applicability to traumatised individuals. I am being conservative, even though I have used hypnosis in the past to treat cancer patients for pain control and medication-related anticipatory nausea. So I do believe that hypnosis is a helpful tool, and I don't want to demonize it. I have become more conservative about hypnosis over time, with reference to trauma, generally because I don't really know how it works and I am afraid it may sometimes do things we don't want it to do. I do think that the relationship between hypnotic susceptibility, dissociation, and suggestibility is real, and therefore I feel nervous about advocating its use with trauma survivors.

Schooler. Following through the logic of your treatment argument: if you need to use systematic desensitisation of the trauma experience in order to have efficacious treatment, and if the individual doesn't remember any of the trauma, then how are you going to be effective in inducing the systematic desensitisation ?

Briere. This question is raised sometimes by clinicians: if you must process traumatic material, but it is not consciously available, how can you process it? Well, first, there may not be any traumatic material there, if it is not remembered. Therefore it could not be processed. On the other hand, if memories of the trauma are not available, remember that the Self-Trauma model allows two pathways to intervention: desensitisation and increasing self capacities. If the material is unavailable due to avoidance — and I suggest that dissociative avoidance is only one of many reasons why memories might not be present — then intervening to increase self capacities may eventually decrease the need for avoidance, and thus material may be more available for processing. This may or may not be enough. When it isn't, there may not be too much you can do for the amnestic individual.

Hyman. Something you raised earlier was that a clear outcome of early childhood abuse is perhaps later rape and other sexual trauma. I want to ask if the correlation goes the other way, if its not the case that we are seeing encoding specificity here. In later trauma it brings to mind the earlier trauma, so it's not that the earlier trauma causes the possibility of a later trauma, but that it brings it back to mind.

Briere. There may be some state dependency here, as per a recent study indicating that depressed college students have better memories of previously depressing material than nondepressed college students. And, clearly, a current trauma may trigger recollection of a previous one. Unfortunately, because we use primarily retrospective methodologies in this area, the directionality of recall is not easily assessed. I think some really interesting research could be done in this area.

Cardeña. Just a quick p.s. to Steve Lynn's comment. I think there is one reason why being conservative might have risks. Irving Kirsch and collaborators did an analysis of cognitive behavioural alone and cognitive behavioural with hypnosis, and found that the latter was very noticeably a better treatment. Granted, we don't have a similar study for the treatment of trauma, and we should get the data.

Briere. I agree with you. That was a great study, and I'll admit I was very impressed with the improvement associated with the addition of hypnosis. Of course, as you say, the target wasn't trauma-related. It only showed that under certain circumstances hypnosis might be helpful. I really don't argue that hypnosis cannot be helpful in lots of areas. I just don't think we are ready to use it in this area.

Creamer. Just to change the subject completely, and to come back to the strengths of treatment. I agree with what you see as the main components of treatment, and in terms that I'd use such as anxiety management and exposure treatment. In terms of PTSD, I often see the need for a third stage of addressing the processing with cognitive restructuring, addressing the meaning of the event for the person.

Briere. I agree completely, I just didn't have time to address cognitive interventions to any extent. As Patti Resick notes, desensitisation alone may be insufficient when it doesn't change the cognitive structure or schema. I think that, not just with PTSD, modern cognitive behavioural approaches do cognitive restructuring along with some kind of exposure treatment. And, I think that what a lot of people are doing when they treat child abuse survivors is using cognitive therapy principles.

REFERENCES

Resick, P.A. & Schnicke, M.K. (1993). *Cognitive processing therapy for rape victims: A treatment manual.* Newbury Park, CA: Sage.
Kirsch, Irving, Montgomery, Guy & Sapirstein (1995). Hypnosis as an adjuct to cognitive-behavioural psychotherapy: A meta-analysis. *Journal of Consulting and Clinical Psychology, 63,* 214–220.

3

ACCURACY OF ADULT RECOLLECTIONS OF EARLY CHILDHOOD ABUSE

Cathy Spatz Widom

The University at Albany (SUNY)
135 Western Ave.
Albany, New York 12222

1. INTRODUCTION

Over the last two decades, there has been a dramatic increase in the number of reports retrospectively linking childhood abuse to a variety of short- and long-term effects. Typically, adolescents or adults are asked about a history of abuse in an interview or on a questionnaire designed to elicit this information retrospectively. However, considerable controversy exists about the validity of information obtained from retrospective self-reports (Berliner & Williams, 1994; Briere & Conte, 1993; Della Femina, Yeager, & Lewis, 1990; Herman & Schatzow, 1987; Kruttschnitt & Dornfeld, 1992; Lindsay & Read, 1994; Loftus, 1993; Widom, 1989c; Williams, 1994). Although many researchers argue that estimates based on adult retrospective reports are probably underestimates (Finkelhor, 1993), others have argued that retrospective reports may contain many false positives (Nash, 1992).

Although debates about the accuracy of autobiographical recall have a long history, there seems to be general acceptance that memory is at least partly reconstructive (Fivush, 1993; Neisser, 1967; Radke-Yarrow, Campbell, & Burton, 1970). As Fivush (1993, p. 2) has pointed out "it becomes difficult to determine whether an individual is recalling the actual details of a particular experience or reconstructing what must have occurred based on general event knowledge."

A significant risk of distortion and loss of information is associated with the recollection of events from childhood. If asked to recall childhood events, it is possible that respondents forget or redefine their behaviors in accordance with later life circumstances or their current situation. It is also possible that a person might redefine someone else's behavior in light of current knowledge. Unconscious denial (or repression of childhood traumatic events) may also be at work in preventing the recollection of severe cases of childhood abuse. Furthermore, given society's disapproval of various forms of family violence, a person may be unwilling to reveal such private information in the context of an interview setting. Thus, for a variety of reasons, there may be considerable slippage in accuracy in retrospective reporting. As Brewin, Andrews, and Gotlib (1993, p. 94) pointed out:

Recollections of Trauma, edited by Read and Lindsay
Plenum Press, New York, 1997

Obtaining the retrospective recall of childhood events appears, therefore, to be a flawed process that can be shaped by both internal and external factors. Social influences, childhood amnesia, and the simple fallibility of memory all impose limitations on the accuracy of recall, and fear of the consequences of disclosure may further disadvantage this process.

What other factors might affect the accuracy of retrospective reporting? There may be gender differences in reporting or willingness to report childhood sexual abuse for a variety of reasons. Female psychiatric patients were more likely to report histories of sexual abuse than males (Brown & Anderson, 1991; Carmen, Rieker, & Mills, 1984), females were more likely to reveal childhood sexual assault experiences to therapists than males (Jacobson & Richardson, 1987), and females reported greater risk of being a victim of sexual assault than males (Burnam, Stein, Golding, Siegel, Sorenson, Forsythe, & Telles, 1988). Social pressures against reporting early childhood sexual experiences, out of embarrassment, may lead to greater reluctance among males to report, whereas it may be socially more acceptable for females to report such histories. On the other hand, some of the apparent under-reporting may be associated with the small number of male victims of sexual abuse in most studies (Finkelhor, 1990).

Researchers have also speculated that age at the time of the abuse experience may affect the accuracy of memory and the likelihood of recall or reporting. For example, Herman and Schatzow (1987) reported a strong association between degree of reported amnesia and age of onset and duration of the abuse. Women who reported no memory deficits were generally those whose abuse had begun or continued well into adolescence. The most severe deficits were usually associated with abuse that began in early childhood, often in the preschool years, and ended before adolescence. In one of the few prospective studies, Williams (1994) reported that women who were younger (ages 0–6 years) at the time of the abuse were less likely to report the experiences than women who were older at the time (ages 7–12 years). On the other hand, Loftus (1993) and others (Wakefield & Underwager, 1992) have suggested that to have no recall of earlier abuse is uncommon, and that, unless the event occurred before the age of three, they believe it is unlikely that a child would forget a truly traumatic event. Although dealing with children and not adults, Leippe, Manion, and Romanczyk (1991) designed a laboratory situation in which the experimenter engaged in interpersonal "touching" with a group of children who were later asked to recall the details of the event. Interestingly, memory errors of 5–6 year olds were primarily restricted to failure to report touches that did occur, rather than reporting touches that did not occur.

This chapter describes a study that examined the accuracy of adult recollections of childhood sexual and physical abuse using a sample of individuals with officially documented and substantiated cases of childhood victimization (sexual and physical abuse and neglect) and a matched control group. Although most research on the accuracy of memories of childhood abuse focuses on sexual abuse, the design of this study permits an examination of the accuracy of retrospective reports of both types of childhood experiences—sexual and physical abuse. The combination of two sets of findings places this examination of the accuracy of adult recollections in the context of a broad perspective. This chapter represents a condensation of two articles in the journal *Psychological Assessment* on adult recollections of childhood physical abuse (Widom & Shepard, 1996) and sexual abuse (Widom & Morris, in press). After a brief introduction, this chapter reports on (1) the accuracy of self-report measures of childhood sexual and physical abuse by comparison to "known groups"; (2) the extent to which accuracy varies by the age of the child at the time of the abuse; (3) the predictive efficiency of the measures of abuse;

and (4) construct validity. To facilitate understanding of the findings, the methods involved in selecting subjects and in assessing both childhood sexual and physical abuse are described first. Then, the findings for each type of childhood victimization (sexual and physical abuse) will be presented separately. Finally, there is a general discussion and conclusion at the end of the chapter.

Following Fivush (1993, p. 2), accuracy of adult recollections of early childhood abuse is operationally defined "as agreement between the individual's recall and either an objective record of the event or social consensus from other participants of the event as to what occurred." Here, the "objective record of the event" refers to the fact that the cases of childhood abuse involved here were substantiated by the courts at the time. Though this design characteristic represents a strength, there are also limitations to this design which should be noted at the outset. First, this study does not permit determination of the extent of false positives, since it is not possible to determine whether individuals who self-report childhood abuse, but who do not have an official record of abuse, are reporting accurately or not. In many instances, it is likely (and expected) that childhood abuse occurred and was not officially reported. Thus, some of the respondents without official records of abuse, will answer "yes" to these questions, introducing ambiguity. The working assumption underlying this research is that these self-reports are valid, until some empirical evidence contradicts that assumption. It should also be pointed out that not all of the abused respondents will acknowledge their early childhood experiences. Finally, there may be some ambiguity associated with the respondent's cognitive appraisal of these childhood experiences, and some ambiguity will remain simply because of memory problems, denial, or social desirability pressures not to report. Unfortunately, these limitations effect most research in this field, with the possible exception of some laboratory analogue studies where behavior and social interactions can be monitored and assessed with more control.

2. THE STUDY

2.1. Design

The data employed in these analyses are part of a research project based on a cohorts design study (Leventhal, 1982; Schulsinger, Mednick, & Knop, 1981) in which abused and neglected children were matched with non-abused and non-neglected children and followed prospectively into young adulthood. Characteristics of the design include: 1) an unambiguous operationalization of abuse and neglect; 2) a prospective design; 3) separate abused and neglected groups; 4) a large sample; 5) a control group matched as closely as possible for age, sex, race and approximate social class background; and 6) assessment of the long-term consequences of abuse and neglect beyond adolescence and into adulthood.

The prospective nature of the study disentangles the effects of childhood victimization from other potential confounding effects. Because of the matching procedure, the subjects are assumed to differ only in the risk factor: that is, having experienced childhood sexual or physical abuse or neglect. Since it is not possible to randomly assign subjects to groups, the assumption of equivalency for the groups is an approximation. The control group may also differ from the abused and neglected individuals on other variables nested with abuse or neglect. (For complete details of the study design and subject selection criteria, see Widom, 1989a.)

In the first phase of this research, a large group of children who were abused and/or neglected approximately 20 years ago were followed-up through an examination of official juvenile and criminal records and compared with a matched control group of children (Widom, 1989b). The rationale for identifying the abused and neglected group was that their cases were serious enough to come to the attention of the authorities. Only court substantiated cases of child abuse and neglect were included here. Cases were drawn from the records of county juvenile and adult criminal courts in a metropolitan area in the Midwest during the years 1967 through 1971. To avoid potential problems with ambiguity in the direction of causality, and to ensure that temporal sequence was clear (that is, child abuse or neglect ——> subsequent outcomes), abuse and neglect cases were restricted to those in which children were less than 11 years of age at the time of the abuse or neglect incident. Thus, these are cases of early childhood abuse and/or neglect.

Physical abuse cases included injuries such as bruises, welts, burns, abrasions, lacerations, wounds, cuts, bone and skull fractures, and other evidence of physical injury. Sexual abuse charges varied from relatively non-specific charges of "assault and battery with intent to gratify sexual desires" to more specific charges of "fondling or touching in an obscene manner", sodomy, incest, and so forth. Neglect cases reflected a judgment that the parents' deficiencies in child care were beyond those found acceptable by community and professional standards at the time. These cases represented extreme failure to provide adequate food, clothing, shelter, and medical attention to children.

A control group was established with children who were matched on age, sex, race, and approximate family social class during the time period of the study (1967 through 1971). Children who were under school age at the time of the abuse and/or neglect were matched with children of the same sex, race, date of birth (+/- 1 week), and hospital of birth through the use of county birth record information. For children of school age, records of more than 100 elementary schools for the same time period were used to find matches with children of the same sex, race, date of birth (+/- 6 months), class in elementary school during the years 1967 through 1971, and home address, preferably within a five-block radius of the abused or neglected child. Overall, there were matches for 74% of the abused and neglected children.

The second phase of the research involved tracing, locating, and interviewing the abused and/or neglected individuals (20 years after their childhood victimization) and controls. The follow-up was designed to document long-term consequences of childhood victimization across a number of outcomes (cognitive and intellectual, emotional, psychiatric, social and interpersonal, occupational, and general health). Two-hour follow-up interviews were conducted between 1989 and 1995. The interview consisted of a series of structured and semi-structured questionnaires and rating scales, including measures of IQ and reading ability and a psychiatric assessment — the NIMH Diagnostic Interview Schedule, Version III Revised (Robins, Helzer, Cottler, & Goldring, 1989).

2.2. The Subjects

These findings are based on interviews with 1,196 individuals (110 cases of physical abuse, 96 of sexual abuse, 520 of neglect, and 543 controls). Of the original sample of 1,575, 1,292 subjects (82%) have been located and 1,196 interviewed (76%). Of the 95 people not interviewed, 39 were deceased, 9 were incapable of being interviewed, and 49 refused to participate (a refusal rate of 3%). Comparison of the current follow-up sample with the original sample indicates no significant differences in terms of percent male, white, abused and/or neglected, poverty in childhood census tract, or mean current age. The interviewed group (follow-up sample) is significantly more likely to have an official criminal arrest record than the original sample of 1,575 (42% in the current sample versus

36% in the original sample). However, this is not surprising since people with a criminal history are generally easier to find, in part because they have more "institutional footprints" to assist in locating them.

The mean age of the sample at the time of the interview was 29.23 (SD = 3.84), with no differences in age between the abused and neglected group and controls. The average highest grade of school completed for the sample was 11.47 (SD = 2.19), although abused and neglected individuals had completed significantly less school (M=10.99, SD=1.99) than controls (M=12.09, SD=2.29). While two-thirds of the control group had completed high school, less than half (48%) of the abused and neglected children at follow-up had done so. Occupational status of the sample was coded according to the Hollingshead Occupational Coding Index (Hollingshead, 1975). Occupational levels of the subjects ranged from 1 (laborer) to 9 (professional). Median occupational level of the sample was semi-skilled workers, and less than 7% of the overall sample was in levels 7–9 (managers through professionals). More of the controls were in higher occupational levels than were the abused and neglected subjects.

Because the interview asks about a history of childhood sexual and physical abuse in a number of different ways, comparisons can be made of self-reported information with information in official case records (recorded at the time of the abuse experience). Percentage accuracy of recall is calculated by comparing self-reported retrospective information with official record information from the earlier time period.

2.3. Measures

Retrospective self-report measures of early childhood sexual and physical abuse were administered in structured interview formats. Copies of the measures are available from the author and complete descriptions of these analyses are provided in Widom and Shepard (1996) and Widom and Morris (in press).

2.3.1. Retrospective Self-Reports of Childhood Sexual Abuse. Several approaches were used to assess a history of childhood sexual abuse. The sexual abuse questions are adaptations of the work of a number of other researchers (Finkelhor, 1979; Lewis, 1985; Russell, 1983). While the content is similar, the structured interview format used here was developed for this study to permit administration by a trained lay interviewer. The goal was to achieve a balance between sensitivity on the part of the interviewer to elicit highly personal and potentially upsetting information and not being perceived as "leading" the subject into an admission of perhaps questionable reminiscences. The four measures are briefly described below:

1. Respondents were presented with a list of explicitly sexual behaviors (ranging from "an invitation or request to do something sexual" to "another person fondling you in a sexual way" to "intercourse") and asked: "Up to the time you finished elementary school (before 6th grade), did you ever have any of the following experiences...?" Responses to individual items are reported here as well as a dichotomous variable which refers to whether the person reported having any of these experiences before they finished elementary school. A positive response to any of these sexual experiences before age 12 is the first measure of self-reported childhood sexual abuse: "any sex before 12".
2. Following the list of sexually explicit questions about early sexual experiences, respondents were "Do you consider any of these experiences to have been sex-

ual abuse?" Responses to this question were considered to reflect the person's cognitive appraisal (or definition) of the event or experience as being childhood sexual abuse, rather than a direct question about whether the event occurred: "considered sex abuse".

3. Following Finkelhor (1979, 1986), childhood sexual abuse is defined as having a sexual experience with a person several years older. The approach used here is based on the person's response to a separate set of questions about whether they had "ever had a sexual experience with anyone 10 years older" and how old they were when this happened for the first time. Following Finkelhor (1979), the cutoff of age 12 was used to coincide with the age frame of the cases of childhood sexual abuse in this sample. Thus, this third approach is based on the person's report that they had sex with a person 10 years older when the event occurred before the age of 12: "sex with older person".

4. At the end of these questions, respondents were asked: "Has anyone *ever* bothered you sexually or tried to have sex with you against your will?" This question was followed-up by a question about the age at which this occurred. This fourth measure of childhood sexual abuse was restricted to events that occurred before age 12, consistent with the age of our subjects at the time of their abuse or neglect experience(s): "sex against will".

2.3.2. Retrospective Self-Reports of Childhood Physical Abuse. Two measures were used to retrospectively assess a history of childhood physical abuse: the Conflict Tactics Scale (CTS) and the Self-Report of Childhood Abuse Physical (SRCAP).

The CTS was developed by Straus (1979) to assess the amount and severity of family violence. Several subscales have been identified: reasoning, verbal aggression, minor violence, severe violence, and very severe violence. When they refer to physical abuse, Straus and Gelles (1990) are using the "very severe violence" (VSV) scale which includes the following items: kick, bite, or hit you with a fist; beat you up; burn or scald you; threaten with a knife or gun; or use a knife or gun. Although the CTS has been used to assess physical child abuse, information on criterion and construct validity is not extensive (Straus & Gelles, 1990).

In the present study, CTS items were framed in the context of an introduction which asked respondents about "...things that your parents or the people in your family might have done when they had a disagreement with you when you were growing up, that is, up to the time *you finished elementary school*." This age limit was imposed to insure that the time period was consistent with official information about the abuse experience. Possible response categories ranged from never to once, twice, sometimes, frequently, or most of the time. Dichotomous summary subscale scores were computed using the five subscales reported by Straus and Gelles (1990).

A second self-report measure of childhood physical abuse (SRCAP) was designed to provide an alternative means to retrospectively assess childhood physical abuse. The SRCAP was introduced with the following statement: "Up to the time you finished elementary school, did anyone...." SRCAP scores reflect the person's response to the following six items: (1) beat or really hurt you by hitting you with a bare hand or fist; (2) beat or hit you with something hard like a stick or baseball bat; (3) injure you with a knife, shoot you with a gun, or use another weapon against you; (4) hurt you badly enough so that you needed a doctor or other medical treatment; (5) physically injure you so that you were admitted to a hospital; and (6) beat you when you didn't deserve it. A dichotomous variable was created to indicate whether the person reported having any of these childhood experiences or none.

3. THE FINDINGS

Findings are presented separately for the two types of childhood victimization, with findings regarding childhood sexual abuse presented first and followed by findings for childhood physical abuse. For both types of early childhood victimization experiences (sexual and physical abuse), four issues are addressed: (1) comparisons of official reports with self-reports; (2) predictive efficiency; (3) differences in recall as a function of age at abuse; and (4) construct validity.

3.1. Childhood Sexual Abuse

3.1.1. Accuracy: Comparisons of Official Reports with Self-Reports. Self-reports of respondents with official histories of childhood sexual abuse were compared to self-reports of respondents who experienced other forms of abuse (physical) or neglect and to those with no official record of having been abused and/or neglected (controls) to determine the accuracy of the four approaches to asking these questions (see Table 1). Overall, 63% of the sexually abused persons reported having at least one of these sexual experiences before age 12, in comparison to 47% of the physically abused and/or neglected group and 45% of the controls. In general, the extent of self-reports of sexual abuse of known victims of childhood sexual abuse is significantly higher than for the physically abused and neglected group and for the controls. In turn, retrospective self-reports of childhood sexual abuse were higher among the physically abused and neglected group than for the controls for three of the self-report measures (considered sex abuse, sex with an older person, and sex against will).

Table 1. Percent self-reporting early sexual experiences by type of abuse

	Sexual abuse (94)	Physical abuse or neglect (572)	Control (515)	Significance
Requested to do something sexual	37.2	24.5	20.0	***ab
Kissed/hugged in sexual way	21.3	24.3	24.1	
Person showed sex organs	40.4	27.6	27.4	*ab
You showed sex organs	22.3	15.9	15.4	
Person fondled sexually	44.1	22.5	16.1	***abc
You fondled another person	15.0	11.4	10.3	
Person touched organs	39.4	21.8	14.8	***abc
You touched organs	22.3	13.7	11.8	*ab
Attempted intercourse	24.5	15.2	11.7	**ab
Intercourse	28.7	15.9	8.0	***abc
Any of the above before age 12	62.8	47.0	44.7	**ab
Considered sex abuse	54.3	24.5	13.8	***abc
Sex with older person	31.9	10.1	5.0	***abc
Sex against will	46.8	20.1	9.5	***abc

[a] Pairwise comparisons of sexual abuse versus physical abuse or neglect, p≤.05
[b] Pairwise comparisons of sexual abuse versus control, p≤.05
[c] Pairwise comparisons of physical abuse or neglect versus control, p≤.05
* p≤.05 **p≤.01 ***p≤.001

Tables 2 and 3 present findings on the accuracy of retrospective self-reports of childhood sexual abuse for females and males, respectively. Several findings in Table 2 should be noted. First, more than two-thirds of the sexually abused females report having any of these sexual experiences before age 12, compared to less than half of the physically abused and neglected (46%) and control (45%) females. Sixty-four percent of the sexually abused females considered the experiences to be sexual abuse, compared to 36% of the physically abused and neglected group and 24% of the controls. More of the sexually abused females reported having sex with an older person (40%) than physically abused and/or neglected (15%) and control (8%) females. Overall, the results in Table 2 indicate good discriminant validity for the four self-report measures of childhood sexual abuse for females.

Although the number of sexually abused males in the sample is small, the pattern of results in Table 3 is different than that for sexually abused females and is noteworthy. First, sexually abused males do *not* report having a higher incidence of these sexual experiences in childhood (42%) than physically abused and/or neglected (48%) or control (45%) males. Second, males who had been officially reported as having experienced sexual abuse reported having "sex against will" and "consider sexual abuse" about as often as physically abused and neglected males, and both groups reported higher rates than for the control males. Interestingly, only 16% of the sexually abused males considered their early experiences to have been sexual abuse, compared to 64% of the sexually abused females.

3.1.2. Age at Onset and Recall. Brewin et al. (1993, p. 86) suggested that individuals were not likely to have had any direct recollection of events in the first five years of their life. "Although the age at which children become able to give verbal reports of significant experiences appears to be around 3 years (Sheingold & Tenney, 1982; Terr, 1988), research with adults has found a falloff in the retrieval of memories for events occurring before the age of 5 years, even when normal retention and forgetting processes are taken into account (Wetzler & Sweeney, 1986)."

Table 2. Percent self-reporting early sexual experiences by type of abuse: Females only

	Sexual abuse (75)	Physical abuse or neglect (259)	Control (242)	Significance
Requested to do something sexual	44.0	29.0	20.7	***abc
Kissed/hugged in sexual way	21.3	21.2	16.5	
Person showed sex organs	45.3	27.2	27.3	**ab
You showed sex organs	24.0	13.5	8.7	**ab
Person fondled sexually	51.4	28.3	19.0	***abc
You fondled another person	17.6	7.8	4.1	***ab
Person touched organs	44.0	23.7	14.9	***abc
You touched organs	24.0	10.8	6.2	***ab
Attempted intercourse	25.3	16.2	9.5	** bc
Intercourse	34.7	14.7	5.0	***abc
Any of the above before age 12	68.0	45.6	44.6	***ab
Considered sex abuse	64.0	35.5	24.0	***abc
Sex with older person	40.0	15.4	7.6	***abc
Sex against will	54.7	27.4	16.5	***abc

[a] Pairwise comparisons of sexual abuse versus physical abuse or neglect,, p≤.05
[b] Pairwise comparisons of sexual abuse versus control,, p≤.05
[c] Pairwise comparisons of physical abuse or neglect versus control,, p≤.05
* p≤.05 **p≤.01 ***p≤.001

Table 3. Percent self-reporting early sexual experiences by type of abuse: Males only

	Sexual abuse (19)	Physical abuse or neglect (313)	Control (273)	Significance
Requested to do something sexual	10.5	20.8	19.4	
Kissed/hugged in sexual way	21.0	26.9	30.8	
Person showed sex organs	21.0	27.9	27.5	
You showed sex organs	15.8	18.0	21.3	
Person fondled sexually	15.8	17.6	13.6	
You fondled another person	5.3	14.4	15.8	
Person touched organs	21.0	20.2	14.	
You touched organs	15.8	16.2	16.8	
Attempted intercourse	21.0	14.4	13.6	
Intercourse	5.3	16.9	10.6	*c
Any of the above before age 12	42.1	48.2	44.7	
Considered sex abuse	15.8	15.3	4.7	***c
Sex with older person	0.0	5.8	2.6	
Sex against will	15.8	14.1	3.0	***bc

[a] Pairwise comparisons of sexual abuse versus physical abuse or neglect, p≤.05
[b] Pairwise comparisons of sexual abuse versus control, p≤.05
[c] Pairwise comparisons of physical abuse or neglect versus control, p≤.05
* p≤.05 **p≤.01 ***p≤.001

Based on this recommendation by Brewin and his colleagues (Brewin et al., 1993), five years of age at the time of the abuse experience was used as the cutoff point for purposes of comparison of accuracy of recall. Surprisingly, there were no differences between children abused before the age of five years and those abused at later ages (6–11) in terms of accuracy of recall (see Table 4), although there was a slight trend for people younger at the time of abuse to recall less often. However, it should also be noted that these are cases of *early* childhood sexual abuse and that much of the existing literature is based on childhood sexual abuse which was reported to occur during early adolescence or older (ages 12–16).

3.1.3. Predictive Efficiency: Relative Improvement over Chance. To what extent are these retrospective reports capturing past events at a level better than one would expect by chance alone? One approach to assessing the power or predictive efficiency of retrospective self-report measures is to calculate the relative improvement over chance (RIOC). Loeber and Dishion (1983) devised the RIOC index to represent the improvement over chance as a function of the range of its possible predictive efficiency. Because it is less

Table 4. Age at childhood sexual abuse and recall (in percents)

	Ages (in years)					
	Overall		Females		Males	
	0-5 (N=15)	6-11 (N=79)	0-5 (N=12)	6-11 (N=63)	0-5 (N=3)	6-11 (N=16)
Any sex before age 12	53.3	64.6	58.3	69.8	33.3	43.8
Considered sex abuse	46.7	55.7	50.0	66.7	33.3	12.5
Sex with older person	26.7	32.9	33.3	41.3	0.0	0.0
Sex against will	40.0	48.1	41.7	57.1	33.3	12.5

Note: Chi-square analyses indicate that none of these differences is significant across the age groups.

sensitive to differences in base rates, one of the advantages of this technique is that it makes it possible to compare predictive efficiency of a variety of predictors or over a range of studies. Optimally, this method should identify individuals who were (valid positives) and were not (valid negatives) abused in childhood. Loeber and Dishion argue that the degree that observed values in these cells deviate from random or chance values provides a more accurate assessment of predictive efficiency than is possible by means of a chi-square measure. Errors occur because self-report scales identify individuals who self-report abuse but who were not abused "false positives" and those who were not identified but who were abused "false negatives". It should, however, be pointed out that "false positives" are not necessarily false. Depending on one's priorities, the percent of false positives or false negatives should be low.

Table 5 presents the results of analyses estimating the predictive efficiency of the self-report measures of childhood sexual abuse for females only. (Because of the small number of sexually abused males, the RIOC results are not reported, but are available on request from the authors). For females, the four measures identify approximately 5–9% of the follow-up sample as valid positives, where the actual base rate is 7.8%. Two measures (any sexual experience before age 12 and considered sexual abuse) produced somewhat more valid positives than the other two measures. Interestingly, the measure with the highest percent of valid negatives was sex with a person 10 years older (77%) and two other measures (sex against will = 68%; considered sexual abuse = 61%) were close. The measure of "any sexual experience before the age of 12" was associated with the highest percent of "false positives" (39%), whereas using the measure of "sex with older person" had the lowest false positives (10%). Overall, the RIOC scores range from 29% (sex with older person) to 45% (considered sexual abuse), meaning that the predictive efficiency is 29–45% better than what would be expected by chance alone.

3.1.4. Construct Validity. Another approach to assessing the usefulness of retrospective reports of childhood abuse is based on the construct validation process, one of the techniques used to establish the psychometric qualities of assessment instruments. In addition to establishing the validity of retrospective self-report measures using "known groups", construct validity attempts to assess how these self-report measures theoretically relate to other variables or indices. That is, there are certain theoretical expectations about the way people who have a history of childhood abuse should behave or manifest certain outcomes. Based on logical relationships, then, tests of construct validity can offer evidence that these measures do or do not measure childhood abuse, without providing definitive proof.

Table 5. Relative improvement over chance: retrospective reporting of sexual abuse for females only (in percents)

Self-report measure	Valid positives	"False" positives	Valid negatives	False negatives	Selection ratio	RIOC	Chi-square	Confidence interval range
Any sex before age 12	8.9	39.2	47.7	4.2	48.1	38.4	13.7***	18.7 - 58.0
Considered sex abuse	8.3	26.0	60.9	4.7	34.4	45.1	33.5***	29.2 - 61.1
Sex with older person	5.2	10.2	76.7	7.8	15.5	29.0	39.8***	16.7 - 41.4
Sex against will	7.1	19.3	67.7	5.9	26.4	38.4	35.5***	23.8 - 53.1

***p ≤ .001

Early adverse experiences, especially sexual abuse, have been implicated as causal factors in the development of a variety of psychiatric disorders (Briere & Runtz, 1988; Brown & Anderson, 1991; Browne & Finkelhor, 1986; Widom, in press; Wyatt, Newcomb, & Riederle, 1993). For example, clinical and research reports have retrospectively linked child sexual abuse to depression and anxiety (Burnam et al., 1988; Lipovsky, Saunders, & Murphy, 1989; Peters, 1984), alcohol and other substance abuse (Ladwig & Anderson, 1989; Miller, Downs, Gondoli, & Keil, 1987; Root, 1989), and self-destructive behaviors and suicide attempts (deWilde, Kienhorst, Diekstra, & Wolters, 1992; Walsh & Rosen, 1988).

Although the follow-up interview assessed a wide range of psychiatric outcomes (Luntz & Widom, 1994; Widom, Ireland, & Glynn, 1995) to validate the retrospective self-report measures of childhood sexual abuse, three outcomes most frequently associated with childhood sexual abuse (depression, alcohol problems, and suicide attempts) were selected for these analyses. Ideally, retrospective reports of childhood sexual abuse will relate to subsequent outcomes similar to the way official reports of childhood sexual abuse relate to these outcomes. While it is clear that all sexual abuse cases do not come to the attention of the authorities and that there are unreported sexual abuse cases in the control group, the pattern of results for documented cases and self-reported cases of sexual should be similar with respect to long-term psychiatric sequelae.

The relationships among these three outcomes (DSM-III-R Depression diagnosis, DSM-III-R Alcohol Abuse/Dependence Diagnosis, and suicide attempts) and childhood sexual abuse using official record information are presented first and then the results using retrospective self-reported information about childhood sexual abuse are presented. Because of gender differences in reporting (described earlier), these findings are reported separately for females and males (see Table 6). Logistic regressions were performed, predicting to DSM-III-R Depression and Alcohol Abuse/Dependence Diagnoses and reports of having made suicide attempts, with controls for race, age, and other types of abuse or neglect[*]. Table 6 shows the coefficient, standard error, significance, and odds ratio for only the sexual abuse variable in the equations. For females, official reports of early childhood sexual abuse predict to Alcohol Diagnosis and suicide attempts in young adulthood, but not to Depression Diagnosis. In contrast, self-reported measures of childhood sexual abuse are strong (and significant) predictors of Depression and Alcohol Diagnoses and suicide attempts in females.

Males who were sexually abused in childhood (according to court records) were not at increased risk for any of the three outcomes (Depression, Alcohol, or suicide attempts), although because of the small number of sexually abused males, power is very limited and these results should be treated with great caution. However, for males, self-reports of having any of these sexual experiences before age 12 "any sex before 12" predicts significantly to Depression, Alcohol, and suicide attempts. In addition, whether the males consider it to be sexual abuse "considered sex abuse" was also associated with Depression Diagnosis and suicide attempts (significant with a one-tailed test).

In sum, there is relatively good discriminant validity for these retrospective reports of childhood sexual abuse for females, and there do not appear to be major differences in recall as a function of age at the time of abuse for this sample. Predictive efficiency is better than chance and there is strong support for the construct validity of the self-report

---

[*] These analyses were repeated with the additional control variable of having parents with alcohol or drug problems and the pattern of results and significance levels did not change.

Table 6. Childhood sexual abuse and expected outcomes by gender

	Females (576)			Males (605)		
	b	S.E.	Odds ratio	b	S.E.	Odds ratio
			Depression diagnosis			
Official report						
Sexual abuse	-.04	.29	0.96	-.57	.76	0.56
Self-report						
Any sex before 12	1.08***	.20	2.94	.75***	.22	2.12
Considered sex abuse	1.10***	.20	3.00	.91**	.30	2.50
Sex with older person	1.09***	.24	2.98	.33	.48	1.39
Sex against will	1.07***	.20	2.92	.94**	.31	2.57
			Alcohol diagnosis			
Official report						
Sexual abuse	.54*	.27	1.72	.07	.54	1.08
Self-report						
Any sex before 12	.64***	.18	1.89	.56**	.18	1.76
Considered sex abuse	.51**	.19	1.66	.57	.32	1.77
Sex with older person	.55*	.24	1.73	.31	.46	1.36
Sex against will	.59**	.20	1.81	.47	.33	1.60
			Suicide attempt			
Official report						
Sexual abuse	1.07***	.31	2.90	.85	.67	2.34
Self-report						
Any sex before 12	1.26***	.25	3.52	.74**	.28	2.10
Considered sex abuse	1.32***	.24	3.75	.61	.38	1.84
Sex with older person	1.52***	.26	4.56	.62	.53	1.87
Sex against will	1.25***	.24	3.50	.45	.40	1.57

Note: Results based on logistic regressions predicting to Depression Diagnosis, Alcohol Abuse/Dependence Diagnosis, or having made a suicide attempt, controlling for race, age, and other types of abuse and neglect. Further details of these analyses are available from the authors.
*p ≤ .05 **p ≤ .01 ***p ≤ .001

measures of childhood sexual abuse for females, although official reports of childhood sexual abuse showed more complicated patterns of outcomes.

3.2. Childhood Physical Abuse

3.2.1. Accuracy: Comparisons of Official Reports with Self-Reports. Depending on the particular subscale (see Table 7), from 60% (Very Severe Violence) to 92% (Minor Violence) of the physically abused group reported physical abuse. There was good discriminant validity for the Severe Violence and Very Severe Violence subscales, with all three groups differing significantly from one another. On the other hand, using the Minor Violence subscale, 92% and 86% of the sexually abused and neglected individuals and controls, respectively, also reported histories of physical abuse, and the three groups did not differ significantly from one another. Based on these results, the remainder of these analyses focus on the two subscales of the CTS (Severe Violence and Very Severe Violence) which appear to have the best discriminant validity. Findings for self-reports of childhood physical abuse did not differ by gender for the CTS or SRCAP scales (described below).

Table 8 presents findings on the accuracy of the SRCAP measure. With one exception, each of the individual items on the SRCAP and the overall SRCAP score discriminates significantly among the three groups, with the physical abuse group (as defined by

Table 7. Accuracy of overall CTS scores by type of abuse (in percents)

| Self-reports | Official reports | | | Significance | |
	Physical abuse	Neglect & sexual abuse	Controls	Overall	Pairwise
Reasoning	83.0	87.9	93.6	***	a,b
Verbal aggression	95.4	94.1	90.3		
Minor violence	91.6	91.5	86.3		
Severe violence	68.9	58.3	43.6	***	a,b,c
Very severe violence	59.8	38.9	20.8	***	a,b,c

*** $p \leq .001$ (two-tailed test), Bonferroni corrected chi square analyses
a=Comparison of physical abuse victims versus control subjects, $p \leq .05$
b=Comparison of neglect & sexual abuse victims versus control subjects, $p \leq .05$
c=Comparison of physical abuse victims versus neglect & sexual abuse victims, $p \leq .05$
N = 1,196

official records) reported the highest percent of childhood physical abuse, followed by the sexual abuse and neglect group. As expected, the lowest percentage of childhood physical abuse was reported by the controls. Almost two-thirds (62%) of the group with official records of childhood physical abuse met the criteria of childhood physical abuse with the SRCAP measure, compared to 42% of the sexual abuse and neglect group, and 25% of the controls. These findings provide evidence for the validity of the SRCAP and clear discrimination between externally documented groups of abused and neglected individuals and controls.

3.2.2. Age at Onset and Recall. Based on the work of Brewin and colleagues (Brewin et al., 1993), five years of age at the time of the abuse experience was used as the cutoff point for this purposes of comparison of accuracy of recall (see Table 9). Surprisingly, there were no differences in terms of accuracy of recall between children abused before the age of 5 and those abused at later ages (6–11). However, it should be noted that these are official cases of *early* childhood physical abuse.

Table 8. Accuracy of SRCAP measure by type of abuse (in percents)

| Self-reports | Official reports | | | Significance | |
	Physical abuse	Neglect & sexual abuse	Controls	Overall	Pairwise
Beat by parent/didn't deserve	56.2	31.1	19.5	***	a,b,c
Hit with bare hand	42.2	23.1	11.4	***	a,b,c
Hit with something hard	31.2	14.9	8.5	***	a,b,c
Injure with weapon	5.5	3.4	0.6	***	a,b
Hurt enough-need doctor	26.4	7.1	1.4	***	a,b,c
Admitted to hospital	13.2	2.3	0.4	***	a,b,c
SRCAP	62.3	41.5	25.3	***	a,b,c

*** $p \leq .001$ (two-tailed test), Bonferroni corrected chi square analyses
a=Comparison of physical abuse victims versus control subjects, $p \leq .05$
b=Comparison of neglect & sexual abuse victims versus control subjects, $p \leq .05$
c=Comparison of physical abuse victims versus neglect & sexual abuse victims, $p \leq .05$
N = 1,196

Table 9. Recall of physical abuse by age at time of abuse (in percents)

	Age at time of physical abuse (in years)	
	0-5 (N=42)	6-11 (N=64)
CTS: severe violence	73.8	65.6
CTS: very severe violence	65.1	56.2
SRCAP	58.1	65.1

Note: Official cases of physical abuse only. None of the differences was significant.

3.2.3. Predictive Efficiency: Relative Improvement over Chance. All three measures identify approximately the same percent of the sample as valid positives (about 5–6%) for childhood physical abuse, where the actual base rate for the sample is 9.2% (see Table 10). However, differences between the measures appear when looking at other characteristics. Both the CTS-Very Severe Violence (CTS-VSV) and the SRCAP identify about the same percents of valid negatives (64% and 60%, respectively) and false positives (28% and 31%), whereas the CTS-SV (Severe Violence) scale identifies a much higher percent of false positives (47%) and a lower percent of valid negatives (44%). All three measures identify about 3–4% of the sample as false negatives, or people who have official records of having been physically abused but who do not self-report a history of abuse according to any of the measures. Overall, the RIOC for the CTS-VSV and the SRCAP is about 40–41%, meaning that predictive efficiency is about 40% better than what would be expected by chance alone.

3.2.4. Construct Validity. Straus and Gelles (1990) reported that children who experienced severe violence were described by their parents to have higher rates of conduct problems and rule violating behaviors than those who did not experience severe violence. In earlier work using official reports of childhood victimization, Widom (1989b) reported a significant relationship between childhood physical abuse and violent criminal behavior. Here, construct validity is assessed using predictions about the consequences of physical abuse for subsequent violent behavior. That is, individuals who self-report physical abuse should have higher rates of arrest for violence and self-reported violence than individuals who do not self-report physical abuse.

Table 10. Relative improvement over chance: retrospective reporting of physical abuse

Self-report measure	Valid positives	False positives	Valid negatives	False negative	Selection ratio	RIOC	Chi-square	Confidence interval range
CTS: severe violence	6.1	46.6	44.4	2.8	52.8	34.1	12.1***	15-7 - 52.4
CTS: very severe violence	5.4	27.5	63.5	3.6	32.9	40.1	38.6***	26.6 - 53.7
SRCAP	5.6	30.7	60.4	3.4	36.3	40.8	34.0***	26.6 - 55.0

*** p ≤ .001

Two measures of violence (official and self-report) were used in these construct validity analyses. The first (official) measure, arrest for violence, is based on information obtained from complete criminal histories collected for these individuals at three levels of law enforcement (local, state, and federal) at two points in time (1986–87 and 1994). Any arrest for violence refers to arrests as a juvenile or as an adult and includes arrests for the following crimes and attempts: assault, battery, robbery, manslaughter, murder, rape, and burglary with injury. The self-report measure of violence refers to the person's response to seven items embedded in a general crime and delinquency scale (adapted from Wolfgang & Weiner, 1989) completed by the respondent during the in-person interview. These items include: hurt someone badly enough for him or her to require medical treatment; threatened to hurt someone if he or she didn't give you money or something else; used a weapon to threaten another person; forced someone to have sex with you; shot someone; attacked someone with the purpose of killing him or her; and used physical force to get money, drugs, or something else from someone.

Information from official reports of childhood physical abuse and self-reported physical abuse (using the CTS and SRCAP) was entered into a series of regression equations predicting to arrests for violence and self-reported violence. Analyses were conducted with dichotomous dependent variables (any arrest for a violent crime versus no arrest for a violent crime and any self-reported violence item). Pure types of officially reported abuse (physical abuse, sexual abuse, and neglect) were introduced into the regression equations (replicating the earlier work of Widom, 1989b), with controls for sex, age, and race. The assumption is that if self-reports of physical abuse (using either the CTS or SRCAP) are valid indicators of childhood physical abuse, then they should predict the same or similar outcomes as found for officially reported physical abuse.

Looking first at the left hand portion of Table 11, it is apparent that officially reported physical abuse is a significant predictor of having an arrest for violence. The self-report measures of childhood physical abuse [CTS: Severe Violence; CTS: Very Severe Violence; and SRCAP] were also introduced into three separate but similar equations. None of the self-report measures of childhood physical abuse predict to arrests for violence. Looking at the right hand portion of Table 11, the results of another series of equations are reported, using the dependent variable of *self-reported violence*, instead of arrests for violence. These results indicate that officially reported physical abuse is not a significant predictor of self-reported violence, whereas each of the self-report measures (both CTS and SRCAP) are significant predictors of self-reported violence.

Table 11. Physical abuse and violence

	Any violent arrest			Self-reported violence		
	b	S.E.	Odds ratio	b	S.E.	Odds ratio
Official						
Physical abuse	.66 *	.36	1.94	.01	.34	1.01
Self-Report						
CTS: severe violence	.03	.17	1.03	1.09 ***	.15	2.97
CTS: very severe violence	.03	.18	1.03	.78 ***	.15	2.18
SRCAP	.16	.18	1.17	.93 ***	.15	2.55

Note: Logistic regressions predicting to any violent arrest and any self-reported violence, controlling for sex, race, age, and other types of abuse or neglect. Further details of these results are available from the author.
* p<.05 ***p<.001

4. DISCUSSION

Taken together, these findings reveal a number of similarities in the accuracy of adult recollections of early childhood sexual and physical abuse, but they also reveal some major differences. There was fairly good discriminant validity for both sexual abuse and physical abuse measures. Individuals who were physically abused, based on official records, retrospectively reported the highest rates of childhood physical abuse in the sample. On the CTS (Severe Violence and Very Severe Violence subscales) and the SRCAP, physically abused individuals reported significantly higher rates of physical abuse than individuals who had experienced sexual abuse or neglect in childhood and individuals who were part of a matched control group. The extent of remembering (that is, the percent of individuals who had been physically abused who reported having been physically abused on one of the measures utilized here) is in line with previous research. These results also reveal that the extent of reporting a history of childhood physical abuse varied dramatically by the criterion (or measure) used.

Similarly, there appears to be good discriminant validity for females for the retrospective self-report measures of childhood sexual abuse used here. This is not the case for sexually abused males. Sexually abused males are more likely to consider that they were sexually abused and to report more often having sex against their will than controls, but so do physically abused and neglected males. Interestingly, more of the physically abused and neglected males report having sex with an older person than sexually abused males, none of whom reported having this experience in childhood.

These findings suggest that the measures of childhood sexual abuse used here have reasonable discriminant validity for females, but much less so for males. This may reflect inadequate measurement techniques or an unwillingness on the part of the males to disclose this information. However, these findings have implications for other researchers and clinicians. For researchers, depending on the proportion of males in a study, results may be influenced in a significant way by under-reporting of childhood sexual abuse, a serious concern for epidemiological research. For clinicians, these findings reinforce the need to develop more sensitive techniques to elicit this information from clinical populations of males.

For both types of childhood abuse, there was substantial underreporting of abuse among known victims of childhood abuse. This is particularly impressive since these are court substantiated cases of childhood abuse. Much attention has been paid to the lack of recall or failure to report histories of childhood abuse among known victims of sexual abuse, but these results indicate that there is also a problem in underreporting of childhood physical abuse. A substantial group of individuals who were physically abused do not report having been physically abused in childhood. Of the people in the sample who had documented cases of physical abuse in childhood, about 60% reported abuse using one of the self-report measures of childhood physical abuse. This means that about 40% of individuals with documented histories of physical abuse did not report. Whether these people did not report (as suggested by Della Femina, Yeager, & Lewis, 1990), because of embarrassment, a wish to protect parents, a sense of having deserved the abuse, a conscious wish to forget the past, or lack of confidence in or rapport with the interviewer, it is not clear. But these findings suggest that a substantial minority would not be included in retrospective self-report assessments of childhood physical abuse. Using a more lenient criterion (such as the CTS-Minor Violence subscale) would capture most of the physically abused people (see Table 7); however, this criterion also identifies 92% of the sexual abuse and neglect cases and 86% of the controls as having been physically abused in childhood. Using the CTS-Minor Violence measure, the rate of "false positives" approaches almost half the sample. These findings illustrate how the rate of false positives is directly related to the measure of childhood physical abuse used. For some purposes, such as in clinical settings, a higher false positive rate may be desirable; for other purposes, a high false positive rate may be unacceptable.

One explanation for the underreporting is that some of these individuals might have been too young at the time of the abuse experience to remember it. These analyses did not reveal differences in accuracy by age at the time of the abuse experience using age five as a cutoff. However, as Radke-Yarrow et al. (1970) pointed out many years ago, information that we remember from childhood may be heavily dependent on information told to us in childhood or later and/or constructed by a parent. It may well be that children who experience sexual or physical abuse (whose cases did not come to the attention of the authorities) would remember their experiences differently. On the other hand, given that these were court substantiated cases, the amount of under-reporting is notable. Unfortunately, by its very nature, family violence occurs "behind closed doors" and this characteristic makes documenting its occurrence problematic and studying the phenomenon difficult, because it often hinges on the report of the victim and there may or may not be physical evidence available.

While this lack of reporting is significant, it may not be surprising viewed in a somewhat different context. Non-reporting of crime victims in the context of victimization surveys has been studied for a number of years (Garofalo & Hindelang, 1977) and problems with respondent embarrassment about the incident or "protective mechanisms", or simply memory decay or forgetting have been described. Because of these problems, National Crime Survey researchers have conducted reliability and validity studies for victimization surveys. In this case, victimization recall has been investigated by comparing crimes disclosed in victimization surveys to crimes found in police records. In this "reverse records check" technique, police records of crimes that have been reported are identified and then victims have been interviewed using standard National Crime Survey methods, to determine if respondents' recall the known victimizations and report it to the interviewer (Lehnen & Skogan, 1981). One such reverse records check study (Turner, 1972) found a relationship between the number of months between the reported incident and the interview and the percent of incidents reported to the interviewer. Turner investigated 206 cases of robbery, assault, and rape from police records. Overall, only 63% of the incidents were reported to the interviewer and the percent reported to the interviewer was strongly related to the time interval: 69% were recalled from 1–3 months prior, 50% from 4–6 months, 46% from 7–9 months, and 30% for 10–12 months. Turner also found that accuracy was a function of the relationship between the victim and the offender: 76% reported when the offender was a stranger, 57% when the offender was "known", and 22% reported when the offender was a relative.

Given that victims of childhood sexual and physical abuse are being asked to recall events from experiences that happened as many as 20 or 30 years earlier, it may be quite understandable that the extent of recall is not perfect. Indeed, despite the fact that one cannot necessarily generalize from the results of these studies of victims of robbery, assault, and rape, it is noteworthy that victim recall for a one-year time-period was as low as 30% (Turner, 1972). Williams (1994) reported recall by approximately 60% of the female childhood sexual abuse victims followed-up in her study. The present findings indicate that 41–67% of female childhood sexual abuse victims retrospectively report childhood

What the underreporting means is that there is a substantial group of individuals with documented histories of childhood sexual and physical abuse who are not reporting this information when it is solicited in a sensitive but not leading interview. Future research needs to determine whether there are characteristics of early childhood experiences (severity, duration, or perpetrator) which are related to non-reporting and to determine whether outcomes for individuals who do not report are better or worse than for those who do report.

In terms of the construct validity of these retrospective self-report measures, particularly of physical abuse, these findings are troubling, suggesting substantial shared method variance. Official reports of physical abuse predict to official reports of violence and self-reports of physical abuse predict to self-reports of violence. While this paper has used official court records (both in terms of documented cases of abuse and arrests for violence) as the criteria against which to assess the validity of these retrospective childhood physical abuse measures, they are not the only criteria possible. For example, medical records of abuse or emergency room contacts might also provide evidence against which to validate physical abuse, although both constitute some level of official processing of these cases. Police records reflect only a sample of all offenses committed by an individual and may include notations of crimes that did not occur as charged. Police have discretion in deciding which subjects to arrest, which arrests to record, and which charges to file. Similarly, official reports of child abuse and neglect are associated with biases, over-representing people of low socio-economic status and more severe cases of abuse and neglect.

Strong relationships were found for retrospective self-report measures of childhood sexual abuse and psychiatric diagnoses of Depression and Alcohol Abuse/Dependence and suicide attempts and for official reports of childhood sexual abuse and Alcohol Diagnosis and suicide attempts in females. The relationship between childhood sexual abuse and depression appears more complicated. Individuals who meet the criterion for a DSM-III-R Depression Diagnosis (current or remitted) are more likely to recall having been sexually abused in childhood, although individuals with official records of sexual abuse followed-up are not at increased risk of becoming depressed. Brewin et al. (1993, p. 84) suggested that "clinical states such as anxiety and depression may have a deleterious effect on all memories, regardless of content, so that psychiatric patients' recall of childhood is likely to be inaccurate." Work is in progress on a paper which focuses on depression and dysthymia as outcomes of childhood victimization in general and in relation to childhood sexual abuse in particular to explore these issues further.

While further attempts should be made to assess the construct validity of these and other measures, researchers should also attempt to utilize information from more than one source when conducting analyses involving child abuse. As Sternberg, Lamb, Greenbaum, Cicchetti, Dawud, Cortes, Krispin, and Lorey (1993, p. 49) concluded, in a study of the effects of experiencing and witnessing domestic violence in Israeli children and controls, "... one cannot discuss the effects of domestic violence without considering the source of information, particularly because the levels of agreement among informants were extremely low." The implication is that, if at all possible, researchers need to use multiple sources of information. Failing that, researchers need to recognize that, similar to the biases associated with official reports of childhood abuse and neglect (Newberger, Reed, Daniel, Hyde, & Kotelchuck, 1977), self-reported childhood victimization may contain systematic biases.

Henry, Moffitt, Caspi, Langley, and Silva (1994) compared the extent of agreement between prospective and retrospective measures across multiple content domains (including residence changes, injuries, reading ability, family characteristics, behavior problems and delinquency) in a large sample of 18-year-old youth who had been studied prospectively from birth. They found reasonable correlations for relatively "objective" information (residence changes, reading skill, height and weight), while psychosocial variables (that is, reports about subjects' psychological states and family processes) had the lowest levels of agreement between prospective and retrospective measures. And, despite significant correlations, the absolute level of agreement between the two data sources was low.

The present results, consistent with the clinical literature based on retrospective self-reports, indicate that the way people define their earlier childhood experiences, whether it is childhood sexual or physical abuse, is extremely important. Empirical findings suggest that a person's cognitive appraisal of life events strongly influences his or her response (Lazarus & Launier, 1978). The same event may be perceived by different individuals as irrelevant, benign, positive, threatening, or harmful. In thinking about the consequences of childhood abuse, it is likely that a child's cognitive appraisal of events will at least in part determine whether they experience the event as negative or neutral. It is also likely that the long-term consequences of these early childhood experiences will be influenced by the way these events are dealt with at the time, including the person's perception of the experiences. One's cognitive appraisal of events may be particularly important for cases of childhood sexual abuse.

The present findings reinforce the importance of considering patients' perceptions of their early childhood experiences, as well as information from collaterals. At the same time, these findings present a challenge to researchers to develop reliable and valid ways to assess histories of childhood victimization. The research question should be: What is the best way to ask questions about childhood victimization to make responses more valid? Hopefully, these findings will be useful to other researchers and clinicians dependent on retrospective self-reported information to obtain histories of childhood victimization.

Henry et al. (1994) concluded that reliance on retrospective reports about psychosocial variables should be treated with caution. They suggested that "the use of retrospective reports should be limited to testing hypotheses about the relative standing of individuals in a distribution and should not be used to test hypotheses that demand precision in estimating event frequencies and event dates" (1994, p. 92). The findings of this chapter support their recommendation to use caution against overly simplistic interpretations that take retrospective reports at "face value".

5. AUTHOR NOTE AND ACKNOWLEDGMENT

Adapted from papers by Widom and Shepard (1996) and Widom and Morris (in press). Correspondence regarding this chapter should be addressed to Cathy Spatz Widom, The University at Albany, School of Criminal Justice, 135 Western Avenue, Albany, New York 12222.

This research was supported, in part, by grants from the National Institute of Mental Health (MH49467) and the National Institute of Justice (86-IJ-CX-0033, 89-IJ-CX-0007, and 93-IJ-CX-0003). The author expresses appreciation to Patty Glynn for help with the statistical analyses reported. Points of view are those of the author and do not necessarily represent the position of the United States Department of Justice.

REFERENCES

Berliner, L., & Williams, L. M. (1994). Memories of child sexual abuse: Response to Lindsay and Read. *Applied Cognitive Psychology, 8,* 379–387.

Brewin, C. R., Andrews, B., & Gotlib, I. H. (1993). Psychopathology and early experience: A reappraisal of retrospective reports. *Psychological Bulletin, 113,* 82–98.

Briere, J., & Conte, J. (1993). Self-reported amnesia for abuse in adults molested as children. *Journal of Traumatic Stress, 6,* 21–31.

Briere, J., & Runtz, M. (1988). Symptomatology associated with childhood sexual victimization in a nonclinical adult sample. *Child Abuse and Neglect, 12,* 51–59.

Brown, G. R., & Anderson, B. (1991). Psychiatric morbidity in adult inpatients with childhood histories of sexual and physical abuse. *American Journal of Psychiatry, 148,* 55–61.

Browne, A., & Finkelhor, D. (1986). Impact of child sexual abuse: A review of the research. *Psychological Bulletin, 99,* 66–77.

Burnam, M. A., Stein, J. A., Golding, J. M., Siegel, J. M., Sorenson, S. B., Forsythe, A. B., & Telles, C. A. (1988). Sexual assault and mental disorders in a community population. *Journal of Consulting and Clinical Psychology, 56,* 843–850.

Carmen, E. H., Rieker, P. P., & Mills, T. (1984). Victims of violence and psychiatric illness. *American Journal of Psychiatry, 141,* 378–383.

Della Femina, D., Yeager, C. A., & Lewis, D. O. (1990). Child abuse: Adolescent records vs. adult recall. *Child Abuse and Neglect, 14,* 227–231.

deWilde, E. J., Kienhorst, I. C., Diekstra, R. F., & Wolters, W. H. (1992). The relationship between adolescent suicidal behavior and life events in childhood and adolescence. *American Journal of Psychiatry, 149,* 45–51.

Finkelhor, D. (1979). *Sexually Victimized Children.* New York: Free Press.

Finkelhor, D. (1986). *Sourcebook on Child Sexual Abuse.* Beverly Hills, CA: Sage.

Finkelhor, D. (1990). Early and long-term effects of child sexual abuse: An update. *Professional Psychology: Research and Practice, 21,* 325–330.

Finkelhor, D. (1993). Answers to important questions about the scope and nature of child sexual abuse. *The future of children, 4,* 31–53. Los Altos, CA: David and Lucille Packard Foundation.

Fivush, R. (1993). Developmental perspectives on autobiographical recall. In G. S. Goodman & B. L. Bottoms (Eds.), *Child victims, child witnesses: Understanding and improving testimony* (pp. 1–24). New York: Guilford Press.

Garofalo, J., & Hindelang, M. J. (1977). An introduction to the National Crime Survey. U.S. Department of Justice, Law Enforcement Assistance Administration, National Criminal Justice Information and Statistics Service, SD-VAD-4 1977. Washington, D.C.: U.S. Government Printing Office.

Henry, B., Moffitt, E. G., Caspi, A., Langley, J., & Silva, P. A. (1994). On the "remembrance of things past": A longitudinal evaluation of the retrospective method. *Psychological Assessment, 6,* 92–101.

Herman, J., & Schatzow, E. (1987). Recovery and verification of memories of childhood sexual trauma. *Psychoanalytic Psychology, 4,* 1–14.

Hollingshead, A. B. (1975). *Four Factor Index of Social Status.* New Haven, CT. (Yale University Working Paper).

Jacobson, A., & Richardson, B. (1987). Assault experiences of 100 psychiatric inpatients: Evidence of the need for routine inquiry. *American Journal of Psychiatry, 144,* 908–913.

Kruttschnitt, C., & Dornfeld, M. (1992). Will they tell? *Journal of Research in Crime and Delinquency, 29,* 136–147.

Ladwig, G. B., & Anderson, M. D. (1989). Substance abuse in women: Relationship between chemical dependency of women and past reports of physical abuse and/or sexual abuse. *International Journal of the Addictions, 24,* 739–754.

Lazarus, R. S., & Launier, R. (1978). Stress-related transactions between person and environment. In Pervin, L.A., and Lewis, M. (Eds.) *Perspectives in Interactional Psychology.* New York: Plenum.

Lehnen, R. G., & Skogan, W. G. (1981). *The National Crime Survey Working Papers. Vol. I: Current and Historical Perspectives.* Washington, D.C.: U.S. Government Printing Office.

Leippe, Manion, & Romanczyk. (1991). Eyewitness memory for a touching experience: Accuracy differences between child and adult witnesses. *Journal of Applied Cognitive Psychology, 76,* 367–379.

Leventhal, J. M. (1982). Research strategies and methodologic standards in studies of risk factors for child abuse. *Child Abuse and Neglect, 6,* 113–123.

Lewis, I. A. (1985). (Los Angeles Times Poll #98). Unpublished raw data. Cited in Finkelhor, D. (1986) Sourcebook on Child Sexual Abuse. (Beverly Hills, CA.: Sage)

Lindsay, D. S., & Read, J. D. (1994). Psychotherapy and memories of childhood sexual abuse: A cognitive perspective. *Applied Cognitive Psychology, 8,* 281–338.

Lipovsky, J. A., Saunders, B. E., & Murphy, S. M. (1989). Depression, anxiety, and behavior problems among victims of father-child sexual assault and nonabused siblings. *Journal of Interpersonal Violence, 4,* 452–468.

Loeber, R., & Dishion, T. (1983). Early predictors of male delinquency: A review. *Psychological Bulletin, 94,* 1, 68–99.

Loftus, E. F. (1993). The reality of repressed memories. *American Psychologist, 48,* 518–537.

Luntz, B. K. & Widom, C. S. (1994). Antisocial personality disorder in abused and neglected children grown up. *American Journal of Psychiatry, 151,* 670–674.

Miller, B., Downs, W., Gondoli, D., & Keil, A. (1987). The role of childhood sexual abuse in the development of alcoholism in women. *Violence and Victims, 2,* 157–172.

Nash, M. R. (August 1992). *Retrieval of childhood memories in psychotherapy: Clinical utility and historical verifiability are not the same thing.* Paper presented at the 100th Annual Convention of the American Psychological Association, Washington, D.C.

Neisser, U. (1967). *Cognitive psychology.* New York: Appleton Century Crofts.

Newberger, E. H., Reed, R. B., Daniel, J. H., Hyde, J. N., & Kotelchuck, M. (1977). Pediatric social illness: Toward an etiological classification. *Pediatrics, 50,* 178–185.

Peters, S. D. (1984). *The relationship between childhood sexual victimization and adult depression among Afro-American and White women.* Unpublished Ph.D. Unpublished dissertation, University of California, Los Angeles.

Radke-Yarrow, M., Campbell, J. D., & Burton, R. V. (1970). Recollections of childhood: A study of the retrospective method. *Monographs of the Society for Research in Child Development: 138, 135,* 5.

Robins, L. N., Helzer, J. E., Cottler, L., & Goldring, E. (1987). *National Institute of Mental Health Diagnostic Interview Schedule (DIS-III-R).* St. Louis, MO: Washington University.

Root, M. P. (1989). Treatment failures: The role of sexual victimization in women's addictive behavior. *American Journal of Orthopsychiatry, 59,* 542–549.

Russell, D. E. H. (1983). The incidence and prevalence of intrafamilial and extrafamilial sexual abuse of female children. *Child Abuse and Neglect, 7,* 133–146.

Schulsinger, F., Mednick, S. A., & Knop, J. (1981). *Longitudinal Research: Methods and Uses in Behavioral Sciences.* Boston: Martinus Nijhoff Publishers.

Sheingold, K., & Tenney, Y. J. (1982). Memory for a salient childhood event. In U. Neisser (Ed.), *Memory Observed* (pp. 201–212). San Francisco: Freeman.

Sternberg, K. J., Lamb, M. E., Greenbaum, C., Cicchetti, D., Dawud, S., Cortes, R. M., Krispin, O., & Lorey, F. (1993). Effects of domestic violence on children's behavior problems and depression. *Developmental Psychology, 29,* 44–52.

Straus, M. A. (1979). Measuring intrafamily conflict and violence: The Conflict Tactics (CT) Scales. *Journal of Marriage and the Family, 41,* 75–86.

Straus, M. A., & Gelles, R. J. (Eds.). (1990). *Physical Violence in American Families: Risk Factors and Adaptations to Violence in 8145 Families.* New Brunswick, NJ: Transaction Publishers.

Terr, L. (1988). What happens to early memories of trauma? A study of twenty children under age five at the time of documented traumatic events. *Journal of the American Academy of Child and Adolescent Psychiatry, 27,* 96–104.

Turner, A. G. (1972). *The San Jose Methods Test of Known Crime Victims.* National Criminal Justice Information and Statistics Service, Law Enforcement Assistance Administration. Washington, D.C.: U.S. Government Printing Office.

Wakefield, H., & Underwager, R. (1992). Recovered memories of alleged sexual abuse: Lawsuits against parents. *Behavioral Sciences and the Law, 10,* 483–507.

Walsh, B. W., & Rosen, P. (1988). *Self-Mutilation: Theory, Research, and Treatment.* New York: Guilford.

Wetzler, S. E., & Sweeney, J. A. (1986). Childhood amnesia: An empirical demonstration. In D. C. Rubin (Ed.), *Autobiographical memory* (pp. 191–201). New York: Cambridge University Press.

Widom, C. S. (1989a). Child abuse, neglect and adult behavior: Research design and findings on criminality, violence, and child abuse. *American Journal of Orthopsychiatry, 59,* 355–367.

Widom, C. S. (1989b). The cycle of violence. *Science, 244,* 160–166.

Widom, C. S. (1989c). Does violence beget violence? A critical examination of the literature. *Psychological Bulletin, 106,* 1, 3–28.

Widom, C. S. (in press). Understanding the consequences of childhood victimization. To appear in: R. M. Reece (Ed.), *The Treatment of Child Abuse.* Baltimore, MD: Johns Hopkins University Press.

Widom, C. S., Ireland, T., & Glynn, P. J. (1995). Alcohol abuse in abused and neglected children followed-up. *Journal of Studies on Alcohol, 56,* 207–217.

Widom, C. S., & Morris, S. (in press). Accuracy of adult recollections of childhood victimization. Part II. Child-
    hood sexual abuse. *Psychological Assessment.*
Widom, C. S., & Shepard, R. L. (1996). Accuracy of adult recollections of childhood victimization: Part I. Child-
    hood physical abuse. *Psychological Assessment, 8,* 4.
Williams, L. M. (1994). Recall of childhood trauma: A prospective study of women's memories of child sexual
    abuse. *Journal of Consulting and Clinical Psychology, 62,* 6, 1167–1176.
Wolfgang, M. E., & Weiner, N. (1989). University of Pennsylvania Greater Philadelphia Area Study. Unpublished
    interview protocol.
Wyatt, G. E., Newcomb, M. D., & Riederle, M. H. (1993). *Sexual Abuse and Consensual Sex: Women's Develop-
    mental Patterns and Outcomes.* Newbury Park, CA: Sage.

COMMENTARY ON ACCURACY OF ADULT RECOLLECTIONS OF CHILDHOOD VICTIMIZATION: STUDY I. CHILDHOOD PHYSICAL ABUSE (WIDOM & SHEPARD), STUDY II. CHILDHOOD SEXUAL ABUSE (WIDOM & MORRIS)

Christine A. Courtois, Post-Traumatic and Dissociative Disorder Program, the Psychiatric Institute of Washington

1. INTRODUCTION

These two studies make a significant contribution to the limited research now available on the accuracy of retrospective reports of childhood victimization, a topic which has generated considerable controversy. Along with the Williams investigation (Williams, 1994, 1995), the Widom studies provide a foundation of prospective research that is needed to counterbalance and assess the validity of retrospective reporting of childhood events of a traumatic nature. The studies are important in that they expand the research base of the field of child maltreatment and its short- and long-term consequences, including the ability to encode, remember, and report abusive events. They are also important in terms of their scope—they anticipate and address many research methodology issues and questions that have come to the fore (Briere, 1992). Finally, their timing is important. These studies were underway before the emergence of the memory controversy and provide information on some of the most pressing and contentious issues such as retrospective overreporting (false positives) versus underreporting (false negatives) of past abuse. This research establishes some middle ground in the controversy: it takes memory issues such as the reconstructive nature of memory into consideration but attends as well to issues and reasons for non-disclosure and motivated forgetting as they pertain to abusive events in childhood.

2. RESEARCH PURPOSE, DESIGN, AND IMPLEMENTATION

2.1. Purpose

The stated purpose of this research is the examination of the accuracy of retrospective reports of childhood physical and sexual abuse using a sample of individuals with officially documented and substantiated cases of childhood victimization and a matched control group.

2.2. Design

The features of the research design include: 1) a prospective cohorts study of a non-clinical sample with a documented abuse history, 2) a control sample matched closely on age, sex, race and approximate social class background, 3) unambiguous and operationalized definitions of sexual and physical abuse and neglect, 4) separate abused and neglected groups (of individuals for whom abuse and neglect occurred before the age of 12, i.e., abuse at a young age), 5) a large sample with a high location and follow-up rate (79% of the original group located, 73% interviewed), 6) assessment of the long-term consequences of abuse and neglect beyond adolescence and into adulthood, 7) a double blind design with structured and semi-structured questionnaires, rating scales, and a psychiatric assessment and 8) assessment of the power or efficiency of the retrospective self-report measures by a) the calculation of a measure of relative improvement over chance and any deviation from random or chance values and b) construct validation of the psychometric qualities of the assessment instruments by analyzing risk history with certain outcomes, e.g., subsequent violent behavior and arrest for crime and delinquency in the physical abuse sample and a subsequent history of depression, alcoholism, and suicide attempts in the sexual abuse sample.

In these two studies, the accuracy of self-report measures of childhood physical and sexual abuse and/or neglect, the extent to which accuracy varies by the age of the child at the time of the abuse, the predictive efficiency of the measures (using relative improvement over chance analyses), and construct validity are analyzed. Accuracy of adult recollections is operationally defined per Fivush (1993, p.2) "as agreement between the individual's recall and either an objective record of the event or social consensus from other participants of the event as to what occurred." It also follows strategies suggested by Brewin, Andrews, and Gotlib (1993) to enhance the reliability of retrospective information by obtaining accounts from other sources of information (collaterals), using structured investigative methods that minimize unrealistic demands on the subject's memory, and comparing independent records with memories of events that occurred after the age of 5 years.

Widom and Shepard (Study I) highlight an issue of considerable significance: the inability of the current design to permit determination of the extent of false positives when corroboration is lacking:

> It is not possible to determine whether individuals who self-report childhood abuse, but who do not have an official record of abuse, are reporting accurately or not. The working assumption underlying this research is that these self-reports are valid, until some empirical evidence contradicts that assumption. Unfortunately, this is a limitation which affects most research in this field, with the possible exception of some laboratory analog studies in which behavior and social interactions can be monitored and assessed with more control (Widom & Shepard, under review, p. 5)

2.3. Implementation

The first phase of the research occurred 20 years ago, when a large group of children with abuse and/or neglect histories that occurred before the age of 12 and was serious enough to have official documentation in juvenile and criminal records were compared with a matched control group of children (as reported in Widom, 1989). The second phase involved tracing, locating, and interviewing the abused and/or neglected cohort and the control cohort 20 years after the original study. Two-hour follow-up interviews consisting of a series of structured and semi-structured questionnaires and rating scales and a psychiatric assessment were conducted between 1989 and 1994 with 1,144 individuals. Different measures and approaches were used to retrospectively assess a history of childhood physical and sexual abuse and/or neglect. Comparisons were them made between the self-reported information and the information contained in the official case records from the past. Percent accuracy of recall was calculated by comparing self-reported retrospective information with the official records.

3. FINDINGS AND DISCUSSION

3.1. Findings

Substantial underreporting of past documented physical abuse (Study I) and sexual abuse (Study II) was found. No significant differences in age at time of abuse and subsequent remembering/reporting were found in either investigation. Racial differences were found in reporting in Study I with whites reporting more physical abuse than African American respondents, but no gender differences were found. In this study, accuracy in retrospective self-reports and good discriminant validity were found for both males and females. In contrast, in Study II, reasonable discriminant validity was found for females, but much less so for males. A significant difference was found between males and females in the extent to which they recalled or reported having experienced childhood sexual abuse. Males were much less likely to remember or report past experiences of sexual abuse and sex against their will (16%) versus 63% and 54% of females, respectively.

3.2 Discussion

Imperfect recall of events that occurred 20 to 30 years in the past is not surprising. What is noteworthy here is the quite substantial percentage of individuals with documented histories of abuse (especially sexual abuse) who did not report the abuse and the significant difference in reporting of sexual abuse between males and females. These findings about male underreporting are consistent with observations in clinical settings and theoretical speculations by researchers that greater gender conflict, stigmatization and shame in boy victims results in a pronounced reluctance to identify past sexual contact as abuse and to disclose it as such. This suggests that studies of males relying on retrospective reports of past sexual abuse should anticipate underreporting and many false negatives. Clearly, much more research is needed and these data suggest a very fertile and important area of inquiry.

The findings of substantial forgetting or underreporting by both males and females are in agreement with the findings of other studies conducted on clinical populations (Briere and Conte, 1993; Gold, Hughes, and Hohnecker, 1994; Herman and Schatzow, 1987; Loftus, Polonsky, and Fullilove, 1994), therapists (Feldman-Summers and Pope, 1994), and community samples (Elliott and Briere, 1995; van der Kolk and Fisler, 1995; Williams, 1994, 1995). The non-remembering and non-reporting for both physical and sexual abuse in these studies provide researchers with additional documentation of these phenomena and suggest that recovered memories are possible (although information about triggers or retrieval cues for such memories are not discussed in Widom's research except for a short discussion about the wording of questions and whether a series of questions or a few critical questions would result in greater recall). Also, except for age at onset of abuse and cognitive appraisal of sexual abuse as variables that might relate to later recollection, no other abuse variables were discussed (it is not clear if they were assessed). As noted above, some abuse aftereffects and diagnoses were used in these studies for the purpose of establishing discriminant validity in the samples; they helped establish validity but otherwise are not discussed as to any additional implications (e.g., alcoholism in the sexual abuse sample as possibly related to blackouts and memory loss).

In these two studies, younger age at time of either physical or sexual abuse was not found to be related to later recollection, consistent with the findings of Loftus, Polonsky, and Fullilove (1994) and Feldman-Summers and Pope (1994) and in contrast to the findings of Briere and Conte (1993), Herman and Schatzow (1987), and Williams (1994, 1995) regarding recollections of sexual abuse. Age at time of abuse as related to later memory loss (and different from normal developmental memory process of infantile and childhood amnesia) therefore remains an issue in need of additional investigation.

By and large, the two Widom studies build upon and extend the Williams' findings concerning memory loss and non-disclosure in a prospective cohort study with a corroborated abuse history, at a rate of approximately 38%. The Widom studies add a further degree of methodological rigor due to the use of a matched control group, male and female subjects, a large sample with a high response rate, and the investigation of physical abuse and neglect in addition to sexual abuse. Despite these obvious methodological improvements, Widom and co-authors do not assess or discuss variables of the index abuse that might impact both forgetting and recall (with the exception of age at onset of abuse and cognitive appraisal of sexual abuse). Unfortunately, no comparison can be made with abuse variables reported by Williams who found that a younger age at the time of the abuse, abuse by someone known to the child rather than by a stranger, and a lack of reported or perceived maternal support for the abused child was associated with the forgetting of abuse for a period of time and with the possibility of later "recovered memories". Williams also reported a range of forgetting strategies reported by her subjects as well as a number of factors related to the stimulation of recall (Williams, 1994, 1995), issues not discussed in the Widom research. As Widom and co-authors report more of the details provided by subjects in the two-hour interviews, perhaps they will have information on variables related to forgetting and variables related to remembering that can then be compared to the Williams' findings.

Taken together, both the Widom and the Williams studies provide substantial documentation of memory loss and/or non-disclosure among adults with documented histories of abuse as children. They thus substantiate the issue of underreporting and the occurrence of recovered memories and provide evidence that these can occur independent of a therapeutic context and influence. The findings are important in their own right yet also point the way for future investigations of the many factors that might be associated with forgetting and recall and also with non-disclosure. Williams concluding comment about her results are equally applicable to those of Widom and co-authors: "While these findings cannot be used to assert the validity of *all* recovered memories of child abuse, this study does suggest that recovered memories of child sexual abuse reported by adults can be quite consistent with contemporaneous documentation of the abuse and should not be summarily dismissed by therapists, lawyers, family members, judges or the women [and men] themselves" (Williams, 1995, p. 670).

REFERENCES

Brewin, C., Andrews, B., & Gotlib, I. (1993). Psychopathology and early experience: A reappraisal of retrospective reports. *Psychological Bulletin, 113,* 82–98.

Briere, J. (1992). Methodological issues in the study of sexual abuse effects. *Journal of Consulting and Clinical Psychology, 60*, 196–203.

Briere, J., & Conte, J. (1993). Self-reported amnesia for abuse in adults molested as children. *Journal of Traumatic Stress, 6*, 21–31.

Elliott, D., & Briere, J. (1995). Posttraumatic stress associated with delayed recall of sexual abuse: A general population study. *Journal of Traumatic Stress, 8*, 629–648.

Feldman-Summers, S., & Pope, K. (1994). The experience of "forgetting" childhood abuse: A national survey of psychologists. *Journal of Consulting and Clinical Psychology, 62*, 001–004.

Fivush, R. (1993). Developmental perspectives on autobiographical recall. In G. S. Goodman & B. L. Bottoms (Eds.), *Child victims, child witnesses: Understanding and improving testimony* (pp. 1–24). New York: Guilford.

Gold, S., Hughes, D., & Hohnecker, L. (1994). Degrees of repression of sexual abuse memories. *American Psychologist, 49*, 441–442.

Herman, J., & Schatzow, E. (1987). Recovery and verification of memories of childhood sexual trauma. *Psychoanalytic Psychology, 4*, 1–14.

Loftus, E., Polonsky, S., & Fullilove, M. (1994). Memories of childhood sexual abuse: Remembering and repressing. *Psychology of Women Quarterly, 18*, 67–84.

van der Kolk, B., & Fisler, R. (1995). Dissociation and the fragmentary nature of traumatic memories: Overview and exploratory study. *Journal of Traumatic Stress, 8*, 505–526.

Widom, C. S. (1989). The cycle of violence. *Science, 244*, 160–166.

Widom, C. S., & Morris, S. (under review). Accuracy of adult recollections of childhood victimization: II. Childhood sexual abuse.

Widom, C. S., & Shepard, R. L. (under review). Accuracy of adult recollections of childhood victimization: I. Childhood physical abuse.

Williams, L. M. (1994). Recall of childhood trauma: A prospective study of women's memories of child sexual abuse. *Journal of Consulting and Clinical Psychology, 62*, 1167–1176.

Williams, L. M. (1995). Recovered memories of abuse in women with documented child sexual victimization histories. *Journal of Traumatic Stress, 8*, 649–674.

QUESTIONS AND ANSWERS

Eth. I have two related clinical questions. The first is, did you collect other kinds of clinical outcome besides the depression, alcohol dependence and suicide attempts? and second did you use the DIS for PTSD diagnosis ?

Widom. Yes, actually we have PTSD, anti-social personality disorder, drug abuse, alcohol abuse, generalised anxiety disorder, depression, dysthymia and you clinicians will be interested to know we included somatization disorder but it just did not work. I'm working on a paper on PTSD and we have published papers on alcohol abuse dependence which came out in the *Journal of Studies in Alcohol* in the last couple of years, and a paper on anti-social personality disorder.

Eth. The data that you chose to show us - why did you select those three ?

Widom. Just because it was confusing enough and because we have published a paper on alcohol abuse, I felt it was critical to do the depression, especially given the Brewin, Andrews and Gotlib paper. I'm hoping to get funding to do the drug analyses.

Schooler. I would like to commend you for the remarkable extent of the research and the care in which you engaged in the matching and just the ambitiousness of the research: I think it's very important data. I have two questions - can we see the final conclusions slide? You conclude that the issue is not whether or not the self-report is valid or not but whether the measures are. It seems to me we have to be very careful in throwing out - I am having trouble not wanting to ask if the reports of childhood physical and sexual abuse are valid or not - that seems to me an awfully big question to dismiss, so I'm having trouble with that implication. Should we really stop asking the question, are these memories valid? The second one is more of an empirical question which is that you have one striking initially counter intuitive finding, which is that self-reports seem to be more predictive of symptoms than actual abuse, and there are all sorts of intriguing interpretations of that, one of which is that if you believe in repression, or forgetting, that forgetting is a good thing. Another possibility is that perhaps those people with more severe abuse are more likely to recall it?

Widom. I am not a memory researcher. What I was saying from the clinical/research perspective that we have now seen, is that there's good discrimination between these groups. It's not as high a percent of the groups and there's major under reporting, I think these are important messages that people in clinical research need to receive. What I think we need to be focusing on now is how to get the best information, to think creatively about getting samples of known victims, and trying to manipulate some of these things to find out the best way to get this information. Frankly, given the consistency of the child development findings, the findings of low agreement that I reviewed at the beginning of the paper which looked at adolescent reports of their own childhood, experiences that had nothing to do with victimisation. If you look at the few studies that have actually tried to compare reports with objective indicators they're all basically finding about the same percentage. You look at the national crime survey, which has been doing this work for many years and people's memories are just not that good. There ought to be more questioning of the validity of college undergraduate students and the assumption that their reports are valid. We need more research on the best way to get as accurate information as we can, but not thinking that we're going to get some pure 100%, because there is so much slippage. Just because my cases had sexual abuse, it may be that there were other experiences also. Science is not pure.

Schooler. I think we have full agreement. What is throwing me is your saying it does not matter if it is valid or not: that statement threw me. I think what you are saying is that we shouldn't ask whether it's valid or not, because no one's memory is 100% valid, is that all you're saying ? Therefore, since no-one's memory is entirely valid, what we should be concerned with is maximising everyone's report. I think we are all in agreement on that.

Widom. Unless there is some hidden thing, I am just saying not be too obsessive about it.

Schooler. We need to be obsessive about the possibility that some people could say that they were abused and they were not.

Widom. That's right. That is the point of the construct validation, that is the point in looking at gender differences. That is the point of looking at race differences. Given this general framework, what are the biases associated with self-report? The question is not are they valid, because we know they are relatively valid but not near 100%. As for your second question, I'm glad you brought that up, because I didn't really have a chance to talk about it as much I would have and should have. Yes, those are very startling findings and in part, the reason for the final implication. But I think you need to look at the context. What is the literature that we have based all the suppositions on? It is a literature which is based on people who are hurting and appraising their childhood as involving some kind of abuse. That's the critical difference in having a prospective design. This suggests to me that it may not be the actual abuse experience, but it may be the way you define it (c.f. Lazarus and cognitive appraisal). It's the way you respond to the situation and define the situation at that point in time or redefine it at a later point in time. Maybe those really are the most meaningful things. Maybe it does not make sense to worry so much any more. In some ways there's good discriminant validity, that's true but not 100%. A colleague went after me because it wasn't near 100%. My feeling is that we should look at everything else we know, look at the early childhood studies. People are not accurate reporters, so I am not troubled by a higher percentage. I can understand this validity data, but it would be much nicer if it was more consistent.

Loftus. That is just a beautiful piece of work as everyone else here recognises. Those age data, I know you want to forget them, but I think they are important for one reason that's already been alluded to by Ira and Robyn, and that is even if there is slop in the actual age of the crime because you've got the age of the petition as your x-axis variable, you can still say that here are some cases where the individual was no older than 3 years old at time of crime, and yet you still had in both the physical and the sexual cases significant levels of "accuracy," so it does make you wonder whether what these people are telling you is what they know to be true, and that's the remember/know distinction that Ira was alluding to and so the reports are not reports of episodic memory, but are reports of knowledge of your past. There may be no way with your current two hour interview to separate that out.

Widom. I realised afterwards Ira came up and we were talking about it and these are issues I had thought about. When you have a child who is sexually abused at 6 months of age because a man puts his finger in her vagina, it is very likely (unless you are a strict Freudian) that she will not remember *unless* there is a big "production" made about that case and the child is told and bad things happen to the family, so that it's not the abuse experience itself but it's the response to the abuse that may be having an effect. We recognise that. I didn't start out trying to do a study of the accuracy of memory. I realised it at a certain point and I thought well great I'm going to do this, but one thing we did do which is relevant is we took the sexual abuse cases, but we could not pursue it the way Linda Williams does, because we could not reveal that we knew they were sexually abused, it was too risky. What we have done is to ask of the people who say they were sexually abused, to what extent does the perpetrator match the perpetrator in the records? This was an attempt to get at some accuracy or concordance with what happened. Surprisingly, of those who reported being abused, there was very good concordance with the perpetrator, which made us feel a little bit better. But they could have been told who the perpetrator was. These are issues we now need to pursue.

Loftus. You mentioned the Della Femina work, and when those discrepancies were brought to the attention of the respondent, they all acknowledged that they did remember the physical abuse but they had failed to report it for a variety of reasons. So, could you speculate if you had done the study in a way you feel was unethical to do and confronted these individuals with their records, whether you would get the under-reporting?

Widom. I think that there is a real balance in doing research on these questions. If one pursues, asking about childhood victimisation in a tenacious way, I suspect you would get a lot more people saying they had been sexually or physically abused. This is a very new field, and we need good research and what we are doing now is starting to expose even the ability to ask these questions. I appreciate your questions.

Carlson. Your paradigm is comparing these reports to some criterion, so you're looking at concordance and a lot of times when one does that one has a very certain criterion. I just wanted to point out that in the case of using legal records as a criterion, we know that we can't really expect it to be the kind of criterion we might have if we knew what had actually happened to people. So when we see a discrepancy between their later retrospective report of what happened to them and these records I think you have to be very careful about slipping into the idea that somehow automatically that it is the report that is not agreeing with the truth of the records. For example, you had some discrepancies between reported violent behaviour toward others as adults and their court arrest records. I can easily imagine people who might be violent and beat up their children, or their wives, or get into bar fights and you ask them about their violent behaviour to other people on the conflict tactics scale - yes I have threatened, punched other people and they would be very high, and you look at the arrest record and, guess what, they never got caught doing any of these things, so there is a discrepancy. My understanding is that if someone is saying they beat people up, I have a hard time imagining they wanted to make something like that up. In my mind I wonder if the arrest record just didn't catch it.

Widom. I worry about all those things. Despite the fact that it's a good size sample, we still have only 110 cases of physical abuse, even though for clinicians 110 cases is a lot, and most people do not worry about power. The question is - is it simply being arrested for violence that has a low base rate, is it a statistical artifact or is it real? I am very troubled by what we seem to have is official predicting to official and self-report, and one of the questions I have is the extent to which we are getting disclosure from these people. We tried to be sensitive, to get this information, but from the field of criminology we know, for example, that there are systematic biases in the extent to which people report known things. We desperately need work in trying to understand the relationship between self report and official report data. I have come under attack because I've said I assume that the self reports are valid. I know that there are going to be people in the control group whose cases did not come to the attention of the authorities, but what is so troubling is the real discrepancy in these findings and what seems to be this method variance and this is not the end of the story. This is just the beginning of the story.

Elliott. I wonder if there's not a more basic explanation, and that is that we don't know if they're reporting to you the index case, so that where we do have people who are under the age of three that were index cases of sexual abuse, we don't know when they said yes to your question if they are talking about that same incident. So that seems to skew anything in terms of the demographic correlation.

Widom. I agree. The only thing that provides any evidence that it's close to the index offence is the fact that perpetrator of those who said they were, matched up quite well.

Elliott. But we don't know if the perpetrator continued to perpetrate.

Widom. Absolutely. Lucy Berliner in a review several years ago and a group of people from Canada, Beitchman et al. (1992), independently in reviewing the literature both concluded that age of onset of sexual abuse experience had not been shown to be consistently related to consequences. Each talked about the difficulty of assessing age of onset, I think what we need is a new prospective longitudinal study by someone who has access to records with more detailed information about the index offence, so that we can look. I, for example, cannot look at severity. My data on severity is not very good or reliable. My study has certain strengths but it has its limitations and it's important to lay those out.

REFERENCES

Beitchman, J.H., Zucker, K.J., Hood, J.E., daCosta, G.A., & Cassavia, E. (1992). A review of the long-term effects of child sexual abuse. *Child Abuse and Neglect, 16,* 101–118.
Della Femina, D., Yeager, C.A., & Lewis, D.O. (1990). Child abuse: Adolescent records vs. adult recall. *Child Abuse and Neglect, 14,.* 227–231.

4

MEMORY ISSUES IN THE DIAGNOSIS OF UNREPORTED TRAUMA

J. Don Read

University of Lethbridge
4401 University Dr.
Lethbridge, AB T1K 3M4
Canada

1. INTRODUCTION

It seems intuitively obvious to many people that if something unpleasant happens to them that they would rather forget, somehow wishing to forget it ought be successful. As the degree of unpleasantness of the event increases, moving it into the realm of perhaps life- or security-threatening experiences, or what might be called traumatic events, it seems all the more obvious that their wish to forget and success at doing so ought to be greater. But, paradoxically, we recognize that the events we generally remember about our past are those that are, in fact, highly salient and unusual which serve as the landmarks and signposts around which we organize the meaning and narratives of our lives. Hence, because traumatic events are also highly unusual and salient it is simultaneously contradictory that we could as easily forget these events as we can other minor, mildly unpleasant and less salient events. Instead, if we are to be successful at forgetting highly unusual, salient, and unpleasant events, the mind needs to be endowed with additional abilities. Hypothetical mental mechanisms like repression and dissociation that will allow us to forget successfully are frequently advanced as likely candidates within the clinical literature (see Lindsay & Read, 1994, 1995; Loftus, 1993; Ofshe & Singer, 1994). The belief that we are able to eliminate from memory the unpleasant events of our lives through these special mechanisms is so highly ingrained in our culture that it has spawned several ancillary beliefs about the operation of memory and these have spilled over into the fields in which we work, some as researchers, some as clinical practitioners, and some who do both. Of course, it may indeed turn out that this core belief relating trauma and successful forgetting has validity. Perhaps so, but in the meantime I will argue that we need to better understand how we can test the claims about memory that are inherent in these beliefs.

To do so, I will provide a context or background from cognitive psychology against which we can look at some beliefs and expectations about memory that are derivatives of the trauma-forgetting relationship described above. I also will provide an empirical con-

Recollections of Trauma, edited by Read and Lindsay
Plenum Press, New York, 1997

text against which we can begin to assess the quantitatively-based claims about the memory difficulties of survivors of childhood sexual abuse (CSA). In doing so, I will specifically question two claims made about memory that are frequently present in the lay and professional literature on the effects of trauma: (1) first, the claim that traumatic events like CSA generate significant, perceptible, gaps or voids in the fabric and continuity of childhood autobiographical memory; and (2), the related idea that the experience of trauma can produce amnesia for the associated event(s) and that subsequent "recovery" of the memory can be taken as hard evidence of the postulated amnestic powers of trauma (and, simultaneously, of the reality of the recovered experience).[*]

Some components of my presentation are based upon existing empirical literature and others from survey work being completed in my laboratory. To assist you in seeing my orientation and biases, a little personal history: My background is in cognitive or experimental psychology. I have completed a wide range of memory research studies usually, but not always, with adults; generally, but not always, in laboratory settings with participants who frequently, but not always, understood they were in a research study, and who usually, but not always, were relatively unstressed by the instructions and tasks at hand, and who approached these tasks in usually, but not always, sober states. The points I make in this chapter arise from basic scientific principles and, after hearing or being reminded of them, I'm sure you will agree there is nothing particularly exceptional in what I have to say.

1.1. Prevalence of the Trauma-Forgetting Belief

In my view, our culture has accepted some aspects of the trauma-forgetting belief relationship so willingly that its derivative beliefs are as readily apparent among among 18-year old undergraduate students as they are among the majority of older adult members of the population. Because the media reflects and contributes to the popular culture around us we can see in both students and older adults beliefs about memory that are currently being played out in therapy, the courtroom, and in science. There have been, of course, surveys of lay belief in memory completed by a number of researchers including Loftus and Loftus (1981) and Garry, Loftus & Brown (1994) and these surveys well document the kinds and frequencies of misperceptions held by the public about the scientific knowledge of memory.

To demonstrate the extent to which beliefs about CSA trauma and memory have been readily incorporated into popular public opinion, 160 undergraduate psychology students were shown this description of a middle-aged woman.

> (A). She hasn't had a happy life because her marriage failed while her two children were quite young. Obtaining adequate food and housing for the family were always difficult for her. She was frequently employed but various problems always arose that caused her to lose her job rather quickly; specifically, physical illness, depression, alcohol, and drug abuse. A psychologist who interviewed her determined that she is bright and motivated but seems to be obsessed with her relationship to her parents who both passed away 15 years earlier, and she has difficulty establishing relationships with new acquaintances.

The description was followed by the question "What do you think caused this woman's problems"?

---

[*] As the reader will learn from Widom's commentary (this volume), an additional claim was challenged in this ASI presentation. For reasons related to complexity and breadth of that work, the reader is referred to the in press paper by Winkielman, Belli, Schwarz and Read for complete details.

Psychology students are more than a little willing to analyze someone's psychological problems because, for many, this activity is exactly what they thought psychology was about (and likely their reason for taking the introductory course). Hence, instead of responding with "There is insufficient information to say anything useful about why this woman", the students happily wrote mini-dissertations based on their psychological analyses.

All students read the core description (A) above; however, a simple experimental manipulation varied in a random manner how much additional information each student received: For one-third of the students (Condition A), no descriptive information beyond the core (A) was given. For the remaining two-thirds, *either* sentence (B) or sentence (C) below had been added to the core:

(B). "Further, she has difficulty remembering portions of recent events in her life; for example, she complains that she can't seem to recall much about what she did two or three months ago."

(C). "Further, she has difficulty remembering some portions of her childhood; for example, she complains that she can't seem to recall much about her life between the ages of 6 and 8."

As you can see, statements B and C are highly similar and both indicate that the woman has perceived problems with her autobiographical memory: in B for recent events and in C for childhood events.

We completed a blind content analysis of the students' written responses and generated seven categories of their, often creative, answers to this problem. However, our real interest was in determining to what extent CSA would be suggested as the primary reason for the woman's distress across the three conditions. For that reason, I focus here only upon answers in which CSA was explicitly offered as the basis of the woman's problems.

1.2. Description of Results

The percentages of students who suggested CSA, sometimes accompanied by physical abuse, as the primary explanation for the woman's difficulties were 11.5%, 7.7% and 52.1% in Conditions A, B, and C, respectively. Statistical analysis revealed that Condition C gave significantly more CSA reasons than did either of Conditions A or B, which were equivalent, X^2 (2, N = 157) = 33.93, $p < .05$, the alpha level used in this research. Hence, it is clear that a single phrase about poor memory for the woman's childhood significantly and greatly influenced the students' hypotheses. I trust it is obvious that I only offer these data as demonstrating the extent to which the trauma-forgetting hypothesis has influenced the popular culture and the ease with which we can tap this belief system. If a single comment about perceived poor childhood memory encourages the hypothesis of childhood sexual abuse in the majority of 18-year olds, it would not be surprising that other beliefs or statements about memory difficulties might also be used to entertain CSA as the basis for someone's difficulties.

2. GAPS IN AUTOBIOGRAPHICAL MEMORY

Ultimately, my interest is with the role that beliefs about memory play in the diagnosis of unreported trauma; that is, the psychological description or diagnosis of adults who are unaware of past trauma in their lives. I recognize that such descriptions and diagnoses are usually made by well-trained clinicians following conscientious and thorough assessments of many features of the client's behaviour. However, it is also well documented that many prominent therapists have placed considerable emphasis upon autobiographical memory problems as supportive of an undisclosed and possibly unknown history of CSA. For example, the symptom checklist approaches recommended by Ratican (1988), Frederickson (1990), Blume (1990), and, most recently, Walker (1994) well support the view that a client's apparent difficulty in recalling some part of childhood may be interpreted by these writers as a significant indicator of CSA. For some of these writers, autobiographical memory gaps have been explicitly assigned highly significant diagnostic roles. Similarly, from the survey work of Poole, Lindsay, Memon, and Bull (1994) we learn that among doctoral-level psychologists in the US and the UK, the presence of memory gaps was one of the 5 most frequently offered presenting symptoms considered an indicator of CSA. And, in a survey of 38 therapists in the Phoenix area by Susan Smith (1991), over 70% said that the presence of such gaps was an indicator of CSA. In two sets of therapeutic notes that I had opportunity to review, the therapists had recorded in the first session the explicit hypothesis that a repressed history of CSA was likely because, for one client, "she didn't seem to remember much about her childhood" and, for the other, the therapist noted that the client "does not remember the house she grew up in very well".

However, I am very pleased that strong claims like these in regard to the diagnostic value of perceived memory gaps are apparently less likely now than they were even a few years ago, an important change due in part, I think, to clinicians like Christine Courtois (1995; also this volume) who have explicitly stated that such perceived gaps should not be used as significant indicators of CSA. If the view is changing, I would like to think that some of the papers in cognitive psychology emphasizing the normal spottiness of autobiographical memory and the need for standardized assessment techniques in general have also played a role.

Nonetheless, I will flesh out the reasons why we need to carefully consider the use of memory gaps and memory difficulties as indicators of an unreported history of CSA. In particular, I will argue that we need a lot more information about the normative characteristics of memory gaps before their presence may be taken as diagnostic features. To do so, we'll look first at the results of some survey work completed at Lethbridge by which we attempt to understand, among other things, the prevalence of self-perceived gaps in autobiographical memory among members of a large public sample not selected for prior history of sexual trauma.

As described earlier, many clinical writers have included an assessment of the coherence and completeness of autobiographical memory as a useful diagnostic related to an undisclosed history of CSA. These writers have concluded that such gaps and holes are indicators of CSA because, presumably, they have believe such gaps were more frequent among clients who later proved to be survivors of CSA than among their other clients. The hypothesis about the presence of gaps is based on the idea that the gaps reflect periods during which a child was victimized and traumatized by sexual abuse. Indeed, it does not seem unreasonable that if children were victimized in abusive ways their attention to and encoding of other aspects of their environment and relationships during the period of victimization might suffer. For the recollection of short-duration emotionally-arousing witnessed events there is good evidence that processing and encoding of the events is disturbed in significant ways (e.g., Christianson, 1992; Read, Yuille & Tollestrup, 1992). And, of course, some have argued that dissociative states during such victimization periods would also serve to reduce encoding of contextual information. To the extent that these kinds of abnormal or impoverished cognitive activities take place, it seems reasonable to anticipate some losses of the type described. In a recent but unpublished PhD dissertation, Vardi (1994, cited in Brown, 1995) apparently did report evidence of greater losses for CSA adult survivors compared to members of a control group.

However, two things have long troubled me about this claim of the presence of such gaps and the hypothetical mechanisms by which they occur. First, other than the use of a simple diagnostic checklist, I have been unable to find any evidence that a standardized test of autobiographical memory has been used by practitioners. This is not to say that there aren't standardized techniques available for getting access to this information because there are (e.g., Kopelman, Wilson & Baddeley, 1989; and mental status exams often have an autobiographical component). However, it appears that most do not use the techniques that are available. Instead, if they follow DSM-IV standards (American Psychiatric Association, 1994) they likely formed a clinical judgment on the basis that the perceived memory losses were "too extensive as to be caused by ordinary forgetfulness"(see Carlson, this volume). This definition, of course, only pushes the problem one step further away because now we must ask how the clinicians assessed "ordinary forgetfulness". Unfortunately, the published research is equally oblique about the basis of this assessment.

As one example of how clients were diagnosed as having significant gaps in autobiographical memory, Colin Ross (1989) asked research participants and clients this one question: "Are there large parts of your childhood after age 5 which you can't remember?" An affirmative response to this question meant that the client was labelled as being amnesic for childhood (see also Ross et al., 1991). It should not surprise us to learn that answers to a single question like this may be influenced by demand characteristics in the situation (see Read & Lindsay, 1994) and is likely of questionable reliability (see Winkielman, Belli, Schwarz, & Read, in press). My concerns here will be with how memory performance is measured and what the background, context, or normative data are to which such measurements might be compared. I appreciate that clinicians argue that "clinical judgment", based upon comparative observations made over years of experience, would be the likely basis of their inferences about a client's gaps in memory. However, a lack of systematic observation and recorded data collection evident in published cases is troubling to me and the validity of such judgments has frequently been questioned (e.g., Dawes, 1994).

The second concern I have is that the published literature related to memory gaps reveals a rather striking inconsistency: Whereas many clinicians have reported that their clients with a history of CSA demonstrate memory gaps, in none of the surveys of the self-perceived consequences of CSA have the survivors volunteered autobiographical memory gaps as a source of psychological distress (e.g., Beitchman, Zucker, Hood, da-Costa, & Cassavia, 1992; Cole & Putnam, 1992; Moeller, Bachmann, & Moeller, 1993; Russell, 1986). The paradox here is that whereas clinicians report having observed such gaps frequently neither the systematic scientific surveys nor the published literature reviews of the sequelae of CSA have reported such gaps, in part perhaps, because they did not ask, and in part because clients apparently did not report them. Of course, one possibility is that CSA survivors are completely unaware of their gaps, hence no distress is caused by the voids and are therefore not reported. If this were true then it is surprising that Ross's CSA clients so readily answered the single question described above. Similarly, the current conceptualization used by many (see Briere, this volume) is that individuals who are unable to recall traumatic incidents of abuse may suffer dissociative amnesia as outlined in the DSM-IV. But, this diagnosis requires that they report the very distress they apparently do not report.

2.1. Survey of Population Beliefs about the Coherence and Integrity of Memory

To explore these issues I will report preliminary results from some survey work that we have undertaken at Lethbridge, work that would not have been completed had I not discussed these issues with Sheila Seelau who was completing a PhD on public beliefs about memory at Iowa State University. Sheila graciously provided me with her questionnaire and allowed me to insert a number of other questions specific to my interests. As a result, we also collected substantial data about memory beliefs about memory but these results will not be detailed here.

We collected two public samples: the first included 209 adult volunteers (minimum age of 18) at a local shopping mall. Each volunteer responded to our displays and came to our office within the mall, and completed the 30-min questionnaire in return for $5. The second sample of 204 was obtained by mailing a questionnaire to all employees at my university that targeted all occupational groups from administrators to grounds people to secretaries and faculty. The return rate was approximately 45%. I do not argue that these samples are representative of the adult Canadian population however, neither do I think that they are particularly unique. As it turned out, the two samples did not generate different data and, in fact, their data were quite similar to those collected from Iowa State undergraduates on my behalf by Sheila Seelau. The survey should be viewed as exploratory only (and a subsequent instrument is being developed to more carefully assess my particular interests, as well as its reliability) and it is in that tentative perspective that they are presented here.

The sample was divided approximately equally with 197 males and 216 females. Overall, the sample ranged in age from 18 to 84 with an mean of 36.2 and a standard deviation of 12.4. The mean ages (and standard deviations) of the male and female samples were 36.5 (13.9) and 35.9 years (11.0). It is important to stress there were neither instructions nor questions in the survey that addressed either sexual abuse or therapy.

2.1.1. Assessment of Autobiographical Memory Gaps. The survey attempted to obtain some baseline assessment of what adults say about the integrity and coherence of their autobiographical memories. To do so, following several pages of demographic and memory belief questions, we first asked our sample whether they believed they had periods of unusually limited memory in their recollection of childhood and beyond.

Specifically, the Yes-No question was: "Can you think of any significant periods in your life for which you seem to have an unusually limited or poor memory? By significant we mean months or years in duration."

If the Yes option was circled, a second question requested detail about relevant ages and the periods of time for which the respondents believed they had unusually limited memory. It is true that some writers have characterized the memory gaps as gaping black holes from which nothing can be recalled, but the more typical description is one of "poor memory" for childhood and our question attempted to tap this quality. Of the total sample, 47.0% reported at least one such period in their lives. For males the overall figure was 50.3% and for females 43.5%, a nonsignificant difference by chi-square [$X^2(1, N=413) = 1.70$]. It is also the case that about 10% reported a second period and another 2% a third and/or a fourth period of unusually limited memory. One might be surprised by these data because we likely assume that virtually everyone would agree that their first year or two of life is unusually limited in recollection. However, on the basis of the respondents' answers to other questions (not to be discussed here), we believe many thought we were asking about periods beyond the very early or infant years, of ages birth to 3. In any event, it is of interest is to ask for what ages are these periods experienced? Figure 1 provides the relationship between the minimum age at the start of any reported period of unusually limited memory and the cumulative percentage of respondents reporting such a period. Data are reported for males and females separately as well as for the total sample.

First, it is clear that if we include all ages beginning with birth that the majority of respondents report a limited period beginning between birth and 3 years of age. However, if we choose a minimum age of, say, 3, we can see that about 20% of all respondents said that they had a limited period of memory beginning at age 3 or beyond. By the minimum age of 5 for example, this percentage has dropped to 15%. To put it another way, 5% of the subjects reported a limited memory period beginning at an age between 3 and 5. These patterns are somewhat easier to see in Figure 2 where the exact percentages of people reporting their first limited periods beginning at specific ages are plotted. Here, for example, 20% of the males reported that they had an unusually limited memory starting at birth whereas about 3% of males say that they had a period beginning at age 10. Summing across ages we again see that a total of about 20% report an unusually limited period beginning at age 3 and beyond.

What is important in Figures 1 and 2 is the finding that a significant minority (20%) of our participants reported significant gaps in their memory beginning after age 3 with additional onset dates occurring through childhood and the teens but with decreasing frequency. At whatever age we choose it should be clear that a client's observation that he or she has a poor memory must be interpreted in the context of the baseline level of such reports. If, for example, a client meeting the characteristics of this sample reports a poor memory for his life between 6 and 9, we should anticipate on these data that perhaps 10% of this population would normally respond in that fashion.

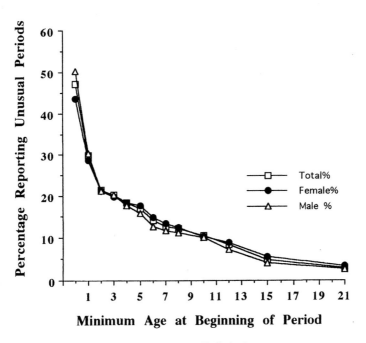

Figure 1. Periods of unusually limited memory.

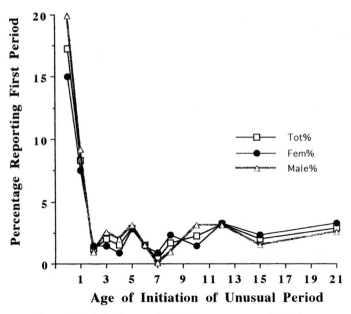

Figure 2. Periods of unusually limited memory: Age of initiation.

2.1.2. Duration of Limited Periods. In Figure 3 the average lengths of these periods of limited memory are plotted by age at the beginning of each reported period. Overall, the average duration is about 4 years and changes unsystematically as the age at which the period begins increases. The longest period reported by a male was 14 years and for females was 18 years.

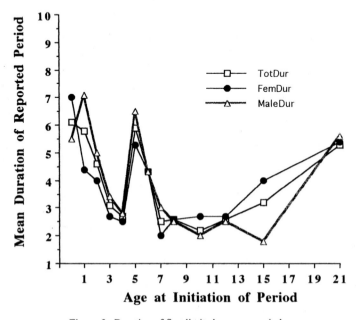

Figure 3. Duration of first limited memory period.

The second finding I find striking is that the functions are essentially identical for male and female respondents and, if anything, males more likely to report a gap than are females. Obviously, this is not a random sample and survivors of CSA may have declined to volunteer at greater rates than non-survivors. However, if we accept well-documented reports (e.g., Finkelhor, 1994) that females suffer CSA at rates well beyond that of males and if such experiences produce perceptible memory gaps, it follows that the female distribution ought to be somewhat higher than the male function. Alternatively, perhaps a solicitation to participate in a survey about memory was uniformly declined by all survivors of CSA because they recognized their memory deficits. But, if they were unaware of their victimization as suggested by the trauma-forgetting hypothesis, their basis for declining presumably would not likely be a result of sensitivity to the memory issue.

Another 10% of the participants reported a second period of limited memory. For the most part, the starting dates for a second period was rarely before the age of 3 (because birth to age 3 was the first period reported) and continued up to ages of at least 21. But this percentage is small throughout and the differences between males and females again nonexistent. However, unlike the first periods reported, the later the starting age of these second periods, the greater the time span they were reported to embrace.

2.1.3. Assessment of Autobiographical Memory "Blank" Periods. A second question asked about periods of time during which they judged their memories for periods of time to be completely absent. The question asked was similar to the earlier question: "Do you believe there are significant periods of time in your life for which you are unable to remember anything at all? By significant we mean months or years in duration". As may be seen in Figure 4, reports of completely blank periods were less frequent than the "unusually limited" periods just described and were reported by only about 5% of the population beyond the age of the first year of life.

2.2. Summary of Respondents' Beliefs about Autobiographical Memory Gaps

These data demonstrate that self-reported gaps in autobiographical memory beyond the age of 4 or 5 may be not typical but they are far from rare. Our participants provided the information within 30 minutes and were not at any time probed about their memories by specific questions that might cue recall or that might yield evidence that could be taken as demonstrating a memory deficiency. As a result, it is suggested that their responses under- rather than over-estimated the frequency of perceived gaps in autobiographical memory. One might argue that the 20% of people who report a significant gap in memory beyond age 3 have gaps because they had, in fact, all been sexually abused. A possibility, but unlikely for two reasons: first, such a claim presumes that there is a "cause" for perceived gaps in childhood memory and that the single cause is CSA. To the extent that claiming a specific cause for what may prove to be simply normal population variability in the "perception" of the completeness of one's memory (much less the actual performance) such a claim excludes many other good reasons suggested by developmental psychologists for difficulties in recalling one's past (e.g., limited opportunities to narrativize daily events through discussion and rehearsal as argued, for example, by Fivush and Hammond (1990), attachment disorders as suggested by Alexander (1993), and extremely long retention intervals). Second, and more cogent, is the near identicality of responses from our male and female respondents. If CSA caused memory gaps then it follows that because females are victimized at a much higher rate than males, considerably higher fre-

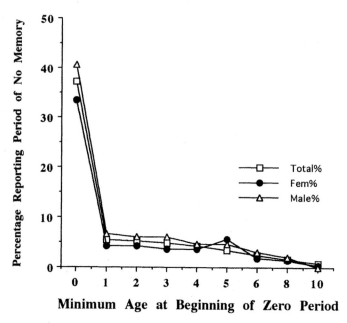

Figure 4. Reported period of no memory.

quencies of reported gaps among adult females than males would be anticipated. There was simply no evidence that this was the case.

However, regardless of the exact frequency of perceived gaps in memory, the reporting of such gaps in non-clinical samples reminds us that if CSA does produce autobiographical memory difficulties, its prevalence rate must exceed by a reasonable amount the background or baseline data in order for the claim to receive support .

3. MEMORY LOSSES SPECIFIC TO CSA

How do we know that abuse memories are rendered unavailable in conscious recall to victims of CSA? Generally, one response is that evidence has been amassed of their "recovery" through various means, for example, spontaneous cuing, hypnosis, and psychotherapy. Another type of evidence is the data gathered through the prospective research methodology taken by Williams (1994a, 1994b, 1995, this volume) and others (see Widom, this volume) by which adults for whom there is documented evidence of CSA are asked about their abuse history. Substantial minorities of these respondents have reported that they believe there were periods of their lives in which they had forgotten the abuse incidents. However, the majority of data taken in support of the claim that abuse memories are unavailable to recall comes from adults identified as survivors of sexual abuse who have retrospectively reported that there were periods of time in their lives during which they remembered little or nothing of the abusive events. The wording of the critical question has varied across studies but Elliott and Briere's (1995) question well captures the common intent. They asked their national survey respondents whether there was ever a time that they had less memory of a traumatic event than they had at the time of questioning. An important difference between these retrospective and the prospective studies de-

scribed above is that for the former the abuse was not documented and usually not corroborated. Together, these reports and the claim that these people now remember the experiences (when they could not before) have been taken as hard evidence that the events
must have been truly unavailable to recall and, therefore, such unavailability was a special
consequence of sexual trauma.

Most importantly, the exact percentages of people reporting these retrospective
memory voids have been proffered as demonstrations of and considered as *prima facie*
evidence of the special power of sexual trauma to produce amnesia for the events. If the
latter claim is accepted, it also follows that the reports are veridical accounts of actual
abuse experiences. Hence many writers have noted that a sizable proportion of CSA survivors report that they previously had no or very poor recollection of the events: for Briere
and Conte (1993) who completed the first and, as it turned out, prescient study in the late
1980's the figure reported was 59%; for Feldman-Summers and Pope (1994) the figure
was 41%; for Loftus, Polonsky and Fullilove (1994) 19%; for Sheiman (1993) 58%; for
Gold, Hughes, & Hohnecker (1994) 30%; for Williams (1995), 16%; and for Elliott and
Briere (1995) 42%. From these statistics have arisen the claims that between 16 and 59%
of CSA survivors experienced a period of time during which they had little or no recollection of the traumatic events or, as characterized by some researchers, had either "complete" or "partial amnesia" during these periods. What should we make of these figures?
For the moment, let's assume, from the data above, that an average 38% of CSA survivors
report that the events were unavailable in memory for significant periods of time.

We can, on the one hand, be impressed that this percentage is well above zero and
accept, at a minimum, the data as evidence of the likely repressive effects of sexually traumatic experiences. Or, we can ask, *compared to what?* Unfortunately, we immediately
recognize that providing a reasonable point of comparison is not going to be simple and is
perhaps one reason other researchers did not seek a baseline or normative level against
which they could compare the reported rates of recovered memories.

3.1. Reports and Descriptions of Recovered Memories

To mimic the retrospective question asked of participants in the other studies mentioned above, we asked participants whether they could recall a circumstance in which
they realized that they had remembered something they believed they had forgotten. The
specific question was "Have you ever recalled an experience or series of related experiences that you had "forgotten" about for some extended period of time? By extended period of time, we mean for weeks, months, or longer." Because a Yes answer strongly
suggests there was a time during which respondents remembered less about an event than
they did when they recalled or discovered the information, Yes responses are hereafter
termed "recovered memories".

We were hopeful that our respondents might recall having had a memory recovery
or discovery experience of a non-trivial event, hence the emphasis upon "extended periods
of time" in the question. Because of the questionnaire's length we only asked for a response in regard to one such experience. Of the total sample, 248 or 60.3% answered Yes
to this question and, of those, 224 went on to give us a written description of what they recalled about the memory recovery experience and the event recovered. Somewhat surprisingly, males (65.3%) were significantly more likely than females (55.6%) to respond
affirmatively [X^2 (1, N=411) = 4.02].

Reading the variety of written descriptions we were struck by the fact that these participants apparently had been quite impressed by their "recovery" experience, so much so

as to be able to recall it when asked to do so without any kind of preparatory reminiscence activity. Following standard content analysis procedures, we read and assigned each of the 224 descriptions to one of 12 content categories. From these we further collapsed the reports (because of cell frequencies less than 3) into six larger categories:. The categories and frequency of report were Everyday Events (35.9%), Childhood Recollections (11.3%), Sexual Abuse (7.3%), Other Trauma (20.6%), Miscellaneous (15.3%), and No Description Provided (9.7%). Clearly, all assignments to these categories reflect our interpretations of the written descriptions. What we might consider either trivial or salient may well have received different assignments by the respondents.

Before describing those categories in more detail, I will first focus upon two types of highly salient events which respondents often reported they had forgotten for substantial periods of time. One memory report that has been taken as strong evidence of the special memory status of sexual abuse trauma is that victims can forget years of sustained abuse, even which that has occurred on a regular, weekly, or even daily basis (e.g., Ofshe & Singer, 1994). Because forgetting of such repeated events would not be predicted by research in cognitive psychology (Lindsay & Read, 1994; Loftus, 1993), we were interested to see whether our respondents would report memory losses of other repeated events in their lives, as a basis of comparison. We were surprised that our respondents sometimes reported they had forgotten recurring events in which they had been involved for lengthy periods of time ranging from 1–9 years, events like music and sport lessons, organized children's activities, vacation trips and so forth. Hence, these reports of the forgetting of sustained but, presumably, non traumatic activities provide existence proofs that, apparently, other kinds of repeated events can also be "forgotten" for long periods of time. Of course, we neglected to ask the parents of those who took violin lessons whether the experience was traumatic to them. The second subset of events of particular interest were significant by virtue of their heavy negative emotional impact and would likely be considered by most clinicians as at least potentially traumatic, if not definitely traumatic. These events included sexual abuse of the respondents when they were children, sometimes sustained in duration, or abuse as an adult, or witnessing of horrific events (e.g., fatal accidents, parental adultery, domestic violence) as well as specific other unpleasant experiences (e.g., corporal punishment, near deaths, etc). On occasion, respondents declined to describe in writing their unpleasant recovered memories saying that the information was too personal and too disturbing to write down. The percentages and numbers of reports in these two categories, the repeated and the traumatic, were 5.65% (n = 14) and 16.94% (n = 42). Of the traumatic, 23 (9.27%) related to sexual abuse and 19 (7.66%) to other kinds of traumatic experiences.

3.2. Actually Forgotten or Not Thought About?

A subsequent question (following a written description of the forgotten and recovered event) asked the participants to clarify what they meant by the term "forgotten". That is, did they believe they had actually *forgotten* the information at that time or simply *had not thought* about it? Given these two choices, 34.4% of the total 248 subjects who reported a recovered memory experience indicated they believed they had actually forgotten the information. The remaining 65.6% reported that by "forgetting" they meant they simply had not thought about the event or events.

If we accept the claims presented by numerous researchers and the implications of the trauma-forgetting hypothesis, we should see some evidence that the traumatic events were more frequently reported to have been truly "forgotten" than the recurring, but, non

traumatic events. To answer this question we looked at the rates at which participants reported that they had actually forgotten (rather than not thought about) each type of experience. Note that our concern is with the percentage of each type of event reported to be
forgotten, not with the absolute percentages because we do not know the base rates of the
two kinds of events. What these participants reported was that the events of an ex-
tended/repeated nature (but neither sexually abusive nor traumatic) were as likely to be
judged as having been truly forgotten (50.0%) as the sexually traumatic events were
(47.8%) and both of these were slightly more likely to have been considered forgotten as
other traumatic experiences (31.6%). These data provide the first suggestion, based on retrospective assessments of whether events were truly forgotten or not, that recovered
memories of sexually abusive experiences may not necessarily be different than other
kinds of salient events

Figure 5 presents the initial 6-category analysis of the written conceptual content of
the respondents' "recovered" memories. The data given here reflect the proportions who
indicated that they had truly forgotten the events in question, rather than simply not thinking about them. As can be seen with this re-classification, most event types are described
as being truly forgotten about 35% of the time, on average. Only the sexual abuse category exceeds the overall average rate by about 15%. This difference is more striking in the
next figure where the data are presented separately for male and female respondents.

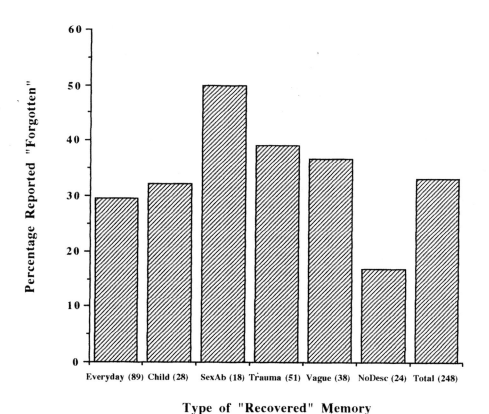

Type of "Recovered" Memory

Figure 5. Percentages of "forgotten" recovered memories.

In Figure 6 we can see that females report a higher rate of forgetting of sexual trauma in comparison to the other categories but the males appear to be particularly unlikely to say they had truly forgotten a sexually abusive experience in comparison to their reported forgetting of other types of experiences. Given the sample size for the male sexual abuse report category ($n = 4$), I would not go beyond the observation that these gender differences data are somewhat supportive of the claims made in the literature about males and females. And, of course, one can always argue that we did not receive reports from survivors who were truly successful in forgetting sexually abusive events because they're not aware that they have such memories. However, one could as easily make the parallel argument that among our respondents there were other non traumatic events that had also been forgotten and of which they were unaware at testing. Recall that there were no references to CSA in our questionnaire. In other words, it is difficult to understand why remembering "memory recovery" experiences would disfavour recollections of abuse. Indeed, one might argue instead that the recollection of recovery experiences related to sexual abuse would be particularly dramatic and memorable.

3.2.1. Reasons for Believing They Had Actually Forgotten. To return to the issue of what evidence our respondents had that they had truly forgotten the events in question, we asked them to select one or more reasons from among four options. Doing so is difficult because they are being asked to comment in an elaborated fashion upon their memory ex-

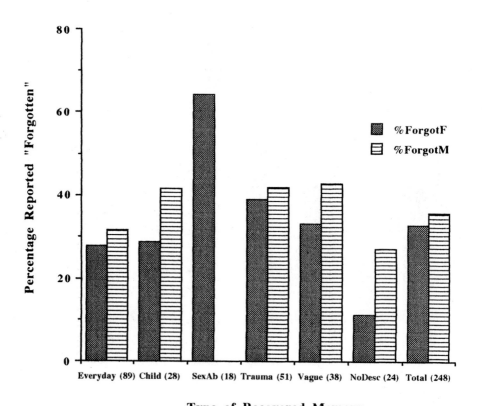

Type of Recovered Memory

Figure 6. Percentage "forgotten" recovered memories: gender.

periences for an event during a period when they claimed to have not remembered the event. However, it is likely that their reasons were the atributions they made on the basis of other characteristics of the memory recovery experience (e.g., surprise, emotional valence, etc.). Schooler (this volume) has described similar cognitive processes involved in memory recovery.

Of the participants who said they had actually forgotten the events, 51.8% reported that they had absolutely no memory during the period of time they thought the information had been forgotten. There was a marginally significant gender difference here with females more likely than males to say they had absolutely no memory, across all events, X^2 (1, $N = 83$) = 3.62, $p < .10$. Another 34.1% took as evidence of forgetting that they had been unsuccessful in trying to remember the events during the critical period of time. To respond in this way suggests that they would have to have had some recollection of the event in order to try to remember and suggests that this corresponds to what many writers have called, quite inappropriately in my view, "partial amnesia". Only 1 person (1.2%) chose the option that indicated her belief that she had amnesia for the event. I thought the very low rate of endorsement of the "amnesia" option interesting because, according to recent work by Elliott and Briere (1995), their respondents frequently volunteered use of the term "amnesia" in regard to their memory recovery experiences. Finally, the remaining participants (18.3%) gave either no reason or idiosyncratic reasons for reaching the belief that they had actually forgotten.

On the other hand, the metamemorial evidence used by respondents to support a claim that they had simply not thought about the events was more varied. The majority (57.6%) of these reasons relate to their observation that there had been no opportunities to think about the event either because there was no occasion to remember, or it was unimportant, or nothing was presented to remind them of it. Some (21.6%) presumed that no one could forget the type of experience they described and another group (25.8%) provided a logical analysis: that because they now remember it, they obviously could not have "forgotten" it. Various other reasons were selected (respondents could choose more than one option) including that the event was not sufficiently important to think about (46.8%), or that nothing served to remind them (34.2%) or they chose not to think about the described event (17.7%). Another 40.5% took as evidence of simply having not thought about it was their belief that they would have remembered had they been asked at the time.

3.2.2. Would a Reminder Have Been Effective to Remember the Event? In this connection, to get at the question of amnesia some researchers have suggested that respondents be asked whether they could have remembered the "forgotten" events had they been directly asked about it during the so-called amnestic period. Accordingly, our next question asked all subjects whether they would have remembered, had they been asked. The results showed an overall affirmative response of 69.7% but when partitioned by their earlier answers to the "forgetting versus not thinking" question, their responses revealed some puzzling inconsistencies. For example, of those who claimed to have actually forgotten, a sizable minority (43.8%) said that they could have nevertheless remembered the event if specifically asked about it. The inconsistency was reduced among those who chose the "not thought about" option because the vast majority (82.4%) thought they would have remembered, but another 17.6% thought they would not have done so. These kinds of responses emphasize the difficulties people have with retrospective metamemorial questions, particularly when we attempt to tease various explanations apart and use terminology that may be inappropriately matched to the participants' experiences.

However, we can with this "would you have remembered if asked" criterion again make comparisons between the claims of having forgotten different kinds of experiences. Figure 7 provides the same six content categories as before but presents the percentages of respondents who thought they would not have recalled, had they been asked. As before, we can see that the event types do not differ substantially on this dependent variable.

3.2.3. A Stringent Criterion of Forgetting. Finally, we can construct a stringent criterion for what some might refer to as amnestic periods during which participants said they truly did not have recall of the specific events. That is, if we take the conjunction of having both originally reported that an event had been forgotten and subsequently indicating that, when asked, they would have been unable to recall the experience we can consider these two responses together as the strongest evidence for periods of time during which events were completely unavailable to memory. Figure 8 presents the percentage of respondents who gave affirmative answers to both questions, separated by event type and gender. There are small and statistically unreliable differences between event types and between genders. Among females the claim of unavailability to memory is as frequent for everyday events as it is for sexually abusive experiences. Males, on the other hand, reported CSA at about one-quarter the rate of females but when they did, they seem unique in that they report no periods during which they truly forgot. This observation is moder-

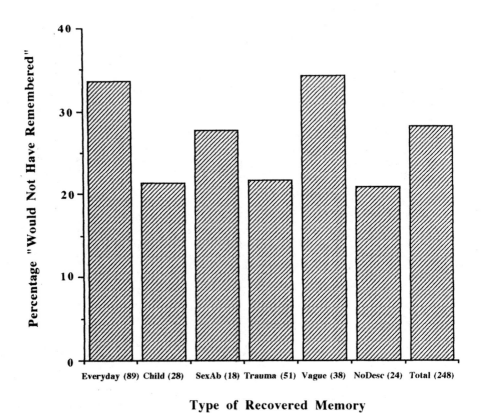

Type of Recovered Memory

Figure 7. Percentage who, if asked, would not have remembered recovered event.

ated by the very small sample size for reports of recovered sexual abuse memories by males.

3.3. Descriptions of Recovered Memory Experiences

We also asked respondents to describe the circumstances in which the memory was recovered or the cues that seemed to provide access to the information they believed they had forgotten. Not surprisingly, a wide variety of bases for remembering were reported, however all respondents included some sort of cuing or experience of having been reminded by seeing a similar event, talking about a similar experience, or being explicitly reminded by someone of the experience. A very small percentage (4.9%) were thought to be entirely spontaneous or unrelated to other environmental events, and only 19.7% were judged to have resulted from efforts to remember or as a product of reminiscing about related topics and events. Another 10.5% reported that something within a dream or flashback reminded them of the event. None of the descriptions suggested sustained efforts to remember as might be found in some therapeutic memory recovery procedures described in the clinical literature and, in fact, only 3 of the 248 recoveries were reported to have taken place in conjunction with some form of therapy. Responses to only one option appeared to differentiate males and females: males were somewhat more likely to report the

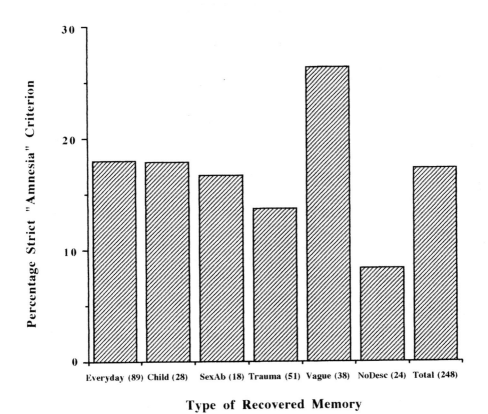

Type of Recovered Memory

Figure 8. Strict amnesia criterion: "forgot" and, if asked, would not have remembered".

role of a visual stimulus as an event that seemed to cue the memory [X^2 (1, N =245) = 2.94, p < .10].

3.4. Implications

In summary, we can say that our adult participants easily recalled an incident that conformed to the "Was there ever a period during which you remembered less about an event than you do now?" kind of question used in earlier research. A substantial proportion of these recovered memories involved what seemed to us to be minor everyday events and general knowledge or personal history facts. But an equally large subset related to negative, and often very traumatic, experiences. As a result, we can conclude that "recovery" experiences are commonplace and seem to have been rather easily recalled by the majority of the survey respondents. However, the data undermine the idea that there is something unique about the memories of CSA in regard to the assessment of periods of time in which an event was remembered less well than it was at the time of our survey.

Second, when asked to indicate whether they had truly forgotten, the majority thought they had not; rather, they stated they simply had not thought about the event. When pressed further as to whether they would have recalled the experience, if asked, the percentage meeting the strict criterion for unavailability was reduced further and revealed few differences between types of experiences. In short, the evidence that these recovered memories followed a period of complete unavailability is reduced from the average of 38% reported by the six studies cited earlier to approximately 18% of the total respondents. As to whether there is evidence that sexually traumatic events are more likely to result in reports of having actually forgotten than other types of life experiences, the answer from these data is that the evidence is minimal or nonexistent. Further, rather than female rates of memory loss of sexual trauma being particularly high, males appear to be particularly low.

Because the survey responses well match, even by a criterion more strict than that used for CSA experiences in previous published research, we may entertain the possibility that our respondents actually suffered from either complete or "partial" amnesia in regard to the wide variety of life events they reported as forgotten . It is obvious that characterizing these everyday memory losses as amnesias emphasizes the inappropriateness of doing so to describe normal memory losses. In my judgment, use of the term "complete amnesia" has often been inappropriate in the earlier studies because the respondents have not demonstrated an absence of recollection in the face of a battery of relevant questions and cues for an event known to have occurred to them. Nor have I seen any normative basis for such classification as might be used to reflect abnormal memory functioning assessed by other psychometric instruments.

In my judgment as well, the use of term partial amnesia" would be equally inappropriate for our data. In many published reports the term "partial amnesia" has been used freely (although Elliott and Briere [1995] caution that its use has no etiologic implications) in regard to descriptions of events that seem no different from those our subjects described and which followed answers to questions that were no different than the ones we posed. If everyday events suffer from memory losses to the same extent as events involving CSA, describing such everyday losses as examples of "partial amnesia" would be odd to say the least. I think many believe it appropriate to apply a medical model to trauma and thereby pathologize memory losses when they relate to trauma (see, for example, Yehuda this volume). However, given the verbal reports of our respondents, the present data would similarly allow the pathologizing of reports of incomplete memory for a wide variety of nontraumatic and mundane events. Could we not then say that we are all partially amnesic for virtually everything we have ever experienced? Would it not be wiser to say that CSA experiences, like most events, are usually "partially remembered"?

I do not dispute the possibility that there may well be, at levels beyond these simple answers to our simple questions, underlying differences that reflect greater losses or greater difficulty in accessing memories for traumatic than mundane events. But, I raise these questions to have us reflect on the need to operationalize what it is that we are calling amnesia, partial or otherwise. When a client is told that he or she has partial amnesia my guess is that the memory problem, if indeed there is one, has been given a new meaning and has been pathologized. The report by Elliott and Briere (1995) to the effect that their survey respondents volunteered use of the term "amnesia" to describe their experiences gives me further pause but greater confidence in arguing that the popular use of these terms themselves has gotten out of control.

4. GENERAL DISCUSSION AND CONCLUSIONS

It bears repeating that I do not argue on the basis of these data that there are no qualitative differences between the memories of traumatic and everyday events or between memories of CSA and other types of trauma. However, given the similarities in our respondents' responses to the same kinds of questions that have been used by other researchers, I believe the task now falls to those making the claims about the special status of trauma memories to demonstrate the qualitative and quantitative differences that separate these kinds of events. As I said earlier, I think these data begin to form a backdrop against which we may evaluate the kinds of absolute numbers reported in the literature. Some interesting work in this direction has recently been completed by van der Kolk and Fisler (1995), as well as by Carlson (this volume).

As an experimental psychologist it is unusual for me to respond to claims about the absolute percentages of mental phenomena, usually reported on through verbal responses, as if the percentages themselves reflect some eternal verity. Instead, I assume the frequency of these kinds of reports may be pushed up or down depending upon a host of personal and contextual variables, not the least of which are the kinds of questions used to elicit the responses. In fact, it is these kinds of manipulations that experimental psychologists use to assess the influence of variables upon verbal reports of inherently subjective phenomena. In that spirit the only claim I would make is that by asking questions similar to those used in some earlier research, the absolute values I reported here are quite similar to those of the earlier reports. I think it obvious that if a claim is made about a specific percentage of people who experienced partial or complete amnesia for an event then that percentage must be compared to some control or baseline value. Otherwise, the reported value is devoid of meaning. It should also be apparent that the baselines for both the perceived presence of gaps in autobiographical memory and for recovered memory experiences are not zero. Unfortunately, an investment has been made by some writers in the specific magnitudes of the previously reported numbers because they can justify particular therapeutic regimens that may involve a client for several to many years. I trust it is obvious that the answer to a single question of the sort used in various research studies should never be the basis of a treatment programme of whatever type or duration (see also Briere, this volume and Courtois, this volume).

Secondly, the more important finding from this exploratory research is that when you hold context, purpose, and question type constant and then assess subjective memory quality across different life event categories, there is little to no evidence that the respondents reported different subjective experiences in regard to their memories for traumatic events, including CSA, than they had for a wide variety of other autobiographical events. And, there is little to no evidence that gender differences exist in these kinds of reports, either in their quantity nor their quality.

Where to go next? If we are of the opinion that pursuing the memory issues make sense then we shall have to devote a lot of energy to a rather tedious task begun by others. Some norms do exist for various psychometric instruments within standard and neuropsychological assessments that are intended to reflect short-term or remote memory functioning often with a concern to the detection of anterograde amnesia as part of the classically studied amnesic syndrome. But these standardized questions are either neutral with respect to a person's life experiences or arise from public, semantic memory, information that we can be reasonably sure most people of a particular age had been exposed to and learned. However, developing norms for personal autobiographical memory is much more difficult because we have little, often no, access to the correct answers. If the client says she does not remember the name of her fourth grade teacher that lack of response might have some meaning in the context of her age cohort all of whom do report a teacher's name. But, generally, when an answer is given, we would have great difficulty assessing its accuracy. Autobiographical memory assessments have, however, been developed by Mike Kopelman and his colleagues (including Alan Baddeley and Barbara Wilson at Cambridge). For these kinds of personal events standardized scores are provided for what the normal person reports as memories from childhood and, eventually, I assume the goal would be to provide such norms for different age groups, presently unavailable.

ACKNOWLEDGMENTS

The research reported herein was supported by the National Sciences and Engineering Research Council and the Alberta Law Foundation.

REFERENCES

Alexander, P. C. (1993). The differential effects of abuse and attachment in the prediction of long-term effects of sexual abuse. *Journal of Interpersonal Violence, 8,* 346–362.

American Psychiatric association (1994). *Diagnostic and statistical manual of mental disorders.* (4th Ed). Washington, D.C.

Anderson, G., Yasenik, L., & Ross, C. A. (1993). Dissociative experiences and disorders among women who identify themselves as sexual abuse survivors. *Child Abuse & Neglect, 17,* 677–686.

Beitchman, J. H., Zucker, K. J., Hood, J. E., daCosta, G. A. & Cassavia, E. (1992). A review of the long-term effects of child sexual abuse. *Child Abuse & Neglect, 16,* 101–118.

Blume, E. S. (1990). *Secret survivors: Uncovering incest and its aftereffects in women.* New York: Ballantine.

Briere, J. & Conte, J. (1993). Self-reported amnesia for abuse in adults molested as children. *Journal of Traumatic Stress, 6,* 21–31.

Brown, D.(1995). Pseudomemories, the standard of science and the standard of care in trauma treatment. *American Journal of Clinical Hypnosis, 37,* 3–29.

Christianson, S.-A. (1992). Emotional stress and eyewitness memory: A critical review. *Psychological Bulletin, 112,* 284–309.

Cole, P. M., & Putnam, F. W. (1992). Effects of incest on self and social functioning: A developmental psychopathology perspective. *Journal of Consulting and Clinical Psychology, 60,* 174–184.

Courtois, C. A. (1995). Scientist-practitioners and the delayed-memory controversy: Scientific standards and the need for collaboration. *The Counseling Psychologist, 23,* 294–299.

Dawes, R. M. (1994). *The house of cards.* Toronto: Maxwell Macmillan Canada.

Elliott, D., & Briere, J. (1995). Posttraumatic stress associated with delayed recall of sexual abuse: A general population study. *Journal of Traumatic Stress, 8,* 629–647.

Feldman-Summers, S., & Pope, K. S. (1994). The experience of "forgetting" childhood abuse: A national survey of psychologists. *Journal of Consulting and Clinical Psychology, 62,* 636–639.

Finkelhor, D. (1994). Current information on the scope and nature of child sexual abuse. *The Future of Children, 4,* 31–53.

Fivush, R., & Hammond, N. R. (1990). Autobiographical memory across the preschool years: Toward reconceptualizing childhood amnesia. In R. Fivush & J. A. Hudson (Eds.), *Knowing and remembering in young children* (pp.223–248). New York: Cambridge University Press.

Frederickson, R. (1992). *Repressed memories: A journey to recovery from sexual abuse.* New York: Simon & Schuster.

Garry, M., Loftus, E. F., & Brown, S. W. (1994). Memory: A river runs through it. *Consciousness and Cognition, 3,* 438–451.

Gold, S. N., Hughes, D., & Hohnecker, L. (1994). Degrees of repression of sexual abuse memories. *American Psychologist, 49,* 441–442.

Kopelman, M. D., Wilson, B. A., & Baddeley, A. D. (1989). The autobiographical memory interview: A new assessment of autobiographical and personal semantic memory in amnesic patients. *Journal of Clinical and Experimental Neuropsychology, 11,* 724–774.

Loftus, E. F., Garry, M., & Feldman, J. (1994). Forgetting sexual trauma: What does it mean when 38% forget? *Journal of Consulting and Clinical Psychology, 62,* 1177–1181.

Loftus, E. F., & Loftus, G. R. (1980). On the permanence of stored information in the human brain. *American Psychologist, 35,* 409–420.

Loftus, E. F., Polonsky, S., & Fullilove, M. (1994). Memories of childhood sexual abuse: Remembering and repressing. *Psychology of Women Quarterly, 18,* 67–84.

Moeller, T. P., Bachmann, G. A., & Moeller, J. R. (1993). The combined effects of physical, sexual, and emotional abuse during childhood: Long-term health consequences for women. *Child Abuse & Neglect, 17,* 623–646.

Ofshe, R. J., & Singer. M. T. (1994). Recovered-memory therapy and robust repression: Influence and pseudomemories. *The International Journal of Clinical and Experimental Hypnosis, XLII,* 391–410.

Polusny, M. A., & Follette. V. M. (1996). Remembering childhood sexual abuse: A national survey of psychologists' clinical practices, beliefs, and personal experiences. *Professional Psychology: Research and Practice, 27,* 41–52.

Poole, D. A., Lindsay, D. S., Memon, A., & Bull, R. (1994). Psychotherapy and the recovery of memories of childhood sexual abuse: U.S. and British practitioners' beliefs, practices, and experiences. *Journal of Consulting and Clinical Psychology, 63,* 426–437.

Ratican, K. L. (1992). Sexual abuse survivors: Identifying symptoms and special treatment considerations. *Journal of Counseling and Development, 71,* 33–38.

Read, J. D., & Lindsay, D. S. (1994). Moving toward a middle ground on the "false memory debate": Reply to commentaries on Lindsay and Read. *Applied Cognitive Psychology, 8,* 407–435.

Read, J. D., Yuille, J. C., & Tollestrup, P. (1992). Recollections of a robbery: Effects of arousal and alcohol upon recall and person identification. *Law and Human Behavior, 16,* 425–446.

Ross, C. A. (1989). *Multiple personality disorder: Diagnosis, clinical features, and treatment.* New York: John Wiley & Sons.

Ross, C. A., Miller, S. D., Bjornson, L., Reagor, P., Fraser, G., & Anderson, G. (1991). Abuse histories in 102 cases of multiple personality disorder. *Canadian Journal of Psychiatry, 36,* 97–101.

Russell, D. (1986).*The secret trauma: Incest in the lives of girls and women.* New York: Basic Books.

Sheiman, J. A. (1993). "I've always wondered if something happened to me": Assessment of child sexual abuse survivors with amnesia. *Journal of Child Sexual Abuse, 2,* 13–21.

Smith, S. (1991). *Survey of 38 therapists specializing in sexual abuse recovery.* Unpublished Master's Thesis, Ottawa University, Phoenix, AZ.

van der Kolk, B., & Fisler, R. (1995). Dissociation and the fragmentary nature of traumatic memories: Overview and exploratory study. *Journal of Traumatic Stress, 8,* 505–525.

Walker, L. E. (1994). *Abused women and survivor therapy.* Washington, D.C.: American Psychological Association.

Williams, L. M. (1994a) Recall of childhood trauma: A prospective study of women's memories of child sexual abuse. *Journal of Consulting and Clinical Psychology, 62,* 1167–1172.

Williams, L. M. (1994b). What does it mean to forget child sexual abuse? A reply to Loftus, Garry, and Feldman (1994). *Journal of Consulting and Clinical Psychology, 62,* 1182–1186.

Williams, L. M. (1995). Recovered memories of abuse in women with documented child sexual victimization histories. *Journal of Traumatic Stress, 8,* 649–673.

Winkielman, P., Belli, R. F., Schwarz, N., & Read, J. D. (in press). Judging childhood memory as worse despite recalling more events: The role of ease of retrieval in memory judgments.

COMMENTARY ON MEMORY ISSUES IN THE DIAGNOSIS OF UNREPORTED TRAUMA

Cathy Spatz Widom, the University of Albany (SUNY), USA

1. DEMAND CHARACTERISTICS AND MEMORY BELIEFS

Don Read provided an interesting discussion of memory issues in the diagnosis of unreported trauma. Read argued that we need to better understand how we can test the claims about memory inherent in the beliefs about trauma and forgetting. He challenged three claims: (1) that traumatic events like childhood sexual abuse generate significant gaps in the continuity of autobiographical memory; (2) that traumatic events can produce amnesia for unpleasant events and that the "recovery" of memory should be taken as evidence of the amnestic powers of trauma; and (3) that the clinical assessment of the integrity of a client's autobiographical memory is reliable and not subject to demand characteristics inherent in the situation for both the client and therapist.

Read provided an example in his presentation in which three students out of 160 answered the question he posed accurately, at least according to his thinking. Read interprets this as an indication that the "trauma-forgetting" hypothesis has influenced popular culture. He argues that if a single comment about a perception of poor childhood memory encourages the hypothesis of childhood sexual abuse in 50% of 18-year olds, it would not be surprising that other beliefs about memory difficulties might also be used to further consider childhood sexual abuse as the basis for someone's difficulties.

However, I do not believe that these results are surprising, given the long history of research in which students meet the expectations of researchers or conform to demand characteristics of the situation (cf. Solomon Asch conformity studies and the Zimbardo prison experiments). In the field of personality, research conducted during the early 1970s demonstrated the power of demand characteristics on students in psychology experiments. In one particular study, students were asked to complete the MMPI as part of the study and then they were given feedback about their personality. After receiving the feedback, the students were asked to evaluate how well they thought the feedback described them. Despite the fact that all the students received the same information (with the order of statements randomised), and not individualised feedback at all, they reported that the feedback was accurate and captured their personalities. At the time, the research raised some ethical issues about deception, but the findings remain instructive.

Ultimately, Read is concerned with the role that beliefs about memory play in the diagnosis of unreported trauma; that is, the psychological description or diagnosis of adults who are unaware of past trauma in their lives. The argument is that gaps in autobiographical memory are supportive of an undisclosed and possibly unknown history of childhood sexual abuse. On the other hand, Read acknowledges that these claims about perceived memory gaps are less common than in the past and that distinguished clinicians like

Christine Courtois have explicitly stated that such gaps should not be used as indicators of childhood sexual abuse.

I also think it is relevant to factor in the influence of contemporary popular culture on what subjects in psychology experiments or "common people" believe. I worry about the effects of stories in the press and other media about these cases, because I am concerned that it will become very difficult to separate "real" consequences of childhood victimisation from "expected" consequences. People who find themselves in trouble may redefine their childhood histories to conform to their current situation. For example, in my own work, we find much stronger relationships between self-reported problem behaviors (depression, alcohol, suicide attempts, violence) and retrospective self-reported childhood victimisation experiences than with official reports. This may reflect that it is the way we define a stressful life event (such as childhood trauma) that has an impact on our behavior, not necessarily the event itself. Certainly, not all people who experience childhood traumatic events go on to manifest consequences in the same manner and there may be some individuals who seem relatively resilient. It is also possible that people who are willing to disclose mental health or other social problems may be more willing to disclose problematic childhood histories. More research is clearly needed on the accuracy of retrospective recall of earlier childhood experiences (see Widom, this volume).

2. ACCURACY OF MEMORY IN GENERAL

Another issue I would like to raise concerns the assumption that people in the studies described by Read are able and willing to describe their experiences and that people can be introspective and accurate. Read's work shows the fallibility of memory in general. While one might assume that virtually everyone would agree that memories of their first 1–2 years of life ought to be unusually limited, only about one-half of Read's (47%) sample reported at least one such period in their lives (this was a non-traumatised sample from the "normal" population). This means that the majority do not report even the first year of life to be without any memory. What does this mean? The presence of such gaps in non-clinical samples such as Read's reminds us that if childhood sexual abuse does produce autobiographic memory difficulties, its prevalence rate must exceed by a reasonable amount the baseline data reported here. One of the points Read makes is the need to interpret memory gaps in the context of a baseline level of such reports. He cites this kind of evidence of the prevalence of self-perceived gaps in autobiographical memory among members of a large public sample who were not selected for prior history of sexual trauma. This is an important reminder to the field.

I am not sure why we assume accuracy in memory, since there is a fair amount of literature elsewhere which indicates that memory is problematic and that there is a substantial amount of non-disclosure — intentional or unintentional. The reality is that there is a lot of slippage. For example, literature from the field of criminology indicates that asking people for information about their criminal behavior is not overwhelmingly accurate and levels of accuracy vary by groups of people. In some work we are currently engaged in, we are comparing the validity of official and self-reported criminal history information. We have found that the extent of accuracy ranges from a low of 63% (for females) to a high of 79% (for males) of people who self-report having been arrested among those with an official record of arrest. One might argue there is some ambiguity involved in an arrest, so using conviction data should eliminate this ambiguity. But, looking at the extent of self-reports about arrests among those with convictions, females still have the lowest levels of accuracy (60%) and males the highest (77%). And the absolute levels of accuracy are not that high. In many cases, this information is fairly recent and not from early childhood. If these are the levels of reporting events which are not necessarily traumatic and most likely did not occur in early childhood, then shouldn't these findings provide perspective on the reports that 16 - 59% of childhood sexual abuse survivors experienced a period of time in which they had reported having little or no recollection of the traumatic event?

An additional issue raised by these comparisons of official and self-reported information is the possibility of gender differences. Read did not find gender differences in reporting a memory gap. If anything, he found that males were more likely to report a gap in their memory than females. Read cautions that this is not a random sample and that survivors of childhood sexual abuse may have declined to volunteer for his study at greater rates than non-survivors. However, other research suggests that survivors may be more likely to volunteer for some types of research or surveys. Read reminds us that there were no comments or questions in the survey that addressed either sexual abuse or therapy. The focus of the survey was on what adults say about the integrity and coherence of their autobiographical memories.

3. DID THE RESPONDENTS REPORT FORGETTING AND RECOVERY OF LIFE EVENTS?

To get at the issue of "recovered memories", Read asked his respondents a question about whether they could recall a circumstance in which they had realized that they had remembered something they believed they had forgotten. Interestingly, Read found that 60% of his sample answered "yes" to that question and that males were more likely to respond affirmatively than females. One wonders whether this reflects a reluctance or sensitivity on the part of females to reveal or disclose this information. Read also found that some respondents reported they had forgotten a series of events in which they had been involved for periods ranging from one to nine years. He interprets this as support for the reports of victims who later remember years of sustained abuse. Read also reported no differences between males and females on either recurrent event experiences or other non-sexual traumatic categories. Males reported childhood sexual abuse at about one-quarter the rate of females, but when males reported abuse, they reported few amnestic periods. For sexual abuse trauma, 63% of the females versus only 14% of the males said they had truly forgotten. As Read points out, there may well be something different about the likelihood of males and females reporting sexually abusive events. It would be interesting to know whether this phenomenon is confined to a subset of people who forgot multiple events or most people who forgot only one event.

In the end, Read argues that "when you hold context, purpose, and question type constant and then assess subjective memory quality across different life event categories, there is little or no evidence that the respondents reported different subjective experiences in regard to their memories for traumatic events, including childhood sexual abuse, than they had for a variety of other autobiographical events". I would suggest that the exploratory empirical research which Read described may represent a very preliminary picture and that further research is needed to determine whether male and female victims of childhood traumatic experiences respond in qualitatively or quantitatively different ways.

4. WHERE SHOULD THE FIELD GO IN THE FUTURE?

I agree with Don Read that we need much more information about the normative characteristics of memory gaps before their presence may be taken as a diagnostic feature. What is normal forgetfulness? None of the surveys report gaps in childhood memory, although some clinicians say this is important in regard to their clients. We need to exert the same level of critical examination of studies with general population samples as we do with studies of other special groups of victims or clients. I would suggest that in the next incarnation of Read's survey, he should change the format so that it takes into account the extent to which the format influences the responses. I would also suggest the use of life events matrices to assist subjects to better remember events that happened in the distinct past.

Finally, I would agree with Read's conclusion that using gaps and voids in autobiographic memory as diagnostic indicators of unreported childhood sexual abuse is a risky venture and one most likely to produce false positives. However, I am not sure that I agree with Read's two final conclusions about the lack of meaning of complete or partial amnesia in some percentage of childhood sexual abuse victims and the influence of demand characteristics on clients and therapists in the therapy situation. I would agree that more and better research and knowledge is needed, but to my mind, Read's own research suggests that common people forget (or temporarily forget) important events in their lives. The research of others mentioned by Read (Briere and Conte, Feldman-Summers and Pope, Loftus, Polonsky, and Fullilove, Williams, Elliott and Briere) indicates that survivors of childhood sexual abuse report a time in which they had reduced or no recollection of the event. I would like to know what determines forgetting and recalling and the relationship of recall to current functioning.

QUESTIONS AND ANSWER SESSION

Hyman. I think in some respects you are asking the right question about what the base line is, but I'm concerned that the events you've asked about are not the right ones. I ask because you drew the conclusions in such a strong form that I wonder whether we should also draw the conclusion that sexual abuse and incidents of forgetting and later remembering aren't any different from your base line events. However, I'm not really clear as to what your events are because you've classified them in chunks of events and I think you might do better if you teased it apart, select your events based on trauma characteristics or lack of trauma characteristics.

Read. Let me provide a few additional examples. We originally completed a content analysis which resulted in 12 different categories of events which we then collapsed into the data for the six categories I showed you. Here are a few examples from three of the collapsed categories I used in my presentation. Some of these examples are quite striking.

"Frequently can't recall large series of experiences related to my 9 years of figure skating. I entirely forget which competitions (major or minor) I had won. I'm sometimes completely blanked as to when I was tested and what exactly happened." - 21 year-old female

"Having unusable (crippled) thumbs as a child. Forgot until in a medical setting dealing with splints and broken limbs, many years later as an adult." - 51 year-old female

Similarly from others, I was astonished to learn that one male recalled that he had forgotten that he had taken piano lessons for 3 years and he was only 18 years old. Another person had forgotten 9 years of violin. Perhaps the parents would have put those experiences in the traumatic category! One of the strong claims that's often made about "robust repression" is that multiple incidents of abuse that occur on a regular basis can be completely forgotten. The reason I show you these examples is that some of these people engaged in repetitive activities for many years and they, apparently, also forgot. As you can see, there were examples of recovered traumatic events that people did report as well.

> "I have forgotten about my mother getting my pets killed - all of them - when I was little. I've also forgotten sexual abuse, for years, until I went to therapy." - 42 year-old female

> "As a teenager I was with a group of 7 or 8 friends riding around in a pickup truck. The driver went around a corner too fast and the truck tipped over on its side. None of us were hurt except for the scrapes and bruises, but we were so scared that our parents would find out we had done something so dangerous and foolish (They didn't - to this day). In my late 20s an old friend from high school talked about it, and I realized that I had completely wiped the incident from my mind." - 47 year-old female

Many other events were the insignificant, general everyday minor kinds of events.

> "The one that jumped immediately to mind was being taken into a room by my hostess and being told that she was placing me in the same room that I'd had last time. I had totally forgotten that I had ever slept in her house. I then remembered that when I was leaving one city to start work in another, I had slept there my last night." - 62 year old female

But you must remember that I'm asking them to report a recollection of having recovered a memory and to do that within the next 30 minutes. My supposition is that their responses and these data likely underestimate the prevalence of this kind of experience. Many of you might say to yourselves that " I know I've had that experience", but if I asked you for the details of it you would likely have difficulty coming up with them. Similarly, some of our subjects said that "recovery" had happened to them frequently, but they couldn't give us a specific example. I do not doubt that there are large qualitative differences between a CSA survivor's recollections in a therapeutic setting and the accounts my respondents provided. However my point is that as I read the survey research, I ask what the basis is for the special claims made about losses of trauma memory. If I can get the same data from a normal group of people recalling everyday or normal life events and experiences then perhaps we should be concerned as to the kinds of questions being asked in those survey studies. That is, perhaps they're asking the wrong questions to get at the kinds of memories they wish to describe.

Hyman. Is this just an autobiographical example of the tip-of-the-tongue phenomena, the times when you cannot think of a name even though you know it and eventually you get it? Is this just the autobiographical correlate of a tip-of-the-tongue experience?

Read. I think probably for some of the insignificant, minor events, it probably is. For example, when they think "oh yes, I saw somebody on TV then I remembered her name, but I didn't think I could have remembered her name earlier", your claim probably is true. But for many of these traumatic events and the recurrent sequential events, I don't think that tip-of-the-tongue adequately characterises these experiences. I think that what they're saying is that they now believe that they were unaware of that information for a substantial period of time, it wasn't just on the tip-of-the-tongue, rather they think the information actually was unavailable. Who knows whether they're correct? We would need to cue people by telling them that their parents said that they had taken violin lessons, and see whether they remember during the specific time they might have later thought they had forgotten. Clearly, the logistics are enormous, the logic so problematic, and the costs so high that none of us is going to take on such a task.

Harrington. Regarding the volunteer subjects that you've used in this survey. Volunteer subjects tend to be higher educated, have higher socio-economic status, higher IQ, are more approval motivated, more sociable, more arousal seeking, more unconventional, and more likely to be female. Some of these characteristics would indicate higher functioning to the degree that volunteer subjects are higher functioning. If there is a special mechanism for traumatic forgetting, you may underestimate the amount of traumatic forgetting in your sample because your volunteers may be less likely to show it. Another way that you can have an artifact is that volunteer subjects try to guess and then act in a way to satisfy the experimental hypothesis. If that is the case, if they guess what your experimental hypothesis is then you can have an overestimate for the amount of gaps for traumatic memory.

Read. I don't disagree with what you say about volunteer subjects and I don't dispute that perhaps our sample respondents are higher functioning although one might wonder about the 200 people who hang out in the mall and are willing to do a survey for five dollars when it takes a half an hour. I don't know if they have a higher socio-economic status. Certainly volunteers may present these problems but it's also the case that the other survey studies I mentioned used volunteers. I also don't dispute the fact that it's possible that very low functioning people probably don't fill out questionnaires. As for whether these volunteers speculated about experimental hypotheses and then tried to serve as samaritans in service of my presumed hypotheses, I guess I would be highly skeptical given the nature of the questionnaire. It had a broad shotgun kind of approach and if people did generate hypotheses, my guess is that they would not likely show much similarity to each other and thus may contribute noise or error variance only.

Loftus. You found that some percentage of your mall sample will say they had an event they forgot, but later remembered and they will say they really mean they forgot; that is, for them they just didn't think about it. Further, they often say that if they were asked about it they would not have remembered it. What do they mean exactly?

Read. I think they believe they really did not have access to the information for some period of time. I also asked them for their reasons as to why they held that belief. Of those who said they "forgot", 51.8% said they had absolutely no memory for the experience during some period of time. Another 34% reported that they had attempted to remember the experiences but had been unable to do so. Those are fairly strong statements. Only 1% characterised their losses as amnesia for the events over some period of time. Another 18.3% said they had simply not thought about it. They can check more than one option for these questions: 57% said the reason they had not thought about it was because there had been no occasion to think about the events, or it was the type of experience one couldn't forget, so it's the kind of thing you would remember. Many people said it was not important to remember it. Some people made a deduction and said, "well, because I can now remember it, it must be the case that I didn't forget it and therefore I simply didn't think about it, or I chose not to think about it, or there was nothing available to remind me." But 40% said the reason they selected "the not thought about" option was because they believe they would have remembered had they been asked.

I think the terms and the questions that we use in this kind of metamemory research (and all of the people engaged in this kind of research have said this from time to time) are very difficult for people to understand. A a result, their answers may seem quite inconsistent. To strengthen the methodology, I doubled up on the criteria for classifying something as having been forgotten by requiring an affirmative response to the forget-did not think about question and a negative response to the "if you had been asked" question. I believe this approach employs a more rigorous definition of forgetting than has been used to answer essentially the same questions in survey studies over the last four of five years.

Williams. Someone just suggested to me that I should point out that those are all activities in which some coach may have molested someone ! That wasn't my idea ! When I first heard you talking about going to the shopping mall to get information, I thought you were going to try to find those people who were lost there. I thought it was very interesting question. What does the general public think about this issue? I'm really of two minds: sometimes I think all those popular psychology books have had an impact on the public but at other times I go to speak to a psychology class who I think will know what I'm talking about and they don't have a clue about false memory. As a sociologist maybe I should do this study, but do we have good data on what the general public's impressions are on this phenomenon, so we might have a better idea what the influence is on individuals in therapy? Maybe there's some data on this.

Read. Actually there are. The earliest study I remember was by Loftus and Loftus in the 1980 *American Psychologist*, which looked at the general question of the permanence of memory. I know that Garry, Loftus & Brown (1994) completed another survey of beliefs about memory. Also Sheila Seelau just finished up her PhD at Iowa State, and her dissertation is about memory beliefs. But it's a valuable point that we have to get some assessment of what the level of public belief is on some of these concepts. Beth Loftus, do you want to say anything about that specific study?

Loftus. I think in general some studies you mentioned and others, do show widespread misconceptions about the nature of memory. Beliefs, for example, that you can use hypnosis to recover things as early as back to birth and sometimes even pre-natal memories. For each question there's a different percentage of people who hold that belief.

Read. As part of this questionnaire we did have a belief section, which I factor analysed and put together as a "beliefs in repression" score. I then correlated those scores with the presence or absence of "recovered memory" experiences from my sample. The correlations were very low, in the range of .15, although statistically significant within a sample of 412 people. One outcome was that a person who held a strong belief in repressed memory phenomena was also more likely to report a memory recovery experience. The highest correlation we obtained was between the reporting of a memory experience and the DES (Dissociative Experiences Scale). The correlation was positive but low, about .2; that is to say, people who report those kinds of dissociative experiences were more inclined to say they also had a memory recovery experience. I also collected DES score on a sample of people under age 18 and the results were absolutely astonishing.

I don't know if they were pulling my leg or not, but teenagers' scores were very high on the DES. What they think is a normal day in their mental life is very striking. I've since learned that the administration of the DES to adolescents poses special problems and that my results are not unusual (E. Carlson, personal communication, June 1996).

Cameron. I think it is very important for us to work across the spectrum of the differences in the disciplines, and I'm happy to see the idea of looking at normal forgetting. However, I think we have to be very careful of generalising over the gap into the clinical situation. Clinicians have not been asking about gaps until recently. People don't ordinarily admit to gaps in memory because they don't think it's important. I had women in my sample who were amnesic earlier and then who were not amnesic. Among the amnesic, as I still think we need to call it, memory losses ranged from dropping out minutes of experience to dropping out a decade or more. For example, a child who was molested by her father remembered many outings but not the moments that were sexual. On the other hand, there was a woman who at age 14 thought her cousin was lying because he reminded her of something they had done the year before in their holiday. To her not having a memory was very normal for that whole length of time, for others it could be five years, and usually could be pinpointed to the time of trauma. When you remember something you forgot, usually it's "gee I just remembered" or "oh my gosh I remember when I was so embarrassed" but with the people who are remembering trauma, not just people who have been sexually abused, but people who have been traumatised in the holocaust, or battles, or seeing a murder or suicide of a parent, these people, when they remember they don't say, "oh gee isn't that interesting?" Many of these women remembered outside of therapy and before they ever went to therapy. You will find they were actively suicidal for weeks after they started remembering, others say they went out and got drunk and weren't sober for a month, or that they cried for two weeks after remembering. We have to be careful about generalising from a normal population who when asked will come up with some gaps that they've never given much thought to. Those differences are really enormous and need to be looked at too.

Read. Let me make clear that you have to make a separation of the kinds of reports we are talking about. I am definitely not saying or suggesting that the reports of the subjects in my studies can be likened to the recollections of CSA survivors. What I'm saying is that the data which are in the literature for CSA survivors upon which claims about memory loss have been based are exactly the same questions I asked of a normal population. So, on the basis of those same questions we obtained response rates at least as high as those reported in the CSA survey work and these suggest to me that the baseline for the "recovery" of life events is not zero.

My point is the claim that 59%, or 16%, or 38% of people forget or are partially amnesic for childhood sexual abuse experiences doesn't mean anything unless we know what the base line is. I am not saying my baseline is necessarily the correct one. It's actually very unusual for an experimental psychologist to even be concerned about absolute percentages. Like most experimentalists, I manipulate variables to assess the impact of those variables, and I look at magnitudes of change. The absolute percentage is usually irrelevant. However, I would assume that the kinds of verbal report we collect in all of these survey studies and in all the clinical interviews can be pushed around by a host of variables such as demand characteristics, question formats, contextual information, as well as the motivations of the questioner and respondent. The absolute percentage of memories recovered from traumatic events is presently not meaningful for me, but if you're going to make strong claims about a specific percentage, you need to know what the baseline is and it certainly isn't zero.

REFERENCES

Garry, M., Loftus, E. F., & Brown, S. W. (1994). Memory: A river runs through it. *Consciousness and Cognition, 3,* 438–451.
Loftus, E. F., & Loftus, G. R. (1980). On the permanence of stored information in the human brain. *American Psychologist, 35,* 409–420.

5

THE LOGICAL STATUS OF CASE HISTORIES

Willem A. Wagenaar

Leiden University
P.O. Box 9555, (Wasenaarseweg 52)
2300 RB Leiden
The Netherlands

1. INTRODUCTION

Much of the discussion on the ontology of forgotten and recovered memories seems to rest upon the interpretation of case histories. I will argue that the logical status of case histories is often poorly understood. As a consequence case histories have the effect of strengthening biases instead of testing theories. I suspect that this problem is introduced through the intertwining of psychology and legal practice. But the difference between science and justice is obvious: while juries and courts of judges use psychological theory to decide about a single case, scientists use single case histories to decide about general theories. If a case history does not allow generalization, it is irrelevant to us, no matter how relevant the trial might have been to those who were involved.

2. KLOK VS. KLOK

Evelyn Klok accused her brother David of sexual abuse that allegedly occurred 31 years ago, when Evelyn was four years of age, and David twelve. The abuse took place when Evelyn was in her bed and the rest of the family had gone to church. David jumped on her, and raped her both vaginally and anally. He hit her on her head, squeezed her arms, pressed the arteries in her neck until she almost fainted, and used the bed rail to immobilize her. Until recently Evelyn had not been aware of these facts.

At the age of 19 Evelyn had ended the relationship with a boy friend, because she could not bear to be touched by him. She became interested in her own past and looked at pictures in her photo album. She discovered a photo of herself at the age of four, and realised that she was looking at a very unhappy girl. She decided to discover why that girl had been so unhappy.

In 1988, at the age of 28, Evelyn consulted the psychiatrist Dr. Westland. In her own story it is suggested that the consultation was related to the earlier problem with her boy friend, but there is no explanation for the nine–year interval. She told Dr. Westland that

Recollections of Trauma, edited by Read and Lindsay
Plenum Press, New York, 1997

David had attempted to abuse her when she was seven or eight. David had not undressed her or himself, but he had pressed himself against her, and he had touched her under her clothes. She remembered that David had an erection and an ejaculation. There was no mention of rape or any type of violence. She had never forgotten this event, but she had made the connection with her current problems only recently. Encouraged by Dr. Westland she wrote a letter to David, who confirmed in his written reply everything she remembered. Subsequently Evelyn arranged a family meeting, in which the whole affair was openly discussed. This seemed to end the case. But, because Evelyn refused to take the prescriptions that Dr. Westland had given her, she decided seven years later to consult another psychiatrist, Dr. Subardjo. There is no explanation for the long delay between the family meeting and Evelyn's first visit to Dr. Subardjo, and we do not know what happened in between.

Dr. Subardjo was a psychiatrist of 72. She suspected that Evelyn had more problems than the relatively mild abuse at the age of seven or eight. In order to uncover Evelyn's hidden memories she used a rather surprising combination of Jungian dream analysis, Rational Emotive Therapy, and Flooding. Evelyn had new sexual contacts in this period, but was unable to establish a lasting relationship. Dr. Subardjo gave her a "self-hypnosis" tape, with which she could put herself into a trance. Supposedly this would help Evelyn to recover memories of her early youth. In this way she started to remember how she was raped by David at the age of four. Dr. Subardjo explained in court that these memories had first appeared as dreams and flashbacks. Her first impression was that these scenes were the products of Evelyn's fantasy. Later Dr. Subardjo became convinced that the images were real memories, but she did not mention any particular grounds for her conviction.

In a letter to her mother Evelyn described how the memories had come back. In the trance-like state, elicited with the help of the self-hypnosis tape, the past was shown to her as in a film. It took many weeks to recover every detail of the film. Then a period started in which she "knew the facts, but did not really feel them." (...) "It takes months of inward struggle to put David at a distance, to find release from the internal memory pains. One must experience a strength, a strength from God, a primordial strength, a strength from the unconscious; at any rate a very pure strength. But the most important was that I wanted this myself, it was my choice." Evelyn went on to explain that she was entitled to her rage, that remembering sexual abuse would promote the healing process, that self-hypnosis was an important tool, which would allow her to go back to her early childhood.

Dr. Subardjo's treatment seemed to have improved Evelyn's condition. As Evelyn was convinced that gaining public recognition of the abuse would complete the healing process, she engaged a well-known lawyer, famous for her defense of women with recovered memories, and for her persistence in claiming damages. Because the statute of limitations in the Netherlands for sexual abuse is 12 years, criminal prosecution of David was not possible. Instead Evelyn decided to sue her brother for damages, up to a sum of Dfl. 50.000, which is an extraordinary sum in our country. The court ordered Evelyn to prove two issues:

a. That she was raped by David at the age of four;
b. That there is a causal relationship between this event and the damage that Evelyn allegedly had sustained.

The evidence for (a) was Evelyn's testimony, David's confession of the later events, and Dr. Subardjo's statement that Evelyn's memories were real. The evidence for (b) was only Dr. Subardjo's statement that Evelyn's present troubles were caused by the alleged abuse 31 years ago. Other evidence available from the file was that Evelyn's sister Irene had been treated for manic depressive disorder.

3. INTERPRETATION OF EVELYN'S CASE

What can be learned from the present case? Some may accept the story as a confirmation of the more general rule that memories to non-existing abuse are implanted by therapists, using dubious and highly suggestive techniques. Others may conclude that Evelyn's story demonstrates how sexual abuse leads to forgetting, followed by psychological suffering at a later age; and how therapeutic treatment helps to recover the lost memories, which subsequently leads to a relief of the trauma. Obviously the case is of no help at all if both types of lessons can be inferred from it.

Why do we have this problem? The vast difference between the two lessons seem to follow from prior assumptions that both sides are making tacitly, viz. that Evelyn was or was not abused. But how do we know this?

It is the court's task to decide, whether Evelyn was abused by David. The abuse is inferred from evidence, such as Evelyn's memories. Scientists who want to use the case to support a theory of where these memories come from, will do just the reverse: they will infer the nature of Evelyn's memories from the fact that she was or was not abused. Both processes of inferential reasoning require a starting point. The court's reasoning requires a prior opinion about the trustworthiness of recovered memories. Often this is established through the testimony of expert witnesses. The scientists' reasoning requires the prior establishment of the truth, which is often achieved through the decision of a court of law. The circularity of the combination of these two processes is obvious. Scientists may convince the court that Evelyn's recovered memories are real. The court convicts David. Then scientists use the case to strengthen their theory of recovered memories. The opposite may also happen: experts convince the court that Evelyn's memories are implanted; the court acquits David, and the scientists use the case as a demonstration of false memories. The selective use of similar case histories allows scientists to support any theory. The selective appreciation of scientists allows courts to reach any conclusion. The composite looks like a travesty of both law and science, but I am afraid this is not an exaggerated representation of the present situation.

What other basis can there be for courts to reach a conclusion about the allegation of sexual abuse, and for scientists to determine the nature of recovered memories? I will elucidate the dilemma by means of the heuristic of anchored narratives, proposed by Wagenaar, Van Koppen, and Crombag (1993).

4. ANCHORED NARRATIVES

Courts of law are confronted with problems that have no logical solutions, because they are underspecified. Underspecification of a problem means that there is not enough information for identifying one and only one answer as the correct solution. An example is: Which animal has wings but is not a bird? The answer is a bat, a flying dog, a pterodactylus, a butterfly, a bee, and many other animals. Without a further specification all these answers are equally good. A similar problem arises when we want to know who abused Evelyn: the answer is David, or his brother Herman, or Evelyn's father, or a large number of others. This diversity is not acceptable to a court of law; in order to convict anybody at all, other possible culprits must be excluded. An underspecified problem does not allow the logical exclusion of alternative answers, but it may be possible to establish probabilities of the various alternatives, so that it may be concluded that one of them is true beyond reasonable doubt. Every legal system in the world is based upon some form of probabilistic solution of underspecified problems.

How are the probabilities of various problem solutions determined? From a vast literature on probabilistic reasoning (cf. Kahneman, Slovic, & Tversky, 1982) we know that people handle probabilities with the use of heuristics that tend to ignore laws of probability, but still work quite well in most everyday situations. The heuristic of anchored narratives is just one example. It poses that judges try to construct a "good" narrative about what happened. A good narrative has a central theme and explains why all the characters acted as they did. But, since the narrative must be more than a novel, it needs to be anchored onto reality by means of evidence. The evidence is presented not only to prove that the story is good, but also that it is true.

The problem with evidence, however, is that it is again nothing but a narrative. The story that David abused Evelyn at the age of four may become more probable through David's written confession that four years later he performed some perverse acts with her. But the evidence is only a story told by Evelyn and David. If we want to improve the status of Evelyn and David's narrative, we should assume that people don't lie about such

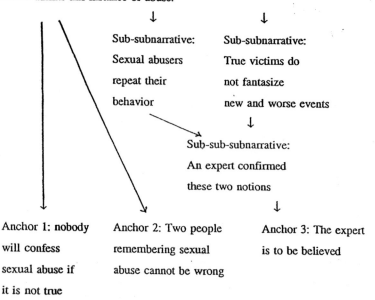

Narrative: Evelyn was raped by David when she was four, but she lost the memories to this event through repression.

↓

Subnarrative: Evelyn remembers being abused by David at the age of seven or eight. David admits this instance of abuse.

↓   ↓

Sub-subnarrative: Sub-subnarrative:
Sexual abusers   True victims do
repeat their   not fantasize
behavior   new and worse events

↓

Sub-sub-subnarrative:
An expert confirmed
these two notions

↓

Anchor 1: nobody   Anchor 2: Two people   Anchor 3: The expert
will confess   remembering sexual   is to be believed
sexual abuse if   abuse cannot be wrong
it is not true

Figure 1. Anchoring structure for part of Evelyn's narrative.

things, or that two people cannot make the same mistake, or something like this. Such an assumption is called a belief. As soon as the court believes that Evelyn and David cannot be both wrong about this, the evidence (Evelyn's and David's story) can be anchored to this belief. Once the story about the abuse at the age of seven or eight is anchored, it can be used to support the accusation of the earlier and more violent abuse. The anchoring chain runs from the allegation, through the story about the abuse at the age of seven or eight, to the anchor, which is the belief that Evelyn and David will not make the same mistake.

This anchoring chain is not very firm, as it contains an unfounded assumption: that the later abuse renders the occurrence of the earlier abuse more probable. What we need is some evidence that sexual abuse is repetitive, and that remembering one true instance of abuse may not lead to fantasizing about other instances. Clearly these two notions can easily be challenged, but an expert psychologist may be found who provides a scientific basis for both beliefs. If both parties accept the authority of the scientific literature, the two statements are anchored. The complex of anchoring chains now seems to prove that Evelyn was abused by David at an earlier age than admitted by David.

It is obvious that in this example the anchors are rather weak. Anchor 1: Some people admit to abuse they never committed. Anchor 2: Sometimes witnesses make the same mistakes. Anchor 3: Some scientific theories are wrong. It is possible to add more sub-sub-subnarratives, such as the absence of any reasons for David to make a false confession, or the generally recognized authority of cited textbooks. But one can always go on having doubts and ask more questions. The obvious result is that, as long as one continues challenging the anchors, no evidence will ever lead to proof of the initial narrative. It is impossible to establish a fact, if one refuses to believe anything at all. When a court reaches a decision, the narrative contained in the charge has apparently been anchored to some beliefs of the judges or members of the jury.

What are these beliefs? For jury members it is impossible to trace the beliefs that have served as anchors. For Dutch courts we are in a slightly better position, because they consist of professional judges who by law are obliged to give reasons for their decisions in written verdicts. Our analyses of these reasons (Wagenaar et al. 1993) show that judges have a tendency to be lenient on beliefs, rather than to require a high degree of certainty.

Probably in most cases the anchoring onto beliefs is not as explicit as demonstrated above. The acceptance of the authority of an expert or of a textbook may easily become an automatism, unless challenged by another expert. The reader may have had the same experience: David's admission of having abused Evelyn when she was 7 or 8 may at first have looked rather ominous for his case. Probably the logical analysis of the anchoring structure uncovered more problems than one had realised originally. It is quite possible that the first impression was based upon another and more risky anchor, namely the belief that who admits one instance of abuse is guilty of any other charge of sexual abuse. "Once a thief, always a thief".

The heuristic of anchored narratives has a number of basic properties. It is assumed that the narrative comes first, and that evidence is only used to anchor it. In legal trials this is not unreasonable, because the narrative is usually produced by the prosecutor or the claimant right at the beginning of the trial. It may get slightly modified during the trial, but it is not the court's task to change it into what really happened. The court only decides whether the alleged events are suffiently supported by evidence. For that reason it is usually only attempted to anchor the one narrative that was presented, not the many other possible narratives that can be imagined. The exception is when the accused or the defendant produces another narrative, claiming that it is equally well or even better supported by the evidence. In Evelyn's case the single story to be anchored is her narrative about the abuse and the recovery of her memories. The contending story is David's claim that Evelyn's memories were implanted through therapy. The heuristic of applying verification vs falsification (Wason & Johnson-Laird, 1972) may lead to the attempt to anchor only Evelyn's narrative, to the neglect of David's version. There are many examples in which the accused was convicted because the evidence was quite overwhelming, even though the falsifying evidence was equally impressive. Many trials involving recovered memories cited by Loftus & Ketcham (1994) are in this category.

Another property of the heuristic of anchored narratives is that the structure of anchoring chains need not be complete. In principle it is necessary to prove at least three things: that there was a criminal act (*actus reus*), that there was a criminal intention (*mens rea*), and that the accused is the culprit (identity). But there is no guarantee that evidence will be offered to support all three issues, or that it is attempted to anchor all the evidence. Imagine that the court in Evelyn's case accepts that she was abused when she was four, and that this was an intentional criminal act (which is not certain if the abuser was a child). The evidence is the testimony about recovered memories being produced by early trauma, anchored onto Dr. Subardjo's authority. But how do we know that David was the culprit, instead of David's brother Herman, or Evelyn's father? In order to accept this we need testimony, not only about the origin of recovered memories, but also about the accuracy of recovered memories. I have seen cases in which this step was simply neglected, so that *actus reus* and *mens rea* were anchored, but identity was not. The heuristic of anchored narratives is, like all heuristics, not a formal process, in which completeness is sought. Rather there seems to be a tendency to seek anchoring for statements that are brought forward, not for all statements that would be required logically in order to prove the charge.

A third property of the heuristic is that narratives may be anchored onto unsafe but implicit beliefs, that would be rejected when stated explicitly. Evelyn's story about abuse by David at the age of seven or eight can only support the allegation if it is anchored to the belief that one experience of sexual abuse does not lead to fantasizing about other instances. The simple reasoning is: Evelyn was right the first time, hence she must be right the second time. However, the fact that she remembered one event spontaneously, and that David never denied it, makes it quite different from the alleged event, which she remembered only with the help of Dr. Subardjo, and which was persistently denied by David. The truth of one instance cannot simply be generalized to the other. There seems to be a tendency to leave beliefs uncriticized unless they are explicitly challenged. Thus the shortest and simplest anchoring constructions are produced that are permitted by the evidence. Longer and more complex anchoring constructions are only produced, when a belief is challenged by one of the parties in the trial. The authority of Dr. Subardjo serves as an anchor, until the other side claims that she is no expert at all. This tendency is helpful, as it leads to fast and efficient problem solving, especially in those areas in which one has already developed some fixed beliefs. It is also risky.

5. CASE HISTORIES IN SCIENTIFIC ARGUMENTS

The theory of anchored narratives claims that judges and juries are forced to use the heuristic, because the problems posed to them are underspecified, and because there is no better way of dealing with underspecified problems. Anchored narratives do not lead to absolutely certain conclusions. But any desired degree of certainty under 1.0 can be attained by a further challenging of beliefs, and that is what good lawyers are supposed to do. Since there is no better way of deciding about single cases, we must accept the remaining small amount of uncertainty.

But are case histories, in which the truth has been established through anchoring, also good arguments in a scientific debate? And can theories be anchored in the same manner as narratives contained in a charge? In this section I discuss the former of the two problems.

Obviously the case of Evelyn is not a good argument to support a theory of forgetting and subsequent recovery. If we believe Evelyn, the case proves that repression and subsequent recovery exist. If, on the other hand, we believe David, the case proves that memories of fantasized abuse can be implanted through suggestive therapeutic methods. Whether the court convicts David or not, is irrelevant here, because it is likely that the conviction would rest upon Dr. Subardjo's expert testimony, that is, upon her belief in the very theory that we are testing.

Can the case be improved, so that the court's decision will be anchored more firmly; or, in other words, are there any cases certain enough for the foundation of a scientific theory? The history of psychology does not look very promising in this respect: theories of repression and dissociation were founded by Freud and Janet, entirely on case histories. The recent literature has effectively brought down such theories, precisely by an attack of the interpretation of the founding case histories. But let us return to the case of Evelyn.

What if David confessed? Would it not confirm Evelyn's allegation? A confession can serve as evidence if it is anchored to the belief that confessions are always true. Unfortunately it is suggested by quite a few cases that suspects can make a confession, even when their confessions are demonstrably false. A confession by David would not solve our problem, unless there is an anchor for the contention that his confession is true.

What if Evelyn's sister Irene also reported that she was abused by David? Obviously this evidence only contributes something new if it is obtained independently of Evelyn's accusation. But Evelyn's stories may have suggested to Irene, who is treated for manic depression, that David is also the cause of her problems. And, even in the case of independence, the evidence needs to be anchored onto the belief that two independent accusations must be true, instead of being caused by the same mechanism of suggestive therapy.

What if it appeared from a medical record that Evelyn had a venereal infection at the age of four? This clearly establishes some form of abuse, because the evidence may be anchored to the conviction that venereal infections cannot occur without sexual contact. Can we now, if Evelyn did not remember the abuse for 31 years, accept the case as a demonstration of forgetting and recovery? A closer look reveals that even the infection does not really help us. It may prove the abuse, but not the abuse by David, nor the claim that Evelyn could not remember it for 31 years, nor even the claim that Evelyn's present story is based on memories dating from 31 years ago. The infection, in combination with a confession by David, may convince a court of law that David abused Evelyn. But it cannot convince us about the existence of total forgetting and recovery. Establishing guilt is entirely different from the establishement of a psychological phenomenon, such as recovery. One may believe that Evelyn was abused by David, even without accepting Evelyn's testimony that she forgot all about it. But total forgetting and subsequent recovery involve a number of claims for which anchors are needed:

- Evelyn formed memories of the abuse;
- These memories became inaccessible for 31 years;
- Therapy helped to recover the original memories.

The evidence about the infection and David's confession do not link these three claims to anchors because it has nothing to do with the claims about Evelyn's memories.

The danger of not anchoring such claims is demonstrated in Williams's (1994) study of remembering a documented instance sexual abuse (index event) after 17 years. To determine whether the event was remembered, the responses of 129 women to an interview about their sexual experiences were examined. Analyses of these responses indicated to Williams that about 38% of the women were judged not to have reported the index event in their recollections. Williams's interpretation in terms of 38% forgetting should be based upon clear answers to two problems already noted in Evelyn's case: were there any initial memories, and were they really inaccessible? The heuristic of anchored narratives allows us to answer the first question only by anchoring onto the belief that sexual abuse occurred in all the cases, and the belief that sexual abuse is always stored in memory. In this particular instance there can be some doubt whether subjects stored that information. Quite a few subjects were at the time below the age of three. For other subjects it is possible that no abuse occurred at all. What if these two categories add up to 38% of the subject group? If Williams' subjects claimed not to remember the abuse, how do we know that they really forgot? The alternative is simply that they remembered the abuse, but did not want to report them to the investigator. Williams' defense is that some subjects reported later instances of abuse, but not the earlier ones. That still does not exclude the possibility that others refused to report their memories. In a study that was somewhat similar to Williams' investigation, Femina, Yeager, & Lewis (1990) reported that many subjects who initially claimed to have forgotten abuse experiences, later confessed that they had always remembered, but had preferred not to talk about them.

Williams' study is in fact based upon a large collection of case studies. In each single case of the claimed 38% it must be checked whether the abuse took place, whether the victim formed memories, and whether the victim really did not remember. It is obvious that none of the cases can provide firm anchors for these contentions. A collection of more than a hundred cases does not cause some averaging out. On the contrary, the problems add up and could have led to the often cited 38%.

Similar collections of case studies have been presented at this symposium by Cathy Widom, Linda Williams, Jonathan Schooler, and Bernice Andrews (all this volume). They suffer from the same weakness that the critical themes are not safely anchored, so that the collections only represent the population of cases in which memory loss and recovery is claimed, not of cases in which it occurred.

It should be noted that the two claims of forgetting and recovery require different types of anchors. Even if the initial formation of a memory and the subsequent forgetting are safely anchored, it still needs to be proven that the recovered story is based on memories, not on suggestion. This is important, as the victim's memories will be used as legal evidence. Let us take Evelyn's case as an example again. Assume that she had a venereal infection at the age of four. Now we still have only her word for it that David was the culprit. This is based upon her recovered memories, but why should we believe that these memories are accurate? Because childhood memories are not 100% reliable, why should Evelyn's childhood memories be an exception? It is easy to imagine that Evelyn's more recent memories of abuse by David at the age of seven or eight, have painted David as an abuser in the rather vague recollection of the earlier event. Because there is no other proof of David's involvement, we are forced to anchor onto the belief that recovered memories are more accurate than ordinary childhood memories. To me that seems an unsafe anchor. As a further illustration it may be remembered that some of Williams' (1994) subjects remembered the abuse of 17 years ago, even though they were at the time no more than 2 years old. Is it not likely that these memories were based on stories that were told to them, rather than on the experiences themselves, and that those stories are not more accurate than the memories of the story tellers?

My conclusion thus far is that case histories cannot logically provide a proof of existence of forgetting and recovery of abuse memories. Every demonstration of forgetting and recovery involves a circularity: the principles that are supposedly demonstrated have to be assumed before the case can be interpreted.

6. TESTING THEORIES THROUGH THE ANCHORED NARRATIVES HEURISTIC

Can the anchored narratives heuristic, that seems to work quite well when a court of law decides about a single case, also be used to decide about the existence of forgetting and recovery in general? In what ways is evidence in a trial different from evidence supporting a scientific theory? Some theorists believe that both science and courts proceed through some form of Bayesian decision making. I have demonstrated elsewhere that this position is wrong. It may be true that science proceeds through Bayesian updating of opinions (which I doubt), but courtroom decisions are definitively different (cf. Wagenaar et al. 1993). Is it possible that they both proceed through the heuristics of anchored narratives?

The theory of recovered memories is a good example of the problem. The anchoring structure starts with the narrative (theory) that memories of childhood trauma can be totally forgotten and recovered many years later. The evidence for this consists of empirical data, that are anchored to some basic beliefs shared by all or most scientists. I have already concluded that case histories cannot be anchored to safe anchors. But imagine that we obtain other empirical data that are anchored to well-established facts and methodologies. Should the anchoring structure now lead to the acceptance of the theory? I think not.

An important property of anchored narratives is that it considers only one narrative. It does not look actively for alternatives, and it deals with challenges only by extension of the anchoring chains, not by the analysis of other narratives. For instance, the argument that false memories can be implanted (cf. American Psychiatric Association Board of Trustees, 1994) does not logically exclude the existence of forgetting and recovery, and is therefore no direct threat to the anchoring structure. The defense of memory recovery would state that some "bad apples" in the psychiatric community do not prove that all recovered memories are implanted. Even if one of the anchors was the belief that memories cannot be implanted, only an extension of the anchoring chain is needed, in order to reach the belief that some memories cannot be implanted, or that memories of a few people can be implanted but not the memories of many people, or that some extreme therapeutic techniques may lead to memory implantation but that other milder techniques may not have such an effect. And indeed all these arguments are found in the literature. The single structure that is considered by a court of law is usually the one that is proposed by the prosecutor. Not only because it is the one that was proposed first (cf. Pennington & Hastie, 1986; Schünemann & Bandilla, 1989) but also because that structure is legally most relevant. Usually the defense sees it as its task to undermine that structure, not to present another one. Likewise it is the court's task to judge the quality of the proposed structure, not to think of a better one. The data used to strengthen or weaken the proposed structure consist of the evidence contributed by both sides in the legal contest. The court is rarely in the position to produce decisive information on its own initiative.

Why is scientific argumentation different? Science does not usually confine itself to the anchoring structure of one theory only. It considers more alternatives, forms anchoring structures of these alternatives, and compares the quality of these structures. If there is any prior preference given to one of the theories above the others, it is on the basis of the philosophy of "Occam's razor": the simplest anchoring structure is to be preferred. The introduction of new abstract notions is rejected as long as a structure without these notions can be safely anchored. Data that help to strengthen or weaken the structures are not passively received, but actively sought through experimentation. Conditions are defined in which the theories yield opposite predictions. These conditions are then created by means of experimental manipulation, and the results are compared to the predictions. A theory is rejected when the experimental results demolish an essential anchoring chain, or complicate the structure such that the theory must be rejected because of "Occam's razor".

Thus the major properties that distinguish scientific decision making from decision making in the courtroom are: the comparison of multiple anchoring structures, the priority of the simplest structure, and the design of experiments. The case of recovery vs. implantation should be decided through the creation of experimental conditions in which the theories yield opposite predictions. The experimental outcomes will force at least one of the theories to define new and probably longer anchoring chains. In the end one of the theories will have to be dropped because of its lack of anchors, or because of its many unattractive secondary hypotheses. Case histories that lack a reliable anchoring structure cannot supply the type of information that is obtained through proper experimentation.

7. EXPERIMENTS ABOUT REPRESSION

I do not know of any experiments in which childhood trauma was experimentally created in order to study its recollection in later years. Such experiments would be ethically unacceptable, which means that theories are to be tested in other ways. The closest approximation of an experiment is a quasi-experiment, in which conditions are chosen on a post-hoc basis. For instance, if we want to study the effect of age of the victims, we can collect a number of cases and classify them according to age. But the disadvantage is that we cannot make an assessment of the truthfulness of these victims" narratives, because we do not know what really happened. Also we cannot be certain that differences among the age groups are caused by age, instead of some other confounding factor: different types of traffic accidents happen to children of four, as compared to youngsters of 16. These problems are inevitable. All studies on being the victim of a concentration camp regime, of war, of crime, of a traffic accident, etc. lack the control of what happened, and how subjects are divided over various groups. On top of that we cannot assume that these various types of trauma can be used as models of sexual abuse. The usage of real abuse cases only put us in a more difficult situation, because with these cases it is even less certain what really happened.

With these forewarnings in mind I want to discuss the use of sexual abuse case histories as data in quasi-experimental designs. The difference with a single case study, or with studies involving many cases, like the one reported by Williams (1994), is that an experimental variable is introduced in order to test predictions of competing theories, and that Occam's razor can be used to define the preferences. What experimental variable creates a condition in which the theory of repression and its opponent produce different predictions?

The most obvious variable is the occurence or non-occurence of the abuse. Similar studies have been done to test the validity of the polygraph (Carroll, 1988). The cases are classified according to whether the subject was lying or speaking the truth. The test results are then compared between the two groups. Another example is the evaluation of the anatomical dolls test (Jampole & Weber, 1987) in which the test result is plotted against the presence or absence of abuse. In both cases the data are based upon real trials, and the obvious problem is that in neither instance truth is established with absolute certainty. There is even the possibility of circularity, viz. that the truth is partly based on the test, or on information also used by the test. But in both instances one can calculate whether the conclusions are invalidated by allowing a certain degree of error.

We may consider a similar design for repressed memories, in which true and false accusations are separated according to the best available criteria. Imagine the hypothetical classification of 100 allegations of abuse in childhood that have come to trial, presented in Table 1.

This table shows that the base rate of true allegations leads one to accept the charge, irrespective of whether repression was claimed. The base rate masks the diagnostic value of claimed repression, as is demonstrated when the base rate effect is removed by transforming the scores to proportions within rows. This is presented in Table 2.

Table 2 shows that in this hypothetical example the diagnostic value of claimed repression is inverse: when repression is claimed it is more likely than not that the allegation is false. Not claiming repression is diagnostic for truth of the allegation.

The values in the hypothetical example are of course irrelevant. The only purpose is to demonstrate that case studies categorized in this way yield some useful information, even without knowing whether repression exists at all. It might help if the theoretical discussions about repression were stopped for the moment, while selected cases were classified as in Table 2, in order to determine the diagnostic value of the mere claim of repression. The sensitivity for error in the classifications can be evaluated by randomly redistributing various percentages of the cases over the two categories. If the diagnostic value of the repression claim appears to be below 1.0 for every realistic error level, we may even have overcome the problem of not knowing exactly what happened in all these cases.

The two opposing theories about repression and recovery predict quite different outcomes of a quasi-experiment like the one suggested above. The repression theory predicts that repression will be claimed almost only if the allegation is true, and almost never when the allegation is false. The "memory implantation theory" predicts rather the opposite. Examples are presented in Tables 3 and 4.

The finding that claims of repression are diagnostic for truth supports the repression theory. The opposite outcome, that claims of repression are diagnostic for falsehood of the allegation, would support the theory of memory implantation. But I should give a warning here. The theory that true victims claim repression for some reason, even though in fact they never forgot the abuse, leads to the same prediction as the one shown in Table 3.

Table 1. Hypothetical classifications of 100 abuse cases

	Repression claimed	Repression not claimed
Allegation true	50	25
Allegation not true	24	1

Table 2. Proportional transformation of the data presented in Table 1

	Repression claimed	Repression not claimed	Total
Allegation true	67%	33%	100%
Allegation not true	96%	4%	100%
Diagnostic value D	67/96=0.7	33/4=8.2	

Thus the results can be used by a court of law, as far as claims of repression can be used as diagnostic for truth or falsehood of the abuse allegation. The results can never be used in a scientific debate to prove that claims of repression are true. On the other hand these tables may lead to the conclusion that claims of repressed memories are sometimes false. We still do not know whether there were really false memories, because possibly the claimants did not really believe their own memories to be genuine. Hence the contribution of this type of quasi-experiment to the solution of the repression and recovery issue is by definition quite limited.

A more complicated quasi-experimental design is obtained by considering another variable. Imagine a theory that attributes the repression to the repeated character of the abuse. In that case it is predicted that repression is positively correlated to the frequency of abuse reported in the victim's story. The hypothetical data in Table 5 would confirm such a hypothesis.

The basic idea of such an experimental test is that one theory should predict the relationship, while the other does not. Unfortunately, the results in Table 5 are also predicted by the theory that recovered memories are implanted. If some or many in the group of victims who claim repression are led by suggestions of an overzealous therapist, it may happen that these suggestions produce incremental reports of multiple abuse. One might reason that therapists believe that repression indicates frequent abuse and, therefore, they will not rest until they have found it. Thus the introduction of reported abuse frequency will not really help as a test of opposite theories.

The memory implantation theory predicts that memories for exotic events, like sexual abuse before birth, extreme violence towards children without leaving any traces, satanic ritual abuse, abduction by aliens, are paired with the claim of repression and subsequent recovery. Categorizing "normal" and "exotic" cases might lead results shown in Table 6.

It looks as if repression is claimed equally often in normal and extreme cases, but this is of course because the base rates mask the true proportions. After correction for base rates we obtain a clear relationship between extremity of the abuse and the claim of repression. Now it appears that there is a positive relationship between reporting "exotic" abuse and the claim of repression. The interpretation of this result depends entirely upon

Table 3. Hypothetical prediction of memory repression theory

	Scores in 100 cases		Proportions	
	Repression claimed	Repression not claimed	Repression claimed	Repression not claimed
Allegation true	50	25	67%	33%
Allegation not true	1	24	4%	96%
Diagnostic value D			67/4=16.8	33/96=0.3

Table 4. Hypothetical prediction of memory implantation theory

	Scores in 100 cases		Proportions	
	Repression claimed	Repression not claimed	Repression claimed	Repression not claimed
Allegation true	5	70	7%	93%
Allegation not true	24	1	96%	4%
Diagnostic value D			7/96=0.07	93/4=23

the acceptance of 'exotic" claims as true or false. If "exotic" claims are supposed to be un-true, the repression claim is diagnostic for falsehood. If we believe that 'exotic" claims are true, the positive relationship with repression suggests that severe suffering is more likely to be repressed, or even that the culprits of these weird crimes have the power to cause memories to disappear. If one refuses to accept truth or falsehood on such an a priori ba-sis, data as shown in Table 6 are of no help.

The thought experiments presented in Tables 1–6 illustrate the problem quite well: it is difficult to think of experimental variables that can be used in a quasi-experimental de-sign, and that would differentiate between the two theories. Any outcome that was used as an argument in favor of one theory, could be handled equally well by the other.

The only conclusion that can be anchored safely in a quasi-experimental design is, eventually, that claims of repression and recovery can be diagnostic for truth or falsehood of the abuse allegation. This is not very helpful for the advance of psychological theory, because it does not tell us anything about repression and recovery of traumatic memories. Case studies arranged in a quasi-experimental design will most likely be to no avail.

8. THE TRIAL-SCIENCE CIRCULARITY

If the accepted models of testing scientific theories cannot help us to test a theory of repression and recovery, it is understandable that other ways are sought. The appeal to case histories is only a small step from there, and coincides with the tradition of almost a century of psychiatry. But case histories cannot be interpreted without a circular reason-ing, as shown before. In this section I will demonstrate the circularities in more detail.

As shown before, there is the danger that science derives it arguments from court rulings, whereas the rulings were based on that very science. If one wants to use Evelyn's case as a demonstration of the existence of forgetting and recovery, it should be realised that we have only Dr. Subardjo's testimony that Evelyn's memories are real. How did Dr. Subardjo reach that conclusion? She may have used her experience with abuse victims, or she may have relied on some properties of Evelyn's behavior that she assumes to be diag-

Table 5. Hypothetical data on the relationship between claimed repression and reported abuse frequency

	Scores in 100 cases		Proportions	
	Repression claimed	Repression not claimed	Repression claimed	Repression not claimed
Frequent abuse	8	2	80%	20%
Infrequent abuse	9	81	10%	90%
Diagnostic value D			80/10=8.0	20/90=0.2

Table 6. Hypothetical data on the relationship between claimed repression and extremity of case

	Scores in 100 cases		Proportions	
	Repression claimed	Repression not claimed	Repression claimed	Repression not claimed
"Exotic" abuse	9	1	90%	10%
"Normal" abuse	9	81	10%	90%
Diagnostic value D			9/1=9.0	1/9=0.11

nostic for abuse, or as diagnostic for the truthfulness of Evelyn's memories. But how do we know that Dr. Subardjo is experienced? And even if she is experienced, how do we know her diagnostic criteria are valid?

We do not know anything about Dr. Subardjo, except from the fact that she was trained as a psychiatrist about 45 years ago, and that she has experience with three more (alleged) abuse victims. Her knowledge of the literature remained untested. It is probably not possible to prove or disprove her expertise, or to assess the diagnostic value of her clinical insights. But Evelyn's lawyer, established the acceptability of Dr. Subardjo's testimony in a quite different manner, viz. through reference to a Supreme Court ruling. The Dutch Supreme Court ruled that therapists' statements about truth or falsehood of their clients' stories are admissible evidence. "Admissible" is not the same as 'valid", but on the basis of this ruling a therapist's evidence cannot be declared inadmissable because of its known invalidity. The Supreme Court's ruling was not based upon any scientific analysis, but only on the consideration that a court should be allowed to decide for itself whether to accept or reject a therapist's testimony. Thus the status of the therapist as an expert on truthfulness is based on legal arguments, not scientific ones. But, as happened in Evelyn's case, the lawyer may claim that the expert's assessment of truthfulness is to be accepted as valid because of the Supreme Court ruling. This provides a basis for the decision that Evelyn really repressed and recovered her memories of the abuse by David, which in turn establishes the case as a proof of existence.

Another road to circularity occurs when the therapist argues in court that she has much experience with cases of repression, or that there is a vast literature on this topic. Both arguments are circular, because personal experience and literature depend again on case histories, singly or in quasi-experimental designs. The entire clinical literature about repression rests on case studies that entail the same problems as Evelyn's story. How can they help to establish the truth in her case? Even without the interference of the courts the clinical tradition of building science upon case histories is alarmingly circular. Court rulings only add some extra loops to this circle.

An example of circularity created by science itself is the usage of the Diagnostic and Statistical Manual of Mental Disorders (DSM-IV, APA, 1994) as an authorative source in the courtroom. Ideally DSM-IV is compiled on the basis of empirical data, representative, and carefully analyzed. In reality, it is a compromise between scientific conscience and semi-political lobbying. The much acclaimed empiricism consists mainly of case histories that are open to various interpretations. Multiple personality disorder (MPD) or, more currently, dissociative identity disorder, is entered under the pressure of believers in dissociation theory, and supported by case studies interpreted on the basis of this same belief (Van Praag, 1993). When this is achieved it seems as if experts in the courtroom can now refer to critically tested and therefore generally accepted science. In the courtroom, cases of claimed MPD are supported by the scientific standing of the diagnosis. This status is derived from its occurrence in DSM. It was entered in DSM because of the convincing case histories. The case histories were convincing because the concept of MPD is anchored instead of tested; anchoring structures can be quite convincing, even though alternative theories are not tested at all. The court that consults psychiatric experts in order to escape from its own unsafe anchors, will base its judgment on the similarly weak anchors of DSM.

Research about clinical judgment reveals a considerable lack of reliability and validity, which should have warned the courts around the world. Dr. Subardjo and many others do not base their opinion that recovered memories are true on any validated criteria. Instead they use clinical judgment. Even a superficial glance at the literature on the validity of clinical judgment (cf. Dawes, 1994; Ziskin, 1995) reveals that it is probably close to zero. This information can be used to break the circle; but it rarely happens. Authority, experience, literature, and appeal to common beliefs, usually replace the demonstration of validity; and the courts fall for it. If courts base their decision about truth or falsehood of abuse allegations on the opinion of experts, it means that experts replace judges, with no guarantee that their subjective impressions are better than those of judges and jury members.

After the courts have confirmed the experts" opinions, the cases are added to the experts' stock, so that future opinions are given with even more conviction. Neither the scientists, nor the courts seem to realise that they contribute to a process of escalating certainty that hides a validity of almost zero. Not only are people convicted on the basis of mistaken expert testimony; the convictions also help to establish the expertise more firmly.

Flexible definitions of the charge add to the circularity. Consider Evelyn's case again. Is there any chance that facts will eliminate the alleged abuse, repression, and recovery? Imagine that throughout the entire relevant period Evelyn and her parents were abroad, while David stayed with his grandparents in The Netherlands (as happened in many Dutch families). Would this prove that David did not have the opportunity to assault Evelyn, and that for this reason her memories must be false? No it does not. Evelyn could explain that probably the abuse happened when she was two or six, or that Herman was the culprit, etc. There are many cases in which such alternatives were offered and accepted. But it is another instance of circularity. Since Evelyn believes that her memories are true, she will change the anchoring stucture of her narrative, instead of testing her narrative against another one. The truth of the narrative becomes the starting point, not the end result. No fact can affect the theory of repression and recovery, if it is believed that the recovered memories are possibly inaccurate, and need not fit the facts. As long as a case history can be changed at liberty by one who believes in it, the history will always confirm the belief.

9. CAUSALITY

The court requested proof that Evelyn's problems were caused by the alleged abuse. If the causality relationship is to be inferred from case histories, there is a special problem, because they are always retrospective. Studies in retrospect allow conclusions about statistical relationships, not about causal relationships. Causality can only be demonstrated by prospective experimental designs. Establishment of a causal relationship between repression and psychological suffering is particularly difficult, because the repression cannot be demonstrated. There is another lane for circularity here, because those who suffer will seek assistance, and therefore have a bigger chance of discovering and believing repressed memories.

The theory of repressed and recovered memories predicts that repression will cause psychological suffering, and that recovery will alleviate the suffering. But the theory is supported by case studies, at its best; I am not even aware of carefully arranged collections of case studies demonstrating that activation of abuse memories diminishes the suffering. It may be argued by Dr. Subardjo that Evelyn's treatment improved her condition markedly, but this cannot be taken as proof that her problems were caused by the abuse, or by the memories to abuse, or by the repressed memories of abuse. It is equally possible that Evelyn's condition was improved through the extra attention given to her, or the self-hypnotic sessions, or through blaming David for her problems, or through the action taken against David.

The causal relationship between David's behavior and Evelyn's suffering is questionable even when the defense admits the abuse by David, and accepts the mechanisms of subsequent repression and psychological disturbance. Causality is not a dichotomous notion, but a matter of degree. To what degree are Evelyn's problems caused by David? Is it possible that Evelyn is also suffering from the loss of her boy friend? Or from the lack of an intimate relationship? Was she also abused by her brother Herman? And by her father? Is it possible that Evelyn has repressed memories of other abuses, and that they will surface only later? Can Dr. Subardjo guarantee that there are no other repressed memories, apart from the ones relating to David? Many cases have demonstrated that memories of sexual abuse come piecemeal, and that the reported violence is incremental. Perhaps the worst of Evelyn's revelations is still to come. How can a court decide that David is solely responsible, or even that he is more responsible than other abusers yet unknown?

The problem is of course that Dr. Subardjo may testify about psychological theory or other cases known to her, but not about what exactly happened in Evelyn's unconscious. If the theory is strict and the case histories clear, Perhaps what must have happened in Evelyn's case may be inferred. But the theory is pliable and the case histories allow multiple interpretations. Theories that include an unconscious, repression, or multiple personalities, allow a mass of alternative explanations of what happened in Evelyn's head. The possibility that the unconscious has released the memories in a modified form, or still hides some important other memories, will always block the assessment of causality. Any narrative can be anchored if the unconscious and its mysterious ways can be used as anchors. For the application of therapy this might not be a serious obstacle, but for legal factfinding as well as for the testing of scientific theory, it is.

It is probably little realised by the legal community that the relationship between the supposed causes of psychological suffering and type of therapy is rather weak. If the assumption about the cause of one's suffering is correct, the removal of this cause should help more than anything else. Empirical studies of therapy effects do not support this notion, which can only mean that assumptions about causes are often wrong. Dr. Subardjo failed to relate this type of finding, but emphasized her personal clinical insight in the causes of Evelyn's problems. That is, she preferred her own limited set of case histories to experimental therapy evaluation. Selecting a therapist of Dr. Subardjo's type as an expert on causality can hardly lead to a different result; why would she treat Evelyn the way she did, if she did not believe in the causal relationship between repression and psychological suffering as demonstrated by case histories?

I am not arguing that there is no causal relationship between abuse by David and Evelyn's present suffering. But I deny that the relationship can be established on scientific grounds. Case histories are the only basis, and they are not good enough.

10. WHAT TO DO?

Do case histories about recovered memories prove anything at all? Yes, they do. Evelyn's case proves that women tell such stories about sexual abuse. Some other cases prove that courts may convict on the basis of such stories alone, which means that they believe the theory of repression and recovery to be true. Other cases demonstrate that courts may accept the narrative of repression and recovery, even against decisive falsification. A larger collection of case histories may reveal the proportion of cases in which claims of repression and recovery originate during or because of psychotherapy. Case histories may also prove the biased positions of some scientists, or the lack of scientific grounds for some of the claims made in expert testimony. Case histories may even uncover the weakness or unfairness of various systems of criminal justice. But case histories cannot be used for testing a psychological theory about memory recovery.

As the scientific debate seems to revolve around case histories, more than experimental studies, I propose to scrutinize the various materials thoroughly. Any theory based on case histories should be considered untested. Any argument based on case histories should be scrutinized. My expectation is that both sides, those who support the notion of recovered memories and those who don't, would almost be devoid of arguments. It means that the debate is fully open.

But while the debate is pursued there is an a priori preference for theories that meet "Occam's razor" best. Such theories have the simplest anchoring structure, contain the lowest number of subnarratives, and connect to the lowest number of anchors. It is my conviction that the acceptance of repression, dissociation, an unconscious, or accurate recovery of childhood memories requires a large number of extra anchors. Theories based on these notions do therefore not deserve our prior preference.

REFERENCES

American Psychiatric Association Board of Trustees (1994). Statement on memories of sexual abuse, *International Journal of Clinical and Experimental Hypnosis, 42*, 261–264.

Carroll, D. (1988). How accurate is polygraph lie detection? In A. Gale (Ed.), *The Polygraph Test: Lies, truth and science*. London: Sage.

Dawes, R.M. (1994). *House of cards: Psychology and psychotherapy built on myth*. New York: The Free Press.

Femina, D.D., Yeager, C.A. & Lewis, D.O. (1990). Child abuse: Adolescent records vs. adult recall. *Child Abuse and Neglect, 145*, 227–331.

Jampole, L., & Weber, M.K. (1987). An assessment of the behavior of sexually abused children with anatomically correct dolls. *Child Abuse and Neglect, 11*, 187–192.

Kahneman, D., Slovic, P. & Tversky, A. (1982). *Judgment under uncertainty: Heuristics and biases*. Cambridge University Press.

Loftus, E., & Ketcham, K. (1994). *The myth of repressed memory: False memories and allegations of sexual abuse*. New York: St. Martin's Press.

Pennington, N., & Hastie, R. (1986). Evidence evaluation in complex decision making. *Journal of Personality and Social Psychology, 51*, 242–258.

Praag, H.M. V. (1993). Make-believes, *Psychiatry or the perils of progress*. New York: Brunner/Mazel.

Schünemann, B., & Bandilla, W. (1989). Perseverance in courtroom decisions. In: H. Wegener, F. Lösel & J. Haisch (Eds.), *Criminal behavior and the justice system: psychological perspectives* (pp. 181–192). New York: Springer.

Wagenaar, W.A., Koppen, P.J. van, & Crombag, H.F.M. (1993). *Anchored narratives. The psychology of criminal evidence*. Hemel Hempstead: Harvester Wheatsheaf.

Wason, P.C., & Johnson-Laird, P.N. (1972). *Psychology of reasoning: Structure and content*. London: Batsford (in particular chapter 13).

Williams, L. M. (1994). Recall of childhood trauma: A prospective study of women's memories of child sexual abuse. *Journal of Consulting and Clinical Psychology*, *62*, 1167–1176.

Ziskin, J. (1995). *Coping with psychiatric and psychological testimony*. Los Angeles: Law and Psychology Press.

COMMENTARY ON THE LOGICAL STATUS OF CASE HISTORIES

Sherrill Mulhern, Ecole des Hautes Etudes des Sciences Sociales, 52 bd Raspail, 75006, Paris, France

If it had been presented 25 years ago, Dr. Wagenaar's uncompromising examination of the methods and goals of science and justice and how they interact would probably have provoked an enthusiastic, albeit basically academic debate. Most likely, the case history that he summarized would have been treated as an intriguing curiosity and have elicited a number of questions about how it got into a courtroom to begin with. Today, however, the case of Evelyn and David is all too familiar and his analysis is uniquely challenging because it obliges us to think critically about some of the difficult scientific, social, and legal dilemmas that define the contemporary traumatic memory/recovered memory debate.

Dr. Wagenaar has argued persuasively that case histories cannot be used to decide a scientific theory of memory because they are not generalizable. And I find no logical fault in his argument. However, it was not scientific theories that precipitated and sustained Evelyn's accusations against her brother. It was, at least in part, her identification with a socially negotiated, consensually agreed upon form of "illness behavior" (e.g., Littlewood, 1996). Although the development of a truly scientific theory of memory is certainly a laudable goal, it would be of limited value if we want to better understand Evelyn, David, Dr. Subardjo, and the court's predicaments. For that, we need to know much more about the historical context in which this kind of case and this sort of behavior emerged.

During the past few years, criminal and civil courts in a number of countries have been grappling with the psycho/social consequences of the propagation and clinical application of a novel theoretical model of human memory that was developed by a small group of psychiatrists during the late 1970s to describe a severe form of psychopathology: Multiple Personality Disorder (MPD). This model, which was sanctioned in 1980 by the American Psychiatric Association, in its Diagnostic and Statistical Manual of Mental Disorders, Third Edition (DSM III), had profound legal ramifications. To begin with, Dr. Wagenaar's objections not withstanding, it was perceived to be the product of a scientific revolution in the way that mental disorders are classified. Unlike prior editions, the diagnostic categories that appeared in the DSM III were described as the psychological equivalents of physical diseases. They were said to represent objective, visible phenomena; stable clusters of symptoms that had been specified through the systematic recording, collecting, and comparison of case histories (e.g., Young, 1995).

According to the DSM III, "the essential feature of MPD is the existence within the individual of two or more distinct personalities." Personalities are described as fully integrated, complex psychological units; discrete volitional mental entities that are the repositories of memories of events that have been experienced by those individuals who exhibit the disorder but that their "original" personalities do not remember. These hidden memories only become conscious when these individuals' subpersonalities take control over their overt behavior. The text implies that, in so far as subpersonalities are created during

childhood, endure over time, and have unique memories, behavior patterns, and social relationships, the histories that they reveal can be treated as creditable autobiographical accounts. Clinicians are advised that hypnosis is an effective tool which can be used to
facilitate an individual's transition from one personality to another. Significantly, this is
the only time that the word hypnosis appears in the DSM III description of the disorder.

Official DSM III endorsement of MPD came at a time when North American public
and professional appreciation of the reality and social impact of domestic violence, particularly violence against women and children, had risen dramatically. Beginning in the
early 1960s, parental maltreatment and neglect of children—which had traditionally been
considered socio/economic problems—were re-defined as a diagnosable, treatable, and ultimately preventable medical disorder. In 1962, a group of pediatricians published a landmark paper, the Battered Child Syndrome, that presented medical evidence that a
significant proportion of the infants treated in hospitals for alleged accidental injuries had
actually been repeatedly brutalized by their caretakers (e.g., Kempe, Silverman, Steele,
Droegemueller, & Silver, 1962). The authors asserted that child abuse was not a by-prod-
uct of poverty, low intelligence, alcoholism and serious mental disorders, noting that the
problem frequently arose among people with good educations and stable financial and social backgrounds. Consequently, they concluded that psychiatric factors were probably of
prime importance in the pathogenesis of the disorder; that abusive parents were mentally
ill. During the next few years, the rapid dissemination of this discovery by the mass media, particularly in North America, precipitated the emergence of a vibrant socio/economic
sector specialized in child protection that included distinctive educational programs, journals, professional conferences, research grants, etc (e.g., Scheper-Hughes & Stein, 1987).

Just as organized institutional response to the medicalized problem of child abuse
was beginning to take shape, a second, even more compelling set of social issues was
thrust into American public awareness: incest and the sexual assault and exploitation of
women and children. However, unlike the problem of child battering, sexual abuse first
emerged as a political issue, raised by a cohort of feminists activists who had begun establishing shelters for women who were victims of rape and/or domestic violence (e.g., Armstrong, 1994).

In 1971, the first feminist analysis of incestuous child sexual abuse was presented by
a professional social worker, Florence Rush, at a landmark conference on rape organized
in New York City. Drawing on her case files, the few available studies that had been published by Freudian analysts and the American Humane Society's 1966 statistics on sex
crimes against children—which revealed that 97% of offenders were male and that 90% of
their victims were females—she argued that the intra-familial sexual abuse of female children by males was the lynch pin of male power over women. Males coerced their victims
into silence by shaming them—placing responsibility for child rape directly on the purportedly seductive behavior of the victims and by threats of physical violence and possible
pregnancy. Furthermore, there was no social space in which female victims could reveal
their experiences and be taken seriously. Male demands for silence within the family unit
were reinforced by psychoanalytic theory which suggested that female disclosures of incestuous experiences were in fact fantasies. According to Rush, the reality of incestuous
sexual abuse experienced by females was avoided and deformed by psychiatric practice
that liberally cited the psychoanalytic myth of consent—that is that women want to acquire a man, or to have a penis.

Rush (1971) asserted that "although women—young women and even children—do
not talk freely about their molestation, there are few who consciously, or otherwise, consistently avoid the subject. For women who have not been believed or had the opportunity

to confront their molester (with adult support), there is always a sense of unfinished business; there is always humiliation and rage. When the subject of sexual abuse of children received some media exposure as a result of feminist discussions on the radio, in lectures and in articles, many women approached me and finally found an opportunity to ventilate their long-festering secret."

Feminists exhorted adult victims of intra-familial sexual assault to speak out. They demanded that society recognize these "survivors" of patriarchal oppression as competent witnesses to their pasts, and that the accused perpetrators of child sexual abuse be arrested, tried before a court of law, convicted, and jailed (e.g., Armstrong, 1994). Although the original feminist initiative effectively raised public awareness about incest and was instrumental in ensuring that child sexual abuse was officially recognized in the innovative Child Abuse Prevention and Treatment Act that was passed by the United States Congress in 1974, during the ensuing years, activists and professional child abuse intervenors, who rallied to the feminist cause, soon discovered that political theories are not easily translated into genuine social change.

During the 1970s, although child sexual abuse had been legally defined and publicly denounced as a particularly heinous crime, child welfare professionals were often confounded when they attempted to bring suspected offenders to trial. As a rule the only witnesses to the proscribed events were the victim and the perpetrator. Unlike physical abuse, sexual abuse does not necessarily generate material evidence. Furthermore, when children are victimized they rarely disclose their experiences immediately. Consequently, even in cases where children have been raped, by the time an investigation begins, valuable physical evidence has often disappeared. All that remains to bring before the court is a traumatized, reluctant child telling a story.

This same problem was actually exacerbated when adult survivors attempted to obtain reparation for years of suffering. Even in cases where corroborative evidence emerged, prevailing statutes of limitations generally prevented victims from bringing their aggressors to court. By the end of the decade, it appeared that the legal barriers, which had been designed ostensibly to protect the innocent, were actually vindicating the guilty.

Given this unique socio/political context, the American Psychiatric Association's specification and endorsement of MPD as an independent diagnostic entity was of particular import both to survivors and the courts. The DSM III description of the disorder explicitly stated that "child abuse and other forms of severe emotional trauma in childhood may be predisposing factors." In other words, it affirmed that individuals who either exhibit or who come to exhibit subpersonalities as a result of hypnotic therapy are frequently victims of a crime. Moreover, in so far as the condition was presented as the natural, behavioral expression of an inborn psycho/physiological mechanism—i.e. it is not produced iatrogenically by therapy—when a case of alleged child abuse was brought to court, both the diagnosis of subpersonalities and the narratives that the latter produce could arguably constitute admissible corroborative evidence that a particular crime had indeed been committed.

Recently, some of the principal theoreticians of contemporary MPD have protested that the disorder has been singled out for criticism unfairly, arguing that, in so far as it meets current professional standards of validity and reliability, it should be treated just like any other psychiatric disorder (e.g., Ross, 1996). However, this objection fails to take into account the substantial body of literature that documents the fact that in all cultures, psychological "illness entities" are produced, evolve, and are abandoned through ongoing overt and covert social negotiation (e.g., Angel & Thoits, 1987). Although, the DSM III was widely accepted as a scientific document, the diagnostic categories that figured in the manual were produced by the same complex social process.

Each time a particular pattern of dramatic or unconventional behavior is specified by an authoritative cultural elite and promulgated as the expression of an illness, its adoption by individuals experiencing subjective distress and concomitant acceptance by members of their immediate social network as both meaningful and non-volitional, invariably produces profound, often unanticipated social, political and legal repercussions. Before a new pattern can be accepted, it must be learned. The frequency and prevalence of an emerging pattern of "illness behavior" is generally directly related to its exposure through real and fictional media instances (e.g., Littlewood, 1996). For example: throughout the 20th century there were certainly thousands of individuals who could have come to understand themselves as multiples and to have been satisfactorily diagnosed as such according to DSM III criteria. However, they did not and were not because from the social perspective being "multiple" did not "mean" anything. The novels, movies, articles in professional journals and the popular press, as well as the prime time television news programs that dealt with the emerging MPD model during the late 1970s and early 1980s, clearly document the fact that from the very beginning, multiple personality was not only perceived as a unique disorder, it was presented as such by experts in the field (e.g., American Broadcasting Companies, Inc., 1983).

For example: just two years after MPD was sanctioned in the DSM III, a number of the principal architects of the diagnosis, including Cornelia Wilbur, George Greaves, Myron Boor, David Caul, Richard Kluft, and Frank Putnam, were cited by Elliot (1982) in an article published in the Journal of Psychiatry & Law, in support of the proposition that the criminal justice system should consider that MPD constituted formal proof that child abuse had occurred. Although the author recognized that some experts allowed that the disorder could be triggered by other forms of trauma, apparently he was impressed by, among others, Wilbur's declaration that "Yes, MP is proof of child abuse," and Putnam's observation that "multiple personality is in fact a psychiatric disorder that has a relatively specific precipitant, incestuous sexual abuse, and begins in childhood." He concluded that "because of the extremely high incidence of abuse in cases of MPD, the burden of proof will be on the child's caretakers to explain what other trauma may have served as causal factor in the development of the disorder."

At first glance, it might appear that MPD is not really relevant to Evelyn's case. After all, her therapist never claimed that she was a multiple, only that she recovered memories of her brother's criminal assaults during therapy. In fact, if she had entered therapy prior to 1994, Dr. Subardjo would probably have had some difficulty choosing a suitable DSM diagnosis to describe her patient's psychological condition. Evelyn apparently did not manifest a recognizable personality shift during her therapy, so she would not even have qualified for a diagnosis of Dissociative Disorders Not Otherwise Specified (DDNOS). She appeared, however, to have been amnestic for a violent rape perpetrated ostensibly by David when she was only four years old, although curiously she had continuous memory of an apparently less traumatic incident that occurred three years later. If her amnesia for the earlier assault had terminated abruptly, she might have qualified for the diagnosis of Psychogenic Amnesia. However, according to her case history, that memory was reconstructed out of bits and pieces of intrusive affect and images, over an extended period of time. On the other hand, if Evelyn had entered treatment after the 1994 DSM IV revisions of the dissociative disorders had been published, Dr. Subardjo would have immediately recognized that her patient was suffering from a classic case of a disorder that—its evocative label not withstanding—had just come into existence: Dissociative Amnesia (formerly Psychogenic Amnesia). In other words, both Dr. Subardjo's description of her patient's condition and to a large extent Evelyn's understanding of herself were determined as much by the historical moment when she entered therapy as by her psychological symptoms.

It is important to keep in mind that in each successive edition of the DSM, the clusters of symptoms that were selected to specify the different dissociative disorders clearly reflected a subtle intermingling of patients' behaviors, the beliefs and diagnostic techniques of the clinicians who observed them, and the socio/political context in which they emerged. There is good evidence that the clinical application of the DSM III and DSM III-R theories of multiple personality between the late 1970s and the early 1990s inadvertently gave rise to the novel class of "illness behavior" that is illustrated by Evelyn's case. And that the radical re-specification and re-labeling of Psychogenic Amnesia in the 1994 DSM IV as a chronic psychological condition was, at least in part, an effort to accommodate this behavior's developing psycho/social impact.

Up to this point I have described MPD essentially as a contemporary, North American phenomena. However, its theoretical roots can be traced back to a series of models of human memory that were elaborated in Europe during the late 19th century. Although the successive re-specifications of the DSM dissociative disorders category were motivated as much by socio/political considerations as clinical observations, they were expressed in the historically sanctioned language of psychiatry. Since to a great extent the descriptions that actually appeared in the manuals were produced by selectively recombining segments of these earlier models, a brief review of this older material is warranted here. Those theories that are most relevant to the current debate are Pierre Janet's clinical theories of hysteria, dissociation, and traumatic memory and Sigmund Freud's successive theories of hysterical neurosis. I will begin with Janet because many contemporary authorities on MPD acknowledge him as their theoretical forefather and because his 1907 book, The Major Symptoms of Hysteria, served as a reference for the task force that defined the DSM III Dissociative Disorders category.

Early in his career, inspired by Théodule Ribot's clinical descriptions of double consciousness and periodic memory, and Jean Martin Charcot's description of hysterical neurosis in both male and female patients, and his own extensive observations, Janet (1889) theorized that the unity of the self as expressed in personality is best understood, not as a given, but as an achievement in that an individual's physical and social unity are complemented by a temporal unity that is provided by memory. He observed that while in somnambulistic trance hysterics almost invariably exhibited secondary personalities that appeared to remember traumatic events; "fixed ideas" that were unavailable to them in their normal waking state. Moreover, while in these secondary states many of their intractable somatic symptoms, that were characteristic of the disorder, disappeared. As his clinical work progressed, Janet (1911) noted that because of their severe memory deficiencies, the psychological examination of hysterics was particularly difficult. The narratives that they produced were consistently incomplete and contradictory; information that emerged during one session, was often negated during the next. Although he insisted that these patients should not simply be dismissed as simulators, he observed that "it is not possible to rely on their narratives to reconstruct the history of their lives or that of their illness."

In his major work, L'Etat Mental des Hystériques (1911), Janet reported that the characteristic amnesias exhibited by hysterics could be classified in three, traditionally accepted, major categories: systematized amnesia—in which a patient lost a certain class of memories, or group of interrelated ideas that constituted a logical system; localized amnesia—in which the lost memories were all related the same period of the patient's life; and generalized amnesia—in which the patient, after a series of violent psychological attacks or periods of sleep, lost all memory of the events that had occurred throughout his or her life. However, he completed this list, by adding a fourth category: continuous amnesia—which he described, not as a loss of historical memories, but as an ongoing alteration in the manner in which hysterics acquire memories in the first place; a disorder in the manner in which these individuals perceived events; a chronic inability to focus attention.

For Janet, relief of hysterics' psycho/physiological symptoms was not necessarily contingent on recovering dissociated traumatic material. He demonstrated that because of their unique sensitivity to hypnosis and suggestion, it was often possible to re-construct their subconscious fixed ideas in less traumatic forms that could then be reintegrated into normal conscious memory. He concluded that when these patients underwent distressing or traumatic events, an underlying, hereditary, nervous disorder prevented them from representing them in unified memory. Because of this condition, hysterics were singularly vulnerable to a wide variety of human experiences including hemorrhages, chronic illness, infectious diseases, physical and psychological exhaustion or trauma, violent emotions, etc.

He observed that they were particularly sensitive around the age of puberty when most of life's difficulties come to a head: choosing a career and the problem of finding employment, the turmoil of sexuality, and in some cases religious issues. Although their fragile psychological condition might go unrecognized for a period of time, the accumulated weight of their heterogeneous disturbing experiences would inevitably lead to a form of mental "disaggregation" characterized by a tendency towards a permanent and complete doubling of the personality, which in turn precipitated the development of the disparate constellation of physical and psychological symptoms that characterized hysteria.

At this point, Janet scholars might legitimately object that the preceding summary of his theory of hysteria is both woefully incomplete and highly selective. Although they would be correct, I have chosen to focus my remarks on essential components of his theory that—between the mid 1970s and the mid-1990s—were rarely, if ever mentioned by the architects of the contemporary model of MPD, who claimed to be Janet's theoretical successors. Significantly, these constituent elements of the psychopathological condition which he defined as a chronic doubling of the personality were not included in the DSM III description of the disorder. What I am suggesting is that, although Janet repeatedly demonstrated that extreme suggestibility is a defining psychological characteristic of individuals who exhibit double personalities, this seminal observation was excluded from the DSM III clinical specification of MPD because the social impact of Freud's psychoanalytic theory of hysteria had made it politically unacceptable. In the end, the critically under-specified model of illness behavior that made headlines both in the clinical and legal literature and the popular press of the early 1980s, and that was presented and perceived as a viable solution to some of the heretofore insurmountable barriers that prevented most adult survivors from suing their abusers, functioned as a blueprint for social disaster.

Whereas Janet's theories of dissociation, trauma, and hysteria can be understood as extensions of the work of his predecessors, his contemporary, Sigmund Freud fundamentally revised the theories and practices that he had observed in Paris, while studying with Janet's predecessor and collaborator, Jean Martin Charcot, at the Salpêtrière hospital. For example: whereas French clinicians had urged caution when working with the narratives produced by hysterics, Freud was much less circumspect. In a 1896 study (republished in 1952), drawing on his work with 18 hysterics, he reported that, although they initially resisted his therapeutic efforts, after being treated with his technique of psychoanalysis, all of these patients ultimately produced memories of childhood sexual assault. He concluded that the emotional quality of their abreactions confirmed the facticity of their reminiscences, and that once the shroud of amnesia that enveloped their memories of childhood sexual trauma had been lifted, and the details of their experiences had been cathected with affect and brought back into unified conscious memory, hysterics would be cured.

Initially, Freud argued that he had made a significant discovery. However, contrary to his expectation, he was soon forced to admit that he was unable to bring any of his patients' analyses to a real close. Even when he encountered a partial success, he could explain it without referring to his initial theory. In an often cited 1887 letter to his friend, Willem Fliess (republished in 1950), Freud expressed his disappointment and surprise that all of his patients ended up recovering identical memories. If his theory was correct, given that all of his patients ultimately identified their fathers as their abusers, it would imply that the fathers of all hysterics, including his own, had to be accused of being perverse. He asserted that it was inconceivable that all hysterics had undergone exactly the same experiences. However, he added that his clinical work had led him to the fundamental insight that "there are no indications of reality in the unconscious, so that one cannot distinguish between truth and fiction that has been cathected with affect." In other words, although hysterics might exhibit violent emotions while abreacting recovered memories, this in itself did not constitute proof that these reminiscences were historically true. Although, after his sojourn in France, Freud was clearly aware of hysterics' unique vulnerability to suggestion, he rejected the possibility that his personal preoccupations with his own father might have had a determining influence on his patients' converging stories. Instead he concluded that what he had been observing was his hysterical patients' "elaborations of sexual fantasies and that apparently these fantasies invariably seized on the theme of the parents."

During the next few years, Freud abandoned his exploration of hypnotic states and disorders of memory. However, throughout his career, the relationship between parents and their children remained central to his theorizing. In his first etiology of hysteria, he had reduced the broad notion of trauma, that he had inherited from Charcot and the French, and anchored it firmly in the early developmental phase of sexuality (e.g., Barrois, 1988). Subsequently, in accordance with his novel insight, he developed a new theory that asserted that hysterical neurosis is the result of intrapsychic conflict between unacknowledged instinctual sexual drives and the demands of external social reality.

Throughout the first third of the 20th century, Janet continued lecturing and treating patients. However, his theories of the fixated unconscious idea and pathological dissociation were progressively abandoned by the up and coming generation of clinicians because they were closely associated with the use of hypnosis which had become suspect both because it was associated with the increasingly criticized clinical techniques that had been employed by Charcot, and because of a series of legal confrontations in France (Laurence & Perry, 1988) in which hypnotists were accused of "seducing" their patients while the latter were in trance. As might have been expected, young clinicians working in this controversial climate were particularly receptive to Freud's nominally non-hypnotic technique, as well as his ingenious theories.

During the late 19th century, the number of males who were diagnosed with hysteria in France was about equal to the number of females. This fact is often overlooked because the latter were far more frequently represented in the drawings and photographs produced both by clinicians and the popular press of the period. It is important to note that Janet and his contemporaries, following the lead of Charcot, had re-defined the gender specific model of hysteria, that they had inherited from their 18th century predecessors, in a gender neutral form that reflected not only their clinical observations but the political philosophy of equality and citizenship advocated by the ideologues of the new French "République" (e.g., Edelman, 1995). However, their unique understanding of the neurosis was gradually set aside largely because Freud's theory—that hysteria is the result of re-pressed infantile sexual desires that are directed towards parents—effectively revived the archaic gender specific, sexual etiology of the disorder (e.g., Micale, 1995). In time, as the radical feminists of the early 1970s so persuasively argued, the commonplace clinical in-terpretation of his theory proved to be devastating to female victims of childhood sexual assault. For most of the 20th century any woman who disclosed a memory of incest risked being repudiated as a confabulating hysteric by psychoanalytically inspired psychiatrists, who routinely dismissed factual accounts of exploitation and humiliation as imaginary constructions driven by repressed, unconscious sexual desires (e.g., Rush, 1980).

Unfortunately, as we have seen, the feminist analysis of child sexual abuse and con-comitant demand that the courts act on survivors' straightforward, unmediated narratives of childhood victimization, suffered from a fatal lack of political and historical realism. The ensuing crisis forced activists to reconsider their original animosity toward the psy-chotherapeutic establishment. In 1980, the American Psychiatric Association ratified, in a sense, a growing rapprochement between disillusioned feminist social theorists and the therapeutic perspective—which implied that personal change was a necessary prerequisite to any eventual political change—by coincidentally voting to eliminate the misogynic di-agnosis of hysterical neurosis and re-assigning the most significant psychological symp-toms that had formerly been associated with that syndrome to the autonomous dissociative disorder MPD. The new diagnostic entity was inspired by Janet's unified theory of hys-teria, but it was distinctly politically correct in so far as no mention was made of his ob-servations of these patients' vulnerability to suggestion and confabulation.

Unlike 19th century hysterics, who—although they had been portrayed as victims of trauma—were understood to be suffering from a chronic nervous condition, late 20th cen-tury multiples were consistently depicted as psychological virtuosos. According to the ex-perts, these creative geniuses, who were endowed with enviably high I.Q.s, used their extraordinary auto-hypnotic skills as an effective defense against grotesque child abuse (e.g., Wilbur, 1984). Although the DSM III had formally defined multiple personality as a severe mental disorder, when they emerged from the clinical milieu multiples were ex-alted socially as heroines. For example: in her booklet. United We Stand: A Book for Peo-ple with Multiple Personalities, psychologist and sexual abuse expert, Dr. Eliana Gil (1980) claimed that "multiplicity is not a form of mental illness." She advised readers, who might have the feeling that they were multiples, that first they must accept that "be-ing a multiple was a gift that allowed you to survive. Not everyone can become a multiple. Those of you that could become multiples were luckier. Usually, multiples are very intelli-gent and very creative."

The unique social status conferred on multiples allowed members of an emerging segment of the mental health establishment—that was trying to shed the stigma of having been complacent about male sexual violence— to establish themselves as privileged me-diators and guarantors of the legitimacy of adults survivors' accounts of incestuous child abuse. Because multiples apparently had no memory of their victimization and were gen-erally unaware of the existence of their alter personalities prior to diagnosis, unlike the adult survivors envisioned by the radical feminists, these individuals needed therapists in order to know themselves (e.g., Kluft, 1991). In contrast to the acrimonious, politically ac-tive, feminist incest survivors of the 1970s, who spoke out as adults and demanded the overthrow of the patriarchy, multiples, with the help of therapists, spoke of their pain and of barbarous abuse in the terrified voices of innocent children (e.g., Mulhern, 1995).

In 1984, when the First International Conference on Multiple Personality/ Dissocia-tive States convened in Chicago, theoreticians of MPD candidly recognized that multiples are hypnotic virtuosos. However, no mention was made of the fact that this defining char-acteristic could have a decisive impact on the content of the narratives that they produced through their alter personalities. On the contrary, experts encouraged conference partici-pants to accept that even the most extraordinary memories produced by their patients were historically accurate.

For example: during the inaugural plenary session, Cornelia Wilbur (1984), who was acknowledged as the single most influential clinician working in the field, told the following story:

> How would you like to be exposed to multiple murders as an infant and a child? Since your grandfather formed the first Klan, and your father formed the second Klan, and the family lit-erally owned the town. And if anybody moved in that didn't agree with them they promptly moved out; because they were harassed or advised to leave. There were only about 100 people living in the town which was surrounded by rich farms, all of which were owned by the Klan. I don't know how many murders this child saw. I haven't even tried to keep track of the ones she's reported, but in talking to her about it she tells me that that group of individuals, in that part of the United States, killed every single black person that came within their purview, and they killed a great many itinerant whites that were itinerant farm workers, including the chil-dren.

> Now we know of course that a great many people disappear in this country and are never seen again, and one of the ways that this happens is that groups like this destroy them in rituals, dismember them, and then put the dismembered parts in these large burners on the farms that are used to burn trash from the harvest. Such as burners that burn corn husks and even the bones burn in these burners because they're extremely hot so that there is no evidence, except of course the reported evidence of this multiple personality.

> Now she herself, later on in her life still as a child around the age of 8 was forced to take the knife that slit the throat of the individual who was being destroyed. And she reports that every single time she was forced to do this, her hand was held by her father, who proceeded to push the knife down, and she proceeded to pull the knife back. She was not as strong as he was of course and so the person had their throat cut, and blood was caught in jars, and often times, everyone shared in drinking the blood. These are ritual slayings and on occasion they would cut off a piece of everyone and pass it around for everyone to take some, in order to eat it, this again was part of the ritual slaying.

> She told one doctor that one of the slayings took place in Florida in a very famous condomin-ium club, and he said, "that's impossible, you couldn't possibly get a dead body out of there." And she said, "Oh no?" She said, "I'll tell you how." She said, "You know these very large very expensive containers of golf clubs? You take all of the golf clubs out and you can get a dismembered body in. If you don't believe it, try it."

Wilbur's presentation of her patient's appalling story was riveting. However, instead of reminding her audience (which included a sizeable contingent of patients) that—be-cause her patient was highly hypnotizable and thus singularly prone to confabulation—her uncorroborated account of organized, mass murders and ritual cannibalism should be treated with extreme circumspection; instead of pointing out that—farm trash burners and golf club containers not withstanding—crimes on this scale would necessarily generate some enduring material evidence; instead of advising that extreme narratives should be vigorously investigated and corroborated by law enforcement and confirmed by the crimi-nal justice system before they are endorsed publicly as historical facts; she insisted that "since we know of course that ritual clan killings do take place in this country, and since this woman is older, and since these things took place about thirty years ago, I don't think that we can possibly deny the truth of her descriptions, these are not allegations, they're descriptions of behaviors that she was forced to participate in and which, were to her, extremely abusive. So that not only do we have physical abuse, psychological abuse, sexual abuse, but we have an abuse in which the child is forced to participate in gruesome activities that are extremely destructive to that child's ego and development."

During the second half of her presentation, Wilbur (1984) complemented this first case history with a second, which both reinforced her assertion that clinicians should accept the narratives that multiples produced in therapy as accurate historical accounts, and suggested that there was a direct link between the sadistic quality of the abuse which her patient had ostensibly experienced and her prodigious psychological symptoms. In the second case history the victim was a woman who, as a child, had been interned with her brother in the Nazi concentration camp of Buchenwald. According to Wilbur

She was taken there at the age of one, and when she was three, her brother told her that they were going to run away. And she loved her brother, and he was very protective of her, so she said fine. So they ran away. The Nazi's sent the dogs after them and she saw her brother dismembered by the dogs. I don't know anything about her from then until she was 17 and was in Finland. How she managed to survive to escape or anything else, I don't know. But I do know that she's multiple.

Now some multiples who have been through terrifying circumstances like the woman I told you about that saw the multiple murders and this lady have fragmented, which is a kind of thing that happens in multiple personality when the trauma is so overwhelming that a single bit personality appears to deal with the overwhelming trauma.

According to what I have been able to learn, the woman in Buchenwald has supposedly about 200 personalities of which about at least 50 of them or more are fragments, individual, individuals who appeared to deal with one single traumatic incident. The woman who saw the multiple murders, I asked her, you know, "Do you have any idea how many alters you have?" And she shook her head and she said, "All I know is 5 times 258." And I said, "Well what does that mean?" She said, "Well they occur in groups of 5 and the groups of 5 deal with a certain kind of traumatic situation." I would suppose that those groups of 5 might come together first and be one, in terms of the fusion of personalities. But she said, "A great many of them only were there once; for one specific situation that was so terrifying that nobody else could deal with it." And here is your explanation. We have a woman who actually has, what we might say, call fragmented, instead of developing alters which deal with a type of trauma.

In so far as both of these women exhibited the same psychological symptoms, by associating the two cases Wilbur clearly insinuated that the moral authority that society accords to narratives produced by victims of the Holocaust could and should be accorded to her first patient's uncorroborated account of ritual mass murder. In addition, her talk as well as those presented by other experts during that first international conference, demonstrated that—the DSM III's formal description of the disorder not withstanding—there was a radical difference between the theoretical model of multiple personality which was actually being implemented in the late 20th century clinical milieu in the United States and the 19th century model of double personality and hysteria which had been developed by Janet and his contemporaries in France.

Whereas the latter focused on the unique psycho/physiological constitution of hysterics which made them vulnerable to a variety of relatively commonplace, albeit disturbing events, the poly-fragmented MPD model focused on the trauma itself. It hypothesized a direct relationship between the barbarous quality and quantity of multiples' childhood experiences on the one hand, and the number of personalities and the complexity of the personality systems that they exhibited, on the other. Experts argued that psychological dissociation could be charted along a continuum which ran from normal dissociative experiences, like highway hypnosis, to poly-fragmented MPD (e.g., Putnam, 1989).

Unfortunately, the case histories—like those summarized by Wilbur—that were used to elucidate this model, suggested that the hypothesized continuum was paralleled by a moral hierarchy of multiplicity. Paradoxically, instead of being perceived to be more profoundly impaired by the disorder, poly-fragmented, super-multiples were perceived to be more authoritative. This perception was reinforced by experts like Wilbur, who—after summarizing sensational case studies—repeatedly referred to their patients as their teachers; as portraits in courage. As a result, these clinical case studies were subtly transformed into morality tales.

Although poly-fragmented, super-multiples may not have been typical of the disorder, they were presented as exemplary by recognized experts, both in professional conferences and, more importantly to the mass media. During the early 1980s, practically every local and national television documentary program, that focused on MPD, featured one or more of the most respected theoreticians working in the field, as well as one or more patients, each of whom reported 30 or more personalities, and all of whom were described as having experienced brutal child abuse. At no time, in any of these programs, did any of the experts ever suggest that both these patients' vulnerability to suggestion and the demand characteristics of the theoretical model of psychopathology, that they had been induced to accommodate behaviorally during treatment, could have had a decisive influence on their reported symptoms as well as the content of their professed autobiographical traumatic memories.

In the years following the publication of the DSM III, the numbers of diagnosed multiples in North America rose dramatically, as did attendance at professional meetings and continuing medical education programs that focused on the disorder. By 1986 more than four hundred papers, presentations, books, articles, radio, and television programs, workshops, and seminars had appeared, including three major international conferences (e.g., Greaves, 1986). Although the new diagnosis seemed to be a resounding success, audio transcripts of presentations made at professional meetings revealed a disturbing trend. The numbers of personalities reported by a significant number of patients was rising and the contents of their recovered memories was becoming increasingly bizarre. In 1986, an informal survey of participants at the Third International Conference on Multiple Personality/Dissociative States (e.g., Braun & Gray, 1987) found that—over and above their recovered memories of violent child abuse—approximately 25% of multiples were recalling that they had been tortured in ritualized satanic sex-orgies where adults and children had been murdered and cannibalized.

The potentially political impact of these fantastic stories was enormous because by the mid-1980s, the influence of the MPD model had spread throughout the child abuse prevention and the adult survivor movements. By this time, a number of surveys had been published which suggested that hundreds of thousands of women had been victims of childhood sexual abuse. Furthermore, hypnosis researchers had confirmed that high trance capacity was proportionally distributed across the entire population. Once the link between child abuse and MPD had been established, experts treating the disorder had pointed out that, since they regularly encountered dissociating patients, who were clearly not multiple but who were suffering from a form of traumatically induced psychogenic amnesia, and since it was presumptive that all dissociative disorders shared similar mechanisms, in all probability, there were an enormous number of undiagnosed multiples in the psychiatric population—both in and out of treatment (e.g., Greaves, 1984). This reasoning incited many mental health professionals to suspect that dissociated memories of child abuse, particularly sexual abuse, might be responsible for a wide variety of psychological problems.

Paradoxically, at a time when experimental researchers in hypnosis had repeatedly demonstrated through controlled studies that the apparent enhancement of a subject's memory when in hypnoid states is actually a powerful illusion and that hypnotized subjects tend to spontaneously confabulate information (e.g., Orne, 1959, 1979; Spiegel, 1974, 1978, 1980), evolving clinical wisdom intimated that the special authority that was afforded to the accounts of extreme violence which multiples, with the help of therapists, reconstructed through their subpersonalities from intrusive images and affects, could be extended to similar material which non-multiples directly experienced in dissociated states of consciousness, such as dreams, guided imagery, hypnotic regression, and flashbacks (e.g., Loftus, 1980). In addition, some mental health professionals, working with women experiencing chronic psychological distress, had begun hypothesizing that even when their clients were unable to recover explicit traumatic memories, they could still have been victims of childhood incest (e.g., Bass & Davis, 1988). These clinical assumptions, which were sanctioned to a large extent by the MPD model of memory, were particularly problematic because by 1986, recovered memories of child sexual abuse had begun entering the courtroom. Adults, who had recovered heretofore unsuspected memories of childhood incest during therapy, had begun arguing that, because they had been amnestic for the abuse, the courts should toll the prevailing statute of limitations and allow them to sue their alleged abusers (e.g., Ernsdorff & Loftus, 1993).

Given this volatile social and legal climate, one might have expected that the task force of experts assigned to revise the DSM III dissociative disorders category—which included the author of the aforementioned 1986 survey of MPD and satanic cult involvement—would have included among their revisions at least a mention of the fact that there was some evidence that some of the memories recovered by a significant number of patients diagnosed as MPD might not be historically accurate. However, when it appeared in 1987, although the extensively revised description of the disorder did note that over half of recently reported cases of MPD reported more than 10 personalities—instead of recommending that clinicians exercise caution when doing memory work with their patients' ever extending list of alter personalities, it advised that both hypnosis and amobarbital could be used to elicit transitions from one personality to another.

Unlike the DSM III, that had defined both original personalities and subpersonalities as a fully integrated, complex psychological units, the DSM III-R (1987) defined personality as "a relatively enduring pattern of perceiving, relating to, and thinking about the environment, and one's self." Furthermore, it subsumed under the same term: personality, both personalities, which were described as patterns that were "exhibited in a wide range of important social and personal contexts," as well as personality states, which were described as "patterns that were not exhibited in as wide a range of contexts." Moreover, according to the revised definition, individuals who exhibited only one distinct personality and one or more personality states qualified for the same diagnosis as individuals who exhibited two or more distinct personalities. Unfortunately, this formulation is so vague that both inexperienced clinicians and their patients could plausibly confuse relatively enduring personality states with relatively enduring altered states of consciousness, an error which would significantly impact both the ongoing process and the outcome of therapy.

This erosion of the theoretical model, which effectively extended the diagnosis over a substantially larger clinical population, had serious social and legal implications because the revised description of MPD explicitly reinforced the causal link between the embodiment of a personality on the one hand, and abuse or other forms of severe trauma in childhood on the other, which had only been postulated in the DSM III.

At this point it is important to remember that many of the individuals who entered treatment for MPD toward the end of the 1980s, brought along rather unusual cultural baggage. Since the late 1960s, rumors of clandestine satanic cult activity had become something of an epiphenomena in American popular culture (Lyons, 1970; Victor, 1993). Throughout the 1970's and the early 1980's—stimulated both by organized middle-class reaction to the promiscuous life style and exotic religious pursuits that had been championed by the hippie counter-culture movement, and mass-media coverage of the murdering rampage of Charles Manson's gang—the tabloids and a number of Christian fundamentalist publications had exhibited a predilection for feature stories about the exploits of covert Satanists, who were held responsible for an outbreak of cattle mutilations and a series of bizarre or unexplained murders (Ellis, 1990; Balach & Gilliam, 1991).

The trend spawned a series of paperback books, including two purported autobiographical accounts of satanic cult involvement: The Satan Seller (Warnke, 1972) and Michelle Remembers (Padzer & Smith). The first volume was written by a born-again, Christian evangelist who claimed that, before he found Jesus, he had been a satanic high priest, possessed of supernatural powers. According to the author, Satanists constituted a hierarchically organized, international brotherhood that had been secretly running the world for centuries. He provided lurid descriptions of ritual gang rape, blood drinking, and the ceremonial amputation and ingestion of the tips of initiates' little fingers, supplemented by examples of his own supernatural exploits which included casting a spell on a building and burning it to the ground. The second book, co-authored by a psychiatrist and his wife (and former patient), described the young woman's memories of childhood abuse at the hands of a satanic cult, that she had recovered during deep trance states that had begun while she was in therapy with her future husband. According to the text, she had been saved from the grip of Satan himself by a divine intervention of the Virgin Mary. The book included intriguing photographs of diabolical stigmata and celestial ectoplasms hovering over bonfires which ostensibly corroborated her story.

As might have been expected, the authors of both of these novels enjoyed considerable mass-media attention, and arguably their stories were instrumental in shaping popular beliefs about organized satanic practices. Moreover, in all probability, many of the individuals who were ultimately diagnosed as multiples shared some of these beliefs. However, the repeated invocation of supernatural evidence—the casting of spells and spectral apparitions—which characterized these texts confirmed that they were basically religious documents. In other words, although they may have had a profound impact on certain cultural and religious beliefs, when they appeared, they did not have a significant impact on the functioning of the criminal justice system.

In contrast, although there is evidence that many of the memories of satanic ritual abuse which are produced by poly-fragmented multiples include supernatural elements when they first emerge in therapy, clinicians generally dismiss these elements as hallucinations which covert satanists have cleverly induced in their victims by forcing them to ingest hallucinogenic drugs or by subjecting them to sophisticated mind control techniques (e.g., Mulhern, 1994). As a result, although the case histories of multiples who recovered memories of satanic ritual abuse that were endorsed by mental health professionals during the 1980s were clearly problematic—because they included detailed accounts of extreme, sadistic violence which should have generated some enduring material evidence—they were often accepted as accurate descriptions of real crimes because they ostensibly complied with the laws of physics and because of the victims' unusual psychiatric conditions.

One year after the publication of the DSM III-R, multiples claiming to have been victims of satanic ritual abuse, habitually accompanied by therapists who underscored the seriousness of the heretofore unrecognized social problem, made a spectacular debut on nationally televised talk-shows in the United States (e.g., Rivera, 1988). Even as they spoke, politicians in the State of Washington were preparing landmark legislation that permits the tolling of the statute of limitations in cases of recovered memory of sexual abuse. Clearly, even if the DSM III-R had recommended that clinicians treating multiples totally abandon recovered memory work, it would have not be able to forestall these portentous developments. However, it remains that some mention of these patients' vulnerability to suggestion might have encouraged some clinicians to think more critically about their patients' productions. However, critical thinking was not the order of the day.

During the next few years, extravagant stories of recovered memories of secret ceremonies, bloody rituals, butchered babies, and high-tech mind control experiments filled the halls of hospital units specialized in MPD, newspaper headlines, continuing medical education seminars, talk-shows, churches, and occasionally courtrooms. There were satanic ritual abuse indicators, satanic calendars, a Projective Ideomotor Screening Procedure to Assist in Early Identification of Ritualistic Abuse Victims—that is featured in the American Society of Clinical Hypnosis (1990) Handbook of Hypnotic Suggestions, and Metaphors—and even a satanic Rorschach Test. Critics, including law enforcement officials who had thoroughly investigated but failed to corroborate patients' claims of murder, and child sacrifice, who dared to question this material, were routinely castigated by survivors and therapists alike, who claimed to have clinical evidence that the stories were true.

But what constituted clinical evidence? Invariably, when everything else had been accounted for, the bottom line, the unequivocal proof offered for the veracity of these patients' grotesque memories was that they were MPD. By 1993, as feminist activist Louise Armstrong (1994) wrote in exasperation, "alarm about so-called false memories of incest and satanic or ritual or cult abuse now raged everywhere. And the most spectacular disorder the issue of incest and severe childhood abuse had so far thrown up, Multiple Personality Disorder was everywhere these things were and anywhere they were not."

It would be a gross oversimplification to suggest that the DSM III variant of Multiple Personality Disorder caused the traumatic memory/ recovered memory debate. However, it was clearly instrumental in defining it. During the past two decades, theoreticians of MPD have maintained that the American Psychiatric Association's vote to dismantle hysteria, to disassociate and reclassify the aggregate somatic and psychological symptoms—which Janet had described as distinguishing the disorder—in discrete diagnostic categories, and to individuate the psychological dissociative disorders, has facilitated clinicians' abilities to identify and effectively treat patients' heretofore neglected underlying morbid mental states. These same experts have developed, tested, and re-tested a battery of structured diagnostic instruments which they argue, reliably prove that Dissociative Identity Disorder (formerly Multiple Personality Disorder) is a legitimate clinical entity. However, they have paid scant attention to the fact that their devices are not simply passive reflectors of the world as it is. Like the experimental tools devised by the laboratory sciences, clinical instruments do not only produce data; they isolate and create phenomena (e.g., Hacking, 1992).

As anthropologist Allen Young (1995) has demonstrated in his recent study of another widely debated clinical entity, PTSD, psychological phenomena are not immutable objects; timeless truths which exist outside of culture. They are "techno-phenomena" which are mediated through ideas, practices, and technologies which have been devised by human beings, at specific places and times, to accommodate specific needs. As we have seen, the ramifications of the pattern of unusual behavior that was defined and promoted by the architects of MPD as a clinical "illness entity" in the late 1970s and early 1980s, were not confined to the clinical milieu. The disorder was socialized as an expedient behavioral idiom of distress which afforded a limited cohort of individuals an intelligible means of expressing personal pain even as it allowed society to contain and control the institutional crisis which had been precipitated by the radical feminist's and child protection movement's recognizably legitimate demands for justice and radical political and legal change.

When examined from a socio/historical perspective, idioms of distress appear as conservative cultural mechanisms that allow communities to translate potentially disastrous conflicts within conventional, appreciated social bounds in which they can be safely examined (e.g., Littlewood, 1996). Although change may be inevitable, it must be processed slowly, in a manner which does not undermine the cultural and institutional fabric of society. In the interim, the dramatic behaviors which are sanctioned within the carefully circumscribed space of idioms of distress generally maintain the status quo by fostering the illusion that things are moving ahead (e.g., Krohn, 1978). However, when the boundaries which contain an idiom of distress breakdown, as they did in the case of MPD, the uncontrolled social propagation of the pattern of behavior which was elicited by the idiom may exacerbate the crisis from which it arose in the first place.

Beginning in the late 1970s, multiples were promoted by representatives of the mental health establishment as visible proof of both the reality of the secret world of incest and child sexual abuse and the fact that its victims suffered profound, lasting damage. However, because of their extraordinary psychological abilities, their hidden subpersonalities were widely regarded as incorruptible unconscious repositories and reliable colporteurs of historical truth. To a great extent, it was the professed historical integrity of the poly-fragmented multiples' recovered memories of extreme childhood abuse which sanctioned the belief that accounts of heretofore unremembered child abuse, which are derived from unconscious traumatic memories which have been recovered by adults experiencing altered states of consciousness, are necessarily more historically accurate than accounts of such events that are derived from continuous, conscious memories which, like other normal memories, are subject to the vicissitudes of time and a host of psycho/social influences. When the linchpin collapsed, the entire edifice fractured. Today, we are left to sort out the pieces.

Much of the contemporary social, political, and legal debate regarding recovered memories is constructed on the premise that the same psycho-social factors operate in a wide and disparate variety of cases: The 1990 case of a 35-year-old poly-fragmented multiple who (while embodying in rotation 127 different alter personalities) co-constructed with her therapist over a 3.5-year period horrifying accounts of skinning babies; the 1995 case of a 25-year-old woman who did not report, when interviewed by a researcher, a sexual molestation that occurred when she was a small child; the 1977 case of a woman of 50 who, when hearing that her daughter has been assaulted, suddenly remembering having been assaulted herself when she was a college undergraduate; Evelyn's case of recovered memories of early childhood rape. The assumption that all such cases reflect the operation of the same psycho/social factors is simply not true. Although the narratives produced in these cases may in fact contain elements which accurately reflect experienced events, they can only be fully understood when they are replaced in their respective socio/historical contexts.

Dr. Wagenaar may find it ironic that I have responded to his presentation with the sociological equivalent of a case history. However, as he noted in his conclusion, although case histories may not be used for testing scientific theories, we can still learn from them because they can help us uncover weaknesses in the various social systems through that we produce, elaborate, and propagate the theoretical models by that we organize and structure our lives. Today, in courtrooms around the world, hundreds of Evelyns, Davids and Dr. Subardjos are telling stories of remembered and remembering violence. Each of these stories has been profoundly influenced by a complex network of social and psychological factors. Although the preceding commentary highlighted only a few, select aspects of the history of one of these factors: the socialization of the DSM III theoretical model of Multiple Personality Disorder, it is my belief that a thorough analysis of this entire history has as much to contribute to the resolution of their conflicts as a scientific theory of memory.

REFERENCES

American Broadcasting Companies, Inc. (1983). *20/20 : The People Inside Me*. Denver, CO: Journal Graphics, Inc.

Angel, R. & Thoits, P. (1987). The Impact of Culture on the Cognitive Structure of Illness. *Culture, Medicine and Psychiatry, 11*, 465–494.

APA (1980). *Diagnostic and Statistical Manual (DSM-III)*. Washington, D.C. American Psychiatric Association.

APA (1994). *Diagnostic and Statistical Manual (DSM-IV)*. Washington, D.C. American Psychiatric Association.

Armstrong, L. (1994). *Rocking the Cradle of Sexual Politics: What happened when women said incest*. New York: Addison-Wesley Publishing Company.

Balch, R.W. & Gilliam, M. (1991). Devil worship in western Montana: A case study in rumor construction. In Richardson, J.T., Best, J. & Bromley, D.G. (Eds.), *The Satanism Scare*. New York: Aldine de Gruyter.

Barrois, C. (1988). *Les Névroses Traumatiques*. Paris, Dunod.

Bass, E. & Davis, L., (1988). *The Courage to Heal*. New York: Harper & Row Publishers.

Braun, B.G. & Gray, G. (1987). Report on the 1986 mpd questionnaire - MPD and cult involvement. *Fourth International Conference on Multiple Personality/ Dissociative States*. Alexandria, VA: Audio Transcripts Va-383–87.

Edelman, N. (1995). *Voyantes, Guérisseuses, et Visionnaires en France: 1785–1914*. Paris: Albin Michel.

Elliot, D. (1982). State Intervention and Childhood Multiple Personality Disorder. *The Journal of Psychiatry and Law, 10*, 441–456.

Ellis, B. (1990). Cattle mutilation: Contemporary legends and contemporary mythologies. *Perspectives on Contemporary Legend Conference*. Sheffield, England.

Ernsdorff, G.M. & Loftus, E.F. (1993). Let Sleeping Memories Lie? Words of caution about tolling the statue of limitations in cases of memory repression. *The Journal of Criminal Law and Criminology, 84:1*, 129–174.

Freud, S. (1950). Letter of 21, September, 1887. In Bonaparte, M., Freud, A. & Kris, E. (Eds. & Trans.), *The origins of psychoanalysis: Letters to Wilhelm Fliess, drafts and notes: 1887–1902*. New York: Basic Books.

Freud, S. (1952). Zur ätiologie der hysterie. *Weitere bemerkungen über die abwehr-neuropsychosen*. GW, I. London: Imago. (Original work published, 1886).

Gil, E. (1990). *United We Stand: A book for people with multiple personalities*. Walnut Creek, CA: Launch Press.

Greaves, G. (1986). Book Review. *ISSMP&D Newsletter, 4:3*, 3.

Greaves, G. (1984). Editorial. *International Society for the Study of Multiple Personality Newsletter, 2:2*, 4.

Hacking, I. (1992). The Self-Vindication of the Laboratory Sciences. In Pickering, A. (Ed.), *Science and Practice and Culture*, (pp. 29–64). Chicago: University of Chicago Press.

Janet, P. (1911). *L'Etat Mental des Hystériques*. Paris: Alcan.

Janet, P. (1889). *L'Automatisme Psychologique*. Paris: Félix Alcan.

Kempe, C.H., Silverman, F.N., Steele, B.F. Droegemueller, W. & Silver, H.K. (1962). The Battered-Child Syndrome. *The Journal of the American Medical Association, 181*, 17–24.

Kluft, R.P. (1991). Clinical Presentations of Multiple Personality Disorder. *The Psychiatric Clinics of North America, 14:13,* 605–630.

Krohn, A. (1978) Hysteria the Elusive Neurosis. *Psychological Issues, Monograph 45–46, 11, 1/2.*

Lawrence, J.R. & Perry, C. (1988). *Hypnosis, Will and Memory.* New York: The Guilford Press.

Littlewood, R. (1996). Psychopathology, Embodiment and Religious Innovation. In Bhugra, D. (Ed.), *Psychiatry and Religion: Context, Consensus and Controversies.* (pp. 178–197). London: Routledge.

Loftus, E.F., Loftus, G.R. (1980). On the permanence of stored information in the human brain. *American Psychologist, 35,* 409–420.

Lyons, A. (1970). *The Second Coming.* New York: Dood, Mead & Company.

Micale, M.S. (1995). *Approaching Hysteria.* Princeton, NJ: Princeton University Press.

Mulhern, S. (1994). Satanism, Ritual abuse and Multiple Personality: A socio/historical perspective. *The International Journal of Clinical and Experimental Hypnosis, 62:4,* 265–288.

Mulhern, S. (1995). Inceste au Carrefour des Fantasmes et des Fantômes. In Castro, D. (Ed.), *Incestes* (pp.). Paris: l'Esprit du Temps - Psychologie.

Orne, M.T. (1979) The use and misuse of hypnosis in court. *International Journal of Clinical and Experimental Hypnosis, 27,* 311–341.

Orne, M.T. (1959) The nature of hypnosis: artifact and essence." *Journal of Abnormal Social Psychology, 58,* 277–299.

Padzer, L. & Smith, M. (1980). *Michelle Remembers.* New York: Pocket Books.

Putnam, F.W. (1989). *Diagnosis and Treatment of Multiple Personality Disorder.* New York: The Guilford Press.

Rivera, G. (1988). *Devil Worship: Exposing Satan's underground.* New York: Journal Graphics, Inc.

Ross, C.A. (1996). *Dissociative Identity Disorder.* New York: John Wiley & Sons, Inc.

Rush, F. (1980). *The Best Kept Secret: The sexual abuse of children.* New York: McGraw-Hill Book Company.

Rush, F. (1971). *The Sexual Abuse of Children: A feminist point of view.* Paper presented at the New York Radical Feminist Rape Conference, April, 1971.

Scheper-Hughes, N. & Stein, H.F. (1987). Child Abuse and the Unconscious in American Popular Culture. In Scheper-Hughes, N. (Ed.), *Child Survival* (pp.). Netherlands: D. Reidel Publishing Company.

Spiegel, H. (1980) Hypnosis and evidence: help or hinderance? *Annals of the New York Academy of Sciences, 347,* 73–85.

Spiegel, H. (1974) The grade 5 syndrome: the highly hypnotizable person. *The International Journal of Clinical and Experimental Hypnosis, 22,* 303–319.

Victor, J.S. (1993). *Satanic Panic: The creation of a contemporary legend.* Chicago: Open Court.

Warnke, M. (1972). *The Satan Seller.* New Jersey: Logos International.

Wilbur, C. (1984). Multiple Personality and Child Abuse: An Etiologic Overview. *First International Conference on Multiple Personality/ Dissociative States.* Alexandria, VA: Audio Transcripts Va-1A-127–84

Young, A. (1995). *The Harmony of Illusions.* Princeton, NJ: Princeton University Press.

QUESTION AND ANSWER SESSION

Brewer. The anchoring analysis seems fine for what goes on in court. You make a hard line distinction between science and case histories. But in your work on your own autobiographical memory you have found that low frequency events are better remembered than high frequency events. How can you say that such an observation does not belong to science ?

Wagenaar. You should not confuse case histories and N=1 studies. The N=1 study is to test a theory, unlike case studies. You may argue that even experimental tests are based on some beliefs, but my answer is that these beliefs are made explicit, and that they are shared by all experimenters.

Schooler. It is useful to consider the assumptions that underlie case histories, and I agree that case studies are only as good as the anchors on which they are based. I also agree that courts add a lot of complexity to science because they have different objectives. If we base science on case outcome, we have a problem. But science is also based on beliefs; you don't prove things, you only reject a null hypothesis. Some experiments prove nothing because the proper controls are missing. Some case histories have proved to be extremely helpful. From H.M. we learned a lot about short term and long term memory; the split brain patients were useful in understanding the differences between the two hemispheres. Case studies are helpful in the advancement of science, just as experimentation.

Wagenaar. I agree only partly. The fact that some experiments lack the proper controls means only that one should design better experiments. It is no excuse for accepting case histories without the proper controls. I am not saying that case histories cannot prove anything at all; my argument is that case histories lack the natural anchoring provided by classical experimentation. The number of anchors needed to accept a case history as proof of anything at all is surprisingly large. In the case of Evelyn, described in my talk, it is even impossible to produce anchors that would turn the story into a proof of the existence of recovered memories.

Hyman. If you throw out case histories, then neurology, biology, and evolutionary theory is gone. Theories predict that certain things will happen; then we find a case that confirms the prediction, which is as clear a corroboration as an experiment. Bill Brewer's point should be well taken; case studies can cause us to throw out an entire theory, if the theory says that the observation was not supposed to happen.

Wagenaar. I disagree that my position leads to the rejection of entire disciplines. If a theory predicts that some events should happen, one would accept observations of such events only if they had been properly anchored. Neurologists, biologists, and astronomers collect observations, but not without generally accepted theories; instead usually the anchors are challenged and the observations rejected. The systematic observation of the stellar world by astronomers resembles systematic experimentation, more than collecting case histories.

Shuman. If what you say is correct, then what can a treating clinician know in the way of historical accuracy and what does this suggest about the appropriate role of the treating clinician in judicial proceedings? I don't think clinicians should fold up their tent and go home. I think that there is scientifically and ethically an appropriate role and that role is to describe the history that is provided to you by the patient, to describe your assessment of the mental status of the patient and your grounds for a diagnosis, to describe the treatment that you provided and how the patient has responded and so on. I think that if you avoid issues of causation that you are ethically and scientifically on appropriate grounds.

Wagenaar. I agree completely, but the problem is that the courts want our opinion on matters of causation. In Evelyn's case the court wanted to know whether her suffering was caused by the alleged abuse many years ago. The issue of the loss of memory due to traumatic experiences and the later recovery of memory cannot be addressed on the basis of case histories, unless the expert is prepared to establish causality between some trauma and the loss of memory, between recovery and a luxating event. If we claim, like Jonathan Schooler (this volume), that we have discovered some reliable cases of recovered memories, we are implicitly making these causal judgments. I would never do that.

6

CLINICAL AND EXPERIMENTAL APPROACHES TO UNDERSTANDING REPRESSION

Chris R. Brewin

Royal Holloway
University of London
Egham, Surrey TW20 0EX
United Kingdom

1. EXPLANATIONS OF OBSERVED FORGETTING

Clinicians working with survivors of traumatic experiences have frequently noted the existence of psychogenic amnesia and the recovery of additional memories during clinical sessions, although amnesia for significant parts of a traumatic event is probably only found in a minority of cases. Recently, surveys of women in therapy for the effects of childhood sexual abuse and other problems have found that a substantial proportion, varying from around 20–60%, report periods of forgetting some or all of the abuse (e.g., Briere & Conte, 1993; Elliott & Briere, 1995; Herman & Schatzow, 1987; Loftus, Polonsky, & Fullilove, 1994; van der Kolk & Fisler, 1995). Follow-up studies of children with documented abuse also find that abuse is sometimes not reported when the children are re-interviewed some years later, both under conditions in which they are explicitly asked about these events (Bagley, 1995) and in which they are not (Williams, 1994). A national survey of the experiences of American psychologists (Feldman-Summers & Pope, 1994) also found reported periods of forgetting in 40% of those reporting abuse.

Clinicians have generally atttributed this forgetting to psychological defence mechanisms, particularly repression and dissociation. In discussing repression, it is necessary to begin with a description of the original formulation of the concept and of its relation to other clinical phenomena involving psychogenic forgetting. In 1895 Breuer and Freud noted "...it was a question of things which the patient wished to forget, and therefore intentionally repressed from his conscious thought and inhibited and suppressed" (p. 61). There are many indications that Freud was uncertain about whether repression should be thought of as a process that is unconscious from the outset ("primary repression"), to be contrasted with a conscious act of suppression, or whether repression should be considered as an unconscious process that only develops following a period of deliberate suppression ("repression proper" or "after-expulsion"). This uncertainty has remained with the field ever since.

Recollections of Trauma, edited by Read and Lindsay
Plenum Press, New York, 1997

The other major defence mechanism associated with forgetting is dissociation, the focus of theorizing by Janet in the last century (Janet, 1889). A dissociative state is an altered state of consciousness in which ordinary cognitive or motor functioning is impaired. For example, there appears to be a spectrum of dissociative states involving greater or lesser degrees of awareness of the current environment. Thus, in therapy sessions, dissociative states may range from a reduced ability to hear or see the therapist, a transient sense of depersonalisation or derealisation, or an out-of-body experience, to a complete loss of awareness of time and space. Sometimes these states are accompanied by "flashbacks," a term I use to include a spectrum of intrusions from fragmentary sensorimotor experiences to the sensation of vividly reliving a past event in the present. Other dissociative states involve what appears to be a separate personality. Although dissociation does not invariably involve amnesia, lack of memory for events experienced in different states is common.

Although repression and dissociation are often not clearly distinguished, there appears to be an important difference between theoretical descriptions of "after-expulsion" and dissociation. Ordinarily, autobiographical memories are more or less accessible to being retrieved into "working memory," a short-term, limited capacity store in which memories can be readily rehearsed and edited. A memory that has once been consciously available but has simply become repressed following deliberate attempts to forget is in principle no different to any other autobiographical memory, although the probability of it being retrieved is by definition very low. Once retrieved, however, the new information is presumably free to be edited and to interact with the rest of accessible autobiographical memory. Retrieval of a dissociated memory, on the other hand, is expected to be accompanied by changes in consciousness that disrupt working memory. The memory often has a stereotyped repetitive quality that endures over multiple retrievals, and access to the new information does not guarantee the possibility of interaction with the rest of the autobiographical memory system. In these respects it would appear to have many of the characteristics of an informationally encapsulated, modular process being run off.

Both repressive and dissociative forgetting imply the presence of cognitive mechanisms that specifically inhibit the activation of representations of the traumatic event and prevent them from entering working memory. In contrast, Loftus (Loftus, Garry, & Feldman, 1994) suggested that the forgetting of trauma is no different from the forgetting of everyday events, and that no special mechanisms are required to explain it. Forgetting can be accounted for by the normal processes of interference, or of the gradual decay of an unrehearsed memory trace, resulting in a progressive decrease in the probability of it being retrieved.

A third explanation for the apparent "forgetting" and then recall of childhood trauma has been promulgated by the False Memory Syndrome Foundation (FMSF) in the U.S. and by its counterpart in the U.K., the British False Memory Society (BFMS). It has been suggested that at least some of the memories of child sexual abuse (CSA) recovered in therapy may not be veridical, but may be false memories "implanted" by therapists who have prematurely decided that the patient is an abuse victim and who use inappropriate therapeutic techniques to persuade the client to recover corresponding "memories." A less extreme scenario would involve therapists who had a strong bias to explain problems in terms of early abuse encouraging clients to explore the possibility of repressed memories without due acknowledgment of the fallibility of memory and the power of suggestion. The false memory societies have claimed that there are many cases known to them in which previously happy families have been disrupted by accusations of abuse that were only triggered by an adult child entering therapy with a poorly-trained or "fringe" practitioner. Various other experimental psychologists, clinicians, and members of the scientific advisory boards of the false memory societies have now also warned about the likely unreliability of "memories" recovered in this way (Kihlstrom, 1995; Loftus, 1993; Merskey, 1995; Pope and Hudson, 1994; Wakefield & Underwager, 1992).

Which of these explanations is more likely to be correct? Are all correct? Can any be ruled out? A major consideration is plausibility. Members of the scientific advisory boards of the false memory societies have argued that it is implausible that many of these memories of abuse apparently recovered after long periods of time correspond to actual events because: (a) the content is either stereotypical, conforming to therapists' preconceptions about the causes of psychological disorder, or highly unusual, for example of Satanic rituals with human sacrifices; (b) the age at which the events are supposed to have occurred may precede the development of explicit event memory; (c) there is typically no independent corroboration of the events; (d) therapists may hold inaccurate beliefs about the accuracy of memory and may employ procedures such as hypnosis or guided fantasy that increase the risk of imaginary scenes and images being interpreted as actual events; and (e) the conditions under which recall occurs, for example within therapy sessions, may be stereotyped, again reflecting therapists' preconceptions.

Equally, more plausibility would accrue to the view that recovered memories typically do correspond to actual events if it could be shown: (a) the content of most recovered memories concerns a variety of events known to occur with reasonable frequency, and is not limited to CSA; (b) the age at which the events are said to have occurred extends beyond the period of infant amnesia; (c) corroboration occurs with reasonable frequency given the nature of the alleged incidents; (d) well-trained therapists not using inappropriate techniques also report clients recovering memories; and (e) recall is not stereotyped but occurs under a variety of conditions.

Given that forgetting of actual trauma is agreed to occur, the plausibility of competing accounts of forgetting depends in part on whether (a) clients report active attempts to forget memories or banish them from consciousness, and (b) hypothesized defence mechanisms such as repression and dissociation have parallels in everyday cognitive processing. It is therefore worth asking if there is evidence for inhibitory processes in cognition, and whether there is any support for the notion that a subgroup of individuals might demonstrate specific problems in the learning and recall of negatively valenced stimuli. In the rest of this chapter we consider the clinical and experimental evidence relevant to these issues.

2. CLINICAL AND SURVEY EVIDENCE

2.1. Content of Recovered Memories

Several surveys have now been published that indicate the kinds of conditions surrounding memory recovery and the content of the memories. Morton et al. (1995) reviewed the frequency with which, according to records kept by the false memory societies, recovered memories involved reports of Satanic or ritual abuse (SRA). The American data were abstracted from a report produced in Summer 1993 by the director of the False Memory Syndrome Foundation. This indicated that 11% of callers mentioned such abuse when asked an open-ended question, and 18% when asked a closed question. The British data were derived from inspection of around 200 records made available by the director of the BFMS. In this sample 6% of callers to the BFMS volunteered information that memories involved SRA. A subsequent survey of around 400 BFMS members

(Gudjonsson, in press) obtained a 70% response rate, with approximately 70% of responders agreeing that recovered memories were involved in the accusations, 20% not being sure, and 10% denying that recovered memories were involved. Thus clear indications about the possible involvement of recovered memories were only obtained from about half the membership. Data from this survey were reanalyzed by Andrews (in press) to enable them to be directly compared with those obtained from previous surveys. Seven percent of respondents agreed that accusations involved SRA when asked a closed question about it.

Andrews et al. (1995) sent questionnaires to approximately 4,000 chartered psychologists in the UK and obtained a response rate of 27%. Almost half of the 810 with relevant caseloads who replied reported they had had a patient retrieve a memory from total amnesia (i.e., the patient reported no knowledge of the event prior to memory recovery) while in therapy with them. Respondents were also asked whether they had come across a client alleging Satanic ritual abuse, whether or not this involved a recovered memory. Fifteen percent of respondents replied they had had at least one such client.

The Andrews et al. survey also inquired about memories for non-CSA events. Over a quarter of the respondents reported having clients recovering such memories in the past year. Because the vast majority had at least 1 client reporting CSA, it was possible that these memories were exclusively related to that experience, and arose only in the course of recovering CSA memories. To control for this possibility, respondents who had no CSA clients were distinguished from the rest. The proportions with clients with non-CSA recovered memories were fairly similar in the two groups - 29% with CSA clients and 21% with no such clients. Other studies have similarly reported the existence of non-CSA recovered memories (Feldman-Summers & Pope, 1994). A current interview study of therapists is collecting more detailed information about such memories, and preliminary data will be reported during this conference (see Andrews, this volume).

2.2. Age of Memory

There is currently some dispute about the earliest age at which episodic memories of significant childhood events may be retained and later retrieved. Some reports put this as early as the third year of life (Howes, Siegel, & Brown, 1993; Usher & Neisser, 1993). In any event, there is agreement on the paucity of evidence for later retrieval of verbal memories from the first two years of life, and on the rarity of memories from the third year of life. It is also important to distinguish between memories for single events falling within the period of infant amnesia, and memories for a series of events that commenced within the period of infant amnesia but continued for several years. Whereas the former are highly implausible, the latter may be more readily explained as involving guesses about the age of onset without necessarily casting doubt on the validity of the pattern of events described.

Morton et al. (1995) reported that, according to the American FMSF data, 26% of allegations involved abuse that had begun when the child was aged 0–2. However, only 6% of allegations involved abuse that ended before age 5. In the British data 4% of allegations involved abuse that ended before age 5. This figure has since been confirmed by Gudjonsson (1995).

2.3. Corroboration

Some authors (e.g. Pope & Hudson, 1995) demand stringent evidence of the authenticity of a memory before they are willing to concede that it has been recovered after a period of amnesia. Feldman-Summers and Pope (1994) asked their respondents for any corroborative evidence for recovered memories of abuse. Forty-seven percent reported some corroboration, for example the abuser acknowledged some or all of the remembered abuse, someone who knew about the abuse told the respondent, or someone else reported abuse by the same perpetrator.

Despite the problems arising from the relatively recent appreciation of the extent and importance of child sexual abuse, and the fact that such events often occur in secret, Pope and Hudson argued that independent, documented evidence is required if the concept of the recovery of forgotten memories of trauma is to be accepted at all. In fact there are reports of individual cases where documentary corroboration of forgotten trauma has been reported (Schooler, 1994). Such evidence is also available from Williams' (1994) follow-up study of women with documented histories of CSA. In her sample, approximately one in six of the women who recalled the abuse at interview said that there had been a period when they had completely forgotten the abuse. When current accounts of the abuse and the original records were compared, Williams (1995) reported that the accounts of women with recovered memories were just as accurate as those of women who had always remembered the abuse. Further examples of independently verified recovered memories were presented at this conference by Schooler, Andrews, Dalenberg, and Bendiksen.

2.4. Therapists and Their Practices

At least three studies have provided confirmation that some therapists hold beliefs that run contrary to what we know about memory. One survey of around 860 hypnotherapists and family therapists attending conferences and workshops in the United States was mainly concerned with beliefs about hypnosis (Yapko, 1994). The other investigated 145 US and 57 UK psychologists' practices and experiences as well as more general beliefs concerning memory recovery of sexual abuse in childhood (Poole, Lindsay, Memon, & Bull, 1995). Both surveys also found a high proportion of respondents endorsing the belief that recovered memories can be false. In Poole et al.'s study the British respondents (who were all chartered clinical psychologists) were less likely than their U.S. counterparts to use memory recovery techniques such as hypnosis and age regression, although both groups had similarly high rates of respondents reporting memory recovery in at least some clients.

The majority of the respondents in the Andrews et al. survey believed that false memories were possible, although the proportion with this belief (67%) was smaller than in the other two surveys asking this question (91%, Poole et al., 1995; 79%, Yapko, 1994). Twenty percent of those who had experienced recovered memories in their own practice thought they had also encountered examples of false memories. The majority of respondents also believed that recovered memories were sometimes or usually accurate (although a small minority believed they would always be so) - a question not asked in the other surveys. Use of hypnotic regression was reported by 10% of respondents, but was more common in Poole et al.'s survey.

2.5. Conditions of Recall

A central issue is whether recall occurs exclusively during therapy sessions, or after the onset of therapy, as opposed to before therapy. Feldman-Summers and Pope (1994) found that although over half of memories were recovered in the context of therapy, 44% of their respondents stated that recovery had been triggered exclusively in other contexts.

Andrews et al. (1995) reported that the most common context in which CSA memories were recovered was prior to any therapy, with nearly a third of respondents reporting that clients had recovered memories in this context. Just under a quarter had clients recovering CSA memories in therapy with them, and around one in five in therapy with someone else.

Of equal importance is the way in which memories are recovered. For example, Loftus et al. (1994) distinguished between recall from total and partial amnesia, finding the former somewhat more common than the latter in their sample. Similarly, Harvey and Herman (1994) described composite clinical cases illustrating partial amnesia, in which some knowledge of abuse was retained although there was forgetting of many salient facts and episodes, and profound amnesia, in which the autobiographical fact of abuse was forgotten along with the specific episodic memories. Harvey and Herman emphasized the complexity of traumatic forgetting and the fact that recall is rarely an all-or-none phenomenon.

In order to investigate the subjective aspects of memory recovery in more depth, Elaine Hunter, Bernice Andrews and I have recently carried out an interview study of 16 women currently or previously in therapy for the effects of CSA. A separate conference poster (this volume) presents the results in greater detail. The women were questioned in detail about the extent of any amnesia, the quality of the memories recovered, the context of memory recovery, and coping strategies employed both at the time of the remembered events and currently. We too found evidence for partial amnesia (6 cases), profound amnesia (6 cases) and no amnesia (4 cases). Table 1 shows that there were no gross differences between the groups in the age at which the abuse occurred, the frequency of abuse, or the identity of the abuser, although there was a slight tendency for amnesia to be associated with an earlier onset, more episodes, and (in the case of profound amnesia) parental CSA. Some rather more clear-cut differences did emerge, although these should be treated with extreme caution given the very small number of subjects in the groups.

Table 1 suggests that the individuals who had reported no amnesia differed from the other groups in that none of their parents had suffered from a mental illness and there was little evidence of other parental abuse. One respondent with no apparent amnesia for abuse reported repeated physical abuse from her stepfather, an out-of-body experience when the sexual abuse occurred, but a separate period of global amnesia in which she could remember no events occurring between ages 3–5 years. In contrast, two thirds of respondents in the other groups reported that at least one parent had a mental illness, and parental abuse of one sort or another was more likely.

Amnesia was also associated with the occurrence of flashbacks, a common feature of post-traumatic stress disorder (Brewin, Dalgleish, & Joseph, 1996; van der Kolk & Fis-

Table 1. Characteristics of recalled abuse associated with different levels of amnesia

	No amnesia N=4	Partial amnesia N=6	Profound amnesia N=6
Onset after 10 years	50%	17%	17%
3 episodes or fewer	50%	17%	33%
Parental sexual abuse	0%	0%	33%
Parental mental illness	0%	66%	66%
Other parental abuse	25%	50%	33%
Flashbacks	0%	50%	66%
Dissociative strategies	25%	50%	66%

ler, 1995). Flashbacks are unlike ordinary autobiographical memories because people experience in an intense and detailed way the sensory, motor and emotional components of the memory, and these details remain remarkably constant with repetition of the flashbacks. During the flashback the subjective sense of time changes so that the event appears to be happening now rather than belonging to the past. The second way in which these memories differ is that they cannot be deliberately accessed through a normal search of autobiographical memory. Rather, people learn which internal or external cues are likely to trigger them, and develop strategies to increase or decrease the probability of accessing the memories by manipulating their exposure to the relevant cues.

According to the dual representation theory of post-traumatic stress disorder (Brewin et al., 1996), flashbacks represent the activation of records of the detailed, nonconscious cognitive processing accorded to traumatic experiences. It is widely recognised that flashbacks are highly aversive experiences and that many individuals are strongly motivated to prevent their continued activation following a trauma, succeeding in this for periods of months or years. It is conceivable that partial or profound amnesia develops in order to eliminate internal cues that would be likely to trigger distressing flashbacks.

2.6. Attempts to Forget

The survey by Hunter, Brewin and Andrews revealed numerous reports of dissociative strategies, which Table 1 suggests to have been more commonly associated with amnesia. These took three forms. One was an out-of-body experience (3 respondents), in which during the assaults the respondent experienced them as happening to a separate corporeal entity, either her or someone who looked like her. This did not necessarily reflect a deliberate coping strategy. The second form was a conscious attempt to "blank out" or "distance" memories of the assaults during or after they had happened (3 respondents). The third strategy involved deliberately creating an imaginary world to which the respondent could escape and where they would be safe, either during or after the abuse (2 respondents).

Attempts to forget are also characteristic of the vast majority of trauma survivors, who similarly report in detail the strategies they use to banish upsetting thoughts and images from their minds (Briere, 1992; Herman, 1992). Successful behavioural treatment of post-traumatic stress disorder frequently involves countermanding these instructions and having clients choose to remember in detail all aspects of the traumatic experience (e.g., Rothbaum & Foa, 1996). It is also now recognised by cognitive-behaviour therapists that the effects of exposure to a feared stimulus may be blocked by distraction or cognitive avoidance (e.g. Rachman, 1980). Influential cognitive-behavioural theories now explicitly contain the idea that mental activity can be used to block feared images or thoughts, and considerable efforts are now made to diagnose and prevent cognitive avoidance at an early stage.

2.7. Summary

From the clinical observations reviewed it is apparent that there are indications that at least some recovered memories may not correspond to actual events. Some memories contain unusual content and refer to events that occurred at an age preceding the development of verbal memories. Some memories occur within a therapy context and cannot be corroborated, and some practitioners appear to have important misconceptions about the nature of memory. At the same time the data from these surveys suggest that many recovered memories are not susceptible to this kind of explanation. Memory recovery appears to be a remarkably robust phenomenon, occurring in and out of therapy and involving a wide variety of different types of event. Studies of poorly trained practitioners might however reveal a different pattern.

Of particular value is the clinical evidence that memory recovery may take several forms. Amnesia may be partial or profound, forgetting may appear more similar to repression or dissociation, and recovered memories may be in the form of flashbacks or ordinary autobiographical memories. This suggests that several different kinds of underlying cognitive process are likely to be necessary to explain such diverse phenomena. In search of such processes we now turn to the experimental literature.

3. EXPERIMENTAL EVIDENCE

Loftus (1993) and Lindsay and Read (1994, 1995) reviewed relevant literature on autobiographical memory, eyewitness testimony, reality monitoring, suggestibility, and studies concerning the fallibility and malleability of memory, concluding that the creation of false memories within therapy is a possibility that must be taken seriously. The likelihood of suggestive influences leading to memory errors is increased by the perceived authority and trustworthiness of the source of suggestions, repetition of suggestions, their plausibility and imagibility, and lowering of memory-monitoring response criteria (Lindsay & Read, 1995). As noted by these authors, such features may characterise a type of therapy that they term "long-term, multifaceted, suggestive memory work," and they review a considerable amount of evidence supporting the view that this type of therapy could indeed give rise to false memories.

I have no argument with these conclusions, and concur that such procedures are inappropriate and not in the interests of clients or their families. Rather than review this evidence in detail, I intend to discuss areas of experimental cognitive psychology that, although perhaps equally relevant, have been relatively neglected in the false memory debate.

3.1. Experimental Evidence for Inhibitory Processes

One could be forgiven, after reading some commentators, for concluding that repression was an outlandish notion believed in only by gullible clinicians and with no analogue in experimental research. In fact this does not seem to be the case, providing we define repression somewhat more narrowly than usual as a decrease in the level of activation, and hence of the accessibility of a specific representation in memory, produced by an active inhibitory process. At the most general level, we may note that an efficient nervous system depends on a balance between levels of activation in different systems, increased or decreased by facilitatory and inhibitory connections respectively. Moreover, the inhibition of behavioural responding is a very important aspect of the biological response to conditioned stimuli signalling fear or frustration (Gray, 1982). Other distinguished neuroscientists have suggested that repression and related phenomena can be explained by the inhibitory effects of fear on central cue-producing responses in the brain (Miller, 1995).

Inhibition in the cognitive system has been discussed by numerous researchers who investigate the topics of attention and memory. In a manner analogous to neuronal interactions, there is evidence for lateral inhibition of related constructs in memory. One example is retrieval-induced forgetting (Anderson, Bjork, & Bjork, 1994). In the study phase, subjects study several categories, each with a set of examples (e.g. Animal-Horse). In the second phase subjects practice retrieval of half the items from the studied categories, by completing category-plus-exemplar stem cue tests (e.g. Animal-Ho___). Following a retention interval, there is an unexpected recall test in which subjects are cued with the category name and asked to remember as many exemplars as possible. Under these conditions subjects recalled more of the practised items but at the expense of unpractised items from the same categories - recall of these unpractised items was impaired relative to recall of items from baseline categories in which no items were practised. Subsequent studies using this paradigm have suggested that there are active inhibitory processes serving to reduce the level of activation of unpractised items from practised categories (Anderson & Spellman, 1995).

Likewise, Simpson and Kang (1994) investigated the naming of words that were related to alternative meanings of a homograph prime. When subjects were first exposed to a prime-target pair exemplifying one meaning of the homograph, they were subsequently slower to name a target related to the other meaning of the homograph, compared to a target unrelated to the homograph. The previous context was effective in reducing the accessibility of words related to one meaning of the homograph, even when this was the dominant meaning. Simpson and Kang concluded from the results of several studies that these inhibitory processes were restricted to situations where there was potential interference between competing meanings, and where the subject made a commitment to one of the meanings in the form of a response. Initially, all competing meanings would be activated, but this would be followed by the suppression of unwanted or irrelevant meanings. For another example of work suggesting that the retrieval of weakly activated information is assisted by a centre-surround mechanism that inhibits the activation of competing items but has no effect on unrelated items, see Dagenbach, Carr and Barnhart (1990) and Carr and Dagenbach (1990).

However, inhibitory effects are not limited to stimuli that are already associated by virtue of prior learning. In their analysis of the neural substrate of attentional processes, Posner and Peterson (1990) distinguished between a posterior system that orients to objects in the external world and generates perceptual awareness, and an anterior system that orients to the meaning of internal stimuli such as percepts and guides selection for action. Rafal and Henik (1994) suggested that the anterior attentional system is able to maximise the efficiency of goal-directed behaviour by exercising inhibitory control over automatic processes.

For example, Tzelgov, Henik, and Berger (1992) investigated the effect of expectations on the Stroop test, in which subjects have to name the colour in which a word is printed and ignore the word itself. Generally, colour naming is speeded when the colour and the word are congruent (red-red) and slowed when the colour and the word are incongruent (red-green), relative to neutral trials in which the colour and the word are unrelated. This is usually interpreted as due to automaticity effects in word reading. Under conditions in which an incongruent word is highly probable, however, subjects appear able to inhibit word reading and increase the speed of colour naming, relative to a control condition in which incongruent words are unexpected, although automaticity effects are not entirely abolished.

Studies of semantic priming typically involve presenting a prime stimulus and measuring subjects' response to a semantically related or unrelated target word. Neely (1977) and others demonstrated the existence of very rapid, automatic facilitatory effects, occurring at prime-target intervals of less than 250 msec. At longer prime-target intervals, however, experimenter-induced expectations and instructions were able to produce either facilitatory or inhibitory effects, suggesting the operation of strategic processing.

Other inhibitory effects have been shown in the negative priming paradigm (Tipper, 1985). This involves the presentation of primes that have to be ignored, followed by target trials in which subjects are required to respond to the previously ignored stimulus. It has been reliably shown that responding to the target stimulus is slower when it has been ignored on a previous trial. For example, an ignored picture of a cat can impair the subsequent processing of a semantically related word such as dog.

These examples of selective attention are closely related to the phenomenon of directed forgetting. This paradigm involves comparing the recall of stimuli that subjects are instructed either to remember or to forget. There are several methods used to designate some material as to-be-forgotten (TBF) and some material as to-be-remembered (TBR). Midway through presentation of a word list, for example, subjects may be instructed to forget the first half of the list and remember the second half of the list. This would constitute a global instruction to forget, because all the items that had been associated were to be forgotten.. Another method involves designating stimuli as TBR or TBF by instructions given after the presentation of the entire list (e.g. forget the animal names). This would constitute a specific instruction to forget, because only a subset of the associated items were to be forgotten. In a surprise recall test of the entire list, subjects given global or specific instructions to forget recall fewer stimuli in the TBF set than in the TBR set. In a recognition test, however, the difference between TBF and TBR items disappears.

Geiselman, Bjork, and Fishman (1983) conducted an ingenious experiment demonstrating that the directed forgetting effect could not be explained by differential rehearsal of TBF and TBR items, and hypothesized that a cue to forget inhibits access to the TBF items. Because recognition performance was unimpaired, they concluded that the inhibition induced via the forget cue took the form of retrieval inhibition. Other evidence suggests that this inhibition can be lifted by presentation of some of the TBF items.

3.1.1. Summary. Bjork (1989), Rafal and Henik (1994), Hasher and Zacks (1988), Tipper (1985), and others propose that selective attention is a highly flexible, goal-based system consisting of facilitatory and inhibitory processes that operate in concert to produce effective and efficient thought and action. This kind of flexible, targetable inhibitory process may be contrasted with more automatic inhibitory influences that appear to reflect prior learning and act to assist cognitive processing by suppressing related but irrelevant stimuli. The function of both processes is to remove goal-irrelevant information already in working memory and to hinder the access to working memory of irrelevant information. In each case, as proposed by Posner and Snyder (1975), presentation of a stimulus leads to the initial automatic activation of a range of associated representations. This activation is followed by slower facilitatory and inhibitory processes that attempt to limit attention to the most relevant representation by affecting the spread of activation in the network. This is very reminiscent of the observation that subliminally presented primes activate a wider range of associates than supraliminal primes (Dixon, 1981).

What relevance do these paradigms, largely based on responses to verbal stimuli, have to clinical accounts of repression? The first thing to note is the close parallels between the organisation of semantic memory and theories of self-representation. According to Markus and Sentis (1982), Kihlstrom and Cantor (1984), and others, information in memory about the self is organised, similarly to other kinds of information, as a set of related but context-specific knowledge structures. Overlapping representations preserve some consistent features of the self but also contain information relating to the self at different ages and in the performance of different roles. Other aspects of self-knowledge represented in memory include "ought" or "ideal" selves (e.g. Strauman & Higgins, 1988), and perhaps an "undesired self" (Ogilvie, 1987).

In many respects, therefore, self-knowledge may be thought of as a particularly complex area of semantic memory, but one that is organised along similar principles, possibly utilising a hierarchical system of constructs and categories. What aspects of self-knowledge are currently available to a "working self-concept" will depend on similar factors to those that determine the content of "working memory," such as context, current levels of activation, chronic accessibility, and mood. Real life situations may need to be disambiguated by accessing the relevant self-representation in just the same way that homographs have to be related to the most appropriate alternative meaning. What is perhaps unique about the self is the potential for inconsistency and hence competition among alternative self-representations, suggesting a potential role for automatic mechanisms such as retrieval-induced forgetting and centre-surround inhibition.

The role of active attentional facilitation and inhibition is even more clearly seen in individuals' attempts at self-regulation, particularly in mood repair processes. For example, Power and Brewin (1990) showed that presentation of a negative prime led to ordinary subjects taking more time, not less time, to endorse negative adjectives as being self-descriptive. They interpreted this as evidence for an inhibitory process that decreased the accessibility of negative self-representations in order to prevent the induction of a negative mood state.

Psychiatric disorders such as depression, it has been argued, are characterised by the breakdown of these inhibitory processes. Negative information about the self, coexisting with more positive representations (Brewin, Smith, Power, & Furnham, 1992; Kuiper, MacDonald, & Derry, 1983), and negative autobiographical memories, intrude into consciousness at very high frequencies. Both depression (Brewin, Hunter, Carroll, & Tata, in press; Kuyken & Brewin, 1994), and post-traumatic stress disorder (Brewin et al., 1996), are typified by persistent attempts on the part of patients to exclude these memories from consciousness and to reduce the probability of them being reaccessed. As well as the obvious parallel with attentional suppression, the high frequency of instructions to forget upsetting experiences, whether self-generated or provided by others, increases the similarity with directed forgetting experiments.

3.2. Individual Differences in Forgetting

Experimental evidence for inhibitory processes has so far suggested that they constitute a ubiquitous element of cognitive processing. As such, therefore, they are unable to explain why some people may be able to forget traumas whereas others always remember them. It would clearly be of interest to identify a group of people who appear to be particularly good at forgetting negative experiences. Such a group has in fact been identified — they are individuals with a repressive coping style.

Weinberger, Schwartz, and Davidson (1979) defined repressors as individuals who score low on a measure of trait anxiety but high on a measure of defensiveness such as the Marlowe-Crowne Social Desirability Scale (Crowne & Marlowe, 1964). Weinberger et al. proposed a 4-fold classification of individuals differentiated in terms of their coping styles: low anxious (low anxiety-low defensiveness), repressor (low anxiety-high defensiveness), high anxious (high anxiety-low defensiveness), and defensive high anxious (high anxiety-high defensiveness). The basic finding that repressors are characterised by dissociations between self-report and physiological measures of distress, responding strongly physiologically while denying any subjective experience of stress (Gudjonsson, 1981; Weinberger et al., 1979), has since been replicated numerous times.

A series of studies with female undergraduate students has shown that repressors have limited access to negative autobiographical memories. In a free recall task, Davis and Schwartz (1987) found that repressors recalled significantly fewer negative memories from childhood than low anxious or high anxious subjects, and that their age at the time of first negative memory recalled was substantially greater. Using a latency to retrieve paradigm with a cued recall task and including a defensive high anxious subject group, Davis (1987, Experiment 3) found that repressors: were slower at retrieving memories associated with fear and self-consciousness cues than the other three groups; were slower at retrieving memories associated with anger cues than low anxious individuals; were not slower at retrieving memories associated with happiness, sadness and guilt cues.

However, despite plausible prima facie grounds for labeling them as possessing a repressive coping style, until recently no direct evidence has been produced that they in fact have had disturbing or unpleasant experiences in childhood. The possibility had not been ruled out that phenomena such as longer latencies to retrieve negative memories might in fact indicate a childhood that was happier than usual, and thus not constitute evidence for repression. Myers and Brewin (1994) therefore used a semi-structured interview for assessing early experience, developed by Brown and colleagues (e.g., Andrews, Brown, & Creasey, 1990). The interview allows raters to judge reports of childhood experiences according to their own predetermined criteria rather than relying simply on subjects' own judgements about the significance of these experiences. In the interview there are a number of specific questions such as "Did you feel you could go to your parents if you were upset or unhappy?" Independently of whether subjects answer yes or no to this question, specific examples of occasions when they could/could not go to their parents are elicited and form the basis of the interviewer ratings. In this study ratings were checked by an independent judge blind to subjects' group assignment.

Using free recall and cued recall tests on childhood memories, Myers and Brewin replicated Davis' findings that repressors demonstrated longer latencies to report negative memories than the other groups, but that there were no group differences in recall of positive memories. The exclusively female sample of repressors also reported significantly more antipathy, more indifference and less closeness in their relationships with their fathers, thus making it extremely unlikely that they had in fact had happier childhoods than the other groups.

It is still not clear whether repressors' performance on autobiographical memory tasks reflects strategies for manipulating their personal histories or whether it is related to the processing of any negative information. To test whether repressors possess an information processing style that affects more than their own personal histories, Myers and Brewin (1995) carried out an experiment which investigated whether repressors have a selective deficit in intentionally learning and remembering negative experimental material. On the basis of the previous research, it appeared appropriate to construct a story that was concerned with parental relationships. The story concerned a woman's childhood with both positive and negative (examples of criticism and indifference) information about each parent. Personal relevance was enhanced by requiring subjects to process the material in relation to the self. The primary hypothesis was that repressors, compared with non-repressors, would recall less negative information about the father in the story.

The female repressors did not differ from controls in their recall of neutral or positive phrases. They did however show the predicted deficit in recall of negative material concerning fathering as well as impaired recall of the maternal critical phrase but not the maternal indifferent phrase. Data collected subsequently strongly suggested that the failure to find group differences on the maternal indifference phrase was due to its being a less extreme example than the paternal indifference phrase.

3.2.1. Summary. The precise relation of the findings of Myers and Brewin (1994, 1995), and those of others studying the repressive coping style, to the Freudian view of traumatic early experiences leading to repression is not clear at this point. The childhood interview did not result in any dramatic instances of the lifting of repression, but this would have been unlikely given its brevity and the relatively small number of cues provided. At the same time it was not possible to rule out the Freudian hypothesis that there were additional repressed traumatic memories, involving either maternal or paternal behavior, that did not emerge in the interview and that could account for the development of this coping style. An alternative possibility (Dozier & Kobak, 1992; Main, 1990) is that early insensitive or rejecting parenting (of which individuals may have no conscious memory) may have led to deactivation of the attachment system by exclusion of attachment-related information. "Rules consistent with such a strategy restrict subjects' awareness and acknowledgment of negative affect, limit recall of distressing or attachment-related memories, and lead to general or vague descriptions of parents that are not based on actual memories" (Dozier & Kobak, 1992, p. 1474).

In two studies from our laboratory we (Myers, Brewin, & Power, 1996) have established that repressors are superior to non-repressors in their ability to forget negative words when instructed to do so in a directed forgetting task, although they show no differences in their forgetting of positive words. It appears reasonable to conclude that some individuals have particular difficulties in the processing of negative information, and that this may be connected in some way to experiences in childhood. At this juncture we do not know what kind of mechanism is responsible for these effects, or the role played by actual traumatic experiences. The existence of this group of repressors does however suggest interesting possibilities for investigating repression-like effects in the laboratory.

4. INTEGRATING CLINICAL AND EXPERIMENTAL OBSERVATIONS

The clinical data are consistent with the possibility that at least some recovered memories have been manufactured as a result of inappropriate therapy, or because individuals have not adopted sufficiently stringent criteria for distinguishing imaginary from real events. They are also consistent with the possibility that at least some recovered memories correspond more or less to actual events that have been forgotten for long periods of time. The forgetting of traumatic information takes a number of different forms. Amnesia may be total, with no acknowledgment of the autobiographical fact of the abuse having taken place. Some people may have a sense that something bad has happened to them although there is no corresponding explicit memory. In other cases individuals report knowing they were abused but being unable or unwilling to remember any of the circumstances. In still other cases people remember some incidents but are unable to recall others, or are amnesic for particular aspects of an incident. In many cases representations of traumatic experiences appear in principle to be available, but are rendered inaccessible until triggered by a relevant cue.

Nor is there much doubt from the experience of treating trauma victims that substantial numbers of clients actively desire to forget unpleasant experiences. Whether or not their attempts to forget are successful, it seems to be the case that childhood adversity is associated with later memory impairment. Depressed patients with a history of early abuse, compared to those without such abuse, have been found to have difficulty in accessing specific autobiographical memories (Kuyken & Brewin, 1995). In addition to the studies of trauma victims, observations of individuals with early insensitive or rejecting parenting have also revealed evidence for restrictions of subjects' awareness and acknowledgment of negative affect, and impaired recall of distressing or attachment-related memories (Dozier & Kobak, 1992; Main, 1990).

While it is certainly possible that amnesia for some traumatic events reflects interference effects or the simple decay of memory traces, the material we have reviewed also implicates active inhibitory processes in ordinary forgetting. Thus, according to some experimental cognitive psychologists, the notion of repression does not appear necessarily to violate our understanding of ordinary memory. Although we are still far from an adequate cognitive account of repression and dissociation, there do appear to be a number of cognitive mechanisms that may be relevant to understanding these phenomena, particularly repression proper (after-expulsion). Given the ubiquitous reports of individuals actively attempting to cognitively avoid traumatic memories and exposure to repeated traumatic situations, it seems appropriate to begin with the literature on selective attention. Here there is widespread agreement that attention is a flexible process that attempts to ensure an efficient stream of thought by inhibiting the entry into consciousness of activated but irrelevant or unwanted representations. It does not seem unreasonable to hypothesize that the activation of representations involving highly emotionally charged events may lead to subtle changes that individuals can detect even though, because of subsequent inhibition, they may be unaware of their specific content.

This sort of phenomenon may underlie clients' reports that they know something has happened but they cannot say what. It is widely recognised that remembering is often based on simply "knowing" rather than on a specific recollective experience (e.g. Rajaram, 1993). However, these two criteria may not be equally reliable when it comes to establishing the validity of a memory. Recent research shows that judgements of knowing in the absence of recollective experience are more easily influenced by such factors as judgmental strategies and changes in the leniency of response criteria (Lindsay & Kelley, 1996; Strack & Förster, 1995). Similarly, false memories of events recorded in daily diaries are much more likely when recall is determined on the basis of knowing in the absence of a recollective experience (Conway et al., 1996). The implications for therapists are clear.

In many instances recovered memories do involve recollective experiences, sometimes of a vivid and detailed nature. Studies of retrieval inhibition suggest a mechanism to explain how instructions to forget generated by the self or others might lead to profound amnesia for an event, which could subsequently be lifted by exposure to relevant cues. Reports of the circumstances under which memories are recovered do typically furnish appropriate descriptions of cue exposure. What is fascinating about these is how in some cases individuals have previously been exposed to what seem to be highly relevant cues without triggering recall. For example, a memory of CSA was eventually triggered in one of the women interviewed by Elaine Hunter by media reports of sexual abuse in a country that corresponded to the individual's own nationality — similar reports of abuse in the UK, to which she had been exposed for many years, were apparently not specific or powerful enough to have the same effect. Another woman, a mental health professional, attended courses on sexual abuse without recalling her own abuse, memories of which were not triggered until she attended a course on loss.

Johnson (1994) drew attention to the fact that although there were data to support retrieval inhibition as an explanation for amnesia following global instructions to forget, it was a much less plausible explanation for amnesia following specific instructions to forget. In other words, retrieval inhibition may apply to an entire set of items in memory and can explain profound amnesia. In the case of partial amnesia, however, the individual has to forget a subset of items from a larger, interrelated item pool, some of which is accessible to working memory. Because there are associative links between TBF and TBR items, retrieval of TBR material is likely to be accompanied by retrieval of TBF material.

Johnson (1994) argued that once this mixture of TBF and TBR information was in memory, forgetting could not be explained solely by representational processes operating on the storage of information but would additionally require decisional processes operating on the expression of information. For example, the person might encounter discriminatory tags on TBF information which could guide the decisional process. Alternatively, there could be a variety of rules or heuristics governing the retrieval process. This kind of model is consistent with reports of partial amnesia in which clients describe remaining unaware of particular aspects of their trauma by choosing not to remember them. They typically describe a state of mind in which they know that they know something, but prefer to remain in ignorance of it.

At present a plausible cognitive explanation of primary repression, in which forgetting is described as immediate and automatic, appears to be farther off. One possibility worth considering is that dissociative states provide powerful TBF cues by virtue of their association with past episodes involving strategic forgetting. Thus the occurrence of a dissociative state may come to be associated with instructions to forget, with retrieval inhibition being implemented either immediately or at some time over the 24 hours following the episode of dissociation. Events experienced in dissociative states are therefore unlikely to be recalled subsequently unless the dissociative state is reinstated.

Flashbacks can be conceptualised as the experience of the activation of memorial representations of trauma that are based on unconscious cognitive processing rather than on conscious experience ("situationally accessible memories" versus "verbally accessible memories": Brewin et al., 1996). Unlike ordinary autobiographical memories, these representations contain codes that can reinstate sensory, emotional and physiological processes. Although individuals do not have direct access to these memories, they may become aware of the consequences of memory activation, such as intrusive images, feelings of panic, and so on. These representations are therefore by definition dissociated from ordinary memories, but through repeated activation and entry into working memory their content can become integrated with regular autobiographical memories.

The fact that flashbacks are based on memorial representations does not mean that they are necessarily accurate. Cognitive processing of the traumatic event may have been influenced by associative links to relevant previous experiences, particularly traumatic ones. Therefore, flashbacks may reflect several experiences rather than just one, and may have to be interpreted with caution. A dramatic example of this process was provided by a member of the emergency services whom I treated for post-traumatic stress disorder following his attendance at the scene of a particularly brutal murder. Although he had not been present at the murder, he formed an image of this event that appeared to be influenced by a conscious memory of witnessing his father attack his mother when he was 12 years old. Not only did he experience flashbacks based on this image, but he had intrusive imagery of himself attacking a woman in a wood near his home using the same stereotyped motions. This image was so vivid that he paid a visit to the wood to confirm that he was not a murderer.

If flashbacks are to become integrated with regular autobiographical memories, the person must be able to consciously edit and manipulate the information provided by the flashbacks within working memory. That is, they must retain awareness that they are experiencing the flashback, be able to reflect upon the experience as it is happening, and create ordinary autobiographical memories of the experience. In some cases, however, activation of the situationally accessible memories completely disrupts consciousness and orientation in present time and space. Subjectively, individuals are unaware of any reality other than the one which is dissociated. When they finish dissociating and become reoriented in the present, they may be completely ignorant of what was experienced while in that state. In these cases the traumatic experiences remain dissociated and integration in autobiographical memory is not possible.

Dissociated states, whether consisting of flashbacks, depersonalisation, derealisation, out-of-body experiences, absences, or more complex alternative personality states, may be conceptualised as modular, informationally encapsulated processes that are spontaneously triggered by internal or external stimuli. Although the absence of conscious control would seem to rule out the possibility that their levels of activation could be reduced by representational strategies such as retrieval inhibition, inhibition could still theoretically be achieved by post-retrieval decisional processes of the kind discussed above. The principles involved in reducing the impact of dissociated states represent a more complex example of dealing with other kinds of situationally accessible memories, and are put forward in recent cognitive analyses of therapeutic change (Brewin, 1989, 1996). Although individuals may have little direct conscious control over the onset or offset of these states, they can develop hypotheses about the content of the states and the likely internal and external triggers. Structured practice aimed at retaining more information about these states in working memory, and identifying and changing triggering cognitions, may be effective in decreasing the probability of these states being accessed.

Although this discussion has necessarily been speculative, I am firmly convinced that real progress will in the end depend on the kind of integration between clinical observations and cognitive science that I have begun to sketch out. Systematic, repeated clinical observations of unusual phenomena must be taken seriously, even if they contradict knowledge of mental functioning gained in other contexts. Equally, understanding of these phenomena will only be possible when they have been successfully modelled experimentally and related to the neural basis of cognition. Clinicians and cognitive scientists often operate with different models of psychological enquiry, have access to different kinds of data, and have different criteria for what constitutes a good theory (Brewin & Andrews, in press). Nevertheless, the collaboration of both groups is essential to the understanding of complex mental processes such as repression.

REFERENCES

Anderson, M.C., Bjork, R.A., & Bjork, E.L. (1994). Remembering can cause forgetting: Retrieval dynamics in long-term memory. Journal of Experimental Psychology: Learning, Memory and Cognition, 20, 1063–1087.

Anderson, M.C., & Spellman, B.A. (1995). On the status of inhibitory mechanisms in cognition: Memory retrieval as a model case. Psychological Review, 102, 68–100.

Andrews, B. (in press). Can a survey of British False Memory Society members reliably inform the recovered memory debate? Applied Cognitive Psychology.

Andrews, B., Brown., G.W., & Creasey, L. (1990). Intergenerational links between psychiatric disorder in mothers and daughters: The role of parenting experiences. Journal of Child Psychology and Psychiatry, 31, 1115–1129.

Andrews, B., Morton, J., Bekerian, D., Brewin, C.R., Davies, G.M., & Mollon, P. (1995). The recovery of memories in clinical practice. The Psychologist, 8, 209–214.

Bagley, C. (1995). Child sexual abuse and mental health in adolescents and adults. Aldershot: Avebury.

Bjork, R.A. (1989). Retrieval inhibition as an adaptive mechanism in human memory. In H.L. Roediger & F.I.M. Craik (eds.), Varieties of memory and consciousness. Hillsdale, N.J.: Lawrence Erlbaum.

Breuer, J., & Freud, S. (1895/1974). Studies on hysteria. In The Pelican Freud library (Vol. 3), Penguin, Harmondsworth.

Brewin, C.R. (1989). Cognitive change processes in psychotherapy. Psychological Review, 96, 379–394.

Brewin, C.R. (1996) Theoretical foundations of cognitive-behavior therapy for anxiety and depression. Annual Review of Psychology, 47, 33–57.

Brewin, C.R., & Andrews, B. (in press). Reasoning about repression: Inferences from clinical and experimental data. In M.A.Conway (ed.), Recovered memories and false memories. Oxford: OUP.

Brewin, C,R., Andrews, B., & Gotlib, I.H. (1993). Psychopathology and early experience: A reappraisal of retrospective reports. Psychological Bulletin, 113, 82–98.

Brewin, C.R., Dalgleish, T., & Joseph, S. (1996). A dual representation theory of post- traumatic stress disorder. Psychological Review, 103, 670–686.

Brewin, C.R., Hunter, E., Carroll, F., & Tata, P. (in press). Intrusive memories in depression. Psychological Medicine.

Brewin, C.R., Smith, A.J., Power, M., & Furnham, A. (1992). State and trait differences in depressive self-perceptions. Behaviour Research and Therapy, 30, 555–557.

Briere, J.N. (1992). Child abuse trauma. Newbury Park, Ca.: Sage.

Briere, J., & Conte, J. (1993) Self-reported amnesia for abuse in adults molested as children. Journal of Traumatic Stress, 6, 21–31.

Carr, T.H., & Dagenbach, D. (1990). Semantic priming and repetition priming from masked words: Evidence for a center-surround attentional mechanism in perceptual recognition. Journal of Experimental Psychology: Learning, Memory and Cognition, 16, 341–350.

Conway, M.A., Collins, A.F., Gathercole, S.E., & Anderson, S.J. (1996). Recollections of true and false autobiographical memories. Journal of Experimental Psychology: General, 125, 69–95.

Crowne, D.P., & Marlowe, D.A. (1964). The approval motive: Studies in evaluative dependence. New York: Wiley.

Dagenbach, D., Carr, T.H., & Barnhart, T.M. (1990). Inhibitory semantic priming of lexical decisions due to failure to retrieve weakly activated codes. Journal of Experimental Psychology: Learning, Memory and Cognition, 16, 328–340.

Davis, P.J. (1987). Repression and the inaccessibility of affective memories. Journal of Personality and Social Psychology, 53, 585–593.

Davis, P.J., & Schwartz, G.E. (1987). Repression and the inaccessibility of affective memories. Journal of Personality and Social Psychology, 52, 155–162.

Dixon, N.F. (1981). Preconscious processes. Chichester: Wiley.

Dozier, M., & Kobak, R.R. (1992). Psychophysiology in attachment interviews: Converging evidence for deactivating strategies. Child Development, 63, 1473–1480.

Elliott, D.M., & Briere, J. (1995). Posttraumatic stress associated with delayed recall of sexual abuse: A general population study. Journal of Traumatic Stress, 8, 629–647.

Feldman-Summers, S., & Pope, K.S. (1994). The experience of "forgetting" childhood abuse: a national survey of psychologists. Journal of Consulting and Clinical Psychology, 62, 636–639.

Geiselman, R.E., Bjork, R.A., & Fishman, D.L. (1983). Disrupted retrieval in directed forgetting: A link with posthypnotic amnesia. Journal of Experimental Psychology: General, 112, 58–72.

Gray, J.A. (1982). The neuropsychology of anxiety. Oxford: Clarendon Press.

Gudjonsson, G.H. (1981). Self-reported emotional disturbance and its relation to electrodermal reactivity, defensiveness and trait anxiety. Personality and Individual Differences, 2, 47–52.

Gudjonsson, G.H. (in press). Accusations by adults of childhood sexual abuse: A survey of the members of the British False Memory Society (BFMS). Applied Cognitive Psychology.

Harvey, M.R., & Herman, J.L. (1994). Amnesia, partial amnesia, and delayed recall among adult survivors of childhood trauma. Consciousness and Cognition, 3, 295–306.

Hasher, L., & Zacks, R.T. (1988). Working memory, comprehension and aging: A review and a new view. In G.H.Bower (ed.), The psychology of learning and motivation (Vol. 22, pp. 193–225). New York: Academic Press.

Herman, J.L. (1992). Trauma and recovery, Basic Books, New York.

Herman, J.L., & Schatzow, E. (1987). Recovery and verification of memories of childhood sexual trauma. Psychoanalytic Psychology, 4, 1–14.

Howes, M., Siegel, M., & Brown, F. (1993). Early childhood memories: Accuracy and affect. Cognition, 47, 95–119.

Janet, P. (1889). L'automatisme psychologique. Paris: Felix Alcan.

Johnson, H.M. (1994). Processes of successful intentional forgetting. Psychological Bulletin, 116, 274–292.

Kihlstrom, J.F. (1995). The trauma-memory argument. Consciousness and Cognition, 4, 63–67.

Kihlstrom, J.F., & Cantor, N. (1984). Mental representations of the self. In L.Berkowitz (Ed.), Advances in experimental social psychology (Vol. 17). Orlando, Fl.: Academic Press.

Kuiper, N.A., MacDonald, M.R., & Derry, P.A. (1983). Parameters of a depressive self- schema. In J.Suls & A.G.Greenwald (eds.), Psychological perspectives on the self (Vol. 2, pp. 191–217). Hillsdale, N.J.: Lawrence Erlbaum.

Kuyken, W., & Brewin, C.R. (1994). Intrusive memories of childhood abuse during depressive episodes. Behaviour Research and Therapy, 32, 525–528.

Kuyken, W., & Brewin, C.R. (1995). Autobiographical memory functioning in depression and reports of early abuse. Journal of Abnormal Psychology, 104, 585–591.

Lindsay, D.S., & Kelley, C.M. (1996). Creating illusions of familiarity in a cued recall remember/know paradigm. Journal of Memory and Language, 35, 197–211.

Lindsay, D.S., & Read, J.D. (1994). Psychotherapy and memories of childhood sexual abuse. Applied Cognitive Psychology, 8, 281–338.

Lindsay, D.S., & Read, J.D. (1995). "Memory work" and recovered memories of childhood sexual abuse: Scientific evidence and public, professional and personal issues. Psychology, Public Policy and the Law, 1, 846–908.

Loftus, E.F. (1993). The reality of repressed memories. American Psychologist, 48, 518- 537.

Loftus, E.F., Garry, M., & Feldman, J. (1994). Forgetting sexual trauma: What does it mean when 38% forget? Journal of Consulting and Clinical Psychology, 62, 1177–1181.

Loftus, E.F., Polonsky, S., & Fullilove, M. (1994). Memories of childhood sexual abuse: remembering and repressing. Psychology of Women Quarterly, 18, 67–84.

Main, M. (1990). Cross-cultural studies of attachment organization: Recent studies, changing methodologies, and the concept of conditional stategies. Human Development, 33, 48–61.

Markus, H., & Sentis, K. (1982). The self in social information processing. In J.Suls (ed.), Psychological perspectives on the self (Vol. 1). Hillsdale, N.J.: Erlbaum.

Merskey, H. (1995). Editorial. British Journal of Psychiatry, 166, 281–283.

Miller, N.E. (1995). Clinical-experimental interactions in the development of neuroscience. American Psychologist, 50, 901–911.

Morton, J., Andrews, B., Bekerian, D., Brewin, C.R., Davies, G.M., & Mollon, P. (1995). Recovered memories. Leicester: British Psychological Society.

Myers, L.B., & Brewin, C.R. (1994). Recall of early experience and the repressive coping style. Journal of Abnormal Psychology, 103, 288–292.

Myers, L.B., & Brewin, C.R. (1995). Repressive coping and the recall of emotional material. Cognition and Emotion, 9, 637–642.

Myers, L.B., Brewin, C.R., & Power, M.J. (1996). Repressive coping and the directed forgetting of emotional material. Manuscript submitted for publication.

Neely, J.H. (1977). Semantic priming and retrieval from lexical memory: Roles of inhibitionless spreading activation and limited capacity attention. Journal of Experimental Psychology: General, 106, 226–254.

Ogilivie, D.M. (1987). The undesired self: A neglected variable in personality research. Journal of Personality and Social Psychology, 52, 379–385.

Poole, D.A., Lindsay, D.S., Memon, A., & Bull, R. (1995). Psychotherapy and the recovery of memories of childhood sexual abuse: U.S. and British practioners' opinions, practices, and experiences. Journal of Consulting and Clinical Psychology, 63, 426–437.

Pope, H.G., & Hudson, J.I. (1995). Can memories of childhood abuse be repressed? Psychological Medicine, 25, 121–126.

Posner, M.I., & Snyder, C.R. (1975). Attention and cognitive control. In R.L.Solso (ed.), Information processing and cognition: The Loyola symposium. Hillsdale, N.J.: Erlbaum.

Posner, M.I., & Peterson, S. (1990). The attention system of the human brain. Annual Review of Neuroscience, 13, 25–42.

Power, M.J., & Brewin, C.R. (1990). Self-esteem regulation in an emotional priming task. Cognition and Emotion, 4, 39–51.

Rachman, S. (1980). Emotional processing. Behaviour Research and Therapy, 18, 51–60.

Rafal, R., & Henik, A. (1994). The neurology of inhibition: Integrating controlled and automatic processes. In D.Dagenbach & T.H.Carr (eds.), Inhibitory processes in attention, memory, and language (pp. 1–51). San Diego, Ca.: Academic Press.

Rajaram, S. (1993). Remembering and knowing: Two means of access to the personal past. Memory and Cognition, 21, 89–102.

Rothbaum, B.O., & Foa, E.B. (1996). Cognitive-behavioral therapy for posttraumatic stress disorder. In B.A.van der Kolk, A.C.McFarlane, & L.Weisaeth (eds.), Traumatic stress (pp. 491–509). New York: Guilford Press.

Schooler, J.W. (1994). Seeking the core: The issues and evidence surrounding recovered accounts of sexual trauma. Consciousness and Cognition, 3, 452–469.

Simpson, G.B., & Kang, H. (1994). Inhibitory processes in the recognition of homograph meanings. In D.Dagenbach & T.H.Carr (eds.), Inhibitory processes in attention, memory and language (pp. 359–381). San Diego, Ca.: Academic Press.

Strack, F., & Förster, J. (1995). Reporting recollective experiences: Direct access to memory systems? Psychological Science, 6, 352–358.

Strauman, T.J., & Higgins, E.T. (1988). Self-discrepancies as predictors of vulnerability to distinct syndromes of chronic emotional distress. Journal of Personality, 56, 685–707.

Tipper, S.P. (1985). The negative priming effect: Inhibitory effects of ignored primes. Quarterly Journal of Experimental Psychology, 37A, 571–590.

Tzelgov, J., Henik, A., & Berger, A. (1992). Controlling Stroop effects by manipulating expectations for color words. Memory and Cognition, 20, 727–735.

Usher, J.A., & Neisser, U. (1993). Childhood amnesia and the beginnings of memory for four early life events. Journal of Experimental Psychology: General, 122, 155–165.

van der Kolk, B.A., & Fisler, R. (1995). Dissociation and the fragmentary nature of traumatic memories: Overview and exploratory study. Journal of Traumatic Stress, 8, 505–525.

Wakefield, H., & Underwager, R. (1992). Recovered memories of alleged sexual abuse: Lawsuits against parents. Behavioral Sciences and the Law, 10, 483–507.

Weinberger, D.A., Schwartz, G.E., & Davidson, R.J. (1979). Low-anxious, high anxious and repressive coping styles: Psychometric patterns and behavioral responses to stress. Journal of Abnormal Psychology, 88, 369–380.

Williams, L.M. (1994). Recall of childhood trauma: A prospective study of women's memories of childhood sexual abuse. Journal of Consulting and Clinical Psychology, 62, 1167–1176.

Williams, L.M. (1995). Recovered memories of abuse in women with documented child sexual victimization histories. Journal of Traumatic Stress, 8, 649–673.

Yapko, M. (1994). Suggestibility and repressed memories of abuse: A survey of psychotherapists' beliefs. American Journal of Clinical Hypnosis, 36, 163–171.

COMMENTARY ON CLINICAL AND EXPERIMENTAL APPROACHES TO UNDERSTANDING REPRESSION

Arthur P. Shimamura, University of California, Berkeley

Dr. Brewin provides a useful and provocative analysis of clinical and cognitive interpretations of memory disruptions following child sexual abuse. Specifically, he attempts to account for clinical phenomena, such as repression, dissociations, and flashbacks by attributing them to basic cognitive and memory mechanisms. This analysis offers interesting insights concerning the kinds of cognitive investigations that may be helpful in understanding clinical disorders. It also may facilitate the manner in which therapists develop belief systems about memory loss and the psychological experience of reinstated memories.[*] Thus, Dr. Brewin's analysis has strong implications for both the clinical treatment of child sexual abuse and its empirical analysis.

The notion of repression has been a central issue concerning reinstated memories. Brewin suggests that repression can be interpreted in terms of cognitive mechanisms associated with inhibition of information processing. Recently, inhibitory

---

[*] The term reinstated memory is used here to describe instances in which an individual reports a traumatic experience that previously was considered to be out of conscious awareness. Rather than terms such as recovered, repressed or false memory, the term is meant to be neutral with respect to the veridicality of the report (see Shimamura, this volume).

mechanisms have played a significant role in the analysis of memory distortions (see Dagenbach & Carr, 1994; Dempster & Brainerd, 1995; Schacter, 1995). Cognitive phenomena such as suppressed encoding (e.g., Stroop interference, negative priming), directed forgetting, and retrieval inhibition, have been analyzed by cognitive psychologists and described by Brewin under the general rubric of inhibitory mechanisms. Moreover, reduced ability to apply inhibitory mechanisms has been used to explain memory and cognitive performance in special populations, such as young children (Dempster, 1992), elderly adults (Hasher & Zacks, 1988), and patients with frontal lobe lesions (Shimamura, 1994).

Brewin suggests that memory disruptions following child sexual abuse are attributed to increased inhibitory mechanisms applied to memories that are associated with a traumatic experience. In the extreme case, pathologically increased inhibitory mechanisms (e.g., suppressed encoding, directed forgetting) could conceivably prevent traumatic memories from being accessible to conscious awareness. However, such extreme cases are not amenable to experimentation in the laboratory and can only be assessed after the fact. It may, however, be likely that weakened memories due to inhibitory mechanisms cause the subsequent recollection of these memories to appear to have been out of conscious awareness. That is, the facility with which individuals can inhibit information processing may be related to the degree to which individuals report experiences of reinstated memories. This view is supported by the finding that individuals described as "repressors" are better able than "non-repressors" in the ability to inhibit or forget negative words when directed forgetting instructions are given (Myers, Brewin & Powers, in preparation, cited by Brewin). Thus, exaggerated ability to inhibit or forget information may be a psychological characteristic of individuals who claim to have reinstated memories.

Dissociative states are believed to involve cognitive anomalies different from those involved in repression. Dissociative states are assumed to be accompanied by feelings of "depersonalization" or "derealisation." They are considered by Brewin to be related to problems in working memory and conscious awareness. The notion of working memory is evoked because this cognitive process is important for the executive control of information processing that is associated with the encoding, organization, and retrieval of memories. A disruption in working memory, specifically the disruption in the ability to control and monitor information processing, could contribute to the phenomenon of disorganized or dissociative states.

In many respects, dissociative states reflect problems in self-knowledge or what has been termed metacognition (see Metcalfe & Shimamura, 1994). Although not described explicitly by Brewin, problems in metacognition could be related to experiences of a dissociated awareness of self. Indeed, metacognition and consciousness appear to be intricately entwined. Problems in working memory could contribute to dysfunctions in metacognitive processes that are associated with dissociative states. That is, such states could be caused by problems in the monitoring of cognitive processing—such as the monitoring of thoughts, the analysis of the external context, or the appreciation of time. For example, if an individual is experiencing loose, unfocused, or varied ideations, then that individual may not have a strong sense of stability within a time and place context. In the domain of memory disorders following neurological injury, the relationship between metacognition and working memory has been used to characterize patients with frontal lobe lesions (see Shimamura, 1996).

Flashbacks, the clinical phenomenon in which an individual expresses an episode of vividly remembering, almost re-experiencing, a traumatic event, is interpreted by

Brewin in terms of implicit memory or unconscious retrieval. Implicit memory concerns the facilitation or reactivation of memory that can occur automatically and without immediate conscious awareness (see Schacter, 1987; Graf & Masson, 1993). Implicit memory is often described as perceptually driven and reactivated by the reinstatement of contextual information.

An interesting clinical observation described by Brewin is a case in which an emergency service worker was being treated for post-traumatic stress disorder. The individual had experienced a "flashback" memory of having witnessed a brutal murder during his job. Although this individual was at the scene of the crime, he was not an eyewitness to the murder, and thus this "flashback" was spurious. Interestingly, this worker had reported in therapy a recollection of having been a witness to a much earlier episode—an attack of his mother by his father. The images of the "flashback" at the crime scene had similarities to the memory of his mother's attack. This description suggests that flashback memories may be a blending of multiple recollections and not based on a veridical "re-experiencing" of an actual event. That is, such experiences may be influenced by other recollections, which themselves could have been distorted or fabricated. Interestingly, implicit memories have been characterized as free-floating perceptual images that are devoid of the context in which they were experienced. Thus, it may be that cases of flashbacks are related to perceptually-driven implicit memories that are free floating and later become linked to form a sensible scenario.

In summary, clinical and empirical observations described by Brewin suggest that cognitive mechanisms such as inhibition, directed forgetting, working memory, metacognition, and implicit memory can help to explain clinical patterns of repression, dissociative states, and flashbacks. Moreover, the integration of cognitive and clinical psychology offers some important guidelines for therapists and experimental psychologists. In terms of clinical practice, it may be important for therapists to evaluate continually their beliefs about a client's recollections or reports. Also, therapists could benefit from evaluation of their own biases that can arise from one's clinical orientation. Important guidelines for therapists involved in cases of reported child sexual abuse are described in this volume in chapters by Briere and Courtois.

In terms of facilitating experimental analyses, scientists must also be aware of biases and beliefs that can lead to erroneous or exaggerated interpretations of findings. For example, the rather distinct and unusual psychological conditions surrounding child sexual abuse requires experimental psychologists to be more aware about the limitations of studies from the laboratory. Indeed, such scientific investigations will never be able to evaluate completely the validity or invalidity of a reinstated memory (see Shimamura, this volume). However, as Brewin and others have shown, laboratory studies and principles derived from cognitive psychology can offer new and enlightening perspectives on this clinical syndrome. Most importantly, only by cooperation among clinical therapists and experimental psychologists will a thorough analysis of repression and other clinical issues be obtained.

ACKNOWLEDGMENTS

Preparation of this chapter was supported by a grant from the National Institute of Mental Health (Grant MH48757).

REFERENCES

Dempster, F. N. (1992). The rise and fall of the inhibitory mechanism: Toward a unified theory of cognitive development and aging. Developmental Review, 12, 45–75.
Graf, P., & Masson, M. E. J. (1993). Implicit memory: New directions in cognition, development, and neuropsychology. Hillsdale, NJ: Lawrence Erlbaum Associates.
Hasher, L., & Zacks, R. T. (1988). Working memory, comprehension, and aging: A review and a new view (Vol. 22 ed.). San Diego, CA.: Academic Press.
Metcalfe, J., & Shimamura, A. P. (Eds.). (1994). Metacognition: Knowing about knowing. Cambridge, MA: MIT Press.
Schacter, D. L. (1987). Implicit memory: History and current status. Journal of Experimental Psychology: Learning, Memory and Cognition, 13, 501–518.
Schacter, D. L. (1995). Memory distortions: How minds, brains, and societies reconstruct the past. Cambridge, MA: Harvard University Press.
Shimamura, A. P. (1994). Memory and frontal lobe function. In M. S. Gazzaniga (Ed.), The cognitive neurosciences (pp. 803–813). Cambridge, MA: MIT Press.
Shimamura, A. P. (1996). The control and monitoring of memory functions. In L. Reder (Ed.), Metacognition and implicit memory. Hillsdale, NJ.: Erlbaum Press.

QUESTION AND ANSWER SESSION

Stewart. About your analogue research on repressors, I was wondering if anyone has looked within trauma survivors' groups, like maybe a sexual abuse group, with continuous versus some previously forgotten period of memory, and if they've seen whether the people who forget more are higher repressors on this measure ?

Brewin. I am not aware of any studies that have done that. It's completely unclear what relation this repressive coping style has to other clinical accounts of repression: we don't know if there's any relationship to other traumatic memories at all in this particular group. It may have been that there are other sorts of childhood experiences that are relevant, but whether it has any relationship to the classic Freudian notion of repression, we simply don't know. Certainly during the childhood interviews nobody came up with traumatic memories or anything of that kind, but then it's not particularly likely they would have done.

Widom. I really enjoyed your talk. This is totally speculative and off the wall. Repressors have low anxiety and high social desirability, repressors have discrepancies between self report and physiological arousal, repressors have had difficulty accessing or reporting negative autobiographical memories, repressors may have a worse childhood, so that it's not just that they don't have negative childhood experiences, which was your hypothesis. Now there's one glitch in all this. Have you thought about the fact that psychopaths have low anxiety, psychopaths engage in high social desirability, psychopaths have manifest discrepancies between self reported information and physiological arousal? We have some evidence that abused and neglected children are at a higher risk for having a diagnosis of anti-social personality disorder. We also have evidence that abused and neglected children are more likely to have high psychopathy checklist scores in comparison to a group of children without abuse or neglect in their backgrounds. Psychopaths are also high in sensation seeking, which means they engage in high-risk taking behaviors, which means that they expose themselves to traumatic events. So the glitch is that in the one study that you reported it was for females, and although there are female psychopaths the literature is primarily based on male psychopaths. What do you think of these crazy connections?

Brewin. This question has never crossed my mind. They don't act like psychopaths, the repressors were really well behaved, they were the ones who showed up on time, didn't miss the session. It was the low anxious ones who forgot and didn't bother to come because they had something better to do. But there may be different reasons why people might score highly on measures of social desirability. For example, it's been suggested that psychopaths might be trying deliberately to create a false impression about themselves. Whereas the literature suggests that repressors really do think that they don't have angry thoughts about people, that they don't gossip about people, that they would not break the rules if they could get away with it and no-one would ever know. So it's more to do with self-deception than other-deception, and I'm wondering if this could be one way to separate out these two groups.

Fivush. I want to come back to the issue of repressors. I know that in some of her early work Penny Davis reported gender differences with males more likely to show a repressing style and males more likely to include emotional material in their autobiographical reports, and one of the consistent findings in the general literature on autobiographical memory is that women have more detailed and elaborated personal narratives of their past experiences than males do. These differences are small but they are robust. So, I was wondering if you had thought at all about the role of gender role socialization in this whole issue of coping style and how this might play into some of the clinical issues.

Brewin. I think you're right and the chances are it is very important. We have recently looked at male and female repressors, and it appeared that the male repressors didn't behave in the same way as the female repressors do, the effects seem to be limited to the female repressors. We haven't got very large or systematic data on that, it's just an initial impression. When I talked to Penny Davis (personal communication) she said that she found it difficult to find male repressors. I think you're probably right that the process may be different in men and women and it would be wrong to over-generalize from these kinds of findings. We are doing some work in our group at the moment which we hope will enable us to get large numbers of data on both male and female repressors to answer some of these questions.

Brewer. This is directed at an aspect of Chris' talk that hasn't been discussed. He proposed a theory of representation forms for traumatic events: basically, there was a conscious recollective type of representation and then there was another representation which was a kind of raw data that's preserved over a long period of time. I have seen this move in several other areas and you have to be very cautious when you make this move. This position was taken by philosophers studying epistemological issues at the turn of the century, Bertrand Russell being one of them, and the basic line of reasoning is that you're trying to find out things that you can't know for sure. They said we can know for sure about our recollective memory experiences because they are in there as a record, like a Polaroid picture of events that occurred before. What happened in the history of that field, is that other philosophers came up with cases of mistaken autobiographical childhood memories, and they gave up. Then again in the case of flashbulb memory, the argument again was that when a flashbulb memory occurred you got a raw sensory store, based on the strong intuition all of us have about flashbulb memories - they must be real because they're so vivid and so good. More recently we see the same pattern within a subset of people in the clinical area who hear these very vivid memories and they have a strong belief value and one sub-set of people in that area have theorized that what is happening is that we have a repressed sensory store that has now come up. Of course once again, the data are based on the belief value of the person listening. Chris has now, however, tried to provide a theoretical account of this phenomenon as it would apply to the repressed memory case, and so he's got these two forms of memory. But the experimental literature currently tends not to favor a view that you can have this strong sensory store that's preserved, but these are laboratory studies done in non-traumatic cases, and I presume what you do is postulate a special purpose mechanism that causes the sensory kind to stay in. The point of this is just a note of caution, obviously you can postulate the theory but that the trick is that we need to go in beyond the belief value that having the memory yourself or listening to someone, before you can get that view to work and I guess the bottom line here is that's a strong claim and needs to be supported very strongly.

Brewin. If I could have worked out a simpler model to account for the data I would have done. The data are complicated and this is my best shot at trying to account for it. I take your views on board and I will not really be satisfied until I have some kind of independent source of evidence, such as neuroimaging studies, that there is value in looking at things in this way.

Read. I admired the presentation, particularly the integration of the cognitive research which was a striking jump from previous work. What I would like to do is try to get us back to the reports of survivors, related to this issue. I don't think you drew the explicit link, you talked about the individual differences, repressive coping styles and so on, but you didn't explicitly draw the link that people who don't recall experiences of sexual abuse are necessarily more likely to be repressors. But it occurred to me in looking at the data which have been presented in a few studies, Linda Williams' study and the Herman and Schatzow study, in which the age variable was studied, and what you find (and it may be overstating because the data are quite limited) is that there's a declining probability that a person will report amnesia with increasing age of onset of the reported abuse. By the time an individual is beyond puberty, the probability they would report or demonstrate or evidence loss of memory has decreased substantially. Now when you think about it from the perspective of the repressive coping style, one would assume that it is a learned strategy. Then if a repressive coping style is something that's developed as a way of adapting then it should be running the other way; that is to say the older the individual the more likely it is that the repressive coping style would prevent them from remembering, yet we get the exact opposite relationship. I don't know whether there's any developmental studies of the repressive coping measure which would be really interesting. But the question is how can we tie the repressive coping style back to those few studies where there are actual reports and claims of loss of memory ?

Brewin. Yes, the two literatures are really very different. Another problem is that we know very little about this repressive coping style, is it actually a coping style ? As far as I know nobody has done longitudinal follow-up studies showing that if you are a repressor at time A then you'll be a repressor at time B, that is, it may be some more transient response to events. Nor do we know if you would find a similar phenomenon in childhood, which I agree would be very important question to look at. At the moment we really have no idea how to relate these two literatures. It would be interesting to ask people who qualify as having a repressive coping style whether they have ever had experiences of recovered memories, but I'm not all that hopeful that you would find things that would tie the two together in a very direct way. I think there may be other mechanisms involved possibly with response to less traumatic experiences which may be at work here. We talked the other day about neglect in reference to Cathy Widom's data and I think there may be other impacts of other kinds of childhood experiences which may be more relevant here than single traumas.

REFERENCES

Herman, J.L., & Schatzow, E. (1987). Recovery and verification of memories of childhood sexual trauma. *Psychoanalytical Psychology, 48*, 711–721.
Williams, L. M. (1994a). Recall of childhood trauma: A prospective study of women's memories of child sexual abuse. *Journal of Consulting and Clinical Psychology, 62*, 1167–1176.

7

DISPATCH FROM THE (UN)CIVIL MEMORY WARS

Elizabeth F. Loftus

University of Washington
Box 351525
Seattle, Washington 98195-1525

1. THE MEMORY WARS

Over the last few years, our society has been immersed in a motley collection of "Memory Wars," as they were called in a lengthy review of several books on recovered memory published in *Scientific American* (Schacter, 1995). The "memory war" theme was also used to title an editorial that appeared in *Psychology Today* magazine (Neimark, 1996). The editorialist wrote: "You'd think that memory would be the stuff of dry academia, but it turns out to be one of the most illuminating and terrifying stories of our time" (p. 6). And the "war" theme appeared in the title of a book that reprinted a sizzling pair of essays published previously in the *New York Review of Books* by Berkeley professor and Freud scholar, Frederick Crews (1995). In those essays, Crews identified a number of beliefs about human nature that he felt have been propagated by leaders of a well-meaning, but misguided, movement:

> that repression is the normal human response to trauma; that experiences in infancy produce long-term memories that can be accurately retrieved decades later; that adult psychological difficulties can be reliably ascribed to certain forgotten events in early childhood and not others; that sexual traumas are incomparably more susceptible to repression and the formation of neurosis than any other kind; that symptoms are themselves "memories" that can yield up the story of their origin; that dream interpretation, too, can disclose the repressed past; that memory retrieval is necessary for symptom removal; and that psychotherapists can confidently trace their clinical findings to the patient's unconscious without allowing for the contaminating influence of their own diagnostic system, imparted directly or through suggestion (274).

Skepticism about certain beliefs and practices of "repressed memory therapists" must not be taken as skepticism about the existence of childhood trauma. This point is so important, it is worth repeating, and even shouting. Skeptics on the subject of repression have strongly emphasized the enormity of the problem of childhood trauma, and sexual abuse in particular (Lindsay & Read, 1994). One only need to examine documents from the first international war crimes tribunal since the end of World War II, the trial of Bosnian Serb Dusan Tadic, to appreciate the horrible things that human being sometimes do to one another. Tadic, a former cafe owner from the northwestern Bosnian town of Prijedor, was charged with a series of war crimes that occurred between May and August of 1992 at Omarska, a mine complex converted into a concentration camp. The "Indictment" (International Criminal Tribunal, 1995) charges Tadic with participating in the collection, mistreatment, and killings of Bosnian Muslims and Croats. Among other charges, Tadic is accused of taking a woman, referred to in the indictment as "F," to a particular building in the Omarska camp and subjecting her to forcible sexual intercourse. For this he is charged with "Grave Breach," "Violation of the laws or Customs of War" and "Crime against Humanity." In addition to the rapes and murders, Tadic has also been accused of supervising the torture of Muslims, including one charge that he forced one prisoner to emasculate another with his teeth. Tadic has denied all charges (Cohen, 1995). Weschler (1995), writing about the Bosnian horrors, poignantly said: "Yugoslavia today has been turned back into one of those places where people not only seem incapable of forgetting the past but barely seem capable of thinking about anything else" (63).

The "memory wars" are not about those cases of brutalization that have never been forgotten. To make crystal clear the area of concern, it is useful to remind readers that the world's population contains many different kinds of cases. The simplest dichotomy for characterizing these cases is the two-by-two table, a device found helpful by many other scholars. An individual's abuse status could in reality be "not abused" or "abused." And within these two possibilities, the individual might be in one of two recall states, either 1) recalling no abuse or 2) recalling some abuse. The cases of abuse that are never forgotten would fall into one of those quadrants, persons who were in fact abused and do recall it. These might be labeled "true positives." The Bosnian woman, F, might be placed there. So might many of the victims of Father Porter, and many of the women and men in the studies of Williams (this volume) and Widom (this volume).

The 2 × 2 table also has a quadrant for "false negatives", by which I mean people who experienced some horrible trauma and do not recall it. Many of the women and men in the studies of Williams and Widom might also fall here. These studies show that people can have documented experiences and fail to remember or report them years later. The cases sometimes involve sexual or physical abuse, and sometimes other horrifying traumas. One stunning false negative case came to my attention recently. It involved an Vietnamese adult student named Anh Tu Vu who escaped from Vietnam with her family in 1979, when she was only six years old. The story of the escape would exceed anyone's parade of horribles. The families who planned the escape risked being caught and put in prison without hope of release. They made their way to the designated shore hideout through swamps and mud by using a machete to clear paths that were covered by bushes, trees and thorns. They set sail on a small fishing boat on which four times the safe number of people had boarded. They ran out of food and water, and were forced to drink saltwater. Many became seasick and delirious. Some fell off the boat and drowned. The ordeal lasted for months before Anh Tu Vu and her family were safe.

Anh Tu Vu eloquently wrote about her experiences in a paper she submitted for a course on memory that I taught during the Spring of 1996 at the University of Washington. Ahn Tu Vu wrote: "It is my story of what really happened to me and my family when I was six years old. However, these are not my memories. I have never lived a single moment of what I've just retold because I cannot remember a single detail about the entire escape." Anh Tu Vu knew of the details from her many relatives and especially from an

Uncle who had written an autobiography about the escape and the price of freedom that the family paid. "Our names are all in there, so it must have happened."

Anh Tu Vu desperately wants to "remember" these experiences. When I asked her why she wanted to remember, she said it was about appreciating the freedom that had meant so much to her parents that they were willing to die for it. In her paper, she wrote: "An entire part of my life is erased, and I feel sad that I can't share with my parents this journey we endured together. I'll never know what it was like to long for freedom so bad, you would risk everything including your life to get it." Anh Tu Vu's case poignantly reminds us of the false negatives; that is, that there are very powerful cases of trauma that really happened, without accompanying recall.

1.1. Gaps in Recalling

The 2 × 2 table crossing abuse status with recall status must be modified to capture the cases that have been at the heart of the memory wars. We need a category for cases that are characterized by "No recall followed by recall." Of course, some of these No recall/Recall cases reflect genuine cases of abuse, and some reflect "no abuse." Some of these No Recall/Recall cases might be considered "suspicious" because of what has intervened between the state of "no recall" and the state of "recall." The "memory wars" are largely about cases that involve the ingredients identified by Crews: an alleged banishment of horrendous brutalization out of conscious awareness by repression or dissociation or some other special mechanism, and the therapeutic efforts to revive these supposed brutalizations and make their presence mentally known. The promoters of these "repressed memory" beliefs try to bolster their assumptions with what Crew's calls "scientific pretensions" (p. 274). Wounded by such accusations, various respondents to Crews' charges insisted that they do not behave this way, that they caution against using hypnosis and "truth" drugs to dig out memories (Reid, 1995, in Crews, 1995, p. 231) and that they reject the "naive concept of repression" in which memories are hermetically sealed and stored intact for future revelation. Despite belittling repression as a concept, Crews' critics attempted to salvage the situation by referring to the "well-documented" evidence for full or partial amnesia for traumatic events such as combat experiences, natural disasters, and victims of physical and sexual abuse.

One wonders about the meaning of "well-documented evidence" in light of a recent examination by psychiatrist Harrison Pope and his colleagues of 39 studies of 3,636 trauma survivors (Pope, Oliva & Hudson, 1996). The victims had experienced all manner of horrific traumas, including fires, lightning, parental murder, torture, and sexual abuse. None of these victims is reported to have repressed their traumatic experiences. (For a discussion of the types of studies that are sometimes used to support massive repression, and the controversy surrounding the interpretation of those studies, see Pope and Hudson, 1995).

The memory wars continue to be waged in myriad battlegrounds, including courtrooms, academia, psychotherapy circles, policy settings, and feminist circles. In this chapter, I review recent activity in these various arena. The repressed-memory landscape is littered with carnage that is both tragic and unnecessary. When reading about the separate battles, it might be productive to keep a few questions in mind. Is engaging in battle a productive thing to do, or is it creating splits and tears that will be exceedingly difficult to repair? Is it not time to recast the tone from its present black and white extreme to one that appreciates shades of gray? Can't we appreciate that some past practices may have been a mistake, and that it is time to join together to stop them? Can we not collectively get behind a joint effort to devise better methods to tell apart the patients with accurate recovered memories and the patients with illusory ones? After all, uncritical acceptance of every claim, no matter how bizarre or dubious, demeans the genuine, serious cases of sexual abuse. These questions need serious contemplation if we are serious about wanting to help not only the patients, but also their families, the genuine survivors of trauma, and the professionals who care about them.

2. LITIGATION BATTLES

The courtroom battles are, primarily, not about the large numbers of genuine victims who have known of their abuse their whole lives, and perhaps only recently got the courage to tell a trusted friend or therapist about it. Rather, they are mostly about cases like that of Laura B. who claimed that her father, Joel Hungerford, molested her from the ages of 5 to 23, including raping her just days before her wedding. She allegedly totally repressed all memories of her abuse until she entered therapy a couple of years later and the violent ordeals resurfaced.

Repressed memory litigation has expressed itself in myriad forms. The largest class of cases have been brought in the civil courts. In 1989, legislation went into effect in the State of Washington that permitted people to sue for recovery of damages for injury suffered as a result of childhood sexual abuse any time within three years of the time they *remembered* the abuse. The legislature invoked a novel application of the "delayed discovery doctrine," that essentially says that the statute of limitations does not begin to run until the plaintiff has discovered the facts that are essential to the cause of action. The argument in repressed memory cases was that the memory for abuse was hidden away, sometimes for decades, until it was ultimately discovered, and only then did the plaintiff possess the facts that were essential to the cause of action. Now, about half of the states have followed Washington's lead and enacted similar legislation allowing for the tolling of the statute of limitations in cases of massive repression. Several states have adopted the rule without legislation. As a consequence, juries are now hearing cases in which plaintiffs are suing their parents, relatives, neighbors, teachers, and others for acts of childhood sexual abuse that allegedly occurred 10, 20, 30, even 40 years earlier, but were only recently remembered (Loftus, 1993; Loftus & Ketcham, 1994).

The repressed memory cases have sometimes been compared to medical malpractice litigation in which the statute of limitations is sometimes tolled because the cause of action was only recently discovered by the patient. But, as Beaver (1996) points out, in medical malpractice cases, some objective tangible evidence exists to ensure reliable fact finding. In contrast, Beaver notes, the repressed memory cases involve pitting one person's version against another as the basis for liability determination. "This situation does not permit the avoidance of stale and fraudulent (perhaps confabulated) claims that is the central purpose of the statute of limitations" (Beaver, 1996, p 603). Because of "stale claims", weakened memories, lost evidence, and even dead witnesses, these cases can be hard to defend. Typically, defendants try to show the highly suggestive nature of the therapeutic process. Frequently that process of excavating the "repressed" memories involves invasive therapeutic techniques such as age regression, guided visualization, trance writing, dream work, body work, hypnosis, and sodium amytal (truth serum). That these techniques were heavily promoted, especially in the late 1980's and early 1990's appears beyond dispute (Destun & Kuiper, 1996). Numerous research and clinical psychologists have raised grave concerns that these activities are fostering the creation of false beliefs and memories that implicate innocent people.

While, the largest category of cases are those brought by individuals who sue their alleged perpetrators, and hundreds of plaintiffs have brought such suits, there are other types of repressed memory litigation that judges and juries are now deciding. A second wave of lawsuits has been brought by "retractors" who claim that they were led to believe they were sexually molested but now say that they realize their memories are false. As of 1994, some 300 individuals had retracted their sex abuse allegations, and a number of them have sued their former therapists achieving six figure settlements or jury verdicts. The group of retractors may be growing dramatically. One psychiatrist made reference in the American Journal of Psychotherapy to "more than 1000 instances" in which individuals have retracted accusations that "may be regarded on strong grounds as being false" (Merskey, 1996, 334). For a study of retractors and discussion of the evolution of their reported pseudomemories, see Lief and Fetkewicz (1995).

A third set of cases are being brought by people accused on the basis of recovered memories, and these are sometimes referred to as "third party" cases (Slovenko, 1995). These accused persons decide to take the offensive by filing negligence suits against therapists who helped produce abuse accusations. They demand compensation for the psychological upheaval, the ruined reputations and careers, and the breakup of families that inevitably follow the supposed recall of childhood abuse. The Ramona case is the most famous of these. Gary Ramona was sued by his daughter Holly after she recovered memories of repeated brutalization. Gary then sued his daughter's therapists after he became convinced that his daughter's recent accusations of abuse were based on false memories generated by misguided therapy. Ramona's daughter claimed that she had been molested by her father between the ages of 5 and 16, including numerous times with the family dog, Prince, and she unlocked these buried memories in therapy a couple of years later. Ramona sued not only the therapists who treated his daughter, but the hospital where a portion of the treatment took place. A Napa jury awarded Gary Ramona approximately $500,000.

Some cases do not fit neatly in one of the three categories; that is, they are not cases involving underlying accusations against the accused, retractors against their former therapists, or third party litigation against therapists. A most unusual case involved a woman named Patricia Rice (Conklin, 1996). Rice, a 47-year-old housewife and mother of three, went to a hypnotherapist in 1992 for help in losing weight, quitting smoking, and solving her marital problems. In the course of therapy, Rice developed horrific memories of having been sexually abused by her father, vaginally raped with a broom handle by her mother, tortured with electric shock and dragged into ritual killings by a satanic cult. Her delusional memories proved deadly. One day, in June 1992, she was driving her car on Pacific Highway when a "good witch" took control, and she slammed into a car driven by a 54-year-old man, killing him. Rice was charged with manslaughter and found "guilty, but insane." Although she didn't serve time in jail, she was placed under the supervision of the state Mental Health board and ordered never to drive or leave home without board approval. Rice in turn sued her therapist for implanting the grisly delusions about satanic cults that had, she claimed, caused the accident. She was awarded a lump-sum payment of $425,000 and $1,570 a month for the rest of her life.

The class of repressed memory cases that presents particularly great legal challenges are those being tried in the criminal courts. In most states, the statute of limitations for criminal child sex abuse charges has been extended, usually to several years beyond the age of majority, which is 18 in most states. Repressed memory criminal cases thus can and do go forward. Getting access to the process of therapy through the deposition of the therapist and the therapy records is typically not a problem in civil cases where plaintiffs have placed at issue their mental state. They waive their right to confidentiality, and the essential records become available to the defense. But what should happen in the criminal cases where a complainant has not waived those rights yet the defense seeks that information? Here we have the classic tensions between the rights of privacy of a patient who claims to be a victim of a crime or, on other occasions, a witness of a crime, and the sixth amendment and due process rights of the defendant. (See Loftus, Paddock & Guernsey, 1996, for a discussion of the privilege issue).

Invariably in all of these cases, questions arise about the nature of human memory. One memory issue concerns the extent to which extensive horrific trauma can be totally banished from consciousness. But an equally important memory issue concerns the extent to which false memories can be implanted in the minds of individuals who then come to believe they had abusive experiences when they have not.

3. RESEARCH BATTLES

Years ago, before we talked about "memory wars," we talked about "debates." In the Author's Note to our book, The Myth of Repressed Memory, Kathy Ketcham and I ended with a hope that our readers would not construe this as a debate about the reality or the horror of sexual abuse, incest, and violence against children. "This is a debate about memory." That realization appears to have caught on, as evidenced by Schacter's (1996) more extensive comment: "The recovered memories controversy, though a complex affair that touches on issues of incest, family, social mores, and even religious beliefs, is fundamentally a debate about accuracy, distortion, and suggestibility in memory" (251). Schacter nicely separates two critical "memory" questions that have plagued this vitriolic debate, namely the question of whether memories of genuine abuse are ever totally repressed or dissociated and then reliably recovered, and the distinctly different question of whether false memories of abuse can be implanted.

As to the first question, research has shown that some people can forget about single episodes of abuse, and some even forget multiple episodes. But why? "This forgetting is most likely attributable to some combination of normal processes of memory decay and interference, conscious suppression and lack of rehearsal..." (Schacter, 1996, 264). It is even possible that physiological changes might be caused by sexual abuse that play some role in memory disturbance, although this is speculative. What about memory for years of violent, horrific abuse? Some have complained for several years about the lack of cogent scientific evidence regarding repeated brutalization; Schacter stated this concern again, but perhaps more artfully: "...there is as yet little or no scientifically credible evidence that people who have suffered years of violent or horrific abuse after the years of infancy and early childhood can immediately and indefinitely forget about the abuse." He further concludes that the popular idea that forgetting in abuse survivors is caused by a special powerful repression mechanism is still "without a scientific basis" (264). Psychiatrist Joel Paris puts it differently: "....there is scant evidence to support the hypothesis that trauma leads to repression" (1996, 206).

As for the issue of illusory memories of sexual abuse, there are, of course, no experiments proper in which sexual abuse has been implanted. Ethical consideration would preclude the conduct of such studies. However, there are, as Schacter aptly notes, several separate strands of evidence that support the conclusion that some therapists have helped to create illusory recollections of sexual abuse:

> the experimentally documented malleability of memory in response to suggestive influences; evidence that hypnosis can produce compelling but inaccurate pseudomemories; failures to document satanic ritual abuse; recovery of memories for seemingly impossible events (past lives and alien abductions); growing numbers of therapy patients who have retracted their memories; the constructive nature of memory for emotional events, and the risky memory-retrieval techniques advocated by some proponents of recovered memory therapy. (p. 272–273).

In concluding that there is a rational basis for the fear that some therapists have created illusory recollections, Schacter made reference to "the experimentally documented malleability of memory in response to suggestive influences." He specifically cited the work on hypnotically created pseudomemories, including work by Nicholas Spanos and colleagues (1991) that showed that after hypnotic suggestions, some individuals developed memories of being abused in a past life. He also made reference to studies in which wholly false memories have been implanted via the use of suggestive techniques, such as visualization and imagination. I now review some recent findings that bear on this issue. One of the few tangible benefits of the current memory wars is that new scientific studies have been conducted, studies that were directly stimulated by the controversy, studies that hopefully make a more general scientific contribution, and, even more hopefully, have a life in the memory literature long after the last soldier from trenches of the memory wars has been put to rest.

3.1. Research on Memory Distortion

Since the mid-1970's at least, researchers have been investigating how people take their own version of an event and combine it with misinformation that they receive from another source. Memory distortion, it appears, is a fact of life. In these studies, people have recalled nonexistent broken glass and tape recorders, a clean-shaven man as having a mustache, straight hair as curly, and even something as large and conspicuous as a barn in a bucolic scene that contained no buildings at all (Belli, 1989; Chandler, 1991; Loftus, 1979; Lee, 1996; Loftus & Ketcham, 1991; Roediger, Jacoby & McDermott, 1996; Titcomb & Reyna, 1995; Wright, (this volume); Zaragoza, Mitchell & Drivdahl, (this volume)). This growing body of research shows that new, post-event information arriving from another source often becomes incorporated into memory, supplementing and altering a person's recollection. The new information invades us, like a Trojan horse, precisely because we do not detect its influence. Understanding how we can become tricked by exposure to the memories of those around us is central to understanding distortions in autobiographical recollection.

The work on misinformation and its ability to distort memory is but one example of many "memory illusions" that have captured the attention of cognitive psychologists during this century, but have also fascinated physicists and philosophers throughout recorded history (Roediger, 1996). The particular memory illusion that occurs when people think that they experienced something that they only learned about somewhere else can be understood as a failure of source monitoring (Johnson, Lindsay & Hashtroudi, 1993). Perhaps it is not too surprising that people might hear someone else talk about seeing a guy with curly hair and subsequently think that they too saw curly hair. But just how far can you go in terms of tampering with memory? Could you, for example, go beyond simply altering details of actual events, and instead create a entirely false memories for something that never happened? We describe several new paradigms that have revealed the possibly of creating entirely false memories for events that never happened.

3.2. False Memories of a Drug Bust

Can you make people believe that they saw an event two weeks ago that in fact they did not see? Michele Nucci, Hunter Hoffman and collaborators, working in my laboratory, have devised a procedure to implant an entire memory, in this case a memory of a drug bust that was never actually witnessed. The study was conducted in three phases. First subjects watched four videoclips of crime scenes that had been used in prior research (Geiselman, Fisher, MacKinnon, & Holland, 1985). The videoclips depicted a bank robbery, a warehouse burglary, a liquor store hold-up, and a domestic dispute, and each was approximately 4 min. in length. In the second phase, one week later, subjects filled out a questionnaire consisting of multiple-choice questions about each event. There were 10 questions asked about each of the real witnessed events, and 10 questions asked about a non-witnessed "drug bust." More specifically, the subject's attention was directed to an event (e.g., "the bank robbery") and a series of questions followed (e.g., "In the bank robbery scenario, identify the race of the suspect(s): a) White; b) African-American; c) Latino-Hispanic."). The false event was treated the same way, that is, first the subject was directed to think about "the drug bust", and then to answer questions about it, such as this one: "Identify the race of the suspect(s) in the drug bust scenario: a) White; b) African-American; c) Latino-Hispanic." Finally, one week later, subjects were asked to provide open-ended accounts of two of the witnessed scenarios and the non-witnessed but suggested drug bust.

The results revealed that subjects were able to recall something about all of the real events that they had actually witnessed. As for the false event, 64% reported a memory for the drug bust that they never saw. An examination of the mean number of words used to describe the real events, and the false one, revealed that on average subjects used more words to describe the real events. They used an average of over 90 words to describe the real events. In contrast, they used an average of 40 words to describe the false drug bust.

A detailed examination of the elements of the drug bust reports revealed that 76% of the material could be traced to one of the other scenarios, while 24% of the material was brand new, at least in the sense that it could not be directly traced to one of the other scenes. Importing occurred primarily from the warehouse break-in and the liquor store robbery and shooting.

Sample responses from our subjects indicate the mixture of imported and new material. In the following report, material that was imported from the liquor store scenario is left in normal font, and "new" material is italicized:

> A police officer and partner were patrolling the streets by a bar (they were checking locks, etc.) when they heard a gun shot. Someone was shot and the suspect with a gun ran into an alley and hid in a dumpster. *Apparently the shot fired was due to some conflict of interest during the drug deal.* The officer (one of them) then tried to coax the suspect out of the dumpster and he was shot at by the suspect. *There were bystanders at and in the bar (the drug deal was outside)....*

Another subject imported material from the warehouse (in normal font) and added new material (italicized):

There are 3 policemen *who tried to catch a drug dealer and the buyer. They chased them into* a warehouse *and the dealer/buyer gave up but the police shot him anyway.*

Some accounts contain only material that is new, that is, material that cannot be traced to the other scenarios, but might be traceable to some other aspect of the subject's past or imagination:

Memory is very vague of the drug bust. Seems as if there was a woman waiting in a car when the drug bust occurred, a male suspect jumped into the car and told her to drive away.

Can't recall. It takes place during the day and a cop is observing two people interacting. Then a signal is given and the cops make a bust. I'm not sure. I might have seen that on COPS.

This study is consistent with the hypothesis that people can be led, through suggestive questioning, to believe that they have witnessed an event two weeks ago that in fact they never witnessed. Nearly two-thirds of subjects were willing to report that they had seen a drug bust and to offer some description of it. The elements of their descriptions can often be traced to other truly witnessed events, revealing an interesting feature of false memories, namely, that they often contain elements of "truth."

3.3. False Memories of Childhood

One paradigm for studying pseudomemory creation involves an effort to create false memories of events that never happened in childhood. Jacquie Pickrell and I published the results of one study involving 24 individuals who tried to recall events that were supplied by a close relative (Loftus & Pickrell, 1995). Three of the events were true, and one was a research-crafted false event about getting lost in a shopping mall, department store, or other public place. The subjects, who ranged in age from 18 to 53, thought they were taking part in a study of childhood memories. In phase 1, they completed a booklet containing four short stories about events from their childhood provided by a parent, sibling or other older relative. Three events actually happened, and the fourth, always in the third position, was false. The events were described in a single paragraph.

The false event was constructed from information provided by the relative who gave us details about a plausible shopping trip. The relative was asked to provide the following kinds of information: 1) where the family would have shopped when the subject was about five years old; 2) which members of the family usually went along on shopping trips; 3) what kinds of stores might have attracted the subject's interest; and 4) verification that the subject had not been lost in a mall around the age of five. The false event was then crafted from this information. The false events always included the following elements about the subject: 1) lost for an extended period of time, 2) crying, 3) lost in a mall or large department store at about the age of five, 4) found and aided by an elderly woman, 5) reunited with the family.

Subjects completed the booklets by reading what their relative had told us about each event, and then writing what they remembered about each event. If they did not remember the event, they were told to write, "I do not remember this."

When the booklets were returned, subjects were called and scheduled for two interviews. These occurred approximately 1–2 weeks apart. We told the subjects we were interested in examining how much detail they could remember, and how their memories compared with those of their relative. They were encouraged to try to remember the events before the interviews but not given any specific guidance. At the time of the interviews, the event paragraphs were not read to them verbatim, but rather bits of them were provided as retrieval cues. When the subject had recalled as much as possible, they were asked to rate the clarity of their memory for the event on a scale of one to ten, with one being not clear at all and ten being extremely clear.

In all, 72 true events were presented to subjects, and they remembered something about 49 (or 68%) of these. This figure did not change from the initial report through the two follow up interviews. The rate of "remembering" the false event was lower. Seven of 24 subjects "remembered" the false event, either fully or partially, in the initial booklet, but in the follow-up interviews only 6 subjects (25%) remembered the event. There were some differences between the true memories and the false ones. For example, subjects used more words when describing their true memories, whether these memories were fully or only partially recalled. Also, the clarity ratings for the false memories tended to be lower than for true memories produced by those same subjects. Interestingly, there was a tendency for the clarity ratings of the false memories to rise from the first interview to the second. Our results show that people can be led to believe that entire events happened to them after explicit suggestions to that effect. We make no claims about the percentage of people who might be able to be misled in this way, only that these cases provide an existence proof for the phenomenon of false memory formation.

Why are people remembering that they were lost? One possibility is that our subjects may have actually been lost in their lives, perhaps only briefly, and they may be confusing this actual experience with the false memory description that we supplied in the experiment. But it should be kept in mind that our subjects were not asked about ANY experience of being lost. They were asked to remember being lost around the age of five, in a particular location, with particular people present, being frightened, and ultimately being rescued by an elderly person.

Could false memories be created about events that were more unusual than getting lost? Hyman and his colleague have shown that the answer to this question is "yes" (Hyman, Husband & Billings, 1995). Hyman et al. picked more unusual events and tried to implant these in the minds of adult subjects. In one study, college students were asked to recall actual events that had been reported by their parents, and one experimenter-crafted false event. The false event was an overnight hospitalization for a high fever with a possible ear infection, or else a birthday party with pizza and a clown. Parents confirmed that neither of these events had happened, yet subjects were told that they had experienced one of the false events at about the age of five. Subjects tried to recall childhood experiences that they thought had been supplied by their parents, under the belief that the experimenters were interested in how people remember shared experiences differently. All events, both true ones and the false one, were first cued with an event title (family vacation, overnight hospitalization) and an age. Hyman et al. found that subjects remembered something about 84% of the true events in the first interview and 88% in the second interview. As for the creation of false memories, no subject recalled the false event during the first interview, but 20% did by the time of the second interview. One subject "remembered" that the doctor was a male, but the nurse was female, and also she happened to be a friend from church.

In a separate study by these investigators, three new false events were chosen, such unusual events as attending a wedding reception and accidentally spilling a punch bowl on the parents of the bride or having to evacuate a grocery store when the overhead sprinkler systems erroneously activated. In this study subjects were pressured a bit more for more complete recall. In all, subjects remembered something about 89% of the true events during the first interview. Somewhat higher percentages were remembered during the second

(93%) and third (95%) interviews. As for the false events, again no subjects recalled these during the first interview, but 25% did so by the third interview. For example, one subject had no recall of the wedding "accident," stating "I have no clue. I have never heard that one before." By the second interview the subject said: "...It was an outdoor wedding and I think we were running around and knocked something over like the punch bowl or something and um made a big mess and of course got yelled at for it."

In a third study (Hyman & Billings, 1996), the punchbowl false event was used again, in a study designed to explore individual differences in susceptibility to the creation of false memories. In all, subjects remembered something about 74% of the true events in the first interview and 85% in the second interview. As for the false events, only 1% of subjects recalled these during the first interview, but 27% did so by the second interview. One subject, during the second interview, remembered extensive detail about the unfortunate man who got punch spilled on him: "... a heavy set man, not like fat but like tall and big kind big beer belly, and I picture him having a dark suit on, like grayish dark and like having grayish dark hair and balding on top, and uh I picture him with a wide square face and I just picture him getting up and being kind of irritated or mad...." There were two individual differences measured that correlated strongly with the creation of false memories. The first is the Dissociative Experiences Scale (DES). The DES measures the tendency to have dissociative experiences or normal integration of awareness, thought and memory. Also correlated was the Creative Imagination Scale (CIS), which is a measure of hypnotizability, and also can be construed as a self-report measure of the vividness of mental imagery. The latter result is in line with prior research showing that highly-hypnotizable individuals were more likely than "lows" to accept misinformation and report it later as a memory (McConkey, Labelle, Bibb, & Bryant, 1990), and other research showing that individuals who rate highly in vividness of visual imagery are more prone to making source monitoring errors after exposure to misinformation (Dobson & Markham, 1993).

A variation of this procedure has also been used with children whose ages ranged from 3 to 6 (Ceci, Huffman, Smith, & Loftus, 1994). They were interviewed individually about real (parent-supplied) and fictitious (experimenter-contrived) events, and had to say whether each event happened to them or not. One "false" event concerned getting one's hand caught in a mousetrap and having to go to the hospital to get it removed; another concerned going on a hot air balloon ride with their classmates. The children were interviewed many times. As for the false memories, the young children (3–4 years old) assented to them 44% of the time during the first session, and 36% of the time during the seventh session. The false event was remembered at a somewhat lower rate (25% in the first session, 32% in the seventh session) for the older children (5–6 years old). In another study, involving children of the same age but involving more interviews about different fictitious items (i.e. falling off a tricycle and getting stitches in the leg), the rate at which children bought into the false memory increased steadily with more interviews (Ceci, Loftus, Leichtman, & Bruck, 1994).

Taken together, these results show that people will falsely recall childhood experiences in response to misleading information, and the social demands inherent in repeated interviews. The process of false recall appears to depend, in part, on accessing some relevant background information. Hyman and his colleagues hypothesized that some form of schematic reconstruction may account for the creation of false memories. What people appear to do, at the time they encounter the false details, is to call up schematic knowledge that is closely related to the false event. Next they think about the new information in conjunction with the schema, possibly storing the new information with that schema. Now, when they later try to remember the false event, they recall the false information and the underlying schema. The underlying schema is helpful for supporting the false event, in the sense that it adds actual background information and provides the skeletal or generic scenes.

3.4. Imagination Inflation

One process that may play a role in the creation of false childhood memories is imagination. These experimental methods may be inducing subjects to imagine events that they don't recall having happened. To explore the impact of deliberately inducing subjects to imagine a counterfactual past, I and my collaborators have shown that one simple act of imagining a childhood event increases a person's subjective confidence that the event happened to them in the past, a phenomenon we called "Imagination Inflation" (Garry, Manning, Loftus & Sherman, 1996). In this study, subjects were asked about a long list of possible childhood events (e.g., broke a window with your hand) and they told us the likelihood that these events had happened to them as a child. Two weeks later, subjects were instructed to imagine that some of these events had actually happened to them. And, finally, they responded for a second time about the likelihood of that long list of possible childhood events.

Consider one of the critical items. Some subjects were twice asked whether they broke a window with their hand as a child, asked once before and once after the following imagination exercise: "Imagine that it's after school and you are playing in the house. You hear a strange noise outside, so you run to the window to see what made the noise. As you are running, your feet catch on something and you trip and fall." While imagining themselves in this position, subjects answer some questions such as What did you trip on? They further imagine: "As you're falling you reach out to catch yourself and your hand goes through the window. As the window breaks you get cut and there's some blood." While imagining themselves in this predicament, they answer further questions such as What are you likely to do next." How do you feel?

We were most interested in the cases in which subjects initially said that they were unlikely to have had that experience. A one-minute act of counterfactual imagination led a significant minority of these individuals to report greater confidence that the event had happened to them. After engaging in this act of imagination, 24% of subjects increased their subjective confidence that they had broken a window with their hand (compared to 12% who increased when they had not imagined the event.). The other seven critical items used in this study similarly showed increased subjective confidence after imagination.

These findings show that even a single act of imagining a known counterfactual event can increase the subjective likelihood that the event happened in the past. Forming a mental image has also been shown to increase the likelihood that subjects develop a false childhood memory of spilling punch at a wedding reception (Hyman & Pentland, 1996), and to make people falsely believe that they carried out a variety of activities a few weeks earlier (Goff & Roediger, 1996). These studies call to mind the experiences of Christopher Robin Milne, who was immortalized in the children's stories written by his father, A.A. Milne. The fictional Christopher Robin, the young friend of Winnie-the-Pooh, was modeled after A.A.'s son. When Chrisopher Robin, the real one, died at the age of 75, obituaries reported that he had resented the confusing of his childhood with the popular legend: "He could not remember whether it was the real or fictional Christopher Robin who invented the game of "pooh-sticks," dropping sticks from a wooden bridge into a flowing stream" (Associated Press, 1996, p. B6).

A number of psychologists have expressed concerns that imagination activities may be one of the steps down the royal road to creating false memories, and the "imagination inflation" findings should at least make one wonder about the impact of imagination in therapy. Some present-day therapists recommend imagistic work (See Garry et al. for examples). Interestingly, Freud appears to have been fond of something akin to it as well. According to Freud scholar Mikkel Borch-Jacobsen (1996), after giving up on hypnosis, Freud embraced the "pressure technique," which involved pressing the hand on the patient's forehead and asking the patient to evoke an image. When therapists use or recommend imagination strategies for the express purpose of eliciting allegedly buried abuse memories, is it possible that they might create a memory for what was imagined?

3.5. Incorporating Dream Material into Waking Memory

Can dream material be mistaken for reality? University of Florence psychologist Giuliana Mazzoni and I reported three experiments that show that after a subtle suggestion, subjects falsely recognized items from their dreams, and thought these items had been presented during the waking state (Mazzoni & Loftus, in press). The procedure used in these studies involved three phases. Subjects studied a list of items on Day 1. On Day 2, they received a false suggestion that some items from their previously reported dreams had been presented on the list. On Day 3, they tried to recall only what had occurred on the initial list. Subjects falsely recognized their dream items at a very high rate, sometimes as often as they accurately recognized true items. They reported that they genuinely "remembered" the dream items, as opposed to simply "knowing" that they had been previously presented. These findings suggest that dreams can sometimes be mistaken for reality. Dream material might be especially problematic in the hands of a therapist who discusses sexual abuse during the day (causing sexual material to appear in the patient's dreams at night) and then uses dream material as a "resource" to reconstruct supposed past childhood sexual abuse. The danger that these questionable activities might lead a patient to a false belief and memory that sexual abuse actually occurred is more than a passing risk.

3.6. False Feedback Can Induce False Memories of Near Birth

In the typical misinformation study, very specific suggestions are fed to subjects who then occasionally incorporate these into their recollections about past events. In the "false feedback" paradigm, subjects are given false feedback about themselves as part of a manipulation designed to induce them to construct entirely false memories of the past. Drs. Susan DuBreuill, Maryanne Garry and others working in my laboratory have adapted a procedure first used in the Carleton University laboratory of the late N. Spanos (in collaboration with Burgess). The study was designed to simulate certain features that are included in some questionable therapeutic settings. Subjects are given a credible rationale for why they most probably saw a mobile over their cribs on the day after they were born, and why they will probably be able to retrieve memories of the mobile. In the initial research by Spanos and his collaborator Burgess, many subjects reported remembering the mobile, whether they were hypnotized or simply age regressed without hypnosis.

Our adaptation of this procedure used subjects who were interviewed in a therapy clinic room with low light, recliner chairs, and a two-way mirror. They filled out the "Princeton Personality Inventory," which was ostensibly scored by a computer, and were told that they demonstrated the profile of a "High Perceptual Cognitive Monitor." They were further told that this profile suggests that they most probably had visual experiences during a critical period shortly after birth, that they were probably exposed to a colored mobile hung over their cribs in the first few days after birth, the purpose of which was to stimulate coordinated eye movements and visual exploration. They were falsely told that the purpose of the study was to ascertain whether they were born in one of the hospitals that hung such mobiles. To determine this, subjects would under go "guided mnemonic restructuring", a technique for uncovering early infant memories. They were regressed back to the day of birth, and instructed to see themselves as if looking at a mental TV screen, and to describe what they saw. If they reported the mobile, they were urged to focus and provide as much detail as possible. Afterward, subjects were age progressed and they answered questions about their experience, including an assessment of whether they believed their memories were definitely real, probably real, unsure, probably fantasy, or definitely fantasy.

In our research, approximately half the subjects were induced to develop memories not of the first day of life, but of the first day of kindergarten. This was accomplished with parallel false feedback that suggested that they fit the profile of a "High Perceptual Cognitive Monitor" probably due to being exposed to spiral disks hung in the classroom on the first day of kindergarten, designed to stimulate coordinated eye movements and visual exploration. They too were age regressed to ascertain whether they experienced the spiral disks. We hypothesized that subjects might be even more readily induced to falsely remember spiral disks from kindergarten since they would not have metacognitive beliefs about childhood amnesia to keep them from remembering events from this age.

Our preliminary research revealed that over 80% of subjects reported remembering some experience at the target age. In terms of the specific suggested stimulus, approximately 60% claimed some memory of the mobile and 25% claimed some memory of the spiral disk. Thus, the Kindergarten subjects were less likely to create a false memory for the suggested stimulus.

Many of the "memories" were quite detailed. To give the flavor of response, here is one from a "mobile" subject: "There are little paper baby bottles hanging from the ceiling and there's a yellow bow tied to somebody's, um, crib but I don't know why and the crib I'm in is like, um, a clear plastic thing and there's like a red___along the side. And actually I remember there's a mobile. If I'm laying on my back, it's hanging from the left corner. But it seems to be pastel colors. It's nothing bright."

Variations in the false feedback paradigm are now being used in other laboratories. Preliminary reports are consistent with those reported here, namely, that it is possible to induce people to construct false memories and make false memory reports, even to report impossible memories, by giving them a credible rationale for why they might expect to have these specific memories.

To recap, current paradigms have taken the misinformation effect a long way. We and others have succeeded in getting people to harbor entirely false memories of events that didn't happen to them a few weeks ago, events that didn't happen to them as children, and even events that didn't happen on the day after they were born. That is the power of suggestion. Now, in no way does this mean that whenever someone remembers something they have not remembered in some time that the memory must be false, or must have been a product of suggestion. That would be a completely unwarranted interpretation of the false memory research. However, these studies do tell us that suggestion can be powerful in its ability to induce in people a host of unlikely memories, and remind us that suggestive practices should be handled as delicately as one might handle a sharp knife.

Destun and Kuiper (1996) have argued that the misinformation effect has implications for autobiographical memory accuracy in a clinical setting. Presumably their argument would also apply to the more elaborate false memory studies described above. They write: "...given that recovered memory therapy techniques such as journalling encourage clients to rehearse versions of childhood memories that are often deliberately embellished in therapy, it is possible that this rehearsal could lead to clients' increased acceptance and belief in these memories.

By the same token, the passage of time between the episode being remembered and therapy, in combination with the fact that the therapist might be perceived by the client to be in a position of relative authority, might serve to increase the client's acceptance of a memory that is, at least in part, a product of therapist suggestions" (p. 426).

4. BATTLE OVER REPRESSED MEMORY "CRIME VICTIMS"

A burst of gunfire was sent in the direction of one governmental agency over repressed memory claims. The agency had conducted an internal study that, once it received some publicity, was used to bolster the claim that repressed memory therapy might be responsible for significant deterioration in the mental health of some patients. The study was described, for example, in a Canadian newspaper by a popular, articulate columnist writing under the headline: "The taboos of recovered memory" (Wente, 1996, p D7). The columnist described the "victims" of recovered memory therapy pointing out: "These poor women are victims indeed. But of whom?" (Wente, 1996, D7). The study was described in a California newspaper by a leading and lucid columnist who commented on the patients this way: "And since their long-repressed memories have surfaced, they're not healing. They're falling apart" (Jacobs, 1996). Finally, the study was featured in a front-page newspaper story in *The Olympian* with the headline "Victims' therapy called harmful" (Shannon, 1996). The findings of the study were indeed alarming, as the patients did appear to be far worse off after the therapy than before, but as I explain shortly, the study does not "prove" that it was therapy that made patients worse. Unfortunately, the small battle that erupted over publicity that the study received served to distract from its real value, namely, in suggesting to future researchers a novel method for gathering and examining information about repressed memory allegations.

By way of background, a crime victims compensation program in the State of Washington provides for financial, medical and mental health benefits to victims of violent crime. It is one of many states that does so. The Washington program is explicitly a "payer of last resort" which means that an applicant must have already used benefits provided by other insurance. To be eligible for compensation, an applicant must require medical or mental health treatment because of the injuries suffered as a result of a crime.

In the early 1990's, an amendment to the Crime Victims Act allowed for individuals to seek compensation from the State of Washington if they claimed they had repressed their memory for long-ago abuse but now their memories had returned. A document called the "Crime Victims Act" (1994) reveals that the legislature had its own ideas about repression: "Because victims of childhood criminal acts may repress conscious memory of such criminal acts far beyond the age of eighteen, the rights of adult victims of childhood criminal acts shall accrue at the time the victim discovers or reasonably should have discovered the elements of the crime" (p. 4). The Application for Benefits (dated 5/95) informs potential applicants that to be eligible for benefits they must have reported the criminal act to the police (or to a child protection agency) within 12 months of the occurrence or within 12 months of the time it could have been reasonably reported. This clause is what permits financial compensation for victims who only learn much later in life that they had suffered victimization in childhood. Between 1991 and 1995, over 300 individuals had received funds from the State for their "repressed memory" victimization.

Staff employees, including a registered nurse and a Master's of Education, working for the Department of Labor and Industries, reviewed 183 of these claims, ones that were still active in 1995. Of these, 30 were "randomly selected for a preliminary profile" (Parr,

1996a, b); they ranged in age from 15 to 67 (mean age 43), and were almost exclusively Caucasian women. These patients were primarily seeing Master's-level therapists, although in 8 cases an M.D. was involved in the case as the primary therapist, or in conjunction with the Master's-level therapist. Parr (1996a,b) reported that the first memory surfaced during therapy in 87% of the cases (however it is unclear whether this means literally during a therapy session, or during a period when the person was receiving therapy). All 30 were still in therapy three years after their first memory surfaced.

According to Parr's report (1996a,b), before the memories, only 3 (10%) had thought about or attempted suicide; after memories, 20 (67%) had. Before memories, only 2 (7%) had been hospitalized (presumably for psychiatric reasons); after memories, 11 (37%) had. Before memories, only one woman had engaged in self-mutilation; after memories 8 (27%) had.

According to Parr's analysis (1996a,b), all but one of the patients contended they had been abused in satanic rituals. They claimed their abuse began when they were, on average, 7 months old. They said family members were involved in the SRA, that they experienced infant cannibalism, and had to consume body parts, and that they were tortured or mutilated. No mutilation could be corroborated by medical exams.

Parr (1996a,b) also revealed that before entering therapy, the majority (25/30 = 83%) of the patients had been employed, but after three years of therapy, only 3 of 30 (10%) were still employed. Before therapy, 23 of the 30 (77%) were married; within three years of this time, 11/23 (48%) were either separated or divorced. Of the 21 patients who had children, one third lost custody. All 30 were estranged from their extended families.

The financial bottom line, according to Parr (1996a,b) was staggering: The average cost of a non-repressed memory claim was $2,672. By contrast, the average cost for the 183 repressed memory claims was higher: $12,296 (median = $9,296). In four years time, the 325 repressed memory claims of concern had utilized over $2,500,000 in mental health benefits.

To put a "face" on these statistics, consider one case as evaluated and reported by Parr (1996a,b). Terry J was 34 when, in 1992, she filed a repressed memory claim alleging that her grandmother forced her to go with people who molested and raped her. A detailed examination of her medical records revealed that in 1994 she was diagnosed by an MSW as having Multiple Personality Disorder, with at least 3,000 known fragments. Through therapy she had remembered her mother molesting her at age 5. She remembered being mutilated by a "big man in black" at age five. She remembered abuse by her father that involved being forced to keep company with a dead baby. She remembered being forced to eat a baby's heart. She remembered hundreds of physical injuries to her body although none had been substantiated in medical reports. By the time of Parr's report, the State of Washington had spent $29,181.98 on her claim.

What should we make of the Crime Victim Compensation data? One obvious question is why so many cases of satanic ritual abuse? Does this indicate some bias in the sampling process? It certainly does not reflect the proportion of satanic ritual abuse cases in the overall collection of repressed memory claims, that proportion is certainly much smaller. A second question is what to make of the fact that the patients seem to be getting worse rather than better. While this observation appears to be true for the 30 patients in the sample, the data do not prove that it is the therapy that made the patients worse. These patients may have been ones who would have shown dramatic declines in mental health even without any therapeutic intervention at all, or with a different kind of therapy.

After the crime victims' data were publicized, a minor fury erupted in writing, on the internet, and in conference halls. Some individuals, of course, were concerned about the possibility that these patients had been victims of therapy that may have greatly increased their suffering. Although, as I have said, the study does not prove that it is the therapy as opposed to something else that has made these patients worse. Many other individuals who learned about the study complained about the alleged biases of the government employees, or violations of confidentiality of the patients in the sample. Others complained loudly about the seeming lack of random sampling. (Interestingly, this comment about random sampling is rarely heard when mental health professionals write a paper about some unspecified set of their patients, as, for example, did well-known psychiatrist Lenore Terr in a widely cited 1988 report on 20 of her patients). One writer mocked the Crime Victims' findings by writing a parody about patients who get worse after seeing a doctor for lung cancer treatment. (Of course the obvious response to this questionable analogy is to consider the natural history of the disease. With lung cancer we know a great deal about treated versus untreated disease, enough to know that most patients would be smart to choose treatment. For patients with diseases of depression or eating disorders, one cannot make the same claim about the benefits of repressed memory therapy).

Admittedly the concerns about the sampling, about research biases, about confidentiality, may all be quite legitimate. But equally legitimate is the concern about the mental health of the patients, and the most natural question in the world to be asking about these findings is this: Why have these patients worsened after their state-funded therapeutic treatments? The Crime Victims' data cannot tell us definitively why, but the methodology used to gather these data constitutes the germ of a good idea that, with adaptation, could provide valuable information.

The method used by Parr (1996a,b) has advantages over the retrospective surveys of patients or their therapists, since these are so subject to retrospective memory biases. The "crime victims" methodology relies on an examination of medical records and other documentation, and a "counting" of certain outcome measures (e.g., number of hospitalizations, number of suicide attempts, number of divorces). But the study needs to be done again, with proper controls and scientific checks. At the very least greater assurance of random sampling of files is needed. Multiple coders of information and reliability checks would be included in the improved version of this study paradigm. The repressed memory patients may appear to be getting worse, but compared to what? What has happened to other alleged crime victims, say of recent rape, or car jacking, or armed robbery, who pass through the system? Some prominent psychiatrists have worried that the repressed memory therapy is not helping patients. One of them put it this way: "What seems to be happening in the recovered memory saga is not unlike what happened years ago with thalidomide: the premature release of an apparently promising medication produced such disastrous side effects that it had to be withdrawn" (Munro, 1996). An improved study adapted from the initial ideas and contribution produced by Parr and her colleagues (1996a,b) would go a long way towards testing the hypothesis underlying the "thalidomide" analogy.

Assuming a larger, improved study were to find comparable results, we should be deeply distressed. The bizarre events that people reported in Parr (1996a,b) are almost certainly not accurate recollections of real events, especially given that scientific research indicates that adults are unable to recollect experiences from the first two years of life, and that large-scale satanic cults are almost certainly mythical. Such findings would certainly be consistent with the hypothesis that the experience of "recovering" such "memories" is greatly damaging to clients (i.e., marriages and familial relations are disrupted, employment lost, and the incidence of symptoms of extreme psychopathology greatly increased after people recover such memories). Taken together with other evidence of the suggestive power of the "memory retrieval" techniques used by some therapists, these sorts of findings would support concern that such approaches to psychotherapy may grievously harm clients. While the Department of Labor and Industries has chosen not to conduct such a worthy follow-up study at this time, nonetheless the agency is undertaking a campaign to reconsider eligibility guidelines for compensation, and to better monitor the therapies that it funds (Robinson, 1996).

5. BATTLE OF THE PSYCHOTHERAPY BULGE

The memory wars are sometimes cast as a war between clinicians and memory researchers, yet nothing could be farther from the truth. The repressed memory controversy has created splits within the ranks of mental health professionals that threaten to harm the reputation of psychotherapy and ruin past friendships. One clear example can be found in the field of hypnosis. Clinicians are deeply divided over whether hypnosis should or should not be used to dig for buried memories of trauma. In surveys of psychologists in the U.S. and Britain, Poole, Lindsay, Memon and Bull (1995) asked about the techniques that clinicians use to uncover buried memories of abuse. One survey question was put this way: "Some therapists use special techniques to help clients remember childhood sexual abuse. Check any technique that you have used with abuse victims in the past two years." In a second survey, to be sure that the clinicians understood that the technique was to be endorsed only if it had been used explicitly to help clients recall memories of sexual abuse, the wording was modified to make that very clear. In that latter survey, 34% of clinicians reported using hypnosis, while 33% said they disapproved of its use for that purpose. In another survey, U.S. clinicians also demonstrated conflicted feelings about the use of hypnosis for this purpose (Polusny & Follette, 1996). Clinicians were asked to "Please indicate the memory retrieval techniques you use with adult clients who have no specific memory of childhood sexual abuse but who you strongly suspected were sexually abused" (45). Twenty percent said they use hypnosis or trance induction, while 45% said their use was inappropriate for this purpose. The controversy over hypnotically uncovering memories is reviewed more extensively by Lynn (this volume).

It is one thing for clinicians to conduct studies, present data, and trade interpretations of findings regarding hypnosis, and quite another for them to fall into personal attacks over these scientific views. Yet, according to material presented in the Spring 1996 newsletter, the latter is what appears to have happened within the Society for Clinical and Experimental Hypnosis, a prestigious organization for hypnosis researchers. Apparently the awards committee for the organization chose to bestow the prestigious Dorcus Award upon Richard Ofshe and Margaret Singer for an article that they had published in the society's main journal. In the words of the chair of the awards committee: "The paper took aim at a specific subset of therapists who believe that every human disorder... is the product of decades-delayed repressed memories of sexual abuse during childhood" (Perry, 1996, p. 10). The President of the organization, refused to announce the award at the annual meeting, and wrote an editorial attacking the article in the Spring newsletter. "I was so shocked by the choice that I thought it might be a mistake" (Spiegel, 1996, 1). Eleven members sided with the attack on the article claiming biases in the award process (Frischholz, 1996). Subsequently more than 60 individuals expressed their displeasure with the attackers (Adrian et al., 1996), stating "We can disagree with each other about the utility of concepts like repression, dissociation, and the merits of recovered memory therapy. We must be tolerant of this diversity" (p. 7).

One might reasonably ask why mental health professionals, some of whom are exceedingly prominent clinicians, are fighting a war in this fashion?

6. CIVIL WAR IN THE "FORMER FEMINISM UNION"

Gloria Steinem's endorsement is proudly displayed on the cover of E. Sue Blume's book, *Secret Survivors* (1990). It reads: "Explores the constellation of symptoms that result from a crime too cruel for mind and memory to face. This book, like the truth it helps uncover, can set millions free." The book opens to the "Incest Survivor's Aftereffects Checklist" where readers can discover whether they are survivors of incest by comparing themselves to the presented list of symptoms, a long list that included symptoms such as nightmares, headaches, arthritis, alcohol abuse (or total abstinence), depression, inability to trust, total trust, high risk taking, inability to take risks, wearing baggy clothing." The checklist is so all-inclusive that it has been accused of distinguishing only two groups, namely those who are alive and those who are dead. Despite its complete lack of validation, the checklist still managed to gain the endorsement of at least one feminist clinical psychologist advocate who called it a "useful checklist guide for the therapist" (Walker, 1994, 114). Despite its endorsement by prominent feminist spokespersons, *Secret Survivors*, the book and its checklist, has been widely attacked for its misleading information, and its potentially catastrophic advice to women.

In a speech given at the annual meeting of the American Psychological Association, Gloria Steinem (1995) at least acknowledged that false accusations of abuse can damage the true cases, and suggested that we try to look and see what can be corroborated. But why did she feel the need to air at great length the dirty laundry of a family—a father, a mother, a daughter —involved in devastating accusations? Disturbed that a letter written by an uncle in the Freyd family had not been picked up by the media, Steinem read it out loud to thousands during her speech. Its defamatory material did not appear to lead to even a modicum of restraint. Why did Steinem choose to diagnose this family as one probably involved in a continuation of victimization and abuse that started in the past, thus pronouncing individuals whom she had never met guilty of crimes whose authenticity she could not possibly know? Why did she report as fact the highly controversial and disputed claims that multiple disorder patients have alters with different allergies and different eyesight changes due to different curvatures of the cornea? By her own admission, she called a researcher from the New York Times and suggested that the researcher pay attention to the multiple personality disorder patients: "Their reaction to medication changes, their allergies change, their eyesight changes, not because they think it does but because the curvature of the cornea actually changes." Why has Steinem promoted such controversial ideas as widespread ritual sex abuse, and for such questionable beliefs and practices that have devastated the lives of women? Was it her idea to feature a first person account of surviving ritual abuse (Rose, 1993) on the cover of Ms. Magazine, with the exhortation "Believe it! Cult Ritual Abuse Exists." In doing so, has she not helped to damage the cause of feminism that she once so masterfully inspired? But she is not alone on the satanic ritual abuse side of the feminist battlefield. As Nathan and Snedeker so well document, she is joined in her support for the belief in widespread ritual sex abuse by countless psychotherapists, social workers, doctors, lawyers, and writers who "call themselves feminists" (1995, p. 247).

The battle being waged in the "former feminism union" has been eloquently described by Canadian columnist and social activist Donna LaFramboise (1996), in her courageous book, The Princess at the Window. As one deeply committed to principles of reason, fairness and justice, LaFramboise has recognized from the start that actions that might provide an immediate benefit to women, may not be actions that are reasonable, fair and just. Her example to drive this point home is simple but stunningly powerful: Since males aged 15 to 40 commit most of the rapes in our society, it might benefit women as a group if all males within that age bracket were herded into army bases and not permitted to leave until their 40th birthday. The lack of fairness of such an absurd proposal for dealing with the very real problem of rape is immediately apparent: millions of innocent men would be punished. Millions of innocent men would be denied basic fundamental freedoms.

Much of the feminist movement has been about fighting against injustice. When, under the banner of feminism or any other banner, groups of people in our society press for actions that are unjust, it is more than reasonable to feel a strong moral duty to protest. It is not in anyone's interest to substitute one oppressive society for another. Yet many of the actions being advocated under the banner of feminism are not only oppressive, but, according to a major thesis in The Princess at the Window, are self-obsessed, arrogant, intolerant, and are giving female equality a very bad name. Feminism risks generating a backlash like we've never seen before:

> Sooner or later, a society inundated with loony feminist notions is going to slam on the brakes. When that happens, the very idea of feminism, together with all its positive contributions, will become suspect. The general public will harden its heart and grow cynical. It's knee-jerk tendency will be to dismiss all feminist protest out of hand and to declare itself weary of complaints regarding female disadvantage, no matter how justified they might be (7–8).

Other journalists, many of them women, have echoed similar ideas. Neimark (1996) talks of the "misguided feminist cause of other women as victims." Picking up Neimark's ball and running with it, Wente (1996) asks that we recognize that the battle is not about feminism. "It's about reason. Let's hope reason is winning" (p. D7) For all those who truly care about women, about children, about men, about people, these realizations about our culture of victimization must be appreciated at a very deep level, and reason must win..

7. FINAL REMARKS

Although some have suggested that the recovered sex-abuse memory wars are "winding down after a decade of bitter conflict" (Nathan & Haaken, 1996, 29), the battles described in this chapter suggest that the war is still far from over. We continue to have serious problems today, although perhaps some end is in sight. In thinking about where we might be, say 25 years from now, there may be a lesson to be learned from Arthur Miller's (1996) essay "Why I wrote "The Crucible." According to Miller, he wrote the play originally as an act of desperation. He was motivated in great part by the paralysis that had set in among many liberals who, during the hunt for Reds in America, had become fearful of being identified as covert Communists if they protested too strongly the violation of civil rights being pursued by numerous inquisitors. He drew parallels between the Red hunt, led by the House Committee on Un-American Activities, during the 1950's and the witchcraze of Salem during 1962. He was inspired by one man's efforts during the 17th century to set aside his personal concerns and become the most forthright voice against the madness around him. His critics complained about his analogy: "..there never were any witches but there certainly are Communists." (p. 162), he was told. But, the fact of the matter is, during the 17th century, the existence of witches was hardly questioned, and people lost their lives if they doubted this. Back then, anyone could be accused, and even convicted based solely on "spectral evidence." According to Miller (1996, pp. 162–163), spectral evidence meant that "if I swore that you had sent out your 'familiar spirit' to choke, tickle, or poison me or my cattle, or to control my thoughts and actions, I could get you hanged...." Spectral evidence made a "kind of lunatic sense," just as equally invalid evidence made during the Red Hunt of the 1950s. We look back now, and both seem nearly comical. It's hard to conceive of the fear that once so widely pervaded. A quarter century from from now, will we also look back to many of the claims of the 1990's, finding them almost comical, having forgotten the fear and anger and sadness that fueled these sorry Wars?

Earlier in this chapter I posed a few questions for contemplation about these wars. One was about the damaging aspects of doing battle: Is engaging in battle a productive thing to do, or is it creating splits and tears that will be exceedingly difficult to repair? I believe, as the co-signers of one of the hypnosis letters urged, that we must be tolerant of diversity. Many of the battles have been exceedingly unproductive, and past good relationships have been torn apart as a result. The hypnosis professionals provide but a single clear example of this unpleasantness. The splits and tears in families are an order of magnitude worse.

I asked another question: Can't we appreciate that some past practices may have been a mistake, and that it is time to join together to stop them? Fortunately, a number of prominent clinicians have already taken this important step (Courtois, this volume; Briere, this volume).

I asked also: Is it not time to recast the tone from its present black and white extreme to one that appreciates shades of gray? Can we not collectively get behind a joint effort to devise better methods to tell apart the patients with accurate recovered memories and the patients with illusory ones? A few writers have urged professionals to find the middle ground in the recovered-memories debate, to recast the tone from its present black and white extremes to one that appreciates the shades of gray (e.g., Lindsay & Read, 1995; Schacter, 1996, p. 277). They differ in terms of the advice they give for how to accomplish this feat. Schacter urges that risky therapeutic practices need to be stopped and that better methods must be developed to tell apart the patients with accurate recovered memories from the patients with illusory ones. Lindsay and Read (1995) urge the timely realization on the part of therapists that extensive use of memory recovery techniques is ill-advised, but they go on to emphasize that such acknowledgement in no way denies the reality and importance of genuine childhood sexual abuse. Hopefully we can find at least this point of agreement rather quickly: knee-jerk embracing of every abuse report, no matter how bizarre, no matter how extreme the process to extract it, makes a mockery of legitimate cases of grossly inappropriate behavior. My argument is similar to that which was made after a 6-year-old boy was suspended from school for kissing a classmate on the cheek. The friendly boy was charged with sexual harrassment. Public outcry was instantaneous: "It's the adults who are over the line. They apply the term sexual harassment to an incident that is neither sexual nor harassment. In the process, they demean genuine, serious cases of inappropriate sexual behavior in the workplace" (Seattle Times, editorial, 1996).

It is worth giving serious consideration to these questions, and worth figuring out how we can discuss this sensitive subject calmly and rationally. Only then can we hope to minimize the suffering of all victims of the memory wars, all the patients, their families, the genuine survivors of sexual abuse, and the professionals who care deeply about all of them.

REFERENCES

Adrian, C., Andersen, M., Barber, J., Bates, B., Bejenke, C., Bowers, K., Bowers, P., Burrows, G., Chaves, J., Covino, N., Dempster, C., Dengrove, E., Dinges, D., Dywan, J., Erickson, J., Franko, D., Freedman, A., Green, S., Gruenewald, D., Hedenberg, J., Herzog, A., Hopkins, C., Hornyak, L., Karlin, R., Kaushall, P., Kelly, S., Kessler, R., Kihlstrom, J., Kirsch, I., LaClave, L., Laurence, J., Lavoie, G., LeBaron, S., Lert, A., Locke, S., Loftus, E., London, R., Lynn, S., Mulligan, R., Nadon, R., Nash, M., Orne, E., Orne, M., Pettinati, H., Reyher, J., Rhue, J., Rothman, I., Sarbin, T., Sargent, G., Sheehan, P., Singer, M., Strauss, B., Wallace, B., Weinstock, A., Whitehouse, W., Woody, E., Wright, M., Zachariae, R., Zamansky, H., Zeltzer, L., & Zinn, S. (1996, Summer). "Dear Colleagues." *SCEH Focus: A quarterly publication of the Society for Clinical and Experimental Hypnosis*, 7–8.
Associated Press (1996, April 22). Christopher Robin Milne, 75. *Seattle Times*, B6.
Beaver, J. E. (1996). Book Review: The myth of repressed memory. *The Journal of Criminal Law and Criminology*, 86, 596–607.
Belli, R. F. (1989). Influences of misleading postevent information: Misinformation interference and acceptance. *Journal of Experimental Psychology: General*, 118, 72–85.
Borch-Jacobsen, M. (1996, Spring). Neurotica: Freud and the seduction theory. *October 76*, p 15–43.
Blume, E. S. (1990). *Secret Survivors*. NY: Wiley.
Ceci, S. J., Huffman, M. L. C., Smith, E., & Loftus, E.F. (1994). Repeatedly thinking about a non-event: Source misattributions among preschoolers. *Consciousness and Cognition*, 3, 388–407.
Ceci, S. J., Loftus, E. F., Leichtman, M. D., & Bruck, M. (1994). The possible role of source misattributions in the creation of false beliefs among preschoolers. *International Journal of Clinical and Experimental Hypnosis*, Volume XLII, 304–320.
Chandler, C. C. (1991). How memory for an event is influenced by related events: Interference in modified recognition tests. *Journal of Experimental Psychology: Learning, Memory & Cognition*, 17, 115–125.
Cohen, R. (1995, April 27) Bosnian Serb denies all at a War Crimes Tribunal, *New York Times*, A3.
Conklin, E. E. (1996, May 21). Therapy blamed in delusions, death. *Seattle Post-Intelligencer*, B1-B2.
Crews, F. (1995). *The Memory Wars: Freud's legacy in dispute*. NY: The New York Review of Books.
Crime Victims Act (1994, Oct). Crime Victims Compensation Program, Department of Labor and Industries, Chapter 7.68 RCW.
Destun, L. M. & Kuiper, N. A. (1996). Autobiographical memory and recovered memory therapy. *Clinical Psychology Review*, 16, 421–450.
Dobson, M. & Markham, R. (1993). Imagery ability and source monitoring: Implications for eyewitness memory. *British Journal of Psychology*, 84, 111–118.
Frischholz, E. J., Spiegel, H., Greenleaf, M., Finklestein, S., Wickless, C., Fine, C., Brown, D., Gravitz, M., Kluft, R., Coe, W., & Torem, M. (1996, Spring). Letter to the Editor. *SCEH Focus. A quarterly publication of the Society for Clinical and Experimental Hypnosis*, 11–12.
Garry, M., Manning, C., Loftus, E. F., & Sherman, S. J. (1996). Imagination inflation. *Psychonomic Bulletin and Review*, 3, 208–214.
Geiselman, R. E., Fisher, R. P., MacKinnon, D. P., & Holland, H. L. (1985). Eyewitness memory enhancement in the police interview: Cognitive retrieval mnemonics versus hypnosis. *Journal of Applied Psychology*, 70, 401–412.
Goff, L. M. & Roediger, H. L. (1996). Imagination inflation: Multiple imaginings can lead to false recollection of one's actions. Paper presented at the Annual meeting of the Psychonomic Society, Chicago.
Hyman, I.E. & Billings, F.J. (1995) Individual differences and the creation of false childhood memories. Unpublished manuscript, Western Washington University.
Hyman, I. E, Husband, T. H. & Billings, F. J. (1995). False memories of childhood experiences. *Applied Cognitive Psychology*, 9, 181-197.
Hyman, I. E. & Pentland, J. (1996). The role of mental imagery in the creation of false childhood memories. *Journal of Memory and Language*, 35, 101–117.
International Criminal Tribunal for the Former Yugoslavia (1995). Prosecutor of the Tribunal against Dusan Tadic a/k/a "Dule" Goran Borovnica. Indictment.
Jacobs, J. (1996). Suggestion may lead to adult memories of childhood abuse. *San Jose Mercury News*. Reprinted in *The Tacoma News Tribune*, May 28, 1996, A9.
Johnson, M. K. Lindsay, D. S. & Hashtroudi, S. (1993). Source monitoring. *Psychological Bulletin, 114*, 3–28.
LaFramboise, D. (1996). *The princess at the window: A new gender morality*. Toronto: Penguin Books Canada.
Lee, K. (1996). Children's suggestibility: The effect of misinformation vs inconsistent information. Poster presented at the NATO Advanced Study Institute, Port de Bourgenay, France, June (this volume).

Lief, H. I. & Fetkewicz, J. M. (1995) Retractors of false memories: The evolution of pseudomemories. *The Journal of Psychiatry & Law*, 23, 411–436.

Lindsay, D. S. & Read, J. D. (1994). Psychotherapy and memories of childhood sexual abuse: A cognitive perspective. *Applied Cognitive Psychology*, 8, 281–338.

Lindsay, D.S. & Read, J.D. (1995). "Memory work" and recovered memories of childhood sexual abuse. *Psychology, Public Policy, and Law*, 1, 846–908.

Loftus, E. F. (1979). *Eyewitness testimony*. Cambridge: Harvard University Press

Loftus, E. F. & Ketcham, K. (1991). *Witness for the Defense*. NY: St. Martin's Press.

Loftus, E. F. & Ketcham, K. (1994). *The Myth of Repressed Memory*. NY: St. Martin's Press.

Loftus, E. F., Paddock, J. R., & Guernsey, T. F. (1996). Patient-psychotherapist privilege: Access to clinical records in the tangled web of repressed memory litigation. *University of Richmond Law Review*, 30, 109- 154.

Loftus, E. F. & Pickrell, J. (1995). The formation of false memories. *Psychiatric Annals*, 25, 720–724.

Mazzoni, G. A L. & Loftus, E. F. (in press). When dreams become reality. *Consciousness & Cognition*.

McConkey, K. M., Labelle, L., Bibb, B. C., & Bryant, R. A. (1990). Hypnosis and suggested pseudomemory: The relevance of test context. *Australian Journal of Psychology*, 42, 197–205.

Merskey, H. (1996). Ethical issues in the search for repressed memories. *American Journal of Psychotherapy*, 50, 323–335.

Miller, A. (1996, Oct 21). Why I wrote "The Crucible." *The New Yorker*, p 158–164.

Munro, A. (1996). Recovered memories in psychotherapy. *The Canadian Journal of Psychiatry*, 41, 199–200.

Nathan, D. & Haaken, J. (1996, Sept/Oct). From incest to Ivan the Terrible: Science and the Trials of Memory. *Tikkun*, p 29–30, 94–96.

Nathan, D. & Snedeker, M. (1995). *Satan's Silence: Ritual abuse and the making of a modern American witch hunt*. NY: Basic Books.

Neimark, J. (1996, May/June). Dispatch from the memory war. *Psychology Today Magazine*, 6–7.

Paris, J. (1996). A critical review of recovered memories in psychotherapy: Part II- Trauma and Therapy, *Canadian Journal of Psychiatry*, 41, 206–210.

Parr, L. E. (1996a). Repressed memory claim referrals to the nurse consultant. Department of Labor & Industries. Crime Victims Compensation Program. State of Washington. Unpublished manuscript submitted to Mental Health Subcommittee. (CVC Program, PO Box 44520, Olympia Washington 98504–4520. Tel: (360) 902–4945

Parr, L. E. (1996b). Repressed memory claims in the crime victims compensation program. Department of Labor & Industries. Crime Victims Compensation Program. State of Washington. Unpublished manuscript (with contributions from B. Huseby and R. Brown).

Perry, C. (1996, Spring). Letter to the Editor. *SCEH Focus. A quarterly publication of the Society for Clinical and Experimental Hypnosis*, 10.

Polusny, M. A. & Follette, V. M. (1996). Remembering childhood sexual abuse: A national survey of psychologists' clinical practices, beliefs, and personal experiences. *Professional Psychology: Research & Practice*, 27, 41-52.

Poole, D. A., Lindsay, D. S; Memon, A., Bull, R. (1995). Psychotherapy and the recovery of memories of childhood sexual abuse: US and British Practitioners' opinions, practices and experiences. *Journal of Consulting and Clinical Psychology*, 63, 426–437.

Pope, H. G. & Hudson, J. I. (1995). Can memories of childhood sexual abuse be repressed? *Psychological Medicine*, 25, 121–126.

Pope, H. G., Oliva, P. S. & Hudson, J. I. (1996). Can memories of trauma be "repressed?" Unpublished manuscript, Harvard Medical School.

Reyna, V. F., & Titcomb, A. L. (in press). Constraints on the suggestibility of eyewitness testimony: A fuzzy- trace theory analysis. In D. G. Payne & F. G. Conrad (Eds.), *Intersections in basic and applied memory research*. Hillsdale, NJ: Lawrence Erlbaum Associates.

Robinson, K. (1996, Aug 14). It happened one night, I think. *Seattle Weekly*, 9–12.

Roediger, H. L. (1996). Memory illusions. *Journal of Memory and Language*, 35, 76–100.

Roediger, H. L., Jacoby, D., & McDermott, K. B. (1996). Misinformation effects in recall: Creating false memories through repeated retrieval. *Journal of Memory and Language*, 35, 300–318.

Rose, E. S. (1993, Jan/Feb). Surviving the unbelievable: A first-person account of cult ritual abuse, p 40–45.

Schacter, Daniel L. (1995). Memory wars. *Scientific American*, 272, 135–139

Schacter, Daniel L. (1996). *Searching for memory: The brain, the mind, and the past*. NY: Basic Books.

Seattle Times (1996, Sept 29). Editorials: The kiss was just a kiss, B6.

Shannon, B. (1996, June 7). Victims' therapy called harmful. *The Olympian*, A1.

Slovenko, R. (1995). The duty of therapists to third parties. *The Journal of Psychiatry & Law*, 23, 383–410.

Spanos, N. P., Menary, E., Gabora, N., DuBreuil, S., & Dewhirst, B. (1991). Secondary identity enactments during hypnotic past-life regression: A sociocognitive perspective. *Journal of Personality & Social Psychology,* 61, 308–320.

Spiegel, D. (1996, Spring). Presidential column. *SCEH Focus: A quarterly publication of the Society for Clinical and Experimental Hypnosis,* 1–2, 13

Steinem, Gloria (1995, August). Making connections. Speech presented at the American Psychological Association annual Convention, New York.

Terr, L. (1988). What happens to memories of trauma? *American Academy of Child and Adolescent Psychiatry,* 27, 96–l04.

Titcomb, A. L. & Reyna, V. F. (1995). In F. N. Dempster and C. Brainerd (Eds.) *Interference and Inhibition in Cognition,* (pp. 264–294). San Diego: Academic Press.

Walker, L. E. A. (1994). *Abused women and survivor therapy: A practical guide for the psychotherapist.* Washington, D.C.: American Psychological Association.

Wente, M. (1996, May 4). The taboos of recovered memory. *The Globe and Mail,* D7.

Weschler, L. (1995, Nov. 20). Inventing peace. *The New Yorker,* 56–64.

COMMENTARY ON DISPATCH FROM THE (UN)CIVIL MEMORY WARS

Chris R. Brewin, Royal Holloway, University of London, United Kingdom

As all of us attending this meeting are well aware, Elizabeth Loftus has done an enormous amount to alert the clinical and scientific communities to the dangers of using suggestive memory techniques. This has been a most valuable contribution that has provoked wide-ranging scrutiny of the assumptions and methods employed when treating clients thought to have experienced child sexual abuse. Attention has been focused, rightly, on an area where bad clinical practice can have even more damaging consequences than it can do under circumstances where the nature of clients' relationships with close family members is not called into question.

This was a fascinating and impressive presentation in many ways. I was struck by the developments in the study of the implantation of false memories. In the early work, adolescents were persuaded that when they were much younger they had been lost in a shopping mall. These studies seemed to require that the events be described by a trustworthy witness, perhaps someone who was already in a relationship to the participant in which there was a high probability of having shared memories. In this work, the false memories were carefully intermingled with other, true memories, and also contained true details.

Subsequent work by Loftus, Hyman and others has not only replicated this effect with different scenarios, but has shown that many of these features do not seem to be essential for false memory implantation. Simply having participants imagine events, in the absence of witnesses or any concurrent true details, is sometimes sufficient to increase their confidence that the events actually occurred. Reports of earlier and earlier childhood events, stretching back in some cases to the first year and even to the first week of life, were obtained by Malinoski and Lynn (1996) by pushing subjects to use visualisation and concentration to extend their "recall" into infancy.

Exciting though these developments are, there is still some way to go if these experiments are to be considered analogous to what happens in therapy. Typically the experimental approach results in the creation of a "memory" for a single event that supposedly occurred when the participant was aged 6 years or younger. It is clear that the recollections are often partial, and not always very vivid. In contrast, some of the surveys reported at this conference indicate that supposed traumatic memories recovered in therapy frequently involve events occurring at an older age, including adolescence, and may involve repeated events. Recall is often apparently spontaneous, in the absence of obvious suggestive influences. Moreover, many of these events are upsetting, unwelcome, and have profound interpersonal consequences. Although recall is not always particularly vivid, in a substantial number of cases recall is accompanied by the experience of apparently vividly reliving the sensory and motor aspects of the event and by distortions in the subjective sense of time. The powerful nature of these experiences makes them dissimilar to any of the laboratory phenomena obtained to date.

In view of these quite marked differences, it would be interesting to know whether the laboratory research could be pushed still further, while still remaining within the ethical boudaries that constrain work in this area. For example, is it possible to implant a false memory for repeated events, for something the participant did not want to believe, or for an event that, if true, would have negative consequences for the future? This would provide a greater approximation to the clinical reality. What is extremely valuable about the experimental findings, however, is the repeated demonstration that lowering the response criterion for the validity of a memory leads to an increased tendency to accept imaginary events as veridical. This is a clear warning that, in therapy, it is perilous to allow the distinction between memory and imagination to become blurred. Clients should at all times be aware that mental events may or may not correspond to actual experiences, and should not be encouraged to relax the criterion for establishing what is a genuine memory.

The experimental research has also been of value in demonstrating the existence of important individual differences, with 30% or fewer of participants typically accepting the suggestions concerning a false event. Hyman & Billings' (1995) data indicates that those most prone to these errors have high scores on visualisation and on the Dissociative Experiences Scale. It is interesting to speculate whether these participants are adopting a lower response criterion and, if so, why they are doing so. For example, do they come from families that have tended to deny the reality of their feelings and experiences, and to impose an alternative view? Alternatively, do people who score highly on the DES frequently have others alert them to gaps and failures in their memory, such that the experimental situation mirrors common real-life experiences?

Related to the willingness of some subjects to believe they can recall events from the first year of life is work suggesting that a high proportion of experimental subjects believe in the paranormal and think they have had paranormal experiences. A recent study conducted at Royal Holloway by an undergraduate student, Kathy de Beer, found that these beliefs were significantly more strongly endorsed by subjects who also reported experiences of either physical and sexual abuse in childhood. It would be interesting to know if similar reports of trauma are also made by those subjects who are more willing to accept the experimental suggestions concerning imaginary events. In this case it might be instructive to examine the trauma reports of suggestible and non-suggestible participants, with the hypothesis that reports in the former would be less clear, and would attract less corroboration, than those of the latter. An alternative point of view, and one that has previously been voiced in the trauma literature, is that people who have genuinely been traumatised may be more vulnerable to subsequent suggestions concerning imaginary experiences of trauma.

In her paper Loftus cited a recent preliminary study by the State of Washington Department of Labor and Industries in support of her claim that therapy involving suggestive memory techniques and repressed memories may actually make people worse. On the face of it these data are worrying and certainly suggest that a more detailed clinical audit of the scheme is called for. As presented, however, there is simply too much missing information to evaluate the study, and alternative interpretations are likely. For example, there is no information about how claimants were assessed and what measures were used. It is not clear how many therapists were involved, and no evidence is presented that memories surfaced as a result of suggestive memory techniques rather than spontaneously. The very high proportion of bizarre memories, particularly of Satanic ritual abuse, indicates that the sample is unrepresentative of recovered memory cases. For instance, a survey of the members of the False Memory Syndrome Foundation reported by the FMSF in Summer 1993 indicated that only 18% of allegations involved SRA.

The results may also have been influenced by sampling artifacts. These cases were successful claims under the compensation scheme, and hence criteria for accepting claims may be relevant. It may have been the case, for instance, that claims involving recovered memories were more likely to be accepted if there were reports of deterioration following the recovery. We do not know if there were cases of memory recovery followed by a positive outcome among the original claimants. The data concerning average cost are also problematic, since we do not know if the cases involving and not involving recovered memories were matched on relevant clinical variables such as diagnosis, clinical history, etc.

To summarize, there are impressive experimental data that underscore the dangers of failing to distinguish carefully between real and imagined events, and it is clear that a substantial minority of individuals are susceptible to suggestions concerning imaginary events. Who these individuals are is not yet established, but it seems possible that they are suggestible because they have had genuine experiences that correspond to some degree with the suggestions made. Great care is needed, however, in extrapolating from these data to complex therapeutic situations. Previous surveys of therapists, such as that of Poole, Lindsay, Memon, and Bull (1995), enquired about the use of potentially suggestive memory techniques in general but did not establish whether such techniques were used prior to memory recovery in clients with no preexisting knowledge of their abuse. Similarly, the preliminary report from the State of Washington, while giving cause for concern about the operation of this particular scheme, does not in my view permit any more general conclusions to be drawn about therapy involving recovered memories.

REFERENCES

False Memory Syndrome Foundation (1993). Family survey results. Philadelphia, PA.
Hyman, I.E., & Billings, F.J. (1995). Individual differences and the creation of false memories. Unpublished manuscript, Western Washington University.
Malinoski, P., & Lynn, S.J. (1996). The pliability of early memories. Unpublished manuscript, Ohio University.
Poole, D.A., Lindsay, D.S., Memon, A., & Bull, R. (1995). Psychotherapy and the recovery of memories of childhood sexual abuse: U.S. and British practioners' opinions, practices, and experiences. *Journal of Consulting and Clinical Psychology, 63*, 426–437.

QUESTION AND ANSWER SESSION

Mulhern. This last study you presented, I think you are probably already aware of the fact that the concentration of cases surprised a lot of people, myself included, and brought up a lot of questions about the randomness of this sample. We're talking about something that leads to all sorts of problems potentially -we don't know the conditions of the patients over a long period of time though we have some suggestive information here that we have something going on. I think it's tremendously important that we make an effort to specify what we're talking about here particularly when we use a word like "random" - what was the methodology you were using? It may be that this isn't a random sample, or it could tell us something about who is going from not claiming to claiming. There's so much more information we could find if we just had some of this basic data to work with, I feel uncomfortable with it, because although I can understand what you are saying, I would just feel better if I had some of that basic information.

Loftus. I agree with you completely Sherrill. When I first looked at this information I thought how can this be random with all these satanic cases. So I did go back to the nurse consultant and said "tell me exactly what you mean by random"? She is the one who did this, this was her project, it was an internal document distributed at a mental health subcommittee meeting. She said she took the 183 cases, now those are the ones that she reviewed, it's not the whole 325 because some of those had closed already, she was only dealing with the open cases. She reports to me taking every 10th or every 12th case. I don't want to make any claims for this being really random or representative of anything. I do think it is odd too, and it's certainly different from the data that Chris Brewin showed us, which might suggest that 10–20% of certain classes of allegations might involve satanic elements. But just keep in mind that these are a different group of people, they're ones who in many cases have exhausted their insurance and have gone to the crime victim compensation fund.

Mulhern. I understand that, it's just that we are not talking about a mass of cases, it's not 10,000 cases, we're talking about 100 or so cases. Is there any possibility that we could have in the future a firmer specification of what's going on? Is there any idea that they were classified already before she got them? Did she shuffle them? This would give us some basic information, it's not so big that an effort couldn't be made more than just informally saying "well I think I took every 10th case". I'd then feel more comfortable about these things which are coming into the system.

Loftus. There are some efforts under way to do a more formal study. However I invite anyone here who might have some data where you can look at outcome without asking the therapist who did the therapy, what do you think of outcome of your therapy? Maybe there are other crime victim compensation funds in other states where data of this type could be looked at.

Eich. Earlier on you made the comment that sometimes the false memories contain more than just a couple of grains of the truth and I thought I'd throw out a half-baked idea. I do work on anaesthesia and memory and although we mainly deal with adults, sometimes we do watch kids under surgery and it occurred to me that might be a source down the road for certain kinds of bizarre recollections, such that you're surrounded by people wearing strange robes, they sometimes do odd or unpleasant things to you, there's an odd prattle amongst the operating room staff that could be misconstrued by a child, and there's drugs involved so you end up in a twilight sleep. What it basically amount to is that as bizarre as some of those SRA things imply, given that there may be medical records, it might be interesting to check back to see whether anybody had experiences during general anaesthesia during this time.

Loftus. That's interesting because I would have assumed before your comment that the sources of the imported information might be from books or support groups, or group therapy that they engage in, and that those would be the sources of elements that would get imported into these constructions, but you've got another idea that I think would be very interesting to look at.

Williams. I imagine that you're familiar with Kathy Pezdek's recent study about finding the difficulty of implanting a memory of receiving a rectal enema in childhood when one really didn't. Perhaps this has closer ecological value. Do you have any thoughts about how that might fit in?

Loftus. Yes, Kathy Pezdek (personal communication) reported last summer that she with 20 individuals using a "lost-in-mall, spilled-the-punchbowl" type paradigm, had students go out and try to convince their relatives that they were either lost in mall or they had to have a rectal enema. She found that three of these twenty subjects accepted the lost-in-mall suggestion and came up with memories, but none accepted the suggestion from their sibling about the rectal enema. So does this mean it's not possible to convince someone that they had a rectal enema when they didn't? I don't think it means that. I think it may be a lot harder to do that, but I certainly do believe its possible. A couple of aspects of her procedure I would have done different to give this a better test. In at least some of the cases the relatives used for the implantation was younger than the subject. So when your younger sibling says "I was 3 and you were 5, and I heard mommy said you ate too much ice cream and I'm going to give you an enema", are you as likely to accept a suggestion from a younger relative? That's just a minority of her subjects, because most of them were older. The other thing is she had the relatives do the suggesting. In our case we had a common experimenter, Jackie Pickrell. She's a dynamite implanter, she does it stone-faced, doesn't laugh inappropriately, and does it the same every time. I still would need to know about these particular relatives and how good they were at keeping a straight face as they went home and tried to implant the rectal enema memory in their sibling. I would like to see it redone with some of those ideas in mind and then we'd find out more.

Rawls. There's something missing, another person or persons involved, and I don't know if it's validity or reliability, but it really stems from that four-way grid that you put forward, with the true and false negatives and the true and false positives. The focus and the challenge has been to look at that particular grid in terms of experiments that we can make to have clinical validity in the future. It seems to me there's another grid completely missing and you've alluded to one portion only of that grid, there's another person or persons involved and that is the accused - whether that happened or didn't happen. This leads to a an emotional forum. I think the challenge might be to include this other grid in your future experiments if that's possible. But you can't have one half without the other half.

8

CHILDREN'S REPORTS OF PLEASANT AND UNPLEASANT EVENTS

Maggie Bruck,[1] Helene Hembrooke,[2] and Stephen Ceci[2]

[1]McGill University
Montreal, PQ H3A 1B1
[2]Cornell University
Ithaca, New York

1. INTRODUCTION

In the past decade, there has been an exponential increase in research on the accuracy of young children's memories and the degree to which young children's memories and reports can be molded by suggestions implanted by adult interviewers. Several important findings have emerged from this research. On the one hand, the results of a number of studies of children's autobiographical recall or memory for events indicate that children's recall is at times highly accurate and at times quite detailed about a large range of events (e.g., Baker-Ward, Gordon, Ornstein, Larus, & Clubb, 1993; Parker, Bahrick, Lundy, Fivush, & Levitt, in press; poster abstract this volume; Peterson & Bell, 1996). On the other hand there are also a number of studies that highlight the weaknesses of young children's reports of past events when they are interviewed under certain conditions; of particular interest is the suggestibility of children. Until recently, most suggestibility studies examined the influence of a single misleading suggestion on children's recall of an event. Generally, these studies indicated that in a variety of conditions young children are more suggestible than adults with preschoolers being more vulnerable than any other age group (see Ceci & Bruck, 1993, for a review of this literature).

In the past decade, there has been a major paradigmatic shift in this research in an attempt to make it more forensically relevant. Specifically, as more and more children are called to court to provide uncorroborated testimony, especially in cases involving child sexual abuse, social scientists have turned their attention from studying the effects of a single misleading question on children's recall of neutral, nonscripted, and often uninteresting events, to examining the accuracy of children's testimony under a range of conditions that are characteristic of those that bring children to court. One important area of study concerns the effects of different interviewing techniques on the reliability of children's reports. These studies go beyond the examination of how a single misleading question influences children's reports. Rather, they examine the effects of a host of implicit

Recollections of Trauma, edited by Read and Lindsay
Plenum Press, New York, 1997

and explicit suggestive techniques that can be woven into the fabric of the interview through the use of bribes, threats, repetitions of certain questions, and the induction of stereotypes and expectancies (Ceci & Bruck, 1995).

The research that we have conducted at Cornell and McGill Universities has primarily focused on the influence of various types of suggestive interviewing techniques on the reliability of children's reports. Although we have documented a number of conditions that increase children's suggestibility, a major concern that is frequently raised concerning our work as well as that of our colleagues is whether suggestive interviewing techniques only influence children's reports about relatively neutral and unimportant events. In every audience there are those who assert that suggestive interviewing techniques may lower the reliability of emotionally neutral experiences, but not emotionally-laden ones; the latter are held to be impervious to false suggestions.

A second issue concerns the credibility of inaccurate reports. Specifically, it is possible that even though children can be led to make inaccurate reports, nevertheless, their demeanor or the contents of these reports are not perceived as credible by trained (and possibly even untrained) observers.

We address these issues in this paper. First, we will review some of the major findings that have emerged from our laboratory concerning the degree to which children's reports about pleasant and unpleasant events can be tainted by various interviewing practices. Next, we will present new data on the credibility of such reports.

2. SUGGESTIVE INTERVIEWING TECHNIQUES

Our past work has examined the influence of various components of suggestive interviews on the accuracy of young children's reports (Ceci & Bruck, 1995). An overarching dimension that can be used to characterize interviews between children and adults is that of "interviewer bias". Interviewer bias characterizes those interviewers who hold *a priori* beliefs about the occurrence of certain events and, as a result, mold the interview to elicit statements from the interviewee that are consistent with these prior beliefs. One of the hallmarks of "interviewer bias" is the single-minded attempt to gather only confirmatory evidence and to avoid all avenues that may produce negative or inconsistent evidence. Thus, while gathering evidence to support his hypothesis, an interviewer may fail to gather any evidence that could potentially disconfirm his hypothesis. For example, the interviewer does not challenge the child who provides abuse-consistent evidence by saying things like "You're kidding me, aren't you?"or "Did that really happen?" The interviewer does not ask questions that might provide alternate explanations for the allegations (e.g., "Did your mommy and daddy tell you that this happened, or did you see it happen?"). And the interviewer does not ask the child about events that are inconsistent with his hypothesis (e.g., "Who else beside your teacher touched your private parts? Did your mommy touch them, too?"). When children provide biased interviewers' with inconsistent or bizarre evidence, it is either ignored, or else interpreted within the framework of the interviewers' initial suspicions. Note that we are not arguing that it is inappropriate to generate and test suspicions during an interview. The alternative to having no hypotheses is to be completely "in the dark", thus risking the possibility of overlooking forensically significant disclosures. Rather, we are arguing that the preoccupation with a single hypothesis in the absence of a fair test of the most plausible alternative hypotheses is a recipe for disaster.

Interviewer bias can be found whenever an interviewer suspects that he knows the answers before the child divulges them and proceeds to shape the interview to confirm his suspicion. When present, interviewer bias can influence the entire architecture of interviews and it is revealed through a number of different component features that are highly suggestive. For example, in order to obtain confirmation of their suspicions, interviewers may not ask children "open-ended" questions, but quickly resort to a barrage of very specific questions, many of which are repeated, and many of which are leading. When interviewers do not obtain information that is consistent with their suspicions, they may repeatedly interview children until they do obtain such information. Thus, in some situations children are interviewed over a prolonged period of time and they are re-interviewed on many occasions about the same set of events.

"Stereotype inducement" is another common feature of biased interviews with children. Here the interviewer gives the child information about some characteristic of the suspected perpetrator. For example, children may be told that a person who is suspected of some crime "is bad" "or does bad things." It is hard to know how frequently this occurs in actual interviews but we have documented elsewhere its occurrence (Ceci & Bruck, 1995).

Interview bias is also reflected in the atmosphere of the interview. Sometimes, interviewers provide much encouragement during the interview in order to put children at ease and to provide a highly supportive environment. Such encouraging statements, however, quickly lose their impartial tone when a biased interviewer *selectively* reinforces children's responses by positively acknowledging statements (e.g. through the use vigorous head nodding, smiling, and statements such as "Wow, that's great!") that are consistent with the interviewer's beliefs or hypotheses, or by ignoring other statements that do not support the interviewer's beliefs. Some interviewers who feel an urgency and responsibility to obtain the desired disclosure may even use threats and bribes. In order to obtain full compliance from the child, interviewers often try to engage the child by co-opting his co-operation, by telling him that he is a helper in an important legal investigation, and sometimes by telling the child that his friends have helped or already told, and that he should also tell, and/or that he will feel better once he has told.

Many of the features of biased interviews can be used in interviews with children by a range of adult interviewers that include parents, teachers, police officers, mental health professionals, and attorneys. In addition, there are some other techniques that are specific to interviews between professionals and children. Although these techniques are not necessarily suggestive, in the hands of biased interviewers they *can* become so (for a discussion of this issues see Ceci & Bruck, 1995). One of these techniques involves the use of anatomically detailed dolls in investigations of sexual abuse. Children may be given these dolls and asked to re-enact the alleged or suspected sexual molestation. It is thought that these props facilitate reports of sexual abuse for children with limited language skills, for children who feel shame and embarrassment, and for children with poor memories of the abusive incident. Another professional technique involves "guided imagery" or "memory work." Interviewers sometimes ask children to first try to remember or pretend if a certain event occurred and then to create a mental picture of the event and think about its details.

In our recent book (Ceci & Bruck, 1995) we have described studies that examined the influence of a number of the interviewing techniques just described. In these studies, children have typically participated in some event and then are interviewed, using one or more of the hypothesized "suggestive" interviewing techniques listed above. These studies often show that such techniques can have detrimental effects on the accuracy of young children's reports—and the effects are cumulative. That is, combinations of such techniques can be more damaging than the use of just one technique.

Although a number of studies indicate that these interviewing techniques can have detrimental effects on the accuracy of young children's reports, the issue has been raised that perhaps these conclusions are specific to events of low-personal interest or of low emotional content; and that perhaps it is very difficult if not impossible to alter children's memories or reports about emotionally charged events, particularly about events that might have negative connotations and that might involve their own bodies. In the present paper, we examine this issue by summarizing the results of some of the studies that have emerged from our own laboratory. Specifically we ask: Do suggestive interviewing techniques have baleful effects on children's reports of both pleasant (positive) and unpleasant (negative) events?

2.1. Influencing Children's Reports of Pleasant and Unpleasant Events

We have found that various interviewing techniques can influence the accuracy of young children's reports about meaningful events—some of which fall on the pleasant end of a continuum and others of which fall on the unpleasant end.

In one study, we examined 3-year-old and 4-year-old children's memories of a just-completed medical examination in which half of the children received a genital examination and half of the children did not (see Bruck, Ceci, Francoeur & Renick, 1995 for results of 3-year old data). After the examination, the children were given an anatomically detailed doll and were asked to show on the doll how the doctor had touched them. In addition, they were provided with props (e.g., a spoon, a stethoscope) and asked to show how the doctor had used these. The wording of some of the questions was misleading for children who had not received a genital examination, though these same questions could be considered to be "correctly leading" for children who *had* received a genital examination ("show me on the doll how the doctor touched your penis"). The results for the 3- and 4-year old children were almost identical. That is, a significant proportion of children showed inaccurate touching. Specifically, the same proportion of 3- and 4-year old children failed to show touching when it had in fact happened (genital condition), and the same proportion showed genital touching when it had not happened (nongenital condition). In the latter situation, had this touching occurred, it might have been painful. That is, a number of children (especially the girls) inaccurately showed the pediatrician inserting his finger or props into their genitalia or buttocks.

In a second study, we suggestively and repeatedly interviewed 7-year-old children about some salient characteristics of a medical examination that had occurred approximately 12 months previously (Bruck, Ceci, Francoeur, & Barr, 1995). During this medical examination the children had received an inoculation which for many was stressful, and which for most was painful during the next few days. As a result of our repeated use of misinformation a year after the procedure, a number of children eventually came to report that our female research assistant rather than their male pediatrician had actually given them their inoculation and an oral vaccine. The results of this study highlight some other deleterious effects of repeating misinformation across interviews on young children's reports: not only did some children directly incorporate the misinformation into their subsequent reports (i.e., they inaccurately reported that the research assistant gave them the shot, or the oral vaccine), but they also made other inaccurate claims that were not suggested but that were inferences based on the misinformation. That is, a number of children falsely reported that the female research assistant had checked their ears and nose. These statements are inferences that are consistent with the erroneous suggestion that the female research assistant had administered the shot, therefore she must have been the doctor, and therefore she carried out procedures commonly performed by doctors. There were also control children who were not given any misinformation or information about who gave them the shot, or the oral vaccine, a year previously. None of the control children made such inaccurate inferences about the research assistant performing a physical examination. Finally, children routinely underestimated their level of pain and crying as a result of erroneous suggestions about how brave and courageous they had been. Thus, young children use suggestions in highly productive ways to reconstruct and at times distort reality about unpleasant events.

Of course, our medical setting studies do not reveal whether it is easier to influence children's reports for unpleasant than for pleasant events. Data from two of our studies do address this concern. In the first study (Ceci, Leichtman, Loftus & Bruck, 1994), parents of preschool children provided us with four true events involving their preschool child: a pleasant event (e.g., a birthday party), an unpleasant event (e.g., death of a pet), and 2 neutral events (e.g., wearing a blue sweater to school). The parents also verified that a list of four false events, devised by the research team, had not occurred to their children. There was a false pleasant event (taking a ride in a hot air balloon), a false unpleasant event (falling off a bike and getting stitches) and two neutral events (waiting for a bus and watching a friend waiting for a bus). We asked our preschool subjects to create images (using visualization techniques) about these real and fictional events. The children were asked to do this for 11 consecutive weeks. Assents to true events were at ceiling, indicating highly accurate affirmation of actual experiences. With time, children began to increasingly assent to fictional events—but their rates of assent for pleasant events (e.g., riding in a hot air balloon) were much higher than those for unpleasant events (e.g., falling off of a bicycle and getting stitches). These results indicate that it may be easier to influence children's reports for pleasant than for unpleasant events, but that the latter is not impossible—it does occur with some frequency.

In a second study (which will be described in greater detail in the next section), we compared children's assents to true and false events that were pleasant and unpleasant. Sixteen preschool children were first asked to tell us about two true events (about which we had details) and about two false events. One of the true events was staged at the school and each subject was a participant. It involved helping a visitor carry a bag of toys and books to the office. During this time, the visitor tripped on a shoelace, hurt her ankle, and asked the child for help. Throughout this paper we label this event as pleasant, positive, or true-helping. The second true event was not staged and varied across all the children: It involved an incident in the past few weeks in which the child had been punished. The details of the event and punishment were furnished by the teacher or the parent. Throughout this paper, this event is labelled as unpleasant, negative or true-punishment. One of the false events involved helping a lady find her lost monkey in the park. This event is labelled pleasant, positive, and false-monkey. The second false event involved an incident about a man coming to the daycare and stealing food. This event is labelled negative, unpleasant, and false-thief. It is important to point out that the last event is not just an "unpleasant" event. This is an alleged criminal event. Unlike the false-monkey event, there are potential consequences for assenting to this event. So even though the child is not an active participant in this scenario, the implications of assent could be very serious.

Children were asked on 5 different occasions whether or not the 4 different events had occurred. In the first interview (baseline) the children were simply asked whether the events had happened; if they assented, they were asked to tell as much as they could remember about it. The next two interviews (abbreviated T2 and T3) included a combination of suggestive interviewing techniques that have been shown to increase children's assents to false events. These techniques included: the use of peer pressure, visualization techniques, repeating misinformation, and selective reinforcement. If children assented, they were asked a number of open-ended and close-ended questions to get them to provide as much detail as possible. If they denied the occurrence of an event, then they were asked to pretend and to answer the open- and close-ended questions. In the fourth interview (T4) the children were asked about the events but this time they were asked to tell their stories to a hand-held puppet (a dog called Cedric). No suggestive techniques were used in this interview, except that the children were asked to pretend if they denied knowledge of the event. The same interviewer questioned the children for the first four interviews. In the fifth interview, they were questioned by a new interviewer who told them that she had heard some things and wondered if they had happened to the child. For example, she said, "I heard something about a lost monkey. Do you know anything about that?"

Interviews were separated by approximately one week. An example of a suggestive T2 interview for a false event is provided.

Interviewer: Do you know what — those kids told me some other neat stuff that happened to them. Do you want to know what else they told me? They told me that..one day they were in the park — and some lady came up to them and told them she had lost her monkey in the park. She asked Susan, and Mark, and Kent to help her find her monkey. So they walked around the park looking all over for the monkey. You know what?...They found the monkey and gave it back to the lady. Have you ever had anything like that happen to you?"

Child: Uh, no.

Interviewer:...The other kids already told me the story — but I want to hear it from you — did you help the lady in the park find her monkey?

Child: Uh, ya.

Interviewer: You did, I thought so. Tell me everything...

Child: She told me to find her monkey and she told me that her monkey went to the high school.

Interviewer: Anything else? (After the interviewer then asks 6 specific questions, she concludes the interview)

Interviewer: It's so wonderful that there are such nice kids like yourself to help people out when they need it. You know it's really important to help people out.

As shown in Figure 1, the repeated interviewing with the suggestive techniques influenced children's assent rates for the two false events as well as for the True-Unpleasant (punish) event where a number of children initially denied that such an event of punishment had occurred. These results show the benefits as well as risks of using such techniques. For children who may not want to talk about unpleasant or embarrassing true events, the use of repeated interviews with suggestive components did prompt children to correctly assent to previously denied events. However, the same pattern is also shown for events that were initially denied but that never occurred.

These new data differ slightly from our previous studies using only visualization techniques. As described above, in the earlier work it was more likely for children to assent to false pleasant than to false unpleasant results. In the newer study, the rate of assents over time

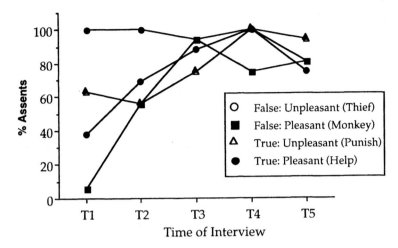

Figure 1. Percentage assents to false and true events over 5 interviews.

is similar for false unpleasant and false pleasant events. There are several possible explanations for these discrepancies. The first is that increasing the suggestiveness of the interview decreases differences between pleasant and unpleasant events. A second possibility is that assent rates for unpleasant events may be higher when the child is thought to be an observer than when she is thought to be a participant. That is, children may be more easily influenced to make inaccurate reports about *seeing* a thief, rather than being hurt in a bicycle accident.

To summarize, suggestive interviewing techniques, which vary in terms of their "suggestiveness," can result in young children making false allegations about pleasant and unpleasant events. Sometimes these false reports involve their own bodies. One study indicates that with milder techniques, it is easier to obtain false reports about pleasant than about unpleasant events. However, it is not known whether the same result would be obtained if the suggestiveness of the interview were increased.

3. CREDIBILITY OF CHILDREN'S REPORTS OBTAINED FROM SUGGESTIVE INTERVIEWS

Although children's reports may be highly influenced by a number of suggestive influences, this does not necessarily mean that the children's reports will appear credible. Of particular concern is whether a juror, or a child development researcher, or a child therapist can differentiate children whose reports are accurate from those whose reports are a product of suggestive interviews. The existing evidence suggests that trained professionals cannot reliably tell the difference between these two kinds of children.

As described above, there have been a number of studies where by virtue of repeated suggestive interviewing techniques, young children have eventually come to assent to a number of false events. These results share a number of features. First, children are not simply parroting verbatim the suggestions of the interviewer, but they elaborate or logically extend the nature of the suggestions (e.g., Bruck, Ceci, Francoeur & Barr, 1995). Second, children's inaccurate reports are often highly elaborate and filled with perceptual details (e.g., Ceci & Leichtman, 1995).

An example is provided by the Sam Stone study (see Leichtman & Ceci, 1995 for details). Here, young children between the ages of 3 and 6 years old were interviewed under a number of different suggestive conditions about a stranger named Sam Stone. The experimenter told some children that Sam Stone was a friend and that he was very clumsy. Over the next few weeks, these children were told numerous stories of Sam Stone's clumsiness. (This technique is called "stereotype induction".) All children in the experiment eventually did meet Sam Stone: he made one visit to their classroom and was introduced to them during story time. The next day, the teacher showed all the children a soiled teddy bear and a ripped book. For the next 8–10 weeks some of the children were provided with repeated misinformation about Sam's visit (e.g., they were asked: "When Sam Stone tore the book, did he do it on purpose or was he being silly?"). Finally, all children were questioned by a new interviewer about what actually happened during Sam Stone's visit ("I wasn't there the day Sam Stone came to your school; would you tell me everything that happened that day?").

There were two major findings. First, children who had received both stereotype induction and the misleading questions made the most false claims about Sam. Second, there were clear age differences. When asked, "Did anything happen to a book?" and "Did anything happen to a teddy bear?" 72% of the youngest preschoolers who had received both stereotype induction and misleading information claimed that Sam Stone did one or both misdeeds, a figure that dropped to 44% when asked if they actually *saw* him do these things. Importantly, 21% continued to insist that they saw him do these things, even when gently challenged. The older preschoolers, though more accurate, still included some children (11%) who insisted they saw him do the misdeeds.

A third important finding was that the children went beyond simple statements of assenting to Sam's misdeeds. They provided a number of false perceptual details as well as nonverbal gestures to embellish their stories of these non-events. For example, children used their hands to show how Sam had purportedly thrown the teddy bear up in the air; some children reported sighting Sam in the playground, or on his way to the store to buy chocolate ice cream, or in the bathroom soaking the teddy bear in water before smearing it with a crayon. Some children claimed there was more than one Sam Stone. And one child provided every parent's favorite false detail; this child claimed that Sam had come to his house to trash his room.

Finally, and most important to the issue of credibility, when highly trained professionals were shown videotapes of children in these studies and asked to judge their believability or credibility, these experts (including mental health professionals, developmental psychologists, and prosecutors) were highly inaccurate. They judged children whose reports were a product of suggestive interviewing as highly credible and believable, whereas those whose reports were more accurate were often judged to be less believable and credible. We have obtained similar results when professionals were asked to rate the credibility of children in some of our other studies (Ceci, et al., 1994a; Ceci et al., 1994b).

In our recent work, joined by our new colleague Helene Hembrooke, we have gone further in our search for potential markers of accurate and inaccurate reports. We hypothesized that perhaps on closer scrutiny there might be linguistic markers of true stories that differentiate them from false stories which emerge from suggestive interviews. For example, we hypothesized that more subtle aspects of children's narratives, such as the total amount of information, or the number of spontaneous unprompted statements, or the cohesiveness (as measured by the use of temporal markers, or by the use of dialogue), or the elaboration (as measured by the use of emotional terms, or by the use of adjectives and adverbs) might differentiate true from false narratives. In addition, we also examined the evolution of children's narratives as they were repeatedly interviewed in order to determine if true and false narratives became more similar with repeated interviewing. Along these same lines, we examined the consistency as well as the inconsistency of children's reports across repeated retellings. Again we reasoned that perhaps children are more likely to repeat the same details for true than for false narratives and that they are less likely to contradict themselves or to change their stories for true than for false stories.

Our selection of dependent or predictor variables was motivated by several different sources. First, a number of studies have indicated that when children's reports are spontaneous (usually in response to open-ended questions such as "Tell me what happened" and, "What happened next?"), their reports are more accurate than when their reports are prompted by direct questions. Thus we predicted that the narratives of the true events would contain more spontaneous statements than the narratives of the false events. Second, because some of our variables have been associated with children's autobiographical narratives (e.g., Fivush, Haden & Adam, 1995), we predicted that they might occur less frequently in children's false narratives. Specifically, we selected several measures of narrative coherence that are thought to define "good" narratives. Specifically, these were: the use of simple and complex temporal markers (references to chronological time or complex temporal relations), the use of dialogue, the use of evaluations or added descriptive material about the events. Third, we examined consistency and inconsistency across interviews because consistency of a child's report is often one of the most important criteria used by professionals in evaluating the reliability of children's allegations of abuse (Conte, Sorenson, Forgarty & Dalla Rosa, 1991) and inconsistency in young children's reports lowers their credibility in the eyes of mock jurors (Leippe, Manion & Romanczyk, 1991).

The procedures for this study were described in the previous section. In that section we showed that with very suggestive interviewing practices, children increasingly assented to both true *and* false unpleasant events, as well as pleasant false events. In addition, the rate of assents for these three types of events were similar to those observed for the pleasant true events (see Figure 1 above). In this section we analyze the narratives that children produced when they assented to each type of event.

First, we analysed the number of details recounted for each event at each interview. One analysis included details that were provided in response to both open-ended questions (i.e., spontaneous statements) and to specific questions. A second analysis only included the spontaneous utterances. The results were similar for both analyses. The results for the first analysis, total number of details, are presented in Figure 2.

Except for the True-Pleasant (Help) event, the children gave few if any details at the first interview. However by the third interview, there were no significant differences in the amount of information (i.e., the total number of details) that the children provided for the two false and for the true-help events. This pattern continued into the fifth interview.

The analyses of the spontaneous utterances (a subset of the total details), revealed that indeed most of the details were provided spontaneously, and that by the third interview the number of spontaneous utterances were similar for the two false and true-pleasant events.

In these analyses and others to follow, the children's narratives of the true unpleasant events are the sparsest. There are several explanations for these results. First, it is possible that for many of the children, there were not that many details to recount (for example, how many ways is there to tell the story of taking a toy outside and being punished for it?). Second, at times, it appears that the children did not want to talk about the incident; some children assented and then denied that the event had actually happened. Most of our discussion will focus on the comparison of the one true (pleasant) event and the two false events.

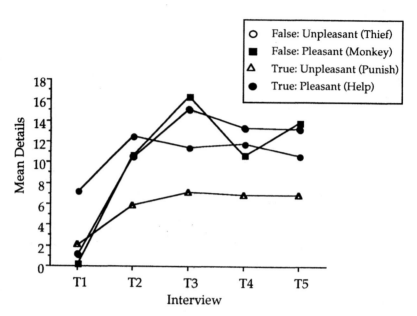

Figure 2. Total number of details in narratives for true and false events.

One of the motivations for repeating interviews, especially with young children, is to provide them with an opportunity to remember important new details that they had not originally reported in the first interview. We examined spontaneous and prompted "reminiscences". A reminiscence is defined as the inclusion of a new detail in an interview that had not previously been reported. There were a number of important findings. First, most of the reminiscences were spontaneous. Analysis of the spontaneous reminiscences (see Figure 3) revealed that reminiscences increased through to the third interview for the false events, but decreased or remained stable after the first interview for the true events. When between-event differences occurred, it was always the case that children provided more reminiscences for false than for true events (particularly at the third and fifth interviews). Thus repeated interviewing does produce new reports regardless of the accuracy of the report, but more reminiscences are sometimes produced for false than for true events.

Our examination of the markers of narrative coherence (e.g., simple temporal markers, complex temporal markers, dialogue) and of elaboration (adjectives, adverbs) revealed similar results. There were rarely any between-event differences on these measures—for example, children used dialogue as frequently in true stories as in false stories. When there *were* differences, it was always the case that the false stories were more coherent than the true stories. Specifically, with time, children's stories became more elaborated (they used more emotional terms, they included more adjectives and adverbs), but this held mainly for the false stories so that by the third interview the false stories contained more elaborate details than the true stories.

Next, we examined the consistency as well as the inconsistency of the children's stories. Consistency refers to the child's mentioning the same detail in more than one interview. In this analysis we examined how frequently children reported an event in one interview that had been reported in a previous interview. Because there were so few assents for false events in the first interview, it is not possible to examine the consistency of de-

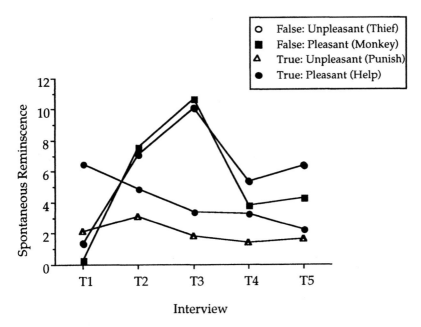

Figure 3. Number of spontaneous reminiscences in narratives for true and false events.

tails in the second interview because none were provided in the first interview. For this reason, we only examined consistency of details beginning at the third interview, asking whether these details had been mentioned in a previous interview. Similarly, we examined how many details in the fourth interview had been mentioned in previous interviews, and how many details in the fifth interview had been mentioned in previous interviews. As can be seen Figure 4, consistency did differentiate true from false stories, with true stories containing more consistent details. However, it is also clear that with repeated interviews, the children's false stories become more consistent such that by the fifth interview there was no statistically significant difference between the proportion of consistent details for the false unpleasant (thief) and the true pleasant (help) events.

Although consistency did differentiate true from false stories, at least in the earlier interviews, inconsistency or contradictions do not. Inconsistency was defined as the children reporting "X" in one interview, but "NOT-X" in another interview. For example, in one interview the child might say that he was by himself, whereas in a later interview, he might say that he was with his friends. The inconsistency analyses were carried out using the same procedures just described for the consistency analyses. As can be seen from Figure 5 the rates of inconsistency were generally low. Importantly, the proportions of inconsistent details were similar across events. Also, as can be seen, across all events, the children became more inconsistent with repeated interviewing.

The foregoing analyses do not reveal whether increases in the inconsistencies for true events reflect children becoming more accurate (that is, they correct previous mistakes) or less accurate. In order to examine the effects of repeated interviewing on the accuracy of children's reports of true events we examined the narratives for the true-help event. Because we staged this event, we were able to verify the accuracy of each statement in the narrative. We omitted the true-punish event from this analysis because we were unable to verify each statement. In undertaking this analysis, we did not count inaccurate mi-

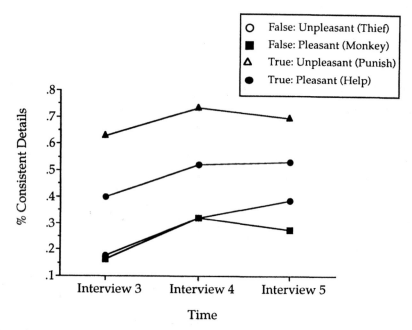

Figure 4. Percentage details consistent with a previous interview in narratives of true and false events.

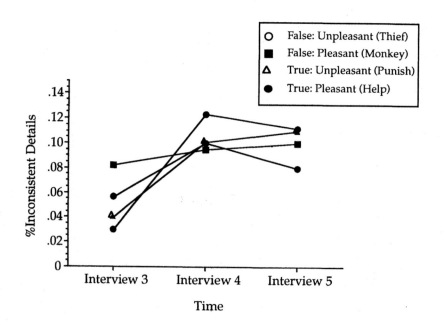

Figure 5. Percentage inconsistent details for narratives of true and false events.

nor details. For example, if the child erred about the appearance or the dress of the visitor (the color of her hair) this was not counted. We only counted inaccurate details that would be of major significance in the interpretation of the event. The following are examples of some of the inaccurate details included in the analysis.

-I called 9-1-1
-She fell many times
-A man came and helped her
-I fell and hurt myself
-She fell down the stairs
-We took her to the hospital.

Overall, given the number of details that children provided in each narrative, their error rates were low. That is the mean error rates at T1, T2, T3, T4, and T5 were: .86, 1.61, 1.38. 1,83 and 1.95 respectively. In addition to counting the number of inaccurate details in each narrative, we also counted the number of narratives that contained at least one inaccurate detail. The latter measure is probably more important because reporting even one of the targeted inaccurate details could have major consequences for the interpretation of a child's entire testimony (e.g., I fell and hurt myself). A number of children provided inaccurate details in their reports, even in the first interview. But, importantly, the number inaccurate reports increased with time. The percentage of reports with inaccurate details for each of the five different interviews was: 32%, 57%, 67%, 70%, and 50%. Repeated interviewing, even when children were provided with correct information about some of the events did not lead to increased accuracy. These data also suggest that increased inconsistency shown in Figure 5 may reflect children changing their accurate reports to inaccurate reports for the true events.

To summarize, we examined the linguistic structure of the children's true and falsely suggested narratives; we examined changes in structure and content of these narratives as a function of repeated interviews. Replicating many of the results of a pilot project involving a different sample of children (Bruck, Ceci, & Hembrooke, 1995), our analyses revealed the following. First, it is the first narrative which was elicited by nonsuggestive techniques that allows the clearest differentiation between true and false stories. This is because children mainly deny the false stories and as a result these contain no details. However, with repeated interviews, the false stories quickly come to resemble the true stories in terms of the number of details provided, the spontaneity of the utterances, the number of new details, inconsistency across narratives, the elaborativeness of the details, and the cohesiveness of the narrative. It is only consistency across narratives that differentiates true from false events; it seems, however, that could become a less potent predictor when children are repeatedly interviewed. When false stories are told as a result of repeated suggestive interviewing, they take on additional qualities that make them seem more believable than true narratives: specifically, after a number of interviews, false narratives contain more descriptive, elaborative and emotional material than true narratives. Interestingly, as children retold the true narratives they became more inaccurate over time.

Finally, returning to the original questions posed at the beginning of this paper, the present results indicate that fine-grained analyses of false narratives produce similar patterns of results for unpleasant events as for pleasant events. Although some might argue that perhaps one might get high rates of assents to unpleasant events when the child is not a participant, it is not entirely clear that our data support this hypothesis. Specifically, although it was only suggested to the children that they might have seen a theft, many of those who did assent falsely reported events that did involve them as participants. Children reported chasing the thief, being chased by the thief, hitting the thief, and similar types of actions. Therefore, it appears that if there are enough suggestive forces children will as easily assent to false unpleasant as to true pleasant events.

4. CONCLUDING REMARKS

We have provided a brief overview of the recent work on the reliability of children's memories and adults' perceptions of their credibility. We have tried to alert the reader to both the misconceptions concerning children's ability to provide accurate reports, and the misperceptions that can be created regarding the credibility of these reports.

Although we have concentrated on the conditions which can compromise reliable reporting, it is also important to acknowledge that under certain circumstances children can be extremely capable of providing accurate, detailed, and useful information. For example, in many of our own studies, children in the control group conditions (who are questioned in nonsuggestive interviews) often recalled events flawlessly. This indicates that the absence of suggestive techniques allows even very young preschoolers to provide highly accurate reports, although they may be sparse in the number of details. Also, mentioned at the beginning of the paper, there are a number of other studies that highlight the strengths of young children's long term memories. What characterizes these studies is the neutral tone of the interviewer, the limited use of misleading questions (for the most part, if suggestions are used, they are limited to a single occasion) and the absence of the induction of any motive or stereotype for the child to make a false report. When such conditions are present, it is a common (although not universal) finding that children are much more immune to suggestive influences, particularly about sexual details.

An important implication of studies that emphasize the strength of children's memories is that they highlight the conditions under which children should be interviewed if one wishes to obtain reliable reports. Again, when children are interviewed by unbiased, neutral interviewers, when the number of interviews as well as the number of leading questions are kept to a minimum, and when there is the absence of threats, bribes and peer-pressure, then children's reports are at considerably less risk for taint. It is these conditions that we must strive for when eliciting information from young children.

REFERENCES

Baker-Ward, L., Gordon, B., Ornstein, P. A., Larus, D., & Clubb, P. (1993). Young children's long-term retention of a pediatric examination. *Child Development*, 64, 1519–1533.

Bruck, M., Ceci, S.J., Francoeur, E., & Barr. R.J. (1995). "I hardly cried when I got my shot!": Influencing children's reports about a visit to their pediatrician. *Child Development, 66*, 193–208

Bruck, M. Ceci, S.J., Francoeur, E., & Renick, A. (1995). Anatomically detailed dolls do not facilitate preschoolers' reports of a pediatric examination involving genital touching. *Journal of Experimental Psychology: Applied, 1*, 95–109.

Bruck, M., Ceci, S.J., Hembrooke, H. (1995). Effects of interviewing procedures on children's narratives for true and false events. Society for Research on Child Development, Indianapolis, Indiana.

Ceci, S. J. & Bruck, M. (1995). *Jeopardy in the courtroom: A scientific analysis of of children's testimony*. Washington, DC: American Psychological Association.

Ceci, S.J., Crotteau-Huffman, M., Smith, E., & Loftus, E.F. (1994a). Repeatedly thinking about non-events. *Consciousness & Cognition*, 3, 388–407.

Ceci, S.J., Loftus, E.F., Leichtman, M. & Bruck, M. (1994b). The role of source misattributions in the creation of false beliefs among preschoolers. *International Journal of Clinical and Experimental Hypnosis, 62,* 304–320.

Conte, J. R., Sorenson, E., Fogarty, L., & Rosa, J. D. (1991). Evaluating children's reports of sexual abuse: Results from a survey of professionals. *American Journal of Orthopsychiatry, 78,* 428–437.

Fivush, R., Haden, C., Adam, S. (1995). Structure and coherences of preschoolers' personal narratives over time: Implications for childhood amnesia. *Journal of Experimental Child Psychology, 60,* 32–56.

Leichtman, M. D., & Ceci, S. J. (1995). The effects of stereotypes and suggestions on preschoolers' reports. *Developmental Psychology, 31,* :568–578

Leippe, M., Manion, A., & Romanczyk, A. (1993). Discernability or discrimination? Understanding jurors' reactions to accurate and inaccurate child and adult eyewitnesses In G. Goodman and B. Bottoms (Eds.), *Child victims, child witnesses: Understanding and improving testimony* (pp. 169–201). Guilford Press: New York.

Parker, J., Bahrick, L., Lundy, B., Fivush., & Levitt, M. (In press). Effects of stress on children's memory for a natural disaster. In C. P. Thompson, D. J. Herrmann, J. D. Read, D. Bruce, D. G. Payne, and M. P. Toglia. (eds.) Eyewitness memory: Theoretical and applied perspectives. Erlbaum

Peterson, C., & Bell, M. (1996). Children's memory for traumatic injury. *Child Development, 67,* 3045–3070.

COMMENTARY ON CHILDREN'S REPORTS OF PLEASANT AND UNPLEASANT EVENTS

Rachel Yehuda, the Mount Sinai School of Medicine, U.S.A

1. INTRODUCTION

The article by Bruck and Ceci provides a brief overview of recent investigations of the reliability of children's memories and adults' perception of the credibility of these memories. Two major conclusions have arisen from this research. First, the studies demonstrate that some experimental manipulations, such as suggestive interviewing, can compromise reliable reporting of both neutral and emotionally charged memories. Second, the findings suggest that adults are generally unable to ascertain whether a child is reporting a true or false memory.

Although the conclusions in this paper as they are stated seem fairly conservative, the results are provocative and have important implications. Indeed, these and similar results have received considerable attention in both the scientific and forensic arena because they are thought to be directly relevant to the question of whether and how to consider child testimony in court. This comment will focus on three major areas. First, some ethical and methodological issues will be discussed. Second, the utility and appropriateness of the findings for the forensic arena will be evaluated. Third, some follow-up research questions will be suggested.

2. ETHICAL AND METHODOLOGICAL ISSUES

It is sometimes argued in court that children alleging sexual or physical abuse have not in fact sustained the abuse they claim to have experienced. Rather, it is often asserted (particularly by the defendants and their expert witnesses) that these children have been led to believe that the abuse occurred as a result of suggestive interviewing or other manipulative techniques. The fact that children can be made to assent to events that never occurred raises some difficult ethical issues regarding the implementation of this type of research.

If one subscribes to the viewpoint that children can be made to assent to events that never occurred, one must also consider the potential impact on the child of believing to have undergone an experience that s/he has not sustained. One might especially question the ethics of studies that are designed to implant false negative memories in children. Certainly if children can internalise false memories, then it is also possible that they can become distressed by these memories — and perhaps even permanently affected by them.

The authors review one study in which 3- and 4-year-old children were examined by their paediatrician. In half of the cases the paediatrician lightly touched the children's genitals. The remaining children had a similar physical exam but in this case the physician did not touch their genitalia. The authors do not indicate whether touching the genitals was something that they had asked the paediatrician to do in the service of the research (i.e., an experimental manipulation), or whether this touching was part of the routine physical (if the latter, then it is not clear whether the manipulation was asking a physician to omit part of a routine examination).

Among the questions that were being asked, the authors were interested in determining whether the children could be made to assent to having had their genitals touched by the paediatrician when in fact they had not been touched. A proportion of the children did assent to having their genitals touched, when in fact they were not touched, when suggestive interviewing techniques were used. One issue that must raised in considering the ethics of such research concerns the long-term effects of suggesting to a child who has not had his/her genitals touched by his/her physician, that his/her genitals had been touched. Furthermore, the results should be more clearly understood in the context of whether the normal procedure of the physical examination involves genital touching or not.

The idea being raised here is that if children can be made to incorporate false memories, the investigators may be editing the child's autobiographical history, and perhaps even instilling ideas in the child — such as that they have been hurt or touched — that have been associated with long-term psychological damage. No mention is made in the paper about whether and how the children may have been "debriefed" in this study (i.e., told the truth about what had actually occurred and also told that they had participated in a study designed to elicit false assertions). Certainly, debriefing a child in and of itself raises several important concerns. For example, how does one go about letting a child know they have been the object of this type of experimentation and what short and long term effects would this have on the child?

It may be that some of the children who were touched by the paediatrician experienced the touching of their genitalia as distressing since they overdramatised and exaggerated the impact of the touch. Although the authors interpret the overdramatisation of the touching as evidence of "inaccurate memory" — since some girls inaccurately showed the paediatrician inserting his finger or props into their genitalia or buttocks — the reasons for this exaggeration are not clear. Perhaps the genital touching was experienced as intrusive (particularly if it was not directly part of or necessary to the physical examination). Perhaps the children had some sense that they were being used, as they were, as part of experimentation and were undergoing the touching gratuitously. Perhaps the small percentage of girls who reported penetration by the physician had been previously abused. There is no way for the authors to know that these subjects had not been abused previously. Even if they had tried to obtain a trauma history from these children, it is not necessarily the case that the informant would disclose or would even be aware of prior abuse. From an ethical and methodological perspective it is important to consider that subjects are not all alike. Some may have prior experiences that might result in seemingly neutral manipulations to be perceived as abusive. Certainly in a child that had a prior history of abuse, the experimental manipulation of a genital exam — or worse yet — the attempt to suggest to a child that touching which did not occur did occur — might be a more damaging game than is intended by the investigators.

Another ethical consideration is that the ideas being permanently instilled in the child are not value-neutral. In fact, some of the studies may be implanting ideas in the child that could be considered detrimental. For example, in one study the intention of the investigators was to see if they could get young children to falsely admit that they helped a stranger find a monkey in the park. This condition was described as "positive" event because it was depicting a situation where the child could be praised for being pleasant and helping — in this case helping a stranger find a monkey in the park is a good thing. In reality, however, talking to strangers in the park and helping them to find lost pets is probably not a positive event, and should probably not be framed as such. For example, it is known that kidnappers and child molesters often use ploys of asking children for "help" to lure them away. Such hypothetical scenarios should only be described in the service of illustrating how unsafe the behaviour of helping strangers can be. One can only wonder what the impact is of having a child believe that s/he participated safely in an activity that is in fact probably not safe in the service of this research.

A final ethical concern to be raised is the issue of informed consent. Certainly the participant (child) cannot be told that s/he is to be part of an experiment that involves using suggestive techniques to cause him/her to assent to situations that did not occur. The question is how much are the parents told about the experiment prior to their consent? It is difficult to believe that parents would wilfully submit to having their children's genitals touched in the service of research or that they would allow their children to be implanted with false truths. If there is full disclosure on consents that parents sign, one wonders to what extent these parents represent a normal sample. How many parents refused to allow their children to participate in such research? Full disclosure also raises the methodological concern of whether and to what extent the parents' knowledge of the protocol will influence the child's response.

3. AREAS FOR FUTURE STUDY

An important observation presented by the authors is that for any given experimental manipulation, there was no single type of response. Rather, responses tended to be heterogeneous. Some children could be made to falsely assent in response to suggestive interviewing, whereas others could not be made to falsely assent. Some children could be made to falsely assent relatively easily (on the first trial), whereas others assented only after repeated trials. Some children could not remember events that had happened to them, whereas other children could report true historical events without distortion. The fact that not all children show homogeneous responses to a standard manipulation suggests that there are important individual differences that underlie these responses. An important key, then, to understanding how suggestive interviewing techniques work lies in a further exploration of these individual differences. As a follow up to this and similar work, it might also be interesting to determine whether possible differences in prior history, and other psychological or sociodemographic factors, increase the probability of "false" memory in children. (However, in suggesting future research, it is understood that this research would be conducted ethically).

The hypothesis underlying this research is that the false assents of children results directly from the experimental manipulation of suggestive interviewing techniques and not the individual differences that may have led to false assents. If this is so, then it should be possible to demonstrate the circumstances that increase the reliability of emotional and neutral experiences. Furthermore, it should be possible to explore how the effects of suggestibility can be prevented or minimised. Until these issues are clarified, it is not immediately obvious that the false assents of children in these studies are in fact directly related to the suggestive techniques.

Should these findings be used in court? Although the research presented by the authors has had wide applicability in criminal litigation, it is certainly not clear what purpose is served by having these results presented in court. What has been appealing from a forensic perspective is the reliability of this research — that is, the research presented by the authors and similar research has generally supported the idea of the infallibility of memory in some children and the ability of suggestive techniques to influence a proportion of children to falsely assent to events that never occurred.

The problem is that proving that memories are sometimes false doesn't mean that memories cannot also be true. For any given individual there is no way of ascertaining whether a particular memory is false or true. What can be concluded from the research is that one can never really know whether a child is telling the truth, lying, distorting, or forgetting an event. This is a conclusion that we might have been able to have reached without the research.

QUESTION AND ANSWER SESSION

Waganaar. We have done a number of studies with consistency, not within witnesses but between witnesses. The study is very simple. You tell two subjects to go to the zoo, and then to come back and give individual statements about what happened at the zoo. Two subjects who did not go the zoo are told to imagine that they had gone to the zoo and then to give independent statements about what they think should have gone on in the zoo. Consistency in the false pairs is much higher than in the true pairs. So in this case, consistency does not correlate with accuracy. When asked to imagine things that are highly stereotyped, non-participants come up with the same stories. When they really went to the zoo, they have such a rich store of details that happened that they pick different things. So although you find consistency to be an indicator of "true", narratives, you may have to be more cautious in the generalizability of these findings.

Brewer. I am not an applied researcher, but I have a suggestion of a possible interviewing strategy. When an interviewer is trying to get information from a child and the child is not forthcoming or spontaneous, perhaps the interviewer should also try questioning the child about another event—an event that is implausible such as " daddy lets me take the car downtown". This strategy would allow the interviewer to compare the evolution of the child's answers to both events—"the suspected event", and the "non-occurring event". These data would allow the interviewer to gauge the child's susceptibility to suggestion.

Bruck. This is an interesting suggestion because it is an example of how interviewers' could test alternative hypotheses, how interviewers could learn about the child's narrative skills, and perhaps about the child's general level of functioning. Of course, the major problem (and probably one that could only be addressed through a training program) would be to ensure that the structure of the interview and the nature of the questions is similar for the "suspected" and for the "implausible" event.

Brewin. In general, children are surrounded by stories, from morning to night; people are telling or reading them stories. So, presumably, at some point, there must be some differentiation going on in their minds between what is a "story" and what is real and between when is it appropriate to tell a "story" rather than the truth. Is it possible that something about your procedures are cueing the children to tell a story rather than what actually happened?

Bruck. First, it is true that we did not tell the children during the interviews that it is important to tell what really happened. We did not challenge the children by asking, "Is this something that really happened or are you telling me a story, or is it something that you saw on TV?". We do not make any claims in this study that the children's reports portray the contents of their memories: that is we do not make any claims about whether the children actually believe that they helped a lady find her monkey in the park, for example. Our study was designed to examine the evolution and structure of narratives that are suggestively produced. But let's consider Brewin's question in the context of therapeutic interviews—ones where children are asked to pretend, where children are asked to "act" or to "play out" various scenarios or themes, and where they are asked to do this repeatedly. It is certainly possible that what some children learn in these settings is that therapy is a place where you come to tell stories and to act out imaginary events. The problem with this is that at some point the stories may be believed by both the child and the therapist. So I think it is really important to consider the risk of various types of techniques that are used in therapy in light of the data that I have presented today.

Lindsay. There have been some questions today about the validity of the data that you have obtained when you have asked professionals to rate the credibility of children's statements on the basis of very short pieces of videotape. But isn't the case that there's some research, where professional interviewers have been given a whole lot of case information and nevertheless had a lot of difficulty?

Bruck. I think you are referring to the work of Mel Guyer and his colleagues. For example, Horner, Guyer, and Kalter (1993a, 1993b) presented an actual case of alleged sexual abuse of a 3-year-old to mental health specialists. These specialists heard a detailed presentation of the court-appointed clinician's findings, which included parent interviews and videotaped child-parent interaction sequences. The case presentation lasted approximately 2 hours, during which time the participants questioned the clinician who evaluated the child and her family. After the presentation, the clinicians estimated the likelihood that sexual molestation had occurred. The range of estimated probabilities of abuse was extreme-many clinicians were confident that abuse had occurred, and many others were just as confident that abuse had not occurred. The same pattern was obtained when the analyses were restricted to a smaller group of experts who were uniquely qualified to assess child sexual abuse. In another study, Realmuto, Jensen, and Wescoe (1990) asked a highly trained child psychiatrist to interview children and then to determine which of them had been sexually abused. Next, videotapes of this psychiatrist's assessments were shown to 14 professionals (pediatricians, psychiatrists, social workers, psychologists, attorneys) each with more than 10 years of experience in the field of child sexual abuse. These professionals were asked to classify the children as either abused or nonabused. Although there was high concordance between the interviewer and these 14 raters in terms of which children they classified as abused and nonabused, the overall rates of accurate classification were low. The point of these studies as well as our own is not to conclude that clinicians are doing a "terrible" job, but rather to highlight how difficult it sometimes is to make decisions in these situations. The work that I talked about today is an attempt to quantify what it is about children's verbal statements that make them seem credible or not-credible.

Before I finish, there have been a number of references to the "ethics" of the research that we and our colleagues are doing. I think it is important to address the specific concerns that a few of you have expressed. In the past, some of the ethical concerns about research such as the type we are doing have been made more explicit. Specifically, we have been criticised for "implanting" false memories in young children, and for including children in studies of "deception". The worry among those who raise this issue is that our procedures are potentially damaging to the child's sense of reality and/or to his self-esteem.

Our colleagues and we have seriously thought about and continue to think about these concerns each time we design studies. In fact, it seems to me that sometimes we spend more time redesigning and reconsidering the design of our studies because of ethical worries rather than methodological ones. I say this to point out the fact that we are indeed sensitive to these issues. Having said that, however, there are also a number of arguments in defence of the types of studies that I have talked about today. First, these studies are designed to measure risks of various interviewing techniques that are commonly used in investigative and therapeutic arenas. We feel that if these techniques are to be recommended for wide-spread use by professionals, then there is a need to evaluate not only their benefits but their risks, too, and to do so under conditions that begin to incorporate the myriad contaminating factors that characterise real world sex abuse investigations. We reasoned that any harm that might be associated with using potentially risky procedures in a strictly controlled experimental environment is insubstantial. After all, these procedures are routinely used by parents and teachers, albeit in a casual and non-systematic manner.

It would be a different matter altogether if our procedures called into question the love of a trusted care giver or diminished a child's self-concept due to false feedback about a central aspect of the identity. We do not come close to doing anything remotely like this, however. Instead, we ask children about everyday events, such as hot air balloon rides, assisting adults in need, and observations of others. We have assured ourselves that our procedures are safe on a number of grounds: First, we have determined from follow-up of the subjects in the many studies that we have carried out (both in medical and in non-medical settings) that our procedures do not appear to have had any observable negative impact either in the short-term or in the long-term. None of the parents have observed any behaviours of concern and the children do not seem to be disturbed in any way that we can detect. Second, as in most studies, our interviewers discontinue children who do not want to participate or who may react poorly in the interview. (The latter is a rare event because in general the children really enjoy participating in our studies.) Finally, children are debriefed whenever there exists a fear of the consequences of their making an inaccurate report. Because of the mild nature of the events we use, this is a rare need. Third, although in some of our studies we have concluded that some of the children have come to actually believe some of the suggestions, long-term follow-up of some of these children suggest that once the interviewing procedures are finished, and with the passage of time, our subjects no longer have these memories. In fact, they either forget the entire suggestion, or when they do remember the suggestion, they will eventually say that it never really happened (Huffman, Crossman, & Ceci, 1996). These findings, of course, are important theoretically as well as practically, because they indicate that perhaps in most cases "false memories" in children are maintained only when there are cues (such as nterviewing or more subtle reminders) for their reinstatement. It is important to remind the audience that the studies in this area have been approved by university and hospital ethics committees. Thus it is not just a researcher's judgment about "morality" that wins the day but rather a consensus of a diverse group of individuals who bring to bear their collective wisdom about the potential risks of the research. In fact, some of the studies that we conducted went through revisions as a result of the ethics committee judgment about the safest manner to conduct such research with young children. Finally, in undertaking this research we have asked ourselves the questions: what are the risks of "doing" this research and what are the risks of not doing it. While the risks are apparent (e.g., potential stress, damage to reality testing), the risks of not doing it are less clear. However, in the past few years, there have been a number of examples of the risks of "not doing" this type of research. For example, the results of our studies and those of our colleagues have provided enough evidence to raise real concerns about the use of anatomically detailed dolls and other types of props in the interviewing of young children. If these studies had not been done, then professionals would blindly continue to use these devices, thinking that they are beneficial and without risk. Not only is this information critically important from the standpoint of accused adults, but we believe that it is also critically important for the many children who might otherwise be led to make false recognitions or false statements as a result of doll-based and other interviewing procedures.

EDITORS NOTE

Questions regarding ethics were not addressed during the Q & A period of Dr. Bruck's lecture but it subsequently became clear that this was an issue for a number of participants (see also commentary by Yehuda, this volume) and we therefore asked Dr. Bruck to comment on it.

REFERENCES

Horner, T. M., Guyer, M., J., & Kalter, N. M. (1993a). Clinical expertise and the assessment of child sexual abuse. *Journal of the American Academy of Child and Adolescent Psychiatry, 32*, 925–931.

Horner, T. M., Guyer, M., J., & Kalter, N. M. (1993b). The biases of child sexual abuse experts: Believing is seeing. *Bulletin of the American Academy of Psychiatry and Law, 21*, 281–292.

Huffman, M.L., Crossman, A.M., & Ceci, S.J. (in press). Are false memories permanent? An investigation of the long-term effects of source misattributions. *Consciousnesss and Cognition.*

Realmuto, G., Jensen, J., & Wescoe, S. (1990). Specificity and sensitivity of sexually anatomically correct dolls in substantiating abuse: A pilot study. *Journal of the American Academy of Child and Adolescent Psychiatry, 29*, 743–746.

9

RELEVANCE OF NEUROENDOCRINE ALTERATIONS IN PTSD TO MEMORY-RELATED IMPAIRMENTS OF TRAUMA SURVIVORS

Rachel Yehuda[1] and Philip Harvey[2]

[1]Mount Sinai School of Medicine
One Gustave L. Levy Pl.
New York, New York 10029-6574
[2]Bronx Veterans Affairs

1. INTRODUCTION

It is now well established that memory consolidation in both animals and humans is influenced by stress-responsive neuromodulators. Recent theories have attempted to apply knowledge about the effect of these neuromodulators on memory, in order to explain the nature of memory-related impairments in trauma survivors with posttraumatic stress disorder (PTSD). However, as will be described in this chapter, most existing theories have not incorporated recent information about biological aspects of PTSD in their formulations. Accordingly, current theories using only extant knowledge of the neurochemistry of stress have not been able to account for several important aspects of memory-related phenomenology in PTSD. For example, current theories do not explain the heterogeneity among trauma survivors in the prevalence of memory-related impairments, nor do they account for how different types of memory-related symptoms can occur over the course of an individual's illness. A consideration of these questions requires knowledge of the biological events that occur at the time of the trauma and during the course of PTSD and an appreciation that these biological events represent an atypical, rather than a normal stress response. Furthermore, as most individuals do not develop long-term PTSD symptoms, current models of memory processing in PTSD must also account for the complex risk factors, other than similar exposures to traumatic events, that give rise to PTSD and PTSD-related memory impairments. This chapter will describe differences in the acute and chronic neurobiological response to trauma in individuals who develop PTSD versus those who do not, and will discuss the relevance of these findings to understanding the biological underpinnings of memory impairments in PTSD. Furthermore, a theoretical formulation of how to explore cognitive impairments in PTSD by considering

Recollections of Trauma, edited by Read and Lindsay
Plenum Press, New York, 1997

possible risk factors for disturbed memory processing in response to trauma will be presented.

2. SYMPTOMS OF PTSD AND THEIR RELATIONSHIP TO MEMORY IMPAIRMENTS

PTSD is a psychiatric disorder that sometimes develops in individuals who have experienced a traumatic event. According to the most current definition in the DSM-IV (American Psychiatric Press, 1994), a traumatic event is one that involves a threat to one's life or physical integrity and that invokes a subjective response of fear, helplessness, or horror. This subjective response is associated with concomitant neurobiological changes that occur in the immediate aftermath of the trauma, which may, in part contribute to the development of symptoms.

The symptoms of PTSD are divided into three clusters: intrusive or reexperiencing, avoidance, and hyperarousal. Intrusive symptoms consist of: 1) having recurrent and unwanted recollections of the event; 2) having distressing dreams of the event; and 3) acting and feeling as if the event were reoccurring (e.g., dissociative flashbacks). Additionally, 4) psychological and 5) physiological distress following exposure to symbolic representations of the event may also occur. Avoidance symptoms include behaviors indicative of actively avoiding reminders of the trauma such as 1) efforts to avoid thoughts, feelings or talk of the trauma; 2) efforts to avoid reminders of the trauma; 3) inability to recall important aspects of the trauma (e.g., psychogenic amnesia); and symptoms of generalized emotional numbing such as 4) markedly diminished interest in normally significant activities; 5) feelings of detachment or estrangement from others; 6) restricted range of affect; and 7) sense of a foreshortened future. Hyperarousal symptoms consist of 1) difficulty falling or staying asleep; 2) irritability or angry outbursts; 3) difficulties with concentration; 4) hypervigilance; and 5) exaggerated startle response. Meeting diagnostic criteria for PTSD requires the concurrent presence of one intrusive symptom, three avoidant symptoms, and two hyperarousal symptoms.

Several of these 17 symptoms of PTSD reflect memory-related impairments. These range from difficulties associated with traumatic memories (e.g., intrusive memories, flashbacks, and amnesias) to more generalized symptoms such as impaired concentration, which can also affect the processing of nontraumatic memory. Furthermore, difficulties associated with traumatic memories can be quite diverse, ranging from reexperiencing of the traumatic event through intrusive recollections to psychogenic amnesia. Some individuals only experience impairments at one end of the memory spectrum. It is not uncommon for the same individual to complain of having too vivid or frequent intrusive recollections of a traumatic event while simultaneously being aware of having forgotten, or being unable to retrieve, important aspects of the event (Fisler & van der Kolk, 1995). The apparent discrepancy between "remembering too much" and "remembering too little" can be easily resolved if these symptoms are understood in a clinical context, rather than from the vantage of experimental memory research. From a clinical perspective, intrusive recollections do not necessarily reflect historical reality. Therefore, their presence is not in conflict with psychogenic amnesias. Likewise, "amnestic" symptoms can be seen as consciously motivated, in the context of attempts to avoid unpleasant re-experiencing.

In fact, the relationship between experienced intrusive memories and the historical reality of the traumatic event which is being remembered does not appear to be an important focus in the field of traumatic stress research. Clinicians and researchers who are concerned with understanding the nature of intrusive recollections and other reexperiencing phenomenon have traditionally not been concerned with the extent to which the traumatic memories reflect the actual traumatic event as it occurred. Rather, intrusive memories are phenomenologically important and clinically significant because they reflect the *psychological* reality of what a trauma survivor has experienced. Although in many cases there is likely to be a strong relationship between the psychological reality and the historical accuracy of a traumatic event, the experience of trauma and the subsequent processing of this experience can indeed leave individuals with incomplete, fragmented or distorted memories and cognitions related to the event. Thus, a trauma survivor may experience intrusive recollections of traumatic experiences that reflect a distorted persepective of an objective reality (Foa et al., 1995). These symptoms are still quite important clinically, and their presence is thought to be a sign that a traumatic event has indeed occurred. However, although the existence of intrusive memories may imply exposure to a trauma (that is likely to be similar if not identical to the one being re-experienced), the content of the intrusive memory does not constitute an historical record.

3. WHAT CAUSES MEMORY-RELATED IMPAIRMENTS OF PTSD?

Until recently, it was assumed that exposure to the traumatic event was the single most important, if not the sole, cause of posttraumatic stress symptoms. However, this assumption has been challenged by recent studies demonstrating that only a subset of those exposed to traumatic events develop chronic PTSD. According to the summary of epidemiological studies in DSM-IV, estimates of the prevalence of PTSD among those exposed to Criterion A stressors range from 3–58% (American Psychiatric Association, 1994). This wide range may reflect the fact that some types of traumatic events are more likely to result in PTSD than others (Kessler, Sonnega, Bromet, Hughes & Nelson, 1995). For example, among those who have experienced torture, such as concentration camp survivors and POWs, the prevalence of PTSD can be quite high with estimates of 50–75% in such samples (Kluznick, Speed, VanValkenberg & Macgraw, 1986). The trauma of rape in women, and combat trauma in men, are also associated with a high prevalence of PTSD in that roughly one half of women (Kilpatrick & Resnick, 1993) and one third of men who undergo these events develop chronic PTSD symptoms (Kessler et al., 1995; Kulka, 1991). In contrast, exposure to natural disasters such as earthquakes, volcanic eruptions and bush fires, is associated with a relatively lower prevalence of lifetime PTSD with estimates ranging from 3.5–16% (McFarlane, 1992; Shore, Vollmer & Tatum, 1989). In considering the diverse prevalence rates of PTSD from epidemiological studies, it is important to note that there may be much variability in people's willingness or ability to provide retrospective reports of both traumatic events and the psychological aftermath of these events. Certain types of events are more likely than others to be recalled or disclosed in a standard research interviews. Prevalence rates may also vary dramatically in normal population samples versus high risk samples in which individuals are recruited because of a known exposure to a particular event.

Despite the complexities involved in obtaining accurate assessments of the prevalence of PTSD it has become clear in recent years that even under the most traumatic conditions some individuals will not develop PTSD. Furthermore, most who develop PTSD will show a remission of their symptoms within several months or years after the traumatic event (Kessler et al., 1995). The limited prevalence of chronic PTSD compared to the prevalence of traumatic events indicates that there are factors other than trauma exposure that influence the development of persistent symptoms following trauma exposure. Accordingly, peritraumatic, posttraumatic, and pretrauma risk factors have each been associated with increased risk for the development of chronic PTSD. Some of these factors include the severity of the trauma (Foy, Sipprelle, Rueger & Carroll, 1984; Yehuda, Southwick & Giller, 1992a); the presence of comorbid psychopathology (McFarlane, 1989); subsequent exposure to reactivating environmental events (Kluznick et al., 1986; Schnurr, Friedman & Rosenberg, 1993; Solomon & Preager, 1992; True et al., 1993; Yehuda, et al., 1995a); history of stress, abuse or trauma (Bremner, Southwick, Johnson, Yehuda & Charney, 1993; Zaidi & Foy, 1994); history of behavioral or psychological problems (Helzer, Robins & McEvoy, 1987); and low IQ prior to the trauma (McNally & Shin, 1995).

One of the more interesting possibilities that has emerged is the idea that there may be genetic (True et al., 1993) or familial (Davidson, Swartz, Storck, Krishnam, & Hammet, 1985) risk factors for the development of PTSD. In a study examining the prevalence of PTSD in monozygotic twins discordant for service in Vietnam, True et al. reported that 30% of PTSD symptoms could be accounted for by heritable factors (1993). Davidson et al. (1985) noted high rates of familial depression and anxiety among combat veterans with PTSD. More recently, it has been demonstrated that the children of parents with chronic PTSD are more likely to develop PTSD in response to traumatic events compared to individuals whose parents experienced similar trauma, but who did not develop chronic PTSD (Yehuda et al., in press).

The limited prevalence of PTSD compared to the prevalence of trauma, and the presence of established risk factors that increase the likelihood for the development of PTSD following exposure to trauma, has had significant implications for understanding the diverse range of phenomenological and neurobiological alterations in trauma survivors (Yehuda & McFarlane, 1995). In essence, these findings have suggested that the experience of trauma may not be the sole explanation for why individuals suffer from PTSD. Rather, explanations about posttraumatic phenomena must include a wider range of predisposing variables, not just the precipitating traumatic event.

In considering the nature of posttraumatic memory impairments, the same issues arise. Although it is tempting to assume that alterations in the processing of traumatic memories result directly from the magnitude of the event, this may not necessarily be true. Thus, the study of memory impairments in PTSD must include an exploration of individual characteristics which could potentially modify the risk or vulnerability for PTSD following exposure to a traumatic event. One way to examine this issue is to study trauma-exposed individuals with and without PTSD. If a particular memory impairment is due to the experience of trauma, then it is more likely to be present in all trauma-exposed individuals (assuming a comparable level of trauma exposure), not just in the subset of those who meet criteria for PTSD. By contrasting memory impairments in trauma survivors with and without PTSD, it is possible to develop a more sophisticated distinction between "normative" memory processing following trauma, and "atypical" memory processing. In studies that do not use a trauma-exposed comparison group without PTSD, it is impossible to determine whether memory impairments observed in relationship to normal controls are a function of the exposure to trauma or due to PTSD. Yet, most published studies exploring cognitive alterations in PTSD have not compared trauma-exposed individuals with PTSD to similarly exposed individuals without PTSD. Nonetheless, these studies have tended to conclude that the observed memory impairments in PTSD subjects are attributable to the experience of trauma.

Studies of the neurobiology of PTSD have made the distinction between trauma survivors with PTSD and trauma survivors without PTSD. As such, it has been possible to describe neurobiological alterations in PTSD as representing specific changes that are distinct from those in similarly exposed trauma survivors. Since many of the biological changes observed in PTSD occur in systems that are intimately involved in memory processing, an understanding of the biological alterations in PTSD may help clarify the nature of cognitive deficits in PTSD. Therefore, a brief review of neuroendocrine findings in PTSD will be presented, and then discussed in the context of understanding how to properly formulate a neurobiology of traumatic memories.

4. NEUROENDOCRINE ASPECTS OF PTSD

Biological examination of trauma survivors has repeatedly demonstrated that individuals with chronic PTSD show differences in several stress-responsive neurochemical systems compared to similarly exposed individuals without PTSD and normal controls. Furthermore, although the systems that have been demonstrated to be affected in PTSD are the same as those that have been implicated in the pathophysiology of other mood and anxiety disorders, they are altered quite differently in PTSD. The two premier examples of the distinct neurochemistry of PTSD are findings of changes in the hypothalamic-pituitary-adrenal (HPA) axis and catecholamine systems. Both of these systems are fundamentally important in human stress responses, and both have been demonstrated to have important roles in normal and stress-related memory processing.

4.1. Hypothalamic-Pituitary-Adrenal Alterations in PTSD

In response to stress, a variety of neuromodulators and neuropeptides in the brain stimulate the release of corticotrophin releasing factor (CRF) (and other secretagogues such as arginine vasopressin) from the hypothalamus, which in turn initiate the release of adrenocorticotrophin hormone (ACTH) from the pituitary and the release of cortisol from the adrenals (Munck, Guyre & Holbrook, 1984; Chrousos & Gold, 1992). The major function of cortisol is to mobilize the body's stress responses, and then help shut down the neural defensive reactions that have been activated by stress (Munck et al., 1984). The stress response is ultimately contained by the negative feedback inhibition of cortisol on the pituitary, hypothalamus, and other sites. Cortisol exerts its actions by binding to glucocorticoid receptors (Svec, 1985). In turn, changes in the number and/or sensitivity of glucocorticoid receptors can influence the body's response to stress (Lowy, Gormley & Reder 1989).

Because high cortisol levels have typically been associated with stress, it was initially hypothesized that cortisol levels would be elevated in PTSD. However, an initial study demonstrated that the 24-hr urinary excretion of cortisol was actually lower in combat veterans with PTSD compared with hospitalized VA patients with other psychiatric diagnoses such as major depression, schizoaffective disorder, bipolar disorder and schizophrenia. To date, four (Mason, Giller, Kosten, Ostroff & Podd,1986; Yehuda et al., 1990a; Yehuda, Boisoneau, Mason & Giller, 1993a; Yehuda et al., 1995a) out of six studies (Pitman & Orr, 1990; Lemiux & Coe, 1994) have demonstrated that urinary cortisol levels were lower in PTSD compared to both similarly exposed trauma survivors without PTSD and nonpsychiatric comparison subjects. Furthermore, a recent epidemiological study conducted on a sample of over 2,000 Vietnam veterans showed that veterans with current PTSD had lower plasma cortisol levels than veterans without PTSD (Boscarino, 1996). An interesting feature of the low average cortisol levels in PTSD is that they are not consistently low over the 24-hr diurnal cycle. On the contrary, PTSD in combat veterans, for example, is characterized by a greater range of cortisol levels as reflected by the lower trough in the face of comparable circadian peak levels (Yehuda, Teicher & Levengood, Trestman, Siever, 1996a).

Following the initial findings of low cortisol, lymphocyte glucocorticoid receptors were found to be increased in number in PTSD compared to normals and other psychiatric groups (Yehuda, Lowy, Southwick, Shaffer & Giller, 1991a; Yehuda et al., 1993a; Yehuda, Boisoneau, Lowy & Giller 1995b). In contrast, glucocorticoid receptors become "downregulated" or decreased in number, in response to stress (Sapolsky, Krey & McEwen 1984). Glucocorticoid receptor numbers are also lower than normal in depressed patients, who tend to have high cortisol levels (Gormley et al., 1985; Whalley, Borthwick & Copolov, 1986).

Lymphocyte glucocorticoid receptor numbers have now been evaluated under basal conditions and following the administration of exogenous steroid (i.e., dexamethasone) in PTSD. Three studies of combat veterans (Yehuda et al., 1991a; Yehuda et al., 1993a, Yehuda et al., 1995b) and one study of adult survivors of childhood sexual abuse (Stein, Yehuda, Koverola & Hanna, in press) showed that glucocorticoid receptor numbers were increased in PTSD compared to non-traumatized subjects without psychiatric disorder. Glucocorticoid receptor number (i.e., Bmax) was found to be decreased following dexamethasone administration in combat veterans with PTSD but not in trauma survivors without PTSD or normal controls (Yehuda et al., 1995b), suggesting that glucocorticoid receptors of PTSD subjects are more sensitive to the administration of the synthetic steroid (Gormley et al., 1985; Yehuda et al., 1995b).

Consistent with both low cortisol and increased glucocorticoid receptor number, the cortisol response to dexamethasone is enhanced in PTSD (Yehuda, Southwick, Krystal, Charney & Mason 1993b; Yehuda et al., 1995b). This response is opposite of the classic nonsuppression of cortisol observed in major depression (Carroll et al., 1981). The hyper-responsiveness to dexamethasone was also present in combat veterans with PTSD who met the diagnostic criteria for concurrent major depression (Yehuda et al., 1993b) but was not present in combat veterans without PTSD (Yehuda et al., 1995b). The finding of an enhanced cortisol suppression to 0.50 mg dexamethasone in PTSD has been replicated by several investigators (Stein et al., in press; Heim & Hellhammer, in press; Goenjin et al., 1996), and has been interpreted as reflecting an enhanced feedback sensitivity of the hypothalamic-pituitary-adrenal axis in PTSD. Recent evidence supporting an enhanced negative feedback sensitivity of the hypothalamic-pituitary-adrenal axis in PTSD has also come from the demonstration of an augmented ACTH response following metyrapone administration in PTSD (Yehuda et al., 1996b).

The enhanced negative feedback model suggests that the primary deficit in PTSD is an increased responsiveness of glucocorticoid receptors at several sites along the hypothalamic-pituitary-adrenal axis (Yehuda, Giller, Southwick & Siever, 1995c; Yehuda, Giller & Mason, 1993c). The enhanced receptor responsiveness results in a stronger negative feedback and attenuated basal cortisol levels and enhanced responsiveness to exogenous steroid (i.e., dexamethasone). This model clearly differentiates the biological stress response in PTSD from that typically associated with stress, and psychiatric disorders such as major depression (Yehuda, Giller, Southwick, Lowy & Mason, 1991b). Whereas chronic stress and depression are associated with a reduced negative feedback inhibition of the hypothalamic-pituitary-adrenal axis and a resultant decrease in stress responsiveness, the biological alterations in PTSD appear to reflect a neuroendocrine system that may be highly responsive to environmental challenge.

4.2. Catecholamine Alterations in PTSD

Activation of the sympathetic nervous system (SNS) is also an important component of the stress response. In response to stress, coordinated sympathetic discharge causes increases in heart rate and blood pressure, thereby allowing a greater perfusion of muscles and vital organs, and increased energy to skeletal muscles by mobilizing blood glucose (Mountcastle, 1973). SNS activation also results in the release of catecholamines (primarily norepinephrine and epinephrine). These and other activities are part of what Cannon originally termed the "flight or fight" response (Cannon, 1914). It is generally the case that the catecholamine system and the hypothalamic-pituitary-adrenal axis work in tandem, and in the brain glucocorticoid and catecholamine receptors are co-localized in many areas such as the locus coeruleus (Harfstrand et al., 1986). Thus, it is not surprising that catecholamine and cortisol levels following stress are typically highly correlated. Interestingly, however, the function of catecholamines and cortisol are synergistic; cortisol's role in stress is to shut down the sympathetic (catecholamine) activation following stress.

The link between catecholamine alterations and trauma was noted in 1918, when investigators noted that combat veterans with "shell shock" had greater increases in heart rate and respiratory rate in responses to sounds of gunfire, and greater increases in subjective anxiety, and blood pressure in response to epinephrine injections compared to healthy controls (Meakins & Wilson, 1918). Several years after Kardiner used the term "physioneurosis" to describe the clinical state of WWII veterans, investigators (Dobbs & Wilson, 1960; Grinker & Spiegal, 1945) wrote of combat soldiers who appeared as if they had "received an injection of adrenaline: and who suffered from chronic stimulation of the SNS." These initial observations prompted a series of studies that demonstrated marked elevations of psychophysiologic parameters during provocation and, in some studies, differences at baseline between combat veterans with PTSD and non-exposed subjects (Kardiner, 1941; Brende, 1982; Blanchard et al., 1986; Malloy, Fairbanks & Keane, 1983; Pallmeyer, Blanchard & Kolb, 1986; Pitman, Orr, Forgue, DeJong & Clairborn, 1987; Orr, Pitman, Lasko & Herz, 1987; Shalev, Orr & Pitman, 1993; Pitman et al., 1990).

Studies focusing on the neuroendocrine underpinnings of SNS activation in PTSD have yielded mixed results. An initial study demonstrated increased urinary norepinephrine and epinephrine in hospitalized Vietnam combat veterans with PTSD compared to other psychiatric groups (Kosten, Mason, Giller, Harkness & Ostroff, 1987). However, a subsequent study failed to reveal differences in norepinephrine and epinephrine in outpatient Vietnam combat veterans with and without PTSD. However, the mean norepinephrine excretion in both groups was quite high (Pitman & Orr, 1990). A third study demonstrated increased urinary norepinephrine, epinephrine and dopamine excretion in Vietnam combat veterans, particularly in those who were inpatients, compared to normal controls (Yehuda, Southwick, Ma, Giller & Mason, 1992b). More recently, Mellman et al. (1995) did not observe significant elevations in urinary norepinephrine and MHPG in Vietnam combat veterans. However, elevations in urinary norepinephrine were reported in residents living near Three Mile Island (Davidson & Baum, 1986). Studies of baseline plasma norepinephrine and its immediate metabolite 3-methoxy-5-hydroxy phenol glycol (MHPG) have generally failed to determine significant differences between PTSD and normal controls (McFall, Murburg & Ko, 1990; Blanchard et al., 1991; Murburg, McFall, Lewis & Veith, 1995). However, these studies used single blood samples of plasma catecholamines which may not adequately characterize the phasic versus tonic releases in catecholamines (Veith & Murburg, 1994). When plasma norepinephrine levels were examined every 30 minutes over a 24-hr period under carefully controlled laboratory conditions, we observed significantly higher levels of plasma norepinephrine in PTSD compared with normal and depressed subjects (Yehuda et al., submitted).

Plasma norepinephrine and MHPG levels have been found to be higher following neuroendocrine provocation (Southwick et al., 1993) or stress testing (McFall et al., 1990) in Vietnam veterans with PTSD compared to nonpsychiatric controls. Of particular interest is that infusion of the selective alpha2-antagonist yohimbine not only produces augmented MHPG responses in Vietnam combat veterans with PTSD, but also induces PTSD-related symptoms such as flashbacks and panic attacks (Southwick et al., 1993). The findings of increased sensitivity of the catecholamine system, then, parallel the HPA axis alterations in demonstrating hyperresponsiveness to neuroendocrine provocation. Investigations of platelet alpha2-adrenergic receptors in Vietnam veterans with PTSD have further supported the idea of catecholamine disturbances in PTSD, and have pointed to the possibility of changes in receptor sensitivity as potentially underlying the catecholamine alterations in PTSD. Fewer total alpha2-adrenergic receptor binding sites per platelets has been observed in Vietnam combat veterans (Perry, Southwick, Yehuda & Giller, 1990; Perry, Giller & Southwick, 1987; Perry, 1994) and traumatized children (Perry, 1994) with PTSD. The finding of fewer alpha2-adrenergic receptors may occur in response to chronic elevations of circulating catecholamines. Perry et al. (1990) demonstrated that epinephrine caused a more rapid degradation of alpha2-receptors in Vietnam veterans with PTSD compared to controls, indicating that the receptors of PTSD subjects were more "supersensitive."

Although the above review demonstrates that catecholamine metabolism is likely altered in PTSD, unlike findings of the hypothalamic-pituitary-adrenal axis in PTSD, it is difficult to draw definitive conclusions about the nature of basal catecholamine alterations in PTSD because of the discrepant findings. It has been traditionally assumed that catecholamine metabolism is increased in PTSD. However, this may reflect the fact that catecholamine release is actually higher in response to provocation, and that PTSD patients may have difficulty achieving a true "basal" or resting state.

An interesting question for future research concerns the relationship between the HPA axis alterations and catecholamine changes (Yehuda, Southwick, Perry, Mason & Giller, 1990b). It has been demonstrated that within the same subjects, cortisol levels are low while catecholamine levels are high (Kosten et al., 1987; see also Figure 1). Thus, one conclusion that can be drawn from these studies is that the normal correlation between catecholamine and cortisol levels is altered in PTSD. This may reflect the fact that the two systems are dissociated in this disorder, or may indicate the failure of one system to exert its usual regulation over the other.

4.3. Biological Studies of the Acute Aftermath of Trauma: Relationship to the Biology of PTSD

The above discussion demonstrates that the neuroendocrine alterations in PTSD are qualitatively and directionally different from those associated with classic stress responses. However, several questions arise in attempting to understand these findings in PTSD subjects. For example, since the neuroendocrine studies summarized above were performed on subjects with chronic PTSD (i.e., trauma survivors who have been symptomatic for years and even decades), it is possible that the alterations observed represent a biological adaptation to chronic symptoms of PTSD, but not the immediate neurobiologi-

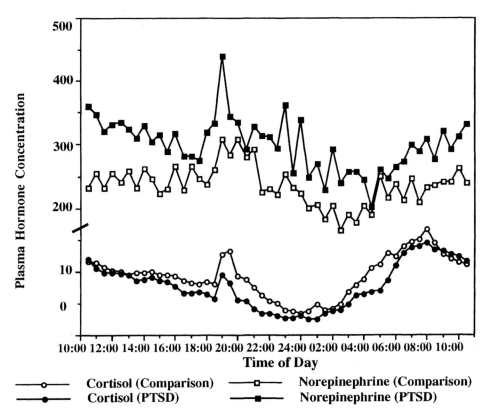

Figure 1. Comparison of Plasma Cortisol and Norepinephrine Over the 24-hr Cycle. Data represent means of cortisol and norepinephrine levels (ug/dl) from 16 normal controls and 15 combat veterans with PTSD. Patients were medication free and free from major medical illness. Blood samples were drawn from subjects after they had followed a monoamine-free diet for 3 days, and while they remained supine, in fasting state as previously described in Yehuda et al., 1996. Part of these data are redrawn from Yehuda et al., 1996.

cal response to the precipitating traumatic event or the earlier adaptation to this event. Furthermore, as it has become increasingly clear that individuals without PTSD do not show similar biological alterations to those with PTSD despite a comparable exposure to trauma, it has become important to consider the possibility that prior and subsequent stressors or risk factors in addition to the focal trauma contribute to the neuroendocrine alterations in PTSD (Yehuda & McFarlane, 1995).

Recent longitudinal studies have begun to explore some of these questions by examining the acute biological response to trauma in those who subsequently do and do not develop PTSD. One study demonstrated that women who are most likely to develop PTSD had lower cortisol levels at the time of the trauma. Low cortisol levels at the time of rape was associated with a prior history of rape, which was the strongest predictor of the subsequent development of PTSD (Resnick, Yehuda, Pitman & Foy, 1995). Interestingly, the severity of the rape (i.e., quantified on the basis of objective characteristics such as whether or not rape involved threat or injury with weapons, multiple penetrations, multiple perpetrators, and/or physical injury) did not predict either cortisol levels or subsequent PTSD. However, rape severity was associated with MHPG responses immediately following rape. As would be predicted, the higher the rape severity, the higher the MHPG response. However, MHPG levels were not associated with the subsequent development of PTSD.

In a second study (McFarlane, personal communication), the cortisol response to motor vehicle accidents was examined in individuals appearing to the emergency room in the immediate aftermath of the trauma. Six months later subjects were evaluated for the presence or absence of psychiatric disorder. In subjects who had developed PTSD, the cortisol response in the immediate aftermath of the motor vehicle was substantially lower, and the cortisol response in those who developed major depression substantially higher, than in individuals who did not develop psychiatric disorder. In the aggregate the two longitudinal studies demonstrate that the acute cortisol responses to trauma in individuals who develop PTSD may be different from those of individuals who do not develop PTSD in response to a similar trauma. Furthermore, the data raise the possibility that the low cortisol levels observed in chronic PTSD reflect more than simply the state of having a chronic illness.

Unfortunately, the two aforementioned studies do not directly address whether or not individuals may have had low cortisol levels before the traumatic event. Thus, it would be premature to conclude that the neuroendocrine findings in PTSD are manifestations of an underlying risk for this disorder rather than describing the consequences of chronic symptoms following trauma exposure. The resolution of this question necessitates prospective studies that assess cortisol levels in subjects before and after they experience traumatic events, which, for obvious reasons, are difficult to perform.

What remains increasingly clear, however, is that it is difficult to ascribe neuroendocrine alterations in PTSD solely to the exposure to traumatic events (Yehuda et al., 1995c). It is even possible that some features of the atypical neuroendocrine response to trauma in those who develop chronic PTSD might be present at the time of the trauma, or even before the traumatic event occurs (and would therefore predispose the individual to specific types of biological responses in following exposure to trauma).

5. SIGNIFICANCE OF NEUROENDOCRINOLOGY OF PTSD TO OUR UNDERSTANDING OF THE PROCESSING OF TRAUMATIC MEMORIES IN PTSD

When we speak about the neurobiology of PTSD, we are clearly dealing with a set of alterations that are present in a subset of individuals who are exposed to traumatic events. Moreover, what is particularly noteworthy about the neuroendocrine alterations is that they are distinct from those that have been described as constituting the classic stress response. Therefore an important question arises concerning the relevance of information about the processing of traumatic memories in nonsymptomatic individuals to understanding how traumatic memories are formed and processed in PTSD, since models of how traumatic memories are normally processed assume a normal stress responsiveness on the part of the subject. To the extent that one posits that memory disturbances in PTSD are qualitatively, not just directionally, different than those observed in individuals who do not develop PTSD, then the larger literature on memory research may have a more circumscribed relevance than if the alterations in PTSD were a direct result of trauma exposure. In the next two sections we will consider how to incorporate what is known about the neurobiologic findings in PTSD into the larger framework of findings about the neurobiology of traumatic memories in order to understand some of the specific issues that arise in considering biological concomitants of PTSD-related memory phenomenology.

5.1. How Stress Normally Modulates Learning and Memory: A Brief Review

Classic studies of learning and memory have demonstrated that a variety of neuropeptides and neuromodulators are intrinsically important in facilitating memory-related processes (for review, see De Wied & Croiset, 1991; McGaugh et al., 1984). These neurochemicals include, but are not limited to ACTH and other derived peptides, catecholamines, vasopressin and other related neuropeptides, and endorphins. In animals, the role of these neuropeptides and neuromodulators have been demonstrated using a variety of experimental paradigms, most notably, the conditioned avoidance test (vanRee & DeWeid, 1988). The basic approach uses avoidance learning, which involves teaching an animal to perform a behavior that it would not normally do because of the threat of stress. For example, a laboratory rat can be taught to cross a barrier in response to a tone in order to avoid an electrical shock. This is done in a series of steps. First the rat is exposed to the tone (called a conditioned stimulus). Five seconds later, the rat receives a shock (called an unconditioned stimulus). In response to the shock the rat will naturally cross over the barrier to avoid the shock. Eventually, the continued pairing of the warning tone and the shock will cause the animal to cross the barrier to avoid the shock. The presumption that learning and memory have occured stems from the animal's ability to cross the barrier prior to the shock. If the tone ceases to be paired with the shock, then eventually the tone will not elicit the conditioned avoidance response. This phenomenon is called extinction. Once the rat has mastered this task, it is possible to examine the effects of each neurochemical separately by manipulating it pharmacologically or surgically, and examining the effect on the rate of learning behavior (e.g., some manipulations can be applied prior to beginning the learning paradigm and some after initial acquisition of the behavior has occured).

Since an electric shock is a classic stressor, a shocked animal will release the neuropeptides and neuromodulators mentioned above and will show an activation of the pituitary-adrenocortical system. In a series of now classic studies, it was demonstrated that the administration of several different types of neuropeptides could enhance learning. For example, exogenous ACTH could facilitate the conditioned avoidance response (i.e., reduce the number of trials it took for the animal to acquire the avoidance behavior), whereas removal of the pituitary increased the number of trials that it took for the animal learned to avoid the shock (Bohus, 1974; DeWied & Croiset, 1991). The administration of exogenous cortisol, however, had the synergistic effect of enhancing extinction (DeWied & Jolles, 1982). The opposite effects of cortisol and ACTH on learning in the rat were conceptualized as reflecting the role of cortisol in terminating the neuroendocrine response to stress and in the suppression of fear-motivated behaviors (DeWied & Croiset, 1991; Bohus, De Kloet & Veldhuis, 1982).

Similar faciliatory effects on learning and memory were observed with catecholamine administration (McGaugh, 1985). Epinephrine in moderate doses enhanced the retention of most learning tasks while removal of the adrenal medulla blocked passive avoidance behavior (Borell, De Kloet, Versteeg & Bohus, 1983). Some (Walker 1958, 1967), but not all (Christianson & Mjorndal, 1985) human studies demonstrated that the administration of small to moderate doses of epinephrine (adrenalin) could also cause memory enhancement (Eysenck, 1982). As discussed earlier in this chapter, the function of catecholamines during stress is to produce arousal (Charney, Deutch, Krystal, Southwick & Nagy, 1993). In a recent study, Cahill et al. (1994) elegantly demonstrated that blocking normal arousal to a series of provocative slides by pretreating normal college students with the drug propranolol prior to having them view the slides, resulted in increasing the rate of retention errors when subjects were subseqeuntly asked to recall details of the slides they had previously viewed. That catecholamines could potentiate learning, and that catecholamine blockade with propranolol could suppress memory for arousing stimuli, have been interpreted as reflecting the importance of arousal to the process of memory consolidation. Although the relationship between arousal and memory consolidation is quite complex, in that too high levels of arousal are actually thought to interfere with memory consolidation (McGaugh et al., 1984), it is widely held that arousal leads to memory consolidation by creating a shift from an organism's baseline which allows new information to be acquired (McGaugh et al., 1984). Arousal during stress may also lead to other types of responses such as focused attention and hypervigilance, which may also affect memory consolidation at the time of a traumatic event (Charney et al., 1993).

The above discussion is not meant to fully describe the biology of learning and memory, which is obviously extremely complex and well beyond the scope of this chapter, but rather to emphasize two specific points. The first, is that there is an intrinsic neurochemical relationship between stress and memory processing that can be observed in both animals and humans. The second point is that whereas some stress-related neuromodulators can enhance learning and memory, other neurochemicals may have opposite effects.

5.2. Current Formulations of Traumatic Memory Formation in PTSD

It has been suggested by some investigators that the intrusive recollections suffered by individuals with chronic PTSD are a result of the high arousal that trauma survivors must have sustained at the time of the trauma (Pitman et al., 1993; Charney et al., 1993). These investigators have argued that exposure to an extremely stressful event can overstimulate certain stress-responsive hormones and neuromodulators (e.g., catecholamines, vasopressin, ACTH) leading to an "overconsolidation" of the memory trace of the event. This overconsolidation, also refered to as "superconditioning" (Pitman et al., 1991) is seen to be manifest in the intrusive recollections that characterizes PTSD patients. Furthermore, these investigators hypothesized that because of the U-inverted dose-response curve that has been typically associated with the effects of arousal on memory, extraordinarily high levels of catecholamines or other neuropeptides at the time of the trauma may interfere with memory consolidation and ultimately lead to amnesias (see also, van der Kolk, 1994).

Although at first glance the idea of overconsolidation appears to address several aspects of the phenomenology of intrusive recollections following trauma, there are several problems with applying this model to PTSD. First, the model does not explain why only some individuals, and not others, develop memory impairments following exposure to similar events. Second, the model does not explain remission and/or re-emergence of memory-related symptoms. Third, although the model attempts to account for how intrusive thoughts and amnesias can both result from increased catecholamine levels, the model does not account for the fact that PTSD patients often have both intrusive thoughts and amnesias. The U-inverted shaped function would predict that trauma survivors have one or the other type of symptom unless their arousal varies over time during the trauma.

In this next section we will propose that these issues can be addressed by accounting for variation in cortisol levels between and within individuals over time.

5.3. How Might Traumatic Memories Be Formed and Processed Differently If Basal Cortisol Levels Were Lower than Usual

In light of the abovementioned findings in PTSD it is logical to consider the possibility that perhaps memory-related impairments in PTSD are due to a failure to release sufficient cortisol at the time of the trauma. Since the role of cortisol in constraining the release of neuromodulators involved in memory consolidation following stress is well known (Munck et al., 1984), it is reasonable to speculate that an attenuated cortisol response during trauma may have consequences for memory-related phenomena in PTSD. Thus, although individuals exposed to traumatic events would show the resultant increase in stress-related neuromodulators (such as catecholamines, vasopressin and some forms of ACTH), a critical determinant of the formation of the traumatic memory might be in how successfully these neuromodulators are terminated by cortisol. Support for this model is derived from the aforementioned studies demonstrating substantial variation in the cortisol response to an acute trauma, and particularly showing an association between lower cortisol at the time of the trauma and the subsequent development of PTSD (Resnick et al., 1995; McFarlane, personal communiation). Differences in cortisol levels in the acute aftermath of trauma (i.e., at the time of encoding the memory) provide a plausible explanation for variation in the encoding of traumatic memory following trauma among trauma survivors. It might be predicted that memories encoded during atypical endocrinological states might be oversalient or fragmented. Carried to its extreme, the overconsolidation model could predict that sufficiently intense neuroendocrine stimulation could create memories of such intensity that they could not be recognized and retrieved by ordinary memory processes. Nonetheless, some processing of the information would have occurred so that the possibility of eventual recovery could not be entirely excluded.

A more complex issue involves the varied symptomatology of memory disturbances and changes in these symptoms over time. However well the memory was formed, it may be retrieved inappropriately (e.g., either in response to triggers of apparently low relevance) or not be accessible. In PTSD, a specific problem arises in trying to explain how it is that the same individual can have both intrusive thoughts and amnestic-like experiences over the course of the posttraumatic phase. Another question concerns how it is possible that the individual can have substantial periods of memory-related symptoms and remissions based on the same disturbances at the time of the trauma. This latter question is potentially applicable to the phenomenon of recovered memories, whether they are accurate or not. To address this question requires that we consider that different neuroendocrine states at the time of memory retrieval may be responsible for the different memory-related phenemonology observed over time in the same individual. That is, to fully account for the neurobiology of memories in PTSD requires a consideration of the biological events that are present in individuals well after a traumatic event has occurred.

The above-described neuroendocrine research has clearly demonstrated that PTSD constitutes an alternative syndrome to the normative response to stress. In particular, basal cortisol levels are not only lower on the average, but also more variable over the diurnal cycle in PTSD (Yehuda et al., 1996a). Correspondingly, the average resting catecholamine levels in PTSD appear to be elevated (Yehuda et al., submitted; see Figure 1). It is plausible to conjecture that corresponding to these basal laboratory findings, the basal cortisol levels are low in PTSD patients but peaks are high. It may be that different types of memory-related symptoms predominate depending on the particular neurochemical "milieu" of the individual at a particular time, in response to either an internal or external trigger. The greater range of basal cortisol levels in PTSD is consistent with more extreme neuroendocrine changes in response to external environmental and/or intrapsychic triggers (Yehuda et al., 1996a). This model is subject to empirical testing, although such tests have not yet been performed.

Implicit in the above approach is that there are individual differences in neurochemical status at the time of encoding and retrieval of traumatic memories. In the next section we discuss the possibility that individual differences in the cognitive processing of both neutral and traumatic memories constitute vulnerability or risk factors for developing PTSD following exposure to a traumatic event.

6. APPLYING RISK STRATEGIES TO THE STUDY OF COGNITION AND PTSD: A THEORETICAL FORMULATION FOR FUTURE RESEARCH

As described in earlier sections of this chapter, one of the most important aspects of the developmental course of PTSD is that less than half of all persons who are exposed to traumatic events develop chronic signs of the memory abnormalities seen in PTSD. As a consequence, it can be concluded that trauma exposure alone does not reliably produce PTSD and that some characteristics of the individual must interact with the trauma in order to result in PTSD. Thus, PTSD can be seen to be a classic application of a diathesis-stress model (Rende & Plomin, 1992), where the stressor is the traumatic event and the diathesis (or vulnerability of the individual) increases the risk for development of PTSD-related memory symptoms following the exposure to the stressor.

As reviewed above, several different factors have been associated with risk for development of PTSD following trauma. It is possible that these factors, especially pretrauma intelligence levels (McNally & Shin, 1995), may be associated with individual differences in the processing of memory information. Several well-recognized disturbances in memory and information processing resemble symptoms of PTSD. Since these disturbances do not depend upon the presence of a traumatic event, an individual who has a tendency or risk for such a condition would be predisposed to react with these characteristic PTSD memory phenomena when exposed to a high salience stimulus such as a traumatic event. For example, a tendency toward obsessive rumination might predispose a person to experience intrusive thoughts; an increased ability to form associations might make it likely that even nonrelevant stimuli would trigger thoughts of the trauma. Indeed, ongoing research in our laboratory is aimed at determining different traits associated with memory processing in trauma survivors with and without memory-related symptoms and/or PTSD. The sections below describe particular tendencies that might predispose individuals toward particular PTSD symptoms following exposure to trauma, and how the presence of such tendencies may ultimately be tested in laboratory studies of trauma survivors.

6.1. Arousal Levels

Basal levels of arousal are known to impact on a variety of cognitive functions (Buchanan & Thompson, 1994). Classical conditioning of startle-response occurs most often in highly aroused animals (Mazurski, Bond, Siddle & Lovibond, 1993) and humans (Lovibond, 1992). Kagan and colleagues have demonstrated that infants who are high in reactivity to environmental events are likely to have more behavioral problems in later life (Kagan, 1994; Robinson, Kagan, Resnick & Corley, 1992). These variations in arousal level may lead to differential appraisal of the salience of events at the time of occurrence or differences in the "tagging" of these events for their frequency of retrievability (Cuthbert & Lang, 1989). In addition, higher arousal levels tend to correlate with greater levels of vigilance and greater tendencies of detection of threat cues in the environment (Cuthbert & Lang, 1989). Basal arousal levels are straightforward to measure with psychophysiological measurement techniques. Trauma survivors who have always been easily arousable might be particularly likely to be more aroused following the trauma, and to associate traumatic memories to arousal, due to their aroused state at the time of the trauma.

6.2. Tendency toward Developing Associations

"Associability" is a well-understood component of language and cognition (Chown, Kaplan & Kortenkamp, 1995). Word pairs that are highly associated (e.g., desk-chair) tend to be more easily remembered and retrieved then word pairs which are not semantically related (desk-blouse) (Palm, 1985). One feature of PTSD is that a variety of environmental stimuli may trigger intrusive memories. If an individual has a greater tendency to form associations between relatively loosely connected stimuli, this may increase the potential field of triggers for traumatic memories. For example, a women raped by a man in a red shirt might be reminded of the rape by a man in a red shirt, or simply by the color red.

Thus, the experience of "everything reminds me of the trauma" constitutes an extraordinarily wide range of triggering stimuli. This hypothesis could be tested by evaluating the processing of neutral stimuli, where the tendency to form associations could be examined in a context unrelated to the traumatic experience (e.g., such as in a paired associates learning test).

6.3. Tendency toward Obsessive Repetition

Recollections of past events are intrusive if they are retained in consciousness for extended periods. Repetitive cognitive processing characterizes other psychiatric conditions, including obsessive-compulsive disorder and obsessive-compulsive personality disorder. Individuals who have a tendency to ruminate over everyday experiences might be more likely to relive a traumatic event in their minds. The general tendency for repetitive responses can be tested by examining over-repetition of correct responses in a simple recall memory test for neutral words.

6.4. Distractibility

PTSD patients may have difficulty focusing on current experiences without the intrusive recollection of a traumatic event. While it is possible that the principal factor that leads to this experience is that of the traumatic memory intruding, it is also possible that the experience is partially based on a general inability to concentrate on current thought content. As described above, the salience of trauma-related memories and the tendency towards excessive focus on these memories makes them primary candidates for intrusion into consciousness when the primary focus of current cognitive operations is lost. Distractibility has been shown in the past to be quite familial (Harvey, 1981; Rose, Miller & Fulker, 1981) and this function has the potential to be transmitted genetically.

6.5. Working Memory Failures

Working memory (Baddeley & Hitch, 1994) refers to the process of keeping information active and available while other cognitive operations are performed on it. A special case of working memory is source monitoring (Johnson, Hashtroundi & Lindsay, 1993), which refers to the ability to distinguish the origin of information in working memory. Deficient source monitoring could result in situations where information that has been retrieved from long term memory, such as in the case of an intrusive traumatic memory, could be confused as information currently occurring in the environment. Such a cognitive failure could result in the "waking flashback" symptoms of PTSD. In general, deficient working memory has the potential to lead to significant problems in the ongoing monitoring and management of current cognitive experiences. In addition to monitoring failures, there are a number of response biases that can operate in source monitoring (Dodson & Johnson, 1993). When normal individuals are confused about the source of information in their memory, their operative response bias is to assume that it must be a memory and not an ongoing event. A bias toward believing that intrusive memories of long-ago events are currently happening could contribute to confusion and "re-experiencing" symptoms of PTSD (Johnson & Weisc, 1994). Deficits in this type of process could lead to ongoing deficits in the ability to discriminate memorial information, possibly intrusive recollections of traumatic events, from ongoing environmental events. The earlier aspects of our model, excessive salience tagging, distractibility, and tendency toward excessive focusing on intruded memories, can interact with failures in working memory or source monitoring to produce some of the memory failures seen in PTSD.

6.6. Future Directions in Traumatic Memory Research in PTSD

The above model can be tested in several ways. Individuals who have the full syndrome of PTSD may differ from individuals who are trauma survivors without PTSD or nontraumatized individuals in their performance on standard tests using stimuli not related to the trauma. Perhaps more interesting would be the comparison of trauma-naive individuals expected to have similar risk factors for PTSD by virtue of their biological relationships to an individual with PTSD, to trauma-naive individuals who are expected to have low risk for the disorder by virtue of being related to a trauma-exposed individual without PTSD symptoms. Differences in performance on cognitive components of the hypothetical risk profile between these two groups could not be due to the consequences of trauma or PTSD and would have to be due to factors related to risk for the disorder.

Since many of these processes may be related to the activity of neuromodulators, the previously described biological alterations in PTSD may reflect these cognitive mechanisms.

7. SUMMARY AND CONCLUSIONS

Most models of memory-related phenomenology in PTSD were developed in the absence of knowledge about the prevalence, course and neurobiology of PTSD. This resulted in a focused consideration of the importance of the traumatic event, and how longlasting changes might arise as a result of biological changes that occured at the time of the trauma. That recent studies have demonstrated that chronic PTSD is a relatively rare phenomenon has required the field to focus on the importance of risk factors for PTSD. Furthermore, because findings of the neurobiology of PTSD have demonstrated that this disorder is characterized by an atypical biological stress response, both in the acute and chronic aftermath of the trauma, it has become necessary to amend previous theories that focused on the uniformity of the stress response and its ability to produce permanent symptoms. Rather, current theories must show how PTSD-related phenomenology may be particularly related to the presence of risk factors and/or the unique characteristics of the biology of this disorder.

ACKNOWLEDGMENTS

The work in this grant was supported by NIMH-49536 (RY), NIMH-59555 (RY) and VA Merit Award (RY). The authors wish to thank James Schmeidler, Ph.D. and Rick Newman, J.D. for their thoughtful comments and suggestions, and Stacey Namm, Karen Connors, and Tamar Duvdevani for their help in manuscript preparation.

REFERENCES

APA task force on laboratory tests in psychiatry (1987): The dexamethasone suppression test : An overview of its current status in psychiatry. *American Journal of Psychiatry 144*:1253–1262.

American Psychiatric Association (1980) *Diagnostic and statistical manual of mental disorders.*, 3rd ed. Washington, DC.

American Psychiatric Association (1994) *Diagnostic and statistical manual of mental disorders.*, 4th ed. Washington, DC.

Baddeley AD, Hitch, GJ (1994): Developments in the concept of working memory. Special section: Working memory, *Neuropsychology, 8(4)*: 45–493.

Blanchard EB, Kolb LC, Pallmeyer TP, Gerardi RJ (1986): A psychophysiological study of post traumatic stress disorder in Vietnam veterans. *Behavioral Research Therapy*, 24:645–652.

Blanchard EB, Kolb LC, Prins A, et al. (1991): Changes in plasma norepinephrine to combat-related stimuli among Vietnam veterans with PTSD. *Journal of Nervous and Mental Diseases, 179*: 371–373.

Bohus B (1974): Pituitary-adrenaline hormaones and the forced extinction of a passive avoidance response in the rat. *Brain Research, 66*:366.

Bohus B, De Kloet ER, Veldhuis HD (1982): Adrenal steroids and behavioral adaptation: relationship to brain corticoid receptors. In Ganten D, Pfaff DW (Eds.), *Current topics in neuroendocrinology: Adrenal action on brain* (pp.107). New York: Springer.

Borrell J, De Kloet ER, Vertseeg DHG, Bohus (1983): Inhibitory avoidance deficit following short-term adrenalectomy in the rat: The role of adrenal catecholamines. *Behavioral Neurobiology, 39*:241.

Boscarino JA (1996): Posttrauamtic stress disorder, exposure to combat, and lower plasma cortisol among Vietnam veterans: Findings and clinical implications. *Journal of Clinical and Consulting Psychology, 64(1)*:191–201.

Bremner JD, Southwick SM, Johnson DR, Yehuda R, Charney DS (1993): Childhood physical abuse and combat-related posttraumatic stress disorder. *American Journal of Psychiatry, 150*: 234–239.

Brende J (1982): Electrodermal responses in posttraumatic syndromes. *Journal of Nervous and Mental Diseases, 170*: 352–361.

Breslau N, Davis GC, Andreski P, Peterson E (1991): Traumatic events and post traumatic stress disorder in an urban population of young adults. *Archives of General Psychiatry , 48*: 216–222.

Buchanan SL, Thomson RH (1994): Neuronal activity in the midline thalamic nuclei during Pavlovian heart rate conditioning. *Brain Research Bulletin, 35(3)*: 237–240.

Cahill L, Prins B, Weber M, McGaugh JL (1994): B-Adrenergic activation and memory for emotional events. Nature, *371(6499)*:702–704.

Cannon WB (1914): Emergency function of adrenal medulla in pain and major emotions. *American Journal of Physiology, 3*:356–372.

Caroll BJ, Feinberg M, Greden JF et al. (1981): A specific laboratory test for the diagnosis of melancholia. *Archives of General Psychiatry, 38*:15–22.

Charney DS, Deutch A, Krystal J, Southwick SM, Nagy L (1993): Psychobiological mechanisms of post-traumatic stress disorder. Archives of General Psychiatry, *50*:294–305.

Chown E, Kaplan S, Kortenkamp D (1995): Prototypes, location, and associative networks: Toward a unified theory of cognitive mapping. *Cognitive Science, 19(1)*:1–51.

Christian S-A, Mjorndal T (1985): Adrenalin, emotional arousal, anmd memory. *Scandinavain Journal of Psychology, 26*:337–248.

Christian S-A, Nilsson L-G (1984): Functional amnesia as induced by a psychological trauma. *Memory and Cognition, 12*:142–155.

Chrousos GP, Gold PW (1992): The concepts of stress and stress system disorders: Overview of physical and behavioral homeostasis. Journal of the American Medical *Association, 267*:1244–1252.

Cuthbert BN, Lang PJ (1989): Imagery, memory, and emotion: A pyschophysiological analysis of clinical anxiety. *Handbook of clinical psychophysiology*. England, John Wiley and Sons.

Davidson LM, Baum A (1986): Chronic stress and PTSD. *Journal of Consulting and Clinical Psychology, 54*:303–308.

Davidson JRT, Fairbank JA (1993): The epidemiology of posttraumatic stress disorder. In Davidson JRT, Foa EB (Eds.), *Posttraumatic stress disorder, DSM-IV and beyond* (pp. 147–172). Washington, DC: American Psychiatric Press.

Davidson JRT, Hughes D, Blazer D, George LK (1991): Posttraumatic stress disorder in the community: An epidemiological study. *Psychological Medicine, 21*:1–9.

Davidson J, Swartz M, Storck M, Krishnam RR, Hammett E (1985): A diagnostic and family study of posttraumatic stress disorder. *American Journal of Psychiatry, 142*:90–93.

De Wied D (1984): Neurohypophyseal hormone influences on learning and memory processes. In Lynch G, McGaugh JL, Weinberger NM (Eds.), *Neurobiology of learning and memory* (pp.289). New York: Guilford.

De Wied D, Croiset G (1991): Stress modulation of learning and memory processes. In Jasmin G, Proschek L (Eds.), *Stress Revisited 2 Systemic Effects of Stress*. Methods Achieve Exp Pathol (pp.167–199). Basel:Karger.

De Wied D, Gaffori O, van Ree JM, de Jong W (1984): Central target for the behavioral effects of vasopressin neuropeptides. *Nature, 308*:276.

De Wied D, Jolles J (1982): Neuropeptides derived from pro-opiocortin: Behavioral, physiological, and neurochemical effects. *Physiological Review, 62*:976.

Dinan TG, Barry S, Yatham LN, Moyabed M, Brown I (1990): A pilot study of a neuroendocrine test battery in posttraumatic stress disorder. *Biological Psychiatry, 28*:665–672.

Dobbs D, Wilson WP (1960): Observations on the persistence of neurosis. *Disorders of the Nervous System, 21*:40–46.

Dodson C, Johnson M (1993): Rate of false source attributions depends on how questions are asked. *American Journal of Psychology, 106(4)*:541–557.

Eysenck MW (1982): *Attention and arousal: Cognition and performance*. Berlin: Springer-Verlag, 1982.

Foa EB, Molnar C, Cashman L (1995): Change in rape narratives during exposure therapy for posttraumatic stress disorder. *Journal of Traumatic Stress, 8(4)*:675–690.

Foy DW, Sipprelle RC, Rueger DB, Carroll EM (1984): Etiology of posttraumatic stress disorder in Vietnam veterans. *Journal of Consulting and Clinical Psychology , 40*:1323–1328.

Friedman MJ, Yehuda R (1995): PTSD and comorbidity: Psychobiological approaches to differential diagnosis. In Friedman MJ, Charney DS, Deutch AY (Eds.), *Neurobiological and Clinical Consequences of Stress: From Normal Adaptation to PTSD*.

Ghazhuddin M, Ghaziuddin N, Stein GS (1990): Life events and the recurrence of depression. *Canadian Journal of Psychiatry; 35*:239–242.

Giller MJ (1991): *Biological Assessment and Treatment of Post-ttaumatic Stress Disorder*. Washington, DC: APA Press.

Goenjian AK, Yehuda R, Pynoos RS, et al (1996): Basal cortisol and dexamethasone suppression of cortisol among adolescents after the 1988 earthquake in Armenia. *American Journal of Psychiatry, 153(7)*:929–934.

Gormley GJ, Lowy MT, Reder AT, et al (1985): Glucocorticoid receptors in depression: Relationship to the dexamethasone suppression test. *American Journal of Psychiatry, 142*:1278–1284.

Green BL, Lindy JD, Grace MC, Leonard AC (1992): Chronic posttraumatic stress disorder and diagnostic comorbidity in a disaster sample. *Journal of Nervous and Mental Diseases, 180*:760–766.

Grinker RR, Spiegal JP (1945): *Men Under Stress*. Philadelphia: Blakiston.

Hamner MB, Diamond BI, Hitri A (1994): Plasma norepinephrine and MHPG responses to excercise stress in PTSD. In MM Murburg (Ed.), *Catecholamine Function in Posttraumatic Stress Disorder: Emerging Concepts* (pp.221–232). Washington, DC: APA Press.

Harfstrand A, Fuxe K, Cintra A, et al (1986):. Glucocorticoid receptor immunoreactivity in monoaminergic neurons in the rat brain. *Proceedings of the National Academy of Sciences USA, 83*:9779–9783.

Harvey P (1981): Distractibility in children vulnerable to psychopathology. *Journal of Abnormal Psychology, 90*(4):298–304.

Heim, C, Hellhammer D (Submitted for publication): *HPA Axis alterations in women (with and without abuse) suffering from chronic pelvic pain.*

Helzer JE, Robins, LN, McEvoy L (1987): Posttraumatic stress disorder in the general population. *New England Journal of Medicine, 317*:1630–1634.

Herman J (1992): *Trauma and Recovery*. New York: Basic Books.

Hoffman L, Watson PB, Wilson G, Montgomery J (1989): Low plasma B-endorphin in posttraumatic stress disorder. *Australian and New Zealand Journal of Psychiatry, 23*:269–273.

Johnson MK, Hashtroudi S, Lindsay DS (1993): Source monitoring. *Psychological Bulletin, 114*(1):3–28.

Johnson MK, Weisz C (1994): Comments on unconscious processing: Finding emotion in the cognitive stream. *The heart's eye: Emotional influences in perception and attention*. San Diego, Academic Press, Inc.

Kagan J (1994): On the nature of emotion. *Monographs of the Society for Research in Child Development, 59*(2–3):250–283.

Kardiner A (1941): *The traumatic neurosis of war*. New York: Hoeber.

Kessler RC, Sonnega A, Bromet E, Hughes M, Nelson CB (1995): Posttraumatic stress disorder in the national comorbidity survey. *Archives of General Psychiatry, 52*:1048–1060.

Kilpatrick DG, Resnick HS (1993): Posttraumatic stress disorder associated with exposure to criminal victimization in clinical and community populations. In Davidson JRT, Foa EB (Eds.), *Posttraumatic stress disorder, DSM-IV and beyond* (pp.147–172). Washington, DC: American Psychiatric Press.

Kluznick JC, Speed N, VanValkenberg C, Magraw R (1986): Forty-year follow-up of United States prisoners of war. *American Journal of Psychiatry, 143*:1443–1446.

Kolb LC (1987): A neuopsychological hypothesis explaining the posttraumatic stress disorder. *American Journal of Psychiatry, 144*:989–955.

Kosten TR, Wahby V, Giller E, Mason J (1990): The dexamethasone suppression test and thyrotropin-releasing hormone stimulation test in PTSD. *Biological Psychiatry, 28*:657.

Kosten TR, Mason JW, Giller EL, Harkness L, Ostroff R (1987): Sustained urinary norepinephrine and epinephrine levels in post-traumatic stress diosrder. *Psychoneuroendocrinology, 12*:13–20.

Kulka RA, Schlenger WE, Fairbank JA, Hough RL, Jordan BK, Marmor CR, Weiss DS (1991): *Trauma the Vietnam War Generation: Report of findings from the National Vietnam Veterans' Readjustment study*. NY: Brunner: Mazel.

Lemiux AM, Coe CL (1995): Abuse-related posttraumatic stress disorder: Evidence for chronic neuroendocrine activation in women. *Psychosomatic Medicine, 57*:105–115.

Lovibond PF (1992): Tonic and phasic electrodermal measures of human aversive conditioning with long duration stimuli. *Psychophysiology, 29*(6):621–632.

Lowy MT, Gormley GJ, Reder AT (1989): Immune function, glucocorticoid receptor regulation and depression. In Miller AH (Ed.), *Depressive Disorders and Immunity* (pp.105–134). Washington, DC: APA Press.

Lowy MT (1989): Quantification of Type I and II adrenal steroid receptors in neuronal, lymphoid, and pituitary tissues. *Brain Research, 503*:191–197.

Malloy PF, Fairbanks JA, Keane TM (1983): Validation of a multimethod assessment of posttraumatic stress disorders in Vietnam veterans. *Journal of Clinical and Consulting Psychology, 51*:488–494.

Mason JW (1975): A historical view of the stress field. *Journal of Human Stress, 6*–12.

Mason JW, Giller EL, Kosten TR, Ostroff RB, Podd L (1986): Urinary-free cortisol levels in post-traumatic stress disorder patients. *Journal of Nervous and Mental Diseases, 174*:145–159.

Mazurski EJ, Bond NW, Siddle DA, Lovibond PF (1993): Classical conditioning of autonomic and affective responses to fear-relevant and fear-irrelevant stimuli. *Australian Journal of Psychology, 45*(3):69–73.

McFall M, Murburg M, Ko G (1990): Autonomic response to stress in Vietnam combat veterans with post-traumatic stress disorder. *Biological Psychiatry*, 27:1165–1175.

McFarlane AC (1984): The Ash Wednesday Bushfires in South Australia: Implications for planning future post-disaster services. *Medical Journal of Australia*, 141:286–291.

McFarlane AC (1989): The aetiology of posttraumatic mobordity: Predisposing and precipitating and perpetuating factors. *British Journal of Psychiatry*, 154:221–228.

McFarlane MC (1992): Aviodance and Intrusion in posttraumatic stress disorder. *Journal of Nervous and Mental diseases*, 180:439–445.

McFarlane AC, Weber D, Clark R (1993): Abnormal stimulus processing in posttraumatic stress disorder. *Biological Psychiatry*, 34:311–320.

McGaugh JL (1985): Peripheral and central adrenergic influences on brain systems involved in the modulation of memory storage. *Annals of the New York Academy of Sciences*, 444:150–161.

McGaugh JL, Liang KC, Bennett C, et al.(1984): Adrenergic influences on memory storage: interaction of peripheral and central systems. In Lynch G, McGaugh JL, Weinberger NM (Eds.), *Neurobiology of learning and memory* (pp.313–332). New York: Guilford.

McNally RJ & Shin LM (1995): Association of itelligence with severity of posttraumatic stress disorder symptoms in Vietnam combate veterans. *American Journal of Psychiatry*, 152(6):936–938.

Meakins JC, Wilson RM (1918): The effect of certain sensory simulation on the respiratory rate in cases of so-called "irritable heart." *Heart*, 7:17–22.

Meaney MJ, Aitken DH,Viau V, Sharma S, Sarieau A (1989): Neonatal handling alters adrenocortical negative feedback sensitivity and hippocampal type II glucocorticoid binding in rat. *Neuroendocrinology*, 50:597–604.

Mellman TA, Adarsh K, Kulik-Bell R, et al (1995): Nocturnal/daytime urine noradrenergic measures and sleep in combat-related PTSD. *Biological Psychiatry*, 38:174–179.

Mountcastle ZB (1973): *Medical physiology*, 13th ed. St. Louis, MO: Moseby Publishing.

Munck A, Guyre PM, Holbrook NJ (1984): Physiological functions of glucocorticoids in stress and their relation to pharmacological actions. *Endocrine Reviews*, 93:9779–9783.

Murburg MM, McFall ME, Lewis N, Veith RC (1995): Plasma norepinephrine kinetics in patients with posttraumatic stress disorder. *Biological Psychiatry*, 38(12):819–825.

Murburgh, MM (1994): *Catecholamine Function in Posttraumatic Stress Disorder: Emerging Concepts*. Washington, DC: APA Press.

Olivera AA, Fero D (1990): Affective disorders, DST, and treatment in PTSD patients: Clinical observations. *Journal of Traumatic Stress*, 3:407–414.

Orr SP, Pitman RK, Lasko NB, Herz LR (1987): Psychophysiological assessment PTSD imagery in World War II and Korean combat veterans. *Journal of Abnormal Psychology*, 102:152–159.

Paige SR, Reid GM, Graham M, Allen MG, Newton JEO (1990): Psychophysiological correlates of posttraumatic stress disorder in Vietnam veterans. *Biological Psychiatry* 27:419–430.

Pallmeyer TP, Blanchard EB, Kolb LC (1986): The psychophysiology of combat induced posttraumatic stress disorder in Vietnam veterans. *Behavior Research Therapy*, 24:645–652.

Palm G (1985): Associative networks and their information storage capacity. *Cognitive Systems*, 1(2):107–118.

Palmer CJ, Ziegler MG, Lake CR (1978): Response of norepinephrine and blood pressure to stress increases with age. *Journal of Gerontology*, 33:482–487.

Perry BD (1994): Neurobiological sequelae of childhood trauma: PTSD in children. In: Murburgh MM (Ed.), *Catecholamine Function in PTSD*. Washington, DC: APA Press.

Perry BD, Southwick SM, Yehuda R, Giller EL (1990): Adrenergic receptor regulation in post-traumatic stress disorder. In EL Giller (Ed.) *Biological Assessment and Treatment of Post-traumatic Stress Disorder* (pp. 87–114) Washington, DC: American Psychiatric Press.

Perry BD, Giller EL, Southwick SM (1987): Altererd platelet alpha2 adrenergic binding sites in post-traumatic stress disorder. *American Journal of Psychiatry*, 144:1511–1512.

Pitman RK (1989): Editorial: Post-traumatic stress disorder, hormones, and memory. *Biological Psychiatry*, 26:221–223.

Pitman RK, Orr SP, Lownhagen MH, Macklin ML, Altman A (1991): Pre-Vietnam contents of PTSD veterans' service medical and personnel records. *Comprehensive Psychiatry*, 32:1–7.

Pitman RK, Orr S (1990): Twenty-four hour urinary cortisol and catecholamine excretion in combat-related PTSD. *Biological Psychiatry*, 27:245–247.

Pitman RK, Orr SP, Forgue DF, DeJong JB, Clairborn JM (1987): Psychophysiologic assessment of posttraumatic stress disorder imagery in Vietnam combat veterans. *Archives of General Psychiatry*, 44:970–975.

Post RM (1992): Transduction of psychosocial stress into the neurobiology of recurrent affective disorder. *American Journal of Psychiatry*, 149:999–1010.

Post RM, Rubinow DR, Ballenger JC (1986): Conditioning and sensitisation in the longitudinal course of affective illness. *British Journal of Psychiatry, 149:*191–201.

Rainey JM, Aleem A, Ortiz A (1987): A laboratory proceure for the induction of flashbacks. *American Journal of Psychiatry, 144:*1317–1319.

Rende R, Plomin R (1992): Diathesis-stress models of psychopathology: A quantitative genetic perspective. *Applied and Preventive Psychology, 1(4):*177–182.

Resnick HS, Kilpatrick DG, Best CL, Kramer TL (1992): Vulnerability-stress factors in development of posttraumatic stress disorder. *Journal of Nervous and Mental Diseases, 180:*424–430.

Resnick HS, Yehuda R, Pitman RK, Foy DW (1995): Effect of previous trauma on acute plasma cortisol level following rape. *American Journal of Psychiatry, 152:*1675–1677.

Reus VI, Peeke VS, Miner C (1985): Habituation and cortisol dysregulation in depression. *Biological Psychiatry, 20:*980–989.

Robinson JL, Kagan J, Reznick JS, Corley R (1992): The heretability of inhibited and uninhibited behavior: A twin study. *Developmental Psychology, 28(6):*1030–1037.

Rose RJ, Miller JZ, Fulker DW (1981): Twin-family studies of perceptual speed ability: II. Parameter estimation. *Behavior Genetics, 11(6):*565–575.

Sapolsky RM, Krey LC, McEwen BS (1984): Stress down regulates corticosterone receptors in a site specific manner in the brain. *Endocrinology, 114:*287–292.

Selye H (1956): *The Stress of Life*. McGraw-Hill Book Co, Inc. New York.

Schnurr PP, Friedman MJ, Rosenberg SD (1993): Premilitary MMPI scores as predictors of combat-related Posttraumatic stress disorder scores. *American Journal of Psychiatry, 150:*479–483.

Shalev AY, Orr SP, Peri P, Schreiber S, Pitman RK (1992): Physiologic responses o loud tones in Israeli post-traumatic stress disorder patients. *Archives of General Psychiatry, 40:*870–975.

Shalev, AY (1992): Posttraumatic stress disorder among injured survivors of a terrorist attack: Predictive value of early intrusion and avoidance symptoms. *Journal of Nervous and Mental Diseases, 180:*505–509.

Shalev A, Rogel-Fuchs Y (1993): Psychophysiology of the PTSD: From sulfur fumes to behavioral genetics. *Psychosomatic Medicine, 55:*413–423.

Shalev AY, Orr FP, Pitman RK (1993): Psychophysiologic assessment of traumatic imagery in Israeli civilian patients with posttraumatic stress disorders. *American Journal of Psychiatry, 150:* 620–624.

Shore JH, Tatum E, Vollmer WM (1986a): Evaluation of mental health effects of disaster: Mt St. Helen's eruption. *American Journal of Public Health, 76:*76–83.

Shore JH, Tatum EL, Vollmer WM (1986b): Psychiatric reactions to disaster: The Mount St. Helens experience. *American Journal of Psychiatry, 143:*590–595.

Shore JH, Vollmer WM, Tatum EL (1989): Community patterns of posttraumatic stress disorders. *Journal of Nervous and Mental Diseases, 177:*681–685.

Siever LJ, Davis KL (1985): Overview: Towad a dysregulation hypothesis of depression. *American Journal of Psychiatry, 41:*1017–1031.

Smith MA, Davidson J, Ritchie JC, Kudler H, Lipper S, Chappell P, Nemeroff CB (1989): The corticotropin releasing hormone test in patients with PTSD. *Biological Psychiatry, 26:*349–355.

Solomon Z, Preager E (1992): Elderly Israeli Holocaust survivors during the Persian Gulf War: A study of psychological distress. *American Journal of Psychiatry, 149:* 1707- 1710.

Southwick SM, Krystal JH, Morgan AC, Johnson D, Nagy LM, Nicolaou A, Heninger GR, Charney DS (1993): Abnormal noradrenergic function in post traumatic stress disorder. *Archives of General Psychiatry, 50:*266–274.

Southwick SM, Yehuda R, Charney DS (in press): Neurobiological alterations in posttraumatic stress disorder: A review of the clinical literature. In: Fullerton CS, and Ursano, RJ (Eds)., *Acute and Longterm Resonses to Trauma and Disaster*, American Psychiatric Press.

Southwick SM, Yehuda R, Giller EL, Perry BD (1991): Alpha2-adrenergic-receptor regulation in major depression and borderline personality disorder. *Psychiatry Residency, 34:*143–203.

Stein MB, Yehuda R, Koverola C, Hanna C (submitted for publication): *HPA axis functioning in adult women who report experiencing severe childhood sexual abuse.*

Svec F(1985): Minireview: Glucocorticoid receptor regulation. *Life Sciences, 35:*2359–2366.

True WR, Rise J, Eisen S, Heath AC, Goldberg J, Lyons M, Nowak J (1993): A twin study of genetic and environmental contributions to liability for posttraumatic stress symptoms. *Archives of General Psychiatry, 50:* 257–264.

van der Kolk BA, Fisler R (1995): Dissociation and the fragmentary nature of traumatic memories: Overview and exploratory study. *Journal of Traumatic Stress, 8(4):*505–525.

Van Ree JM, De Wied D (1988): Behavioral approach to the study of the rat brain. *Discussions in Neuroscience, 32:*190.

Veith RC, Murburg MM (1994):Assessment of sympathetic nervous system functioning in PTSD: A critique of methodology. *Catecholamine Function in PTSD*. Washington, DC: APA Press, pp. 309–334.

Walker, EL (1958): Action Decrement and its relation to learning. *Psychological Review, 65*:129–142.

Walker EL (1967): Arousal and the memory trace. In: DP Kimble (Ed.), *The organization of recall*. New York: The New York Academy of Sciences.

Whalley LJ, Borthwick N, Copolov D (1986): Glucocorticoid receptors and depression. *British Medical Journal, 292*:859–861.

Yehuda R, Antelman S (1993c): Criteria for rationally evaluating animal models of posttraumatic stress disorder. *Biological Psychiatry, 33:*479–486.

Yehuda R, Boisoneau D, Lowy MT, Giller EL (1995b): Dose-response changes in plasma cortisol and lymphocyte glucocorticoid receptors following dexamethasone administration in combat vetrans with and without posttraumatic stress disorder. *Archives of General Psychiatry, 52*:583–593.

Yehuda R, Boisoneau D, Mason JW, Giller EL (1993a): Relationship between lymphocyte glucocorticoid receptor number andurinary-freecortisolexcretioninmood,anxiety,andpsychoticdisorder.*BiologicalPsychiatry,34.*18–25.

Yehuda R, Giller EL, Southwick SM, Siever L (1995c): Hypothalamic-pituitary-adrenal alterations in PTSD. In: Friedman MJ, Charney DS, Deutch AY (eds.), *Neurobiological and Clinical Consequences of Stress: From Normal Adaptation to PTSD*. NY: Raven Press.

Yehuda R, Giller EL, Mason JW (1993c): Psychoendocrine assessment of PTSD: Current progress and new directions. *Progressive Neuropsychopharmacology and biological psychiatry, 17*:541–550.

Yehuda R, Giller EL, Southwick SM, Binder-Brynes K, Schmeidler J, Kahana B (1995a): *The impact of cumulative lifetime trauma and recent stress on current posttraumatic stress disorder symptoms in Holocaust survivors*.

Yehuda R, Giller EL, Southwick SM, Lowy MT, Mason JW (1991b): Hypothalamic-pituitary-adrenal dysfunction in PTSD. *Biological Psychiatry, 30:*1031–1048.

Yehuda R, Kahana B, Binder-Brynes K, Southwick SM, Zemelman S, Mason JW, Giller EL (1995d): Low urinary cortisol excretion in Holocaust survivors with PTSD. American *Journal of Psychiatry, 152:*7–12.

Yehuda R, Levengood R, Schmeidler J, Wilson S, Guo LS, Gerber D (1996b): Increased pituitary activation following metyrapone administration in PTSD. *Psychoneuroendocrinology, 21:*1–16.

Yehuda R, Lowy MT, Southwick SM, Shaffer S, Giller EL (1991a): Increased lymphocyte glucocorticoid receptor number in PTSD. *American Journal of Psychiatry,149:*499–504.

Yehuda R, McFarlane AC (1995e): Coflict between current knowledge about posttraumatic stress disorder and its original conceptual basis. *American Journal Of Psychiatry, 152*(12):1705–1713.

Yehuda R, Resnick H, Kahana B Giller EL (1993d): Longlasting hormonal alterations in extreme stress in humans: Normative or maladaptive? *Psychosomatic Medicine, 55:*287–297.

Yehuda R, Schmeidler J, Elkin A, Houshmand E, Siever L, Binder-Byrnes K, Wainberg M, Aferiot D, Lehman A, Guo LS, Yang RK (in press): Phenomenology and psychobiology of the intergenerational response to trauma. In: Danieli Y (Ed.) *Intergenerational Handbook: Muiltigenerational Legacies of Trauma*. New York: Plenum Press.

Yehuda R, Siever L, Teicher MH, Levengood RA, Gerber DK, Schmeidler J, Yang RK (submitted): Plasma norepinephrine and MHPG concentrations and severity of depression in combat PTSD and major depressive disorder. *Biological Psychiatry*.

Yehuda R, Southwick SM, Giller EL (1992a): Exposure to atrocities and chronic posttraumatic stress disorder in war veterans. *American Journal of Psychiatry, 149*: 333–336.

Yehuda R, Southwick SM, Krystal JM, Charney DS, Mason JW (1993b): Enhanced suppression of cortisol following dexamethasone administration in combat veterans with posttraumatic stress disorder and major depressive disorder. *American Journal of Psychiatry, 150*:83–86.

Yehuda R, Southwick SM, Ma X, Giller EL, Mason JW (1992b): Urinary catecholamine excretion and severity of symptoms in PTSD. *Journal of Nervous and Mental Diseases, 180*:321–325.

Yehuda R, Southwick SM, Nussbaum G, Wahby V, Mason JW, Giller EL (1990a): Low urinary cortisol excretion in patients with PTSD. *Journal of Nervous and Mental Diseases, 178*:366–309.

Yehuda R, Southwick SM, Perry BD, Mason JW, Giller EL (1990b): Interactions of the hypothalamic-pituitary-adrenal and catecholaminergic system in posttraumatic stress disorder. In Earl L. Giller (ed), *Biological Assessment and Treatment of PTSD*, Progress in Psychiatry, APA Press, Washington, D.C., 115–134.

Yehuda R, Teicher MH, Levengood RA, Trestman R, Siever LJ (1996a): Cortisol regulation in combat PTSD and major depression: A chronobiological analysis. *Biological Psychiatry*.

Zaidi LY, Foy DW (1994): Childhood abuse and combat-related PTSD. Journal of *Traumatic Stress, 7:*33–42.

Zager EL, Black PM (1985): Neuropeptides in human memory and learning processes. *Neurosurgery, 17:*355–369.

COMMENTARY ON RELEVANCE OF NEUROENDOCRINE ALTERATIONS IN PTSD TO MEMORY-RELATED IMPAIRMENTS OF TRAUMA SURVIVORS

Ronan E. O'Carroll, Department of Psychology, University of Stirling, United Kingdom

1. INTRODUCTION

"An experience may be so exciting emotionally as almost to leave a scar on the cerebral tissues" (William James, 1890).

Yehuda and Harvey have provided us with a stimulating review of neuroendocrine findings in Post-Traumatic Stress Disorder (PTSD). Furthermore, they have attempted to outline possible mechanisms by which these neuroendocrine abnormalities may be related to disturbances of information processing systems which may, in turn, account for the cardinal features of PTSD. In this commentary, I shall highlight the most important features of this account, as well as critically evaluating relevant aspects of this complex area.

2. THE CONCEPT OF PTSD

There is relatively little coverage of PTSD in this volume. In an attempt to redress the balance, it is important to "step back" and consider the findings of Yehuda and Harvey in relation to the currently accepted concept of PTSD. We must not lose sight of the fact that posttraumatic stress disorder is a concept — nothing more and nothing less. As Mark Creamer reminded us at this conference, over-reliance on the "burgundy bible" of DSM-IV may be misguided. In all probability, there are a diverse number of abnormal chronic reactions to trauma which are currently grouped together under the crude umbrella term of DSM-IV posttraumatic stress disorder. I shall return to the problem of heterogeneity later on in this commentary.

The key neuroendocrine discoveries that Yehuda and Harvey outline are that abnormalities of the Hypothalamic-Pituitary-Adrenal (HPA) axis and the catecholamine system occur in some individuals when they experience a traumatic event, and, in particular, that failure to mount an appropriate cortisol response, coupled with an increase in noradrenergic tone may be predictive of development of chronic PTSD. If these findings are replicated, this represents a major step forward in our understanding of brain-behaviour relationships in PTSD. Identifying a biological marker that predicts the development of a major psychiatric disorder would allow for appropriate targeting of scarce therapeutic resources. However, it is extremely important that these findings are rigorously and independently replicated. At the risk of sounding unduly cautious, a cursory review of research findings in psychiatry reveals that biological markers do not have a particularly impressive track history. However, this problem may be more related to current psychiatric classification rather than underlying biological abnormalities.

3. THE LAYING DOWN AND RECOVERY OF EMOTIONAL MEMORIES

"I can't stop remembering what I don't want to and I can't remember what I do want to." This was a patient's verbatim report to me of his experience of the nature of the memory dysfunction that occurs in PTSD. Yehuda and Harvey propose that a critical determinant of the formation of traumatic memory might be how successfully the activity of stress-related neuromodulators (catecholamines, vasopressin, etc.) is terminated by cortisol. They propose that memories encoded during atypical endocrinological states might be over-salient or fragmented. Furthermore, they propose that varying accessibility of trauma- related memories may be explained by differing neuroendocrine states at the time of retrieval. This is an interesting proposal, and has similarities to the model recently outlined by Schacter, Koutstaal and Norman (1996) in relation to the recovery of traumatic memories. They argue that for stress-related hormones or neuromodulators to be relevant to the recovery of traumatic memories, the neurochemical activity must result in a trace that is potentially available in memory, but rendered temporarily inaccessible by traumatic stress (as opposed to a very weak and permanently unavailable trace). Such a model can be developed along "state-dependent" theory lines, i.e. neuromodulator release during a traumatic event may lead to the temporary inability to remember the trauma. However, a subsequent emotionally arousing experience may trigger the release of neuromodulators, which, if accompanied by other appropriate environmental retrieval cues could activate the formerly inaccessible memory (Schacter et al., 1996). However, while such psychobiological explanations of the recovered memory phenomenon have intuitive appeal, designing appropriate experiments with human subjects to test the model may prove a formidable challenge.

4. THE NORADRENERGIC SYSTEM, THE AMYGDALA AND EMOTIONAL MEMORY

Yehuda and Harvey elaborated the possible role of the HPA axis in their review of possible psychobiological mechanisms in PTSD. However, it may be profitable to review some extremely exciting recent developments implicating the noradrenergic system in modulating the encoding of emotional memories. Yehuda and Harvey briefly described the work of Larry Cahill and colleagues and stated that in their 1994 experiment, propranolol blocked normal arousal to a series of provocative slides resulting in an increased rate of retention errors in college students. However, a fuller account of this key experiment is warranted.

Cahill, Prins, Weber and McGaugh (1994) showed healthy young adults a series of slides with either a neutral or an arousing accompanying narrative (in the arousing narrative, a little boy has a serious car crash and is nearly killed, and in the neutral version, he merely witnesses a minor accident and visits a hospital). The key point is that the slide material is identical in both conditions. Half the subjects received a single 40mg capsule of the beta blocker propranolol one hour before the presentation, the other half received placebo. Importantly, self-ratings of emotional arousal following slide exposure were identical in both the propranolol and placebo conditions. One week later in a "surprise" memory test, it transpired that beta blockade had no effect whatsoever on recall of the neutral material, but there was a selective impairment in recall of the emotive material only in those subjects who had received the beta blocking medication. Cahill et al. (1994) interpreted this finding by suggesting that the noradrenergic system is intimately involved in the normative enhanced recall of emotive material. The work of Larry Cahill, Jim McGaugh and colleagues is outstanding in its ability to link animal and human experimental approaches. Galvez, Mesches and McGaugh (1997) have shown that in animal models, an emotive event (e.g., a painful foot shock) is associated with noradrenergic release within the amygdala of the animal, and they argue that this noradrenaline release from the amygdala acts to modulate encoding of the emotive material. Furthermore, Cahill, Babinsky, Markowitsch and McGaugh (1995) demonstrated in a single case study of a patient with Urbach-Wiethe disease (associated with specific and localised amygdala damage), that this individual demonstrated exactly the same dampening of emotive memory as displayed by healthy young adults following administration of a single beta blocker. The picture that appears to be emerging is that when we process an important, frightening or traumatic event, there is an endogenous release of noradrenaline in our amygdala which modulates the encoding of that event. Such a system would appear to make evolutionary sense in, that when the "fight or flight" mechanism is engaged (e.g., in response to threat), we have a neurobiological mechanism whereby the memory for that event is encoded deeply so as to ensure that it is noted and that we can take avoiding action in the future.

A further piece in the jigsaw of this story was recently reported, again by Cahill et al. (1996). Healthy controls were shown emotive material (emotional videos), while their brain activity was measured by a PET scan. Three weeks later, again in a surprise memory test, recall of the emotive material was assessed. Incredibly, the greater the recall of the emotive material three weeks later, the greater the metabolic activity in the right amygdala of the healthy subjects at the time of stimulus presentation. That is, metabolic activity as measured at the time of encoding almost perfectly predicted recall of emotive material three weeks letter in normal adult subjects. Taken together, the work of Cahill and McGaugh represents a crucial and exciting series of elegant experiments, in both animals and man, implicating the noradrenergic system and the amygdala in emotional memory. However, as Yehuda and Harvey point out, it would be naive to assume a single neurotransmitter system is the key. Multiple systems must interact in order to modulate memory for emotional events and it is probable that some important neuromodulators may not even have been identified as yet.

5. OVERDIAGNOSIS OF PTSD?

Yehuda and Harvey remind us that the majority of individuals who are exposed to severe trauma *do not* develop PTSD. It is easy to lose sight of this fact, given increasing focus on PTSD in professional and general literature and the media. In my opinion, PTSD is an over-diagnosed disorder. There is no doubt at all that many individuals suffer a genuine and significant severe psychiatric disturbance following exposure to trauma, which has been tragically under-recognised in previous years, notably the shameful treatment that traumatised servicemen suffered in World Wars I and II. However, the pendulum appears to have been swinging too far of late. We seem to have created a "PTSD culture" where a major psychiatric disorder is almost expected in individuals who have undergone a traumatic experience, with associated de-briefing sessions hastily organised. It is sobering to look at recent evaluations of the efficacy of such interventions (Bisson & Deahl, 1994; Raphael, Meldrum & McFarlane, 1995). It may be that such well-intentioned therapeutic zeal may, in some cases, do more harm than good (Summerfield, 1995).

If PTSD is over-diagnosed, how does this occur? As Yehuda and Harvey state, to fulfil DSM IV criteria for PTSD, a number of criteria have to be fulfilled, namely A - exposure to a traumatic event, B - symptoms of re-experiencing, C - avoidance and numbing of general responsiveness, D - increased arousal, E - duration of symptoms longer than 1 month and F the disturbance causes significant distress. Some researchers and clinicians seem to equate the presence of intrusive recollections as equivalent to PTSD. This may be due, in part, to over-reliance on instruments such as the revised Impact of Events Scale - IOES (Horowitz, Wilner & Alvarez (1979), which *only* measures intrusions and avoidance. Some workers appear to view a high IOES score as equivalent to a diagnosis of PTSD. However, in order to fulfil the full DSM-IV criteria, categories C - E also have to be fulfilled. Many individuals who have been traumatised do present with some of the features of PTSD, but do not fulfil the full criteria often because they do not fulfil criteria for C, particularly psychogenic amnesia, diminished interest, feelings of detachment or estrangement of others, restricted range of affect, and a sense of fore-shortened future. (See section 7 for details of our ongoing variceal haemorrhage study). The consequences of trauma are not dichotomous (i.e., PTSD versus "normal"). Many individuals *do not* fulfil criteria for PTSD but may well fulfil criteria for other diagnostic disorders, e.g., acute stress disorder, or major depressive episode. Furthermore, the latter diagnosis may lead to more rapid, appropriate and effective therapeutic intervention.

Despite the promising findings of abnormal cortisol responses in patients who then develop PTSD, outlined by Yehuda and Harvey, we do not have a confirmed "laboratory test" for PTSD - it is a disorder that is diagnosed following interview by trained clinicians. Essentially what this means is that PTSD is a diagnosis made via self-report, i.e., the symptom cluster that patients present to us. Given the increasing media attention on PTSD, more and more individuals are presenting, claiming that they have PTSD. Notably, there has been a marked increase in litigation following accidents, whereby individuals claim that the trauma of the accident has led to the development of psychiatric disturbance, and large financial compensation is pursued. We, as clinicians, are not particularly good at differentiating individuals who report genuine symptomatology from those who simulate their distress. While some guidelines have been published trying to help the clinician separate the two (Resnick, 1988), the validity of this differentiation remains open to question. Few clinicians who have been involved in compensation claims would argue with the concern that some individuals may have simulated or exaggerated their symptomatology in order to obtain large financial settlements. It is sobering to note that Blanchard, Hickling, Taylor, Loos, Forneris and Jaccard (1996) found that one of the best correlates of PTSD diagnosis in survivors of motor vehicle accidents was initiation of litigation.

The potential over-reporting of PTSD has the added important effect of minimising the distress, plight and availability of resources for genuine sufferers. Given the popular coverage of the disorder, this is a problem which is not going to go away. If reliable neurobiological markers are awaiting verification, this would be a huge practical step forward.

6. BIOLOGY AND ENVIRONMENT—BI-DIRECTIONAL EFFECTS

A further point which is raised by Yehuda and Harvey, is the interplay between biology and the environment. Many psychologists and sociologists tend to be put off by "biological determinism" - adopting a knee-jerk response that this is too mechanistic, reductionistic, and in some way dehumanising. However, this is an extremely ill-informed view. One of the most exciting aspects of psychobiology is the realisation of bi-directionality of causality i.e., that biological factors (e.g., neural change, endocrine change, neurotransmitter change) can influence behaviour, but also, and equally important, is the opposite, i.e. that environment and experience have a marked impact on neurobiology. Relevant research includes studies of long-term potentiation as a neural model of memory (Bliss & Collingridge, 1993), the effects of changing environment on neuronal development - "environmental enrichment" (Rosenweig, 1984), and finally, and perhaps more relevantly, the recent finding that a history of combat-related trauma can apparently change brain structure (particularly hippocampal volume) in humans (Bremner et al. 1995). We must never lose sight of the fact that the brain influences behaviour, but environment and experience also have marked influences on the brain.

7. MOST PEOPLE COPE WITH THE EXPERIENCE OF TRAUMA

In their review, Yehuda and Harvey highlight that the majority of individuals who experience trauma do *not* develop chronic PTSD. This must surely be correct, as we evolved to survive in a hostile and challenging environment. By way of illustrative example of the argument that most individuals who experience trauma do not develop PTSD, I shall briefly outline a study ongoing in our Liver Clinic at the Edinburgh Royal Infirmary in Scotland. Shalev, Schreiber, Galai and Melmed (1993) proposed that many individuals who experience traumatic medical events may develop PTSD which goes unrecognised, due to the fact that physicians and nurses are not trained in its identification. This prompted our research group to look at the prevalence of PTSD in liver patients who survived variceal haemorrhage. Variceal haemorrhage occurs when, due to cirrhosis of the liver, back-pressure of the blood builds up and varicose veins enlarge at the base of the gullet. Given the build-up of venous back-pressure, these veins often burst, and the person haemorrhages, vomiting litres of blood, and often dies very quickly. Approximately 50% of patients survive. On hearing accounts by survivors, this sounds an extremely traumatic event. A typical scenario would be an individual awakening at home in the middle of the night feeling slightly nauseous, going to the bathroom and suddenly, and unexpectedly, projectile vomiting several litres of blood all over the walls and floor, with the individual being convinced that they are about to die. Our hypothesis was that PTSD would be common in such survivors. We assessed all survivors who had lost more than four units (pints) of blood in such a variceal haemorrhage. Recruitment criteria included full recall of the event, as some patients lose consciousness and have no memory of the bleed. To date, we have assessed 25 such patients using the Structured Clinical Interview for DSM- IV (PTSD section), the revised Impact of Events Scale (Horowitz et al. 1979) and the Hospital Anxiety and Depression Scale (Zigmond and Snaith, 1989). This is an on-going study, but to date we have identified only one individual out of 25 who fulfilled full diagnostic criteria for PTSD i.e., a prevalence rate of 4%. Many of the individuals did have disturbing distressing recollections of the event, but did not fulfil DSM IV criteria for PTSD section C - i.e. psychogenic amnesia, loss of interest, feelings of detachment and estrangement, restricted range of affect, etc. Eleven subjects met criteria for A, 20% for B, 8% for C, 32% for D, 4% for E and 4% for F. This is clearly a small and perhaps non-representative sample and the true prevalence may be much higher than 4%. However, it is clearly important to try and understand why one individual did develop a very severe and distressing, life-crippling degree of PTSD, while the others did not.

8. THE IMPORTANCE OF PREMORBID FACTORS

The preceding section brings us back to a further important point raised by Yehuda and Harvey, namely that explanations about post-traumatic phenomenon must incorporate the possibility that some individuals may be more predisposed to develop a pathological reaction following exposure to trauma, as a consequence of certain pre-morbid characteristics. They cite the extraordinary finding of McNally and Shin (1995) that the lower a Vietnam combat veteran's intelligence level, the more severe were his PTSD symptoms, raising the possibility that higher intelligence may be associated with more effective cognitive coping strategies. (Of course, a plausible alternative interpretation is that those of lower intelligence may get themselves into more serious or severe stress situations). Yehuda and Harvey present PTSD as a classic example of a diathesis-stress model and this leads logically to the attempt to identify vulnerability factors. A recent example of the importance of premorbid characteristics was provided by Deahl, Gillham, Thomas, Searle and Srinivasan (1994). These authors identified psychological morbidity in 62 British soldiers whose duties included the handling and identification of dead bodies during the Gulf War. Importantly, neither prior training nor psychological de-briefing appeared to make any difference to the development of subsequent psychiatric morbidity. Morbidity at nine months follow up, however, was more likely in those with a history of psychological problems and those who believed that their lives had been in danger in the Gulf. This finding was confirmed by Blanchard et al. (1996), in a survey of 158 victims of motor vehicle accidents, who found that a prior history of major depression and fear of dying in the accident were predictive of the development of PTSD. Such results should prompt us to be especially rigorous in identifying "at risk" patients following exposure to trauma. Turning to developmental risk factors, Famularo and Fenton (1994) attempted to identify which factors from early histories of maltreated children were associated with the risk of later developing PTSD. They found that low birth weight, jaundice, poor weight gain and distress when moved were among significant predictors of later PTSD. Such data add support to the argument that the interaction of a vulnerable individual plus extreme trauma may be a good recipe for the subsequent development of chronic PTSD.

Yehuda and Harvey cogently propose a series of pre-existing cognitive styles as possible risk factors for PTSD. For example, they suggest that a pre-morbid tendency towards ready associative learning may lead to ready "triggering" of intrusive memories. If an individual has a tendency to form ready associations between relatively loosely connected stimuli, this may increase the potential field of triggers for traumatic memories. Yehuda and Harvey suggest experiments whereby this hypothesis could be tested by paired-associated learning test paradigms. An added advantage of this particular type of research approach, which Yehuda and Harvey did not point out, is that such a hypothesis predicts *better* performance by patients relative to controls - so called "functional facilitation". This is extremely important, as many clinical studies of memory disordered patients suffer from the "generalised deficit problem" — i.e., that patients tend to perform more poorly than controls on a very wide range of tasks, and it is often difficult to determine whether deficits are due to specific effects of the disorder, or merely reflect general reductions in global cognitive abilities, attention, motivation etc. The novelty in the Yehuda/Harvey proposal is that as a consequence of a tendency towards ready development of associations, it is proposed that such individuals, by nature of their *superior* associative ability, would be more pre-disposed to developing intrusive traumatic memories triggered by loosely related environmental stimuli. (Interested readers may find it profitable to look at the functional facilitation literature in relation to other amnesic disorders, e.g., Kapur, Heath, Meudell & Kennedy (1986)).

Yehuda and Harvey also suggest that a pre-morbid tendency towards obsessive thinking may pre-dispose a person to develop intrusive thoughts about the event following trauma, and also that deficits in working memory, such as deficient source monitoring, could lead to deficits in the ability to discriminate between past events and ongoing environmental events, leading to re-experiencing symptoms. Each of these are intriguing testable hypotheses which should be pursued. However, to return to the heterogeneity problem in PTSD, it seems entirely likely to this commentator at least, that as knowledge develops, it will lead to a fractionation of PTSD into differing sub-types, perhaps along the lines suggested by Yehuda and Harvey, e.g., "PTSD-obsessive subtype" or "PTSD-associative learning subtype", based on clearly outlined models of abnormal information processing systems. The ultimate challenge would then be to link these putative subtypes to differing underlying neurobiological substrates, including degree of arousal and neuroendocrine activity at the time the emotive material was processed. In the target article Yehuda and Harvey propose a three-group-comparison experimental design, PTSD patients versus non-PTSD trauma survivors versus non-traumatised individuals. This is advice which PTSD researchers should heed, as it allows one to control for the effects of trauma exposure. They additionally propose a comparison of trauma-naive individuals, differentiated on the basis of PTSD risk factors. This idea is novel, but in my opinion is too premature to be practicable at present, as we require stronger evidence of robust, reliable and replicable risk factors than we have at present.

9. CONCLUSION

A review chapter by Christianson published 5 years ago stated "If we wish to reach a deeper understanding of how emotion and memory interact, it is necessary to integrate both psychological and biological knowledge" (Christianson, 1992, p.330). Yehuda and Harvey have laid the foundations of a model integrating neuroendocrinology, neuropsychology and clinical symptomatology. It is now up to the rest of us to adopt the approach advocated by Karl Popper, and try to prove them wrong!

10. ACKNOWLEDGMENTS

I would like to thank Norma Brearley for her careful preparation of this chapter, and the Wellcome Trust Grant No. 048090/Z/96 for their financial support.

11. REFERENCES

Bisson, J.I. & Deahl, M.P. (1994). Psychological debriefing and prevention of posttraumatic stress - more research is needed. *British Journal of Psychiatry*, 165, 717–720.

Blanchard, E.B., Hickling, E.J., Taylor, A.E., Loos, W.R., Forneris, C.A. & Jaccard, J. (1996). Who develops PTSD from motor vehicle accidents. *Behaviour Research and Therapy*, 34, 1–10.

Bliss, T.V.P. & Collingridge, G.L. (1993). A synaptic model of memory: long term potentiation in the hippocampus. *Nature*, 361, 31–39.

Bremner, J.D., Randall, P., Scott, T.M., Bronen, R.A., Seibyl, J.P., Southwick, S.M., Delaney, R.C., McCarthy, G., Charney, D.S. & Innis, R.B. (1995). MRI-based measurement of hippocampal volume in patients with combat-related posttraumatic stress disorder. *American Journal of Psychiatry*, 152, 973–981.

Cahill, L., Babinsky, R., Markowitsch, H.J. & McGaugh, J.L. (1995). The amygdala and emotional memory. *Nature*, 377, 295–296.

Cahill, L., Haier, R.J., Fallon, J., Alkire, M.T., Tang, C., Keator, D., Wu, J. & McGaugh, J.L. (1996). Amygdala activity at encoding correlated with long-term, free-recall of emotional information. *Proceedings of the National Academy of Sciences, USA*, 93, 8016–8021.

Cahill, L., Prins, B., Weber, M. & McGaugh, J.L. (1994). b-adrenergic activation and memory for emotional events. *Nature*, 371, 702–704.

Christianson, S.A. (1992). *Handbook of Emotion and Memory: Current Research and Theory*. New Jersey: Erlbaum.

Deahl, M.P., Gillham, A.B., Thomas, J., Searle, M.M. & Srinivasan, M. (1994). Psychological sequelae following the gulf war - factors associated with subsequent morbidity and the effectiveness of psychological debriefing. *British Journal of Psychiatry*, 165, 60–65.

Famularo, R. & Fenton, T. (1994). Early developmental history and pediatric posttraumatic stress disorder. *Archives of Pediatrics and Adolescent Medicine*, 148, 1032–1038.

Galvez, R., Mesches, M. & McGaugh, J.L. (1996). Norepinephrine release in the amygdala in response to footshock stimulation. *Neurobiology of Learning (In press)*.

Horowitz, M., Wilner, N. & Alvarez, W. (1979). Impact of event scale: a measure of subjective stress. *Psychosomatic Medicine*, 41, 209–218.

Kapur, N., Heath, P., Meudell, P. & Kennedy, P. (1986). Amnesia can facilitate memory performance - evidence from a patient with dissociated retrograde amnesia. *Neuropsychologia*, 24, 215–221.

McNally, R.J. & Shin, L.M. (1995). Association of intelligence with severity of posttraumatic stress disorder symptoms in vietnam combat veterans. *American Journal of Psychiatry*, 152, 936–938.

Raphael, B., Meldrum, L. & McFarlane, A.C. (1995). Does debriefing after psychological trauma work. *British Medical Journal*, 310, 1479–1480.

Resnick, P.J. (1988). *Malingering of Posttraumatic Disorders*. In R. Rogers (Eds.), Clinical Assessment of Malingering and Deception (pp. New York: Guilford Press.

Rosenweig, M.R. (1984). Experience, memory and the brain. *American Psychologist*, 39, 365–376.

Schacter, D.L., Koutstaal, W. & Norman, K.A. (1996). Can cognitive neuroscience illuminate the nature of traumatic childhood memories? *Current Opinion in Neurobiology*, 6, 207–214.

Shalev, A.Y., Schreiber, S., Galai, T. & Melmed, R.N. (1993). Post-traumatic stress disorder following medical events. *British Journal of Clinical Psychology*, 32, 247–253.

Summerfield, D. (1995). Debriefing after psychological trauma - inappropriate exporting of western culture may cause additional harm. *British Medical Journal*, 311, 509.

QUESTION AND ANSWER SESSION

Berntsen. Do cortisol levels change with successful treatment?

Yehuda. That's a very good question. We don't have an answer to that question yet, but this issue is being explored in collaboration with Dr. Resick.

Elliott. Can you use the biological tests that you have been talking about to determine whether individuals who have recovered memories, and then developed PTSD to these memories, actually were traumatised?

Yehuda. This has obviously not been studied but it is a great idea to see whether or not individuals with recovered memories are biologically similar to individuals who have been traumatised but never lost their memory for the trauma. Obviously, it would have tremendous clinical and forensic implications if individuals with and without recovered memories, with comparable PTSD symptoms, were similar biologically. It would be even more interesting if somehow we could learn about the underlying neurobiology of individuals who truly were traumatised but who do not remember (e.g., in Linda Williams' (1994) study).

Briere. From what you've said it should be possible to distinguish depression from PTSD as a function of the types of biology you have described. But what might the biology be in individuals with both these conditions, which is quite common?

Yehuda. We might predict that individuals with a "primary" PTSD would look more like the PTSD subjects whereas individuals with a "primary" depression would look more like depressed subjects. Perhaps this is one application of what I've described. However, a less simplistic answer would be that the data that were described in the lecture are really about the fact that there are fundamentally critical individual differences in the way people respond biologically to stress which may predict and influence their clinical course. In contrast, describing symptoms may be a less sensitive way to classify individual responses to stress.

Briere. My other question is that there are people talking about cortisol toxicity with reference to hippocampal damage and memory difficulties. How would you rationalise your findings of low cortisol with hippocampal damage and memory difficulties in PTSD?

Yehuda. Cortisol toxicity is only one way to damage a hippocampus. There are several other ways, such as interfering with the glutamate system or other neurotransmitter systems, etc. Ultimately, high cortisol levels are relevant to hippocampal atrophy only if they can induce glucocorticoid receptors which could initiate the biological responses that are more relevant to hippocampal damage. I presented data showing that glucocorticoid receptors were more sensitive in PTSD patients, and suggested that the receptor alteration is even the primary lesion of the hypothalamic-pituitary-adrenal axis in PTSD. Therefore, one way to understand the hippocampal data in PTSD is to view them as a consequence of a more sensitive glococorticoid receptor activity in the hippocampus. However, the current notion that hippocampal damage in PTSD is a result of high levels of glucocorticoids at the time of the trauma is certainly wrong (even though it is quite popular). Based on the rape data of Heidi Resnick and the motor vehicle accident data of Alexander McFarlane, it is clear that cortisol levels are lower, not higher at the time of the trauma, in individuals who develop PTSD. It should also be mentioned for the sake of completeness that it is possible to damage hippocampal cells in the dentate gyrus with adrenalectomy, which is the absence of cortisol. As our imaging techniques become more sophisticated it will be possible to look at individual regions and get more information on which regions are actually affected in PTSD. If we observe that the atrophy is in the dentate gyrus, then we would learn that this effect is probably related to the lower cortisol levels in PTSD. However I would bet that the hippocampal atrophy in PTSD would be in the CA1 and CA3 regions (Ammon's horn) as a result of increased glucocorticoid receptor sensitivity. Ultimately, it will be possible to clarify this issue.

Hyman. I liked the emphasis on individual differences which I think is lacking in memory research. Could you comment on the applicability of the Yerkes-Dodson Law which suggests an inverted U-shaped function, to your theory. According to the Yerkes-Dodson Law, it may be that low levels of arousal produce different types of PTSD symptoms as high levels of arousal.

Yehuda. Right. But the point here would be that level of arousability following trauma may actually be a risk factor for certain types of symptoms in response to trauma, rather than a consequence of the severity of the trauma.

Noël. Based on the data you presented about cortisol in the immediate aftermath of the trauma, would it be possible to use these data to identify people early on after a trauma and intervene prophylactically?

Yehuda. Ultimately, this would be the best use of this information.

Schooler. On the one hand you seem to be suggesting that the alterations you have described are a result of the trauma exposure, but couldn't it also be that these problems were there before the trauma exposure?

Yehuda. Yes! That's the point. There must be a reason that some people show this type of response to trauma, and at least some aspects of what I have described may have been present to "set the stage" for the enhanced negative feedback observed. Your question brings to mind studies that I did not describe showing cortisol alterations in the children of Holocaust survivors. Many of these adult children also show low cortisol. As a group, these individuals are far more likely to develop PTSD following trauma than other groups. This raises the possibility that some aspects of the HPA findings described are risk factors for the other changes observed.

Powell. Just a small historical point. You mentioned that Freud's patients told him that they had been abused. A lot of people now think that that's a myth, and that in reality only a few of Freud's patients said they had been abused. However, once he heard about one case, he aggressively went after his patients to try to confirm this theory he had come up with. So in effect, he used suggestibility and bad methodology to get his patients to admit to early abuse. I would suggest a number of readings to you to clarify this point.

Yehuda. If the only thing I got wrong was Freud I am in good shape!

REFERENCES

Williams, L. M. (1994). Recall of childhood trauma: A prospective study of women's memories of child sexual abuse. *Journal of Consulting and Clinical Psychology, 62,* 1167–1176.

10

RECOLLECTION

Perspectives on Reinstated Memory and Child Trauma

Arthur P. Shimamura

University of California, Berkeley
Berkeley, California 94720

1. INTRODUCTION

The emotional, clinical, and even legal ramifications of an adult's recollection of childhood trauma have forced memory research into the public limelight. Indeed, decisions related to public policy, ethical practices of clinicians, and child-parent lawsuits have depended in part on what science can tell us about the notion of *reinstated* memories. I use the term *reinstated* memories to refer to instances in which an individual recollects a traumatic experience that previously was not available to conscious or explicit report. The term is meant to be neutral with respect to the veracity of the recollection, especially compared to other terms such as *recovered*, *repressed*, or *false* memories, which by their terminology can appear to be biased toward either the complete validity or complete falsity of a recollection.

The fact that reinstated memories occur cannot be argued. In recent books and articles (see Herman, 1992; Loftus & Ketcham, 1994; Schooler, 1994; Terr, 1994), individuals have reported recollections of severe trauma during childhood and have claimed that such thoughts had lain dormant for years. Of course, the issue raised by clinical and legal ramifications is whether such reinstated memories are true, partly true, or essentially false. Scientific investigations can provide clues to the quality of reinstated memories, can document their frequency, and can even simulate aspects of the experience. Moreover, an understanding of the biological basis of memory function can provide clues to the pattern of memory dysfunction associated with damage to certain brain systems.

It should be noted, however, that scientific investigations *cannot* completely address the veracity of reinstated memories. One limitation concerns the subjective experience of reinstated memories. That is, the feeling that some information was unconscious at an earlier time can only be experienced by the individual who reports that a memory was reinstated. Yet even the individual who experiences a reinstated memory cannot know with certainty that the memory was truly out of conscious awareness. Indeed, the claim that a memory was previously out of conscious awareness must be based on own's belief that the memory was not

Recollections of Trauma, edited by Read and Lindsay
Plenum Press, New York, 1997

previously available to conscious awareness. Failure to remember prior recollections or reluctance to attempt to retrieve traumatic experiences may produce the feeling or belief that some memory was previously out of conscious awareness. Thus, in terms of determining the validity of a reinstated memory, one can only *believe* that an individual is telling the truth and not having problems monitoring his or her prior recollections.

The problem of verifying reports of unconscious memory is not unique to the issue of reinstated memories. In psychiatric disorders, such as psychogenic amnesia and dissociative identity disorder (i.e., multiple personality disorder), the clinician must evaluate the validity of such claims. For example, in cases of psychogenic amnesia, a patient reports to be amnesic for his or her autobiography, including most aspects of personal identity. In cases of dissociative identity disorder, it is often difficult to distinguish a true fractionation of identity from a psychiatric disturbance which elicits role playing. In these cases, it is impossible to determine with certainty whether such a patient is truly amnesic or dissociative or whether the patient is not truthful and trying to escape from personal or legal repercussions or responsibilities. Cases of malingering in putative cases of psychogenic amnesia have been documented (see Kopelman, this volume; Shimamura & Gershberg, 1995).

Compared to psychiatric cases of psychogenic amnesia and dissociative identity disorder, the phenomenon of reinstated memories is more subtle. In reports of reinstated memories, memory lapse is typically specific to a traumatic episode or series of episodes. Clinical disorders such as repression and dissociation have been used to explain the phenomenon of reinstated memories (see Brewin, this volume; Loftus, 1993). Also, the integration of clinical and cognitive factors have provided useful information concerning basic mechanisms that may mediate memory lapses or the feeling of experiencing such lapses (see Brewin, this volume, Lindsay & Read, 1994; Loftus, 1993). For example, poor encoding or memory storage could later affect recollection of a traumatic experience. Also, poor self-awareness of prior recollections (i.e., poor metacognition) could make an individual *believe* that a prior experience was out of consciousness, when in fact it had just not been retrieved recently. Finally, even everyday memories are distorted and integrated with other experiences, and it is sometimes difficult to determine if certain episodes actually occurred the way that they were recollected.

This chapter will explore another scientific domain, cognitive neuroscience, which has recently been integrated with both clinical and cognitive psychology (see also Schacter, Koutstaal, & Norman, 1996). This approach attempts to identify the biological basis of human cognitive function. The two dominant strategies have been to assess performance of brain-injured patients on cognitive tasks and to observe brain activity of normal individuals using functional neuroimaging techniques, such as positron emission tomography (PET) or functional magnetic resonance imaging (fMRI). In the analysis of clinical neurological patients and in the analysis of brain regions that are particularly active during cognitive tests, the field of cognitive neuroscience has provide useful bridges between clinical, cognitive and biological psychology.

To what extent can cognitive neuroscience address the issue of reinstated memories? Based on our understanding of the biological basis of human memory, two neural systems have been shown to be intricately involved in the encoding and storage of information. The first neural system is the prefrontal cortex, which appears to be involved in encoding, organizing and monitoring of on-line information. The second neural system is the medial temporal region, which appears to be important for the storage of new information into existing memory representations. Memory disorders associated with damage to these two neural systems will be discussed. Thereafter, a framework is offered toward a neurobiologically based conception of reinstated memories. Specifically, it is suggested that disruptions in either of these two neural systems during a traumatic experience could potentially fragment encoding and memory of a traumatic experience and make the experience less accessible at a later time. Thus, attempts to reinstate the memory at a later time would likely involve significant reconstruction of the experience and make reinstated memories highly susceptible to distortions and augmentations.

2. THE PREFRONTAL CORTEX

The prefrontal cortex comprise the anterior 28% of the neocortex. In humans, it has been associated with a variety of functions, including attention, emotion, memory, language, and intellectual reasoning (for review, see Damasio, 1993; Milner & Petrides, 1985; Petrides, 1989; Shimamura, 1994a; Stuss, Easkes, & Foster, 1994; Wheeler, Stuss, & Tulving, 1997). Neuropsychological studies of brain-injured patients and neuroimaging studies of brain activity have provided key findings concerning the contribution of the prefrontal cortex to human memory. The pattern of memory disorders associated with prefrontal lesions has been commonly described as an impairment in *working memory*. That is, this brain region appears to be involved in the organization and control of information that is to be stored or retrieved from memory. The role of the prefrontal cortex as a working memory or executive control process has been characterized in various theories of frontal lobe function (see Baddeley, 1986; Fuster, 1995; Goldman-Rakic, 1987, 1995; Moscovitch, 1995; Shimamura, 1994a).

2.1. Selective Attention and Working Memory

The prefrontal cortex acts as an executive control that monitors and organizes information processing (Baddeley, 1986; Shallice & Burgess, 1991; Shimamura, 1995). As such, working memory is closely related to the notion of selective attention. Indeed, it may be suggested that attention is the mechanism by which executive control is implemented. A basic function of working memory appears to be the sustaining of neural activity associated with a percept, after sensory information for that percept is removed. That is, an important role of working memory is the maintenance of information in short-term or immediate memory. Based on animal models of working memory, Fuster (1989) and Goldman-Rakic (1987) have demonstrated that certain cortical neurons in the frontal cortex facilitate the maintenance of neural activity immediately after the offset of a visual stimulus. This process may be central to working memory. Indeed, recent neuroimaging studies suggest that brain regions in frontal and parietal cortex are particularly active during visual short-term memory tasks (Jonides, Smith, Koeppe, Awh, Minoshima, & Mintun, 1993; Petrides, Alivisatos, & Evans, 1995).

Another role of the prefrontal cortex with respect to selective attention is the ability to gate or filter extraneous or irrelevant information. Various tests have been used to assess the ability to filter extraneous information. For example, the Stroop test (Stroop, 1935; see MacLeod, 1991) has been used to assess the influence of irrelevant verbal information during color naming. In this test, subjects are presented color names written in different colors. Responses to name the color of the words is slowed when the word is an incongruous color (e.g., the word RED written in green ink). Perret (1974) reported increased latencies in the Stroop test in patients with frontal lobe lesions. That is, these patients exhibited greater difficulty in disregarding the irrelevant word stimuli. Also,

Petrides and Milner (1982) demonstrated that patients with frontal lobe lesions exhibit impairment in the ability to monitor prior responses. In one task, an array of stimuli is presented and subjects are asked to point to one of the stimuli. On each successive presentation, these stimuli are presented again but in different positions, and subjects are instructed to point to a different stimulus on subsequent trials. Patients with frontal lobe lesions have difficulty monitoring stimuli, and thus often point to the same stimuli on subsequent trials. In a recent neuroimaging study, Petrides demonstrated that activation of the prefrontal cortex occurs during performance on this pointing task (Petrides et al., 1995).

Some recent neurophysiological evidence suggests that the prefrontal cortex is involved in the control of neural activity. Knight and colleagues (Knight, Scabini, & Woods, 1989; Yamaguchi & Knight, 1990) studied scalp evoked potentials in patients with prefrontal lesions. In one study (Knight et al., 1989), the amplitude of middle latency auditory evoked potentials, which are presumed to be generated in primary auditory cortex, was *potentiated* as a result of prefrontal lesions. Thus, there appeared to be a *disinhibition* of posterior cortical activity as a result of prefrontal lesions. In a PET study of normal individuals (Frith, Friston, Liddle, & Frackowiak, 1991), *increases* in activity in the dorsolateral prefrontal cortex were related to *decreases* in activity in posterior cortical regions. Thus, as a result of the extensive reciprocal connections between the prefrontal cortex and other cortical areas, it may be that inhibitory control of many aspects of mental function is provided by this proposed filtering mechanism. Based on this view, a multitude of cognitive disorders would occur as a result of prefrontal lesions, not because different areas of the prefrontal cortex are serving different functions, but because these areas are inhibiting different posterior cortical regions, which themselves serve different cognitive function.

2.2. Organizing Memories

Patients with prefrontal lesions do not always exhibit gross impairment on clinical tests of new learning ability. For example, Janowsky, Shimamura, Kritchevsky, and Squire (1989) demonstrated that patients with prefrontal lesions perform within the normal range on the Wechsler Memory Scale-Revised (WMS-R), a clinical test battery that assesses both verbal and nonverbal memory. Despite relatively good performance on clinical tests of new learning capacity, patients with prefrontal lesions can exhibit impairment on some standard tests of new learning. In particular, these patients exhibit impairment on tests of free recall (Della Rocchetta, 1986; Gershberg & Shimamura, 1995; Janowsky et al., 1989; Jetter, Poser, Freeman, & Markowitsch, 1986; Stuss, Alexander, Palumbo, Buckle, Sayer, & Pogue, 1994). On these tests, a list of items (e.g., words or pictures) are presented, and subjects are asked to recollect as many items from the list as possible. Tests of free recall place heavy demands on internally generated memory strategies, because no cues are presented during testing other than a simple command to recall the information.

The impairment in free recall that occurs as a result of frontal lobe damage appears to be related to problems in the ability to organize and categorize information. During learning, patients with prefrontal lesions are less likely to engage in useful organizational strategies, such as subjective organization or category clustering (Eslinger & Grattan, 1992; Gershberg & Shimamura, 1995; Stuss et al., 1994). Moreover, patients are benefited by providing category cues at the time of learning (Gershberg & Shimamura, 1995) or simply by providing instructions that a list contains semantically related words (Hirst & Volpe, 1988). Category cues and information about the structure of a word list provide organizational benefits that patients with prefrontal lesions apparently cannot glean by themselves.

The prefrontal cortex contribute significantly to the retrieval of information in memory. Patients with prefrontal lesions are benefited by the provision of category cues at the time of retrieval (Gershberg & Shimamura, 1995). Also, patients exhibit significant impairment on tests of verbal fluency in which subjects must retrieve well learned information from semantic memory (Janowsky et al., 1989a). In neuroimaging studies using positron emission tomography (PET), it is possible to identify brain areas that are particularly active during a task. Interestingly, individuals who are engaged in a task involving retrieval of general semantic knowledge exhibit a preponderance of left prefrontal activity, whereas individuals who are engaged in a task involving retrieval of episodic or autobiographical knowledge exhibit a preponderance of right prefrontal activity (Tulving, Kapur, Craik, Moscovitch, & Houle, 1994). Finally, patients with frontal lobe lesions exhibit impairment in the retrieval of names of famous faces (Mangels, Gershberg, Shimamura, & Knight, 1996).

A deficit in the ability to organize information can be related to problems in working memory. Indeed, deficits in memory organization may be caused by increased susceptibility to interference from extraneous memory activations, both at the time of encoding and at the time of retrieval. To test this hypothesis, Shimamura, Jurica, Mangels, Gershberg, & Knight (1995) assessed performance by patients with frontal lobe lesions on a test meant to increase interference. They presented subjects with 12 paired associates (e.g., *thief-crime*; *lion-hunter*) on each of three study-test learning trials. Subjects were tested by giving the first word as the cue for the second word (e.g., *thief- ?*; *lion-?*) Following the three learning trials, subjects were asked to learn a second list in which the cue words used in the first list was paired with new target words (e.g., *thief-bandit*; *lion-circus*). This memory test paradigm is called *AB-AC* paired-associate learning, because the learning of the first paired associate (AB) interferes with later learning of related associates (AC). Although patients learned the first list nearly as a well as control subjects, they exhibited disproportionate impairment when they were required to ignore the first associations and learn new ones.

2.3. Metacognition: Monitoring and Controlling Memory

Metacognition refers to knowledge about one's mental capabilities and the ability to use that knowledge to control and monitor information (see Metcalfe & Shimamura, 1994a). In this sense, metacognition is closely related to executive control processes in working memory. The ability to monitor information processing can be observed under interfering or "memory blocking" situations, such as when information is on the "tip of the tongue." Neurological injury can increase the frequency of tip-of-the-tongue experiences. In severe cases, patients exhibit "anomia" for very common words (see Shimamura, 1994b).

Damage to the prefrontal cortex has been associated with deficits in metacognition. For example, patients with frontal lobe lesions exhibit impaired feeling-of-knowing experiences. Feeling of knowing refers to the sense of familiarity for information that cannot be completely recalled. In one study, patients with frontal lobe lesions and control subjects were asked to rate their feeling of knowing for recently learned information (Janowsky et al., 1989a). Subjects were asked to learn sentences (e.g., *Mary's garden was full of marigolds*). Later, subjects were given a cued recall test for a word in the sentences (e.g., *Mary's garden was full of _____*). If a subject could not recall the word, they were asked to rate their feeling of knowing for the word. That is, they were asked to rate on a 7-point scale how likely they would be able to recognize the word if a multiple-choice test were given. After making their ratings, a multiple-choice test was given to assess their feeling-of-knowing accuracy. Although recall and recognition memory performance were similar between the patient and control subjects, the frontal patients exhibited poor feeling-of-knowing accuracy. That is, they were not able to monitor or make judgments about what was in their memory.

The feeling-of-knowing impairment exhibited by patients with prefrontal lesions may be related to deficits in other tasks that involve memory retrieval and inferential reasoning. One such example is the finding that patients with prefrontal lesions have difficulty making estimates or inferences from everyday experiences (e.g., How tall is the average English woman?; Shallice & Evans, 1978). Such answers are not readily available and typically require search and retrieval strategies. Similarly, patients with prefrontal lesions have difficulty estimating the price of objects (Smith & Milner, 1984). All these deficits—that is, deficits in cognitive estimation as well as in feeling-of-knowing judgments—might be construed as deficits in metacognition (i.e., knowing about what is stored in memory). Such deficits could also contribute to increased memory distortions and confabulations in patients with frontal lobe lesions (see Moscovitch, 1995).

2.4. Source Recollection: Memory for Past Episodes

Source recollection refers to the ability to remember the event or episode in which some information was encountered (for review, see Johnson, Hastroudi, & Lindsay, 1993; Shimamura, 1994). Patients with frontal lobe lesions appear to exhibit a particular impairment in source recollection. In one study, Janowsky et al. (1989b) assessed source memory in patients with prefrontal lesions, age-matched control subjects, and younger control subjects. Subjects learned a set of 20 general-information facts that could not be previously recalled (e.g., *The name of the dog on the Cracker Jacks box is Bingo*). After a 1-week retention interval, fact recall was tested for the 20 learned facts (e.g. *What is the name of the dog on the Cracker Jacks box?*) and for 20 new facts. When subjects correctly answered a fact question, they were asked to recollect the source of the information ("Can you tell me where you learned the answer?"; "When was the most recent time you heard that information?"). Source memory ability was significantly impaired in patients with prefrontal lesions.

Interestingly, source memory impairment also occurs in normal aging. That is, aging has been shown to produce particular problems in the ability to remember where and when some information was learned (Hastroudi, Johnson, Vnek, & Ferguson, 1994; Janowsky et al., 1989b; McIntyre & Craik, 1987; Schacter, Kaszniak, Kihlstrom, & Valdiserri, 1991). Neuronal cell loss associated with normal aging does occur prominently in the frontal lobes (see Haug, Barmwater, Eggers, Fischer, Kuhl, & Sass, 1983), which suggests that source memory impairment in normal aging may also be related to subtle frontal lobe dysfunction.

Remembering source information requires the association of temporal information to factual knowledge (When did I learn that information?). Thus, a critical feature of source monitoring is memory for the temporal order of events. Milner (1971) was the first to report that patients with frontal lobe lesions exhibit an impairment in memory for temporal order. She reported a study of recency judgments, in which subjects are shown a series of stimuli (e.g., words, pictures) and are asked to judge which one of two stimuli was presented more recently (see Milner, Corsi, & Leonard, 1991). In another test of temporal order memory (Shimamura, Janowsky, & Squire, 1990), subjects were presented a list of 15 words one at a time and then asked to reconstruct the list order from a random display of the words. In this list reconstruction test, memory for temporal order was assessed by correlating a subject's judged order with the actual presentation order of the list of words. Patients with prefrontal lesions exhibited impaired memory for temporal order on this test.

3. THE MEDIAL TEMPORAL REGION

3.1. Organic Amnesia

Patients with bilateral damage to the medial temporal region exhibit a profound memory impairment in which new learning ability is severely affected (see Shimamura & Gershberg, 1994; Squire, 1987, 1992). That is, these patients have extreme difficulty remembering facts and events encountered since the onset of amnesia (i.e., anterograde amnesia). The role of the medial temporal region in learning and memory was suggested by studies of the now-famous patient, case H. M., who in 1953 underwent surgery of this brain region for relief of epileptic seizures (Milner, Corkin, & Teuber, 1975). Following surgery, H. M.'s seizure activity was attenuated, but he exhibited a severe anterograde amnesia. Despite this severe impairment in learning, there was no detectable impairment in intellectual, language or social abilities. There was some retrograde amnesia, which refers to impairment of memory for events that occurred before the onset of amnesia. For example, H. M. could not remember the layout of the hospital ward or recognize members of the medical staff. Moreover, he could not recall the death of a favorite uncle who had died three years previously. Yet, following surgery H.M.'s retrograde amnesia was not severe, as indicated by the fact that he performed as well as control subjects on a test of memory for faces of celebrities who became famous prior to 1950 (Marslen-Wilson & Teuber, 1975).

Recent clinical observations of H. M. indicate that memory for ongoing events is still severely impaired. For example, 30 minutes after eating lunch, H. M. could not recall what he had eaten and could not even recall if he had lunch at all. H. M. is aware of his disorder and has reflected upon his impairment as being akin to always "waking from a dream." In other words, he seems to lack continuity in the memory of events across time, even when the events are separated by only a few minutes. Thus, the central feature of H. M.'s memory disorder is anterograde amnesia or new learning impairment (see Corkin, 1984). This impairment affects information received from all sensory modalities and includes impairment of both verbal and nonverbal (e.g., spatial) memory. For example, H. M. has failed to acquire new vocabulary words that have been added to the dictionary since his surgery. He also exhibits severe impairment on laboratory tests of word and picture recall, cued-word learning (e.g., learning word pairs), and recognition memory.

The medial temporal region does not appear to affect on-line, working memory ability. For example, H. M. can perform as well as control subjects on tests of immediate memory, such as digit span tests, in which subjects report a short string of digits immediately after presentation. Also, H. M. can think and solve problems, as indicated by his preserved I.Q. Nevertheless, as soon as information is out of conscious experience, it is not available for conscious recollection. The analysis of H. M.'s amnesia stands as a milestone in our progress to understand memory in the brain. He has provided the crucial evidence for the specific role of the medial temporal region in the process of memory formation and storage. Indeed, analyses of H. M. and other amnesic cases have provided the impetus for many important animal and PET studies on the role of the medial temporal region in learning and memory (see Squire, 1992).

Other neurological disorders that damage the medial temporal region can produce an amnesic syndrome similar to that seen in H. M. For example, tumors, head injuries, or vascular disorders (e.g., strokes) in this region can cause organic amnesia (for review, see Shimamura, 1989; Squire, 1987). Also, some neurological disorders—such as viral infection, ischemia (i.e., loss of blood flow to the brain), or hypoxia (i.e., loss of oxygen to the brain)—particularly damage the medial temporal region. In these disorders, anterograde amnesia is often the outstanding cognitive impairment, though retrograde amnesia can also occur. As in the case of H. M., intellectual abilities and working memory are generally intact.

Neuroimaging studies have corroborated the role of the medial temporal region in learning and memory. For example, in quantitative analyses of magnetic resonance images (MRI), the volume of neural tissue in this region in patients with organic amnesia was found to be 40% less than the volume of tissue observed in images of control subjects (Squire, Amaral, & Press, 1990). Also, in neurologically intact individuals, PET studies have shown increased activation in this brain region during the recollection of recently learned material (Buckner et al., 1995; Squire et al., 1992).

3.2. The Distinction between Explicit and Implicit Memory

One of the most striking finding from studies of patients with organic amnesia is that these patients can perform in an entirely normal fashion on certain kinds of memory tests. These tests involve habit or automatic learning, such as the kind of memory expressed on tests of skill learning, classical conditioning, and "priming" (for review, see Schacter, 1987; Shimamura, 1986, 1993; Squire, 1987, 1992). For example, amnesic patients exhibit considerable retention of perceptual-motor skill on a mirror drawing task in which subjects are required to trace the outline of a star while viewing the star in a mirror (Corkin, 1968). On tests of skill retention, amnesic patients perform as well as control subjects, but they do not appear to have conscious knowledge of having performed the task before. Preserved skill learning has been observed on a variety of perceptual-motor tests (Brooks & Baddeley, 1976; Corkin, 1968).

Amnesic patients have also be shown to exhibit intact performance on tests that involve incremental cognitive skill learning. For example, Cohen and Squire (1980) observed preserved skill learning by amnesic patients on a mirror reading task in which subjects learned to read mirror-reversed words. These patients have also been shown to exhibit incremental prototype learning and the learning of artificial grammars (Knowlton, Ramus, & Squire, 1992; Knowlton & Squire, 1994; Kolodny, 1994). On these tests, amnesic patients appear to acquire central tendencies or probabilistic patterns presented in repeated stimuli. These findings suggest that amnesic patients can modify or tune information processing. These patients, however, fail to distinguish any specific stimulus previously seen from novel but similar stimuli. That is, these patients appear to have a disruption in the binding of learned information to specific contexts (see Chalfonte & Johnson, 1996; Squire, Shimamura, & Amaral, 1986; Shimamura, 1996).

A memory phenomenon known as *priming* is also preserved in amnesia (for review, see Schacter, 1987; Shimamura, 1986, 1993). Priming is an automatic facilitation or bias in performance as a result of recently encountered information. The seminal evidence for preservation of priming in amnesia came from Warrington and Weiskrantz (1968; 1970). Amnesic patients were asked to identify words or pictures that were presented in a degraded form. If the subject could not identify the stimulus, a succession of less degraded versions of the stimulus were shown until identification was successful. When amnesic patients were asked to identify the same degraded words or pictures at a later time, their performance was facilitated by the previous experience; that is, they were able to identify the stimuli more quickly. This priming effect occurred despite failure to discriminate previously presented stimuli from new ones in a recognition memory test.

A variety of priming paradigms have since been used to demonstrate preserved priming in amnesia. For example, in one task words are presented (e.g., MOTEL) to the subject and later cued by three-letter word stems (e.g., MOT). Subjects are asked to say the first word that comes to mind for each word stem (Graf, Squire, & Mandler, 1984). In another task, subjects were presented words (e.g., BABY) and later asked to "free associate" to related words (e.g., CHILD) (Shimamura & Squire, 1984). On these tests, words appear to "pop" into mind, and amnesic patients exhibit this effect to the same level as control subjects. However, when subjects are asked to use the same word stems as aids to recollect words from the study session, control subjects perform better than amnesic patients.

Demonstrations of preserved memory functions in amnesic patients suggest that some memory processes can be dissociated from the brain regions that are damaged in organic amnesia. As reviewed by Squire (1987; 1992), various taxonomies have been used to distinguish the memory forms that are impaired in amnesia from those that are preserved. For example, many distinguish between "conscious" recollection and unconscious or automatic memory. *Explicit* and *implicit* memory have been used to express this distinction (Schacter, 1987). Other similar distinctions include *declarative* versus *nondeclarative* memory (Squire, 1992), *memory* versus *habit* (Mishkin, Malamut, and Bachevalier, 1984), and *propositional* versus *dispositional* memory (Thomas, 1984). Recently, the kind of memory that is impaired in amnesic patients has been described as involving *relational* memory (Cohen & Eichenbaum, 1992). This term is useful because it describes a functional property of the memory process, which is the binding or relating of new information into existing representations (see also, Shimamura, 1996; Squire, Shimamura, & Amaral, 1986).

4. TOWARD A NEUROBIOLOGICALLY BASED CONCEPTION OF REINSTATED MEMORIES

It should be noted first that there is no evidence that victims of psychological trauma experience prefrontal or medial temporal dysfunction. Thus, the neurobiolgically based conception of reinstated memories proposed here is purely speculative. Yet, based on the neuropsychological findings presented here, it is apparent that disruption of either prefrontal or medial temporal processes significantly affects recollection at a later time (for a different but related view, see Schacter et al., 1996). Disruption of prefrontal processes would impair executive control of information processing. Thus, individuals with prefrontal dysfunction would exhibit impairment in monitoring and organizing incoming information. These patients would exhibit increased susceptibility to interference from memory, and thus show increased proactive interference. A faulty working memory also appears to be related to problems in remembering the time and place at which episodes had occurred (i.e., source memory impairment). In addition, disruptions of frontal lobe function during the time of retrieval could reduce the ability to recollect remote information if there are few cues for retrieval. Finally, patients with frontal lobe lesions often exhibit confabulatory behavior, involving spurious and invalid intrusions during recollection (see Moscovitch, 1995).

In terms of medial temporal processes, dysfunction would lead to a failure to learn new facts and events. In particular, medial temporal dysfunction would cause problems in relating new information to existing memory representations. As a result of this failure to bind new information with old information, new information would be fragmented and isolated. Automatic activation (i.e., priming) and general dispositions would remain as preseved as in individuals without medial temporal dysfunction.

Thus, disruption in frontal lobe function would reduce the degree to which an experience is encoded and organized as an encapsulated episode. As a result, source memory or memory for when and where an event occurred would be particularly affected. Although disruption in medial temporal function would not affect working memory processes, it would affect the long-term storage of information and specifically reduce the binding of new information to existing representations. These fragmented memories could be in the form of implicit memory and thus may influence habits and dispositions but may not be accessible in a conscious manner. In sum, as a result of either prefrontal or medial temporal dysfunction, the storage of information would be disrupted in such a way as to reduce the ability to retrieve the information at a later time.

Of course, even in normal recollection fragmentary memory and distortions are common occurences. Thus, the phenomenon of reinstated memories could be explained purely on the basis of normal forgetting processes or psychological dysfunction other than those described here. The point here is that when one considers a neurobiologically based conception, disruption of prefrontal and medial temporal processes are the two likeliest candidates for the phenomenon of reinstated memories. Specifically, disruption of either neural systems contribute to problems in the encoding, storage, and later recollection of experiences. Thus, over and above normal forgetting processes, damage to these neural systems would lead to even more frequent experiences of fragmentary and distorted recollections.

Interestingly, these memory disorders could be modulated by the fact that highly emotional responses act to *increase* attentional and memorial processes (see Cahill, Prins, Weber, & McGaugh, 1994). In particular, noradrenergic activation during emotional or stressful experiences can lead to a transient increase in memory storage (LeDoux, 1995; McGaugh, 1995; Sapolsky, 1994). Thus, in conjunction with disruptions to prefrontal or medial temporal processes these fragments may be unusually strong, yet dissociated or unbound to other memory representations. Such fragmented or free-floating memories could be subject to misplacements in time and spatial context. It seem plausible that the phenomenon of reinstated memories could occur for events that were highly traumatic, because the memories for such experiences would be strongly recorded yet very fragmented and poorly bound to spatial-temporal context. In addition, these fragments may be further suppressed or avoided, due to their unpleasant nature.

It is important to note, however, that by this view aspects of a traumatic episode may *never* have been encoded or stored during the experience. In particular, source information or memory for the context in which an event took place would be weak or lost altogether. *Based on this neurobiological conception it is very unlikely that reinstated memory would be recollected in its veridical and complete form.* Indeed, such memories would be even more susceptible to distortions and augmentations, because the threads that bind a memories to existing knowledge would never have been stitched in the first place.

These neurobiological speculations suggest that reinstated memories would be particularly susceptible to distortions and spurious augmentations. It is plausible, however, that aspects of these recollections are based on past experiences. It is also plausible that such fragmentary memories would lie implicitly, outside the bounds of conscious recollection, for an extended period. However, as mentioned earlier, it is impossible for scientific research to *prove* that any subjective experience, such as an unconscious memory of a traumatic event, had occurred or not occurred. Finally, it is plausible that highly suggestible individuals could be susceptible to the *experience* of having a reinstated memory, even though the experience is completely spurious.

To the extent that disruptions in either prefrontal or medial temporal function mediate the phenomenon of reinstated memory, it can be concluded that such recollections will likely be based on fragmentary knowledge. I suspect that cognitive and brain science will only take us this far in the controversy over the validity of reinstated memories. That is not to say, however, that scientific investigations should not be directed to other important clinical and experimental questions concerning the phenomenon of reinstated memory. Science can address a number of important questions, such as defining appropriate therapies for individuals who experience reinstated memories, assessing psychological symptoms associated with such experiences, and determining ways in which emotional memories are remembered across time. It is hoped that an acceptance of the fact that reinstated memories could be partly true, partly fictional, or totally fictional may defuse contentious and strong arguments which suggest that all reinstated memories are either completely veridical or totally false.

ACKNOWLEDGMENTS

Preparation of this chapter was supported by a grant from the National Institute of Mental Health (Grant MH48757).

REFERENCES

Baddeley, A. (1986). *Working memory*. Oxford, UK: Oxford University Press.
Brooks, D. N., & Baddeley, A. D. (1976). What can amnesic patients learn? *Neuropsychologia, 14,* 111–122.
Buckner, R. L., Petersen, S. E., Ojemann, J. G., Miezin, F. M., & et al. (1995). Functional anatomical studies of explicit and implicit memory retrieval tasks. *Journal of Neuroscience, 15,* 12–29.
Cahill, L., Prins, B., Weber, M., & McGaugh, J. L. (1994). b-Adrenergic activation and memory for emotional events. *Nature, 371,* 702–704.
Cohen, N. J., & Squire, L. R. (1980). Preserved learning and retention of pattern analyzing skill in amnesia: Association of knowing how and knowing that. *Science, 210,* 207–209.
Corkin, S. (1968). Acquisition of motor skill after bilateral medial temporal lobe excision. *Neuropsychologia, 6,* 225–265.
Corkin, S. (1984). Lasting consequences of bilateral medial temporal lobectomy: Clinical course and experimental findings in H.M. *Seminars in Neurology, 4,* 249–259.
Damasio, A. R., & Anderson, S. W. (1993). The frontal lobes. In K. M. Heilman & E. Valenstein (Eds.), *Clinical neuropsychology (3rd ed.)* (pp. 409–460). New York: Oxford University Press.
della Rocchetta, A. I. (1986). Classification and recall of pictures after unilateral frontal or temporal lobectomy. *Cortex, 22,* 189–211.
Eslinger, P. J., & Grattan, L. M. (1994). Altered serial position learning after frontal lobe lesion. *Neuropsychologia, 32,* 729–739.
Frith, C. D., Friston, K. J., Liddle, P. F., & Frackowiak, R. S. J. (1991). A PET study of word finding. *Neuropsychologia, 29,* 1137–1148.
Fuster, J. M. (1995). Frontal cortex and the cognitive support of behavior. In F. B.-R. R. A. P.-A. James L. McGaugh (Ed.), *Plasticity in the central nervous system: Learning and memory.* (pp. 149–160). Mahwah, NJ: Lawrence Erlbaum Associates.
Gershberg, F. B., & Shimamura, A. P. (1995). The role of the frontal lobes in the use of organizational strategies in free recall. *Neuropsychologia, 13,* 1305–1333.

Graf, P., Squire, L. R., & Mandler, G. (1984). The information that amnesic patients do not forget. *Journal of Experimental Psychology: Learning Memory and Cognition, 10*, 164–178.

Hastroudi, S., Johnson, M. K., Vnek, N., & Ferguson, S. A. (1994). Aging and the effects of affective and factual focus on source monitoring and recall. *Psychology and Aging, 9*, 160–170.

Haug, H., Barmwater, U., Eggers, R., Fischer, D., Kuhl, S., & Sass, N. L. (1983). Anatomical changes in aging brain: Morphometric analysis of the human prosencephalon. In J. Cervos-Navarro & H. I. Sarkander (Eds.), *Brain aging: Neuropathology and neuropharmocology* (pp. 1–12). New York: Raven Press.

Herman, J. L. (1992). *Trauma and recovery*. New York: Basic Books.

Hirst, W., & Volpe, B. T. (1988). Memory strategies with brain damage. *Brain and Cognition, 8*, 379–408.

Janowsky, J. S., Shimamura, A. P., Kritchevsky, M., & Squire, L. R. (1989). Cognitive impairment following frontal lobe damage and its relevance to human amnesia. *Behavioral Neuroscience, 103*, 548–560.

Janowsky, J. S., Shimamura, A. P., & Squire, L. R. (1989a). Memory and metamemory: Comparisons between patients with frontal lobe lesions and amnesic patients. *Psychobiology, 17*, 3–11.

Janowsky, J. S., Shimamura, A. P., & Squire, L. R. (1989b). Source memory impairment in patients with frontal lobe lesions. *Neuropsychologia, 27*, 1043–1056.

Jetter, W., Poser, U., Freeman, R. B., & Markowitsch, H. J. (1986). A verbal long term memory deficit in frontal lobe damaged patients. *Cortex, 22*, 229–242.

Johnson, M. K., Hashtroudi, S., & Lindsay, D. S. (1993). Source monitoring. *Psychological Bulletin, 114*, 3–28

Jonides, J., Smith, E. E., Koeppe, R. A., Awh, E., Minoshima, S., & Mintun, M. A. (1993). Spatial working memory in humans as revealed by PET. *Nature, 363*, 623–625.

Knight, R. T., Scabini, D., & Woods, D. L. (1989). Prefrontal gating of auditory transmission in humans. *Brain Research, 504*, 338–342.

Knowlton, B. J., Ramus, S. J., & Squire, L. R. (1992). Intact artificial grammar learning in amnesia: Dissociation of classification learning and explicit memory for specific instances. *Psychological Science, 3*, 172–179.

Knowlton, B. J., & Squire, L. R. (1994). The information acquired during artificial grammar learning. In *Journal of Experimental Psychology: Learning, Memory, & Cognition*

Kolodny, J. A. (1994). Memory processes in classification learning: An investigation of amnesic performance in categorization of dot patterns and artistic styles. In *Psychological Science*

LeDoux, J. E. (1995). Emotion: Clues from the brain. *Annual Review of Psychology, 46*, 209–235.

Lindsay, D. S., & Read, J. D. (1994). Psychotherapy and memories of childhood sexual abuse: A cognitive perspective. Special Issue: Recovery of memories of childhood sexual abuse. *Applied Cognitive Psychology, 8*, 281–338.

Loftus, E. F. (1993). The reality of repressed memories. *American Psychologist, 48*, 518–537.

Loftus, E., & Ketcham, K. (1994). *The Myth of repressed memories*. New York: St. Martin's Press.

MacLeod, C. (1991). Half a century of research on the Stroop effect: An integrative review. *Psychological Bulletin, 109*, 163–203.

Mangels, J. A., Gershberg, F. B., Shimamura, A. P., & Knight, R. T. (1996). Impaired retrieval from remote memory in patients with frontal lobe damage. *Neuropsychology, 10*, 32–41.

Marslen-Wilson, W. D., & Teuber, H.-L. (1975). Memory for remote events in anterograde amnesia: Recognition of public figures from news photographs. *Neuropsychologia, 13*, 353–364.

McGaugh, J. L. (1995). Emotional activation, neuromodulatory systems, and memory. In L. S. Daniel (Ed.), *Memory distortions: How minds, brains, and societies reconstruct the past.* (pp. 255–273). Cambridge, MA: Harvard University Press.

McIntyre, J. S., & Craik, F. I. M. (1987). Age differences in memory for item and source information. *Canadian Journal of Psychology, 42*, 175–192.

Metcalfe, J., & Shimamura, A. P. (Eds.). (1994). *Metacognition: Knowing about knowing*. Cambridge, MA: MIT Press.

Milner, B. (1971). Interhemispheric differences in the localization of psychological processes in man. *British Medical Bulletin, 127*, 272–277.

Milner, B., Corkin, S., & Teuber, H.-L. (1968). Further analysis of the hippocampal amnesic syndrome: 14-year follow-up study of H. M. *Neuropsychologia, 6*, 215–234.

Milner, B., & Petrides, M. (1984). Behavioural effects of frontal-lobe lesions in man. *Trends in Neuroscience, 7*, 403–407.

Moscovitch, M. (1995). Models of consciousness and memory. In S. G. Michael (Ed.), *The cognitive neurosciences.* (pp. 1341–1356). MIT Press, Cambridge, MA, US.

Perret, E. (1974). The left frontal lobe of man and the suppression of habitual responses in verbal categorical behavior. *Neuropsychologia, 12*, 323–330.

Petrides, M. (1989). Frontal lobes and memory. In F. Boller & J. Grafman (Eds.), *Handbook of Neuropsychology, Vol 3.* (pp. 75–90). Amsterdam: Elsevier.

Petrides, M., Alivisatos, B., & Evans, A. C. (1995). Functional activation of the human ventrolateral frontal cortex during mnemonic retrieval of verbal information. *Proceedings of the National Academy of Sciences, 92,* 5803–5807.

Petrides, M., & Milner, B. (1982). Deficits on subject-ordered tasks after frontal- and temporal-lobe lesions in man. *Neuropsychologia, 20,* 249–262.

Sapolsky, R. M. (1992). *Stress, the aging brain, and the mechanisms of neuron death.* Cambridge, MA: MIT Press.

Schacter, D. L. (1987). Implicit memory: History and current status. *Journal of Experimental Psychology: Learning Memory and Cognition, 13,* 501–518.

Schacter, D. L., Kaszniak, A. K., Kihlstrom, J. F., & Valdiserri, M. (1991). The relation between source memory and aging. *Psychology and Aging, 9,* 559–568.

Schacter, D. L., Koutstaal, & Norman, K. A. (1996). Can cognitive neuroscience illuminate the nature of traumatic childhood memories? *Current Opinions in Neurobiology, 6,* 207–214.

Schooler, J. W. (1994). Seeking the core: The issues and evidence surrounding recovered accounts of sexual trauma. Special Issue: The recovered memory/false memory debate. *Consciousness & Cognition: An International Journal, 3,* 452–469.

Shallice, T. (1982). Specific impairments in planning. *Philosophical Transactions of the Royal Society of London B, 298,* 199–209.

Shimamura, A. P. (1986). Priming in amnesia: Evidence for a dissociable memory function. *Quarterly Journal of Experimental Psychology, 38,* 619–644.

Shimamura, A. P. (1989). Disorders of memory: The cognitive science perspective. In F. Boller & J. Grafman (Eds.), *Handbook of neuropsychology* (pp. 35–73). Amsterdam, The Netherlands: Elsevier Sciences Publishers.

Shimamura, A. P. (1993). Neuropsychological analyses of implicit memory: Recent progress and theoretical interpretations. In P. Graf & M. E. Masson (Eds.), *Implicit memory: New directions in cognition, development, and neuropsychology* (pp. 265–185). Hillsdale, NJ: Erlbaum Associates.

Shimamura, A. P. (1994a). Memory and frontal lobe function. In M. S. Gazzaniga (Ed.), *The cognitive neurosciences* (pp. 803–813). Cambridge, MA: MIT Press.

Shimamura, A. P. (1994b). The neuropsychology of metacognition. In J. Metcalfe & A. P. Shimamura (Eds.), *Metacognition: Knowing about knowing* (pp. 253–276). Cambridge, MA: MIT Press.

Shimamura, A. P. (1996). The organization of human memory: A Neuropsychological Analysis. In K. Ishikawa, J. L. McGaugh, & H. Sakata (Eds.), *Brain processes and memory* (pp. 163–171). The Netherlands: Elsevier Science.

Shimamura, A. P., & Gershberg, F. B. (1994). Neuropsychiatric aspects of memory and amnesia. In R. E. H. Stuart C. Yudofsky (Ed.), *Synopsis of neuropsychiatry.* (pp. 261–276). American Psychiatric Press, Inc, Washington, DC, US.

Shimamura, A. P., Janowsky, J. S., & Squire, L. R. (1990). Memory for the temporal order of events in patients with frontal lobe lesions and amnesic patients. *Neuropsychologia, 28,* 803–813.

Shimamura, A. P., Jurica, P. J., Mangels, J. A., Gershberg, F. B., & Knight, R. T. (1995). Susceptibility to memory interference effects following frontal lobe damage: Findings from tests of paired-associated learning. *Journal of Cognitive Neuroscience, 7,* 144–152.

Shimamura, A. P., Salmon, D. P., Squire, L. R., & Butters, N. (1987). Memory dysfunction and word priming in dementia and amnesia. *Behavioral Neuroscience, 101,* 347–351.

Shimamura, A. P., & Squire, L. R. (1984). Paired-associate learning and priming effects in amnesia: A neuropsychological study. *Journal of Experimental Psychology: General, 113,* 556–570.

Smith, M. L., & Milner, B. (1984). Differential effects of frontal-lobe lesions on cognitive estimation and spatial memory. *Neuropsychologia, 22,* 697–705.

Squire, L. R. (1987). *Memory and brain.* New York: Oxford University Press.

Squire, L. R. (1992). Memory and the hippocampus: A synthesis from findings with rats, monkeys, and humans. *Psychological Review, 99,* 195–231.

Squire, L. R., J., O., Miezin, F., Petersen, S., Videen, T., & Raichle, M. (1992). Activation of the hippocampus in normal humans: A functional anatomical study of human memory. *Proceedings of the National Academy of Sciences, 89,* 1837–184.

Squire, L. R., Amaral, D. G., & Press, G. A. (1990). Magnetic resonance measurements of hippocampal formation and mammillary nuclei distinguishes medial temporal lobe and diencephalic amnesia. *Journal of Neuroscience, 10,* 3106–3117.

Squire, L. R., Shimamura, A. P., & Amaral, D. G. (1986). Memory and the hippocampus. In J. Byrne & W. Berry (Eds.), *Neural Models of Plasticity* (pp. 208–239). New York: Academic Press.

Stroop, J. R. (1935). Studies of interference in serial verbal reactions. *Journal of Experimental Psychology, 18,* 643–662.

Stuss, D. T., Alexander, M. P., Palumbo, C. L., Buckle, L., Sayer, L., & Pogue, J. (1994a). Organizational strategies of patients with unilateral or bilateral frontal lobe injury in word list learning tasks. *Neuropsychology*, *8*, 355–373.

Stuss, D. T., Eskes, G. A., & Foster, J. K. (1994b). Experimental neuropsychological studies of frontal lobe functions. In F. Boller & J. Grafman (Eds.), *Handbook of Neuropsychology* (pp. 149–185). Amsterdam: Elsevier.

Terr, L. (1994). *Unchained Memories*. New York: Basic Books.

Thomas, G. J. (1984). Memory: Time binding in organisms. In L. R. Squire & N. Butters (Eds.), *Neuropsychology of Memory* (pp. 374–384). New York: Guilford Press.

Warrington, E. K., & Weiskrantz, L. (1968). New method of testing long-term retention with special reference to amnesic patients. *Nature*, *217*, 972–974.

Warrington, E. K., & Weiskrantz, L. (1970). The amnesic syndrome: Consolidation or retrieval? *Nature*, *228*, 628–630.

Weiskrantz, L., & Warrington, E. K. (1979). Conditioning in amnesic patients. *Neuropsychologia*, *17*, 187–194.

Wheeler, M., Stuss, D., & Tulving, E., (1997). Toward a theory of episodic memory: The frontal lobes and autonoetic consciousness. *Pshychological Bulletin*, *121*, 331–354.

Yamaguchi, S., & Knight, R. T. (1990). Gating of somatosensory inputs by human prefrontal cortex. *Brain Research*, *521*, 281–288.

COMMENTARY ON NEUROPSYCHOLOGICAL FACTORS ASSOCIATED WITH MEMORY RECOLLECTION: WHAT CAN SCIENCE TELL US ABOUT REINSTATED MEMORIES?

Michael D. Kopelman, St. Thomas's Hospital, London, United Kingdom

What Shimamura has given us is a characteristically thorough and lucid account of the ways in which the frontal and temporal lobes contribute to memory, and how lesions in these regions produce differing patterns of memory deficits. There is very little in his account with which any neuropsychologist would disagree. What has been particularly original and ingenious, however, has been his account of how frontal and temporal lobe mechanisms might lead to the forgetting and reinstatement of traumatic memories.

There are two features from Shimamura's presentation which I would particularly want to emphasise. First, Shimamura's work provides a model for investigations of memory and executive function in post-traumatic stress disorder (PTSD), and avoids the need to make use of De Wied's animal work, advocated by Yehuda (this volume). In fact, as has been discussed elsewhere in this conference, that work was largely based on studies of the extinction of passive avoidance conditioning in animals. That is a very poor model for human learning, and when inferences from this work were applied to humans - for example, in the use of DD-AVP (vasopressin) and ACTH as "memory pills" - the results proved very disappointing, except where there was overt evidence of pituitary abnormality (Kopelman & Lishman, 1986). For those who seek models of memory on which to base studies of PTSD, I would very strongly recommend that it is to Shimamura, Schacter, Mayes, and others that they should look.

Secondly, it is notable that Shimamura has discussed this topic without any reference to the word "repression." As discussed in my chapter (Kopelman, this volume), I feel that this word gets in the way. It was used in different senses by Freud in different works, and sometimes within the same work, and the first phase of empirical investigations into the concept between about 1915 and 1945 burned out because of problems of definition. My own prediction is that the present phase of empirical studies will encounter similar problems. For example, Brewin's work (this volume) on the effects of a repressive coping style is extremely interesting, but we cannot be sure how it relates to anyone else's concept of "repression". What Shimamura has done is to provide the groundwork whereby we may be able to apply concepts derived from cognitive studies to an understanding of the interaction between affect and memory. You may feel that this is over-optimistic: 20 years ago, Pribam and Gill (1976) thought that most of Freud's earlier concepts could be accounted for in terms of findings from modern neuropsychology. This was premature. Nevertheless, Shimamura has provided the building blocks, whereby we may be able to use notions concerning frontal control and frontal inhibitory mechanisms to give a better understanding of the effects of trauma upon memory.

I do have a few criticisms, not so much of Shimamura's paper as of the state of theory regarding frontal lobe and "executive" function. First, the emphasis in British and European neuropsychology in establishing dissociations between single-cases, and in North American neuropsychology on doing the same thing but using small groups of patients, sometimes blinds us to the great degree of overlap or commonality between what different regions of the brain do. Secondly, there are relatively low correlations between performance on different measures of "frontal" or executive function, emphasising that the frontal lobes may do many different things. Thirdly, executive function, the supervisory system, and working memory are often poorly defined (and I notice that Shimamura has recently incorporated these notions into his account of the frontal lobes).

The overlap between what the frontal lobes and what other structures do has recently been emphasised in a paper by Wheeler, Stuss and Tulving (1997). Taken by surprise at the recurrent finding from PET activation studies that the frontal lobes are important in encoding and retrieval processes in anterograde memory, these authors reviewed past studies of memory in frontal lobe patients. They found that, without exception, patients with frontal lobe lesions always did worse than healthy controls on learning tests (even where the difference was not actually statistically significant), and this was true not only of studies of free recall, but also of most studies of recognition memory. Likewise, Nicola Stanhope and I, in comparing patients with frontal lobe, temporal lobe, or diencephalic lesions with healthy controls, found that these patient groups performed very similarly on measures of verbal and non-verbal short-term forgetting, on a measure of recall and recognition memory (after "matching" for recognition memory and avoiding initial ceiling or floor effects), and that patients with medial frontal lesions also performed satisfactorily on measures of temporal and spatial memory. On the other hand, the frontal lobe patients showed substantially enhanced performance at recall memory, when the material was semantically organised, and patients with lesions invading the dorso-lateral frontal cortex did indeed do very badly on measures of temporal context memory (for review, see Kopelman, 1996). In brief, although there are important differences, these are relatively subtle, and there are many similarities between the performance of patients with frontal lobe lesions and that of patients with diencephalic or temporal lobe lesions.

Secondly, it can be shown that, for example, Korsakoff and Alzheimer patients do very badly across a number of measures of frontal lobe function, including FAS verbal fluency, fluency for alternating birds/colour words, the Weigl test, card-sorting categories and perseverations, cognitive estimates, and WAIS picture arrangement errors. All these tasks correlate significantly with current IQ, and many of them correlate significantly with age, estimated premorbid IQ, and measures of generalised atrophy on CT brain scan (Kopelman, 1991). However, when the effect of current IQ is partialled out, there are indeed statistically significant intercorrelations in the predicted direction between various of these tasks, but the degree of shared variance is generally only 10 to 15 per cent (Kopelman, 1991). This suggests that these various tasks are measuring differing aspects of frontal function.

Thirdly, our models of frontal, supervisory, or executive function tend to be somewhat crude. First, the notion of executive or supervisory function needs tight definition to avoid an accumulation of tests, all measuring somewhat different things, as just discussed. Secondly, there is a danger of circularity in the development of such models. We know that patients with frontal lesions have difficulty in organising and planning memory processes, so we set up a model to account for this: we then find that patients with frontal lobe lesions have difficulty in organising and planning memory processes, but that cannot be used as evidence to validate the model. Thirdly, as the authors of these models are well aware, there is a danger of anthropomorphism - the supervisory pilot in the cockpit of the frontal lobes. These criticisms have been made many times by various authors (e.g., Della Sala & Logie, 1993; Stuss, Eskes, & Foster, 1994; Kopelman, 1994), and Shimamura deliberately attempted to avoid them by pointing out that he was seeking specific mechanisms, rather than postulating some over-riding supervisory or executive system.

As I mentioned, these are criticisms more of the current state of theory regarding executive and frontal lobe function rather than of Shimamura's paper. However, they do need to be grappled with, and they are by no means easy to resolve. What Shimamura (this volume) has given us is a very thorough and clear account of the current state of understanding of what the frontal lobes and temporal lobes do in memory; and he has, thereby, provided us with the ground-rules whereby we can attempt to apply such notions to the immensely important issue of the effects of trauma upon memory.

REFERENCES

Della Sala, S & Logie, R.H. (1993). When working memory does not work: the role of working memory in neuropsychology. In H. Spinnler & F. Boller (eds) *Handbook of neuropsychology, vol 8*, Elsevier Science Publishers, Amsterdam, pp1–62.

De Wied, D. (1984). The importance of vasopressin in memory. *Trends in Neuroscience, 7*, 62–64.

Kopelman, M.D. (1991). Frontal lobe dysfunction and memory deficits in the alcoholic Korsakoff syndrome and Alzheimer-type dementia. *Brain, 114*, 117–137.

Kopelman, M.D. (1994). Working memory in the amnesic syndrome and degenerative dementia. *Neuropsychology, 8*, 555–562.

Kopelman, M.D. (1996). Comments on Mayes & Downes (1996): What do theories of the functional deficit(s) underlying amnesia have to explain? *Memory*, in press.

Kopelman, M.D. & Lishman, W.A. (1986). Pharmacological treatments of dementia (non-cholinergic). *British Medical Bulletin, 42*, 101–105.

Pribram, K. & Gill, M. (1976). *Freud's "Project" re-assessed*, London, Hutchinson.

Stuss, D.T., Eskes, G.A. & Foster, J.K. (1994). Experimental neuropsychological studies of frontal lobe functions. In F. Boller & J. Grafman (eds) *Handbook of neuropsychology, Vol 9*, Elsevier Science BV.

Wheeler, M.A., Stuss, D.T., & Tulving, E. (1997). Toward a theory of episodic memory: The frontal lobes and autonoetic consciousness. *Pyschological Bulletin, 121*, 331–354.

QUESTION AND ANSWER SESSION

Lindsay. Something you said was that frontal development goes on pretty late in childhood, which is one of the reasons that seven-year-olds are so different from five-year-olds in terms of impulsivity control and so on. So if one were wildly speculating on the frontal lobe story, you'd often see these fragmentation and context problems with young children. Consistent with that we know that when young children are tested in source monitoring tests, they can do well in some, but in some conditions will do differentially more poorly than adults even when they are matched on recognition on a source monitoring test. Also we know that divided attention tasks or secondary tasks produce dissociations that in some way mimic what you see with frontal patients, so for example if you have people do a distracting task while the study material is being presented, you can have them be just as good at recognising the studied items as people who didn't do the distracting task, but if you ask them which of two people said it or something that requires them to be able to integrate different aspects of the event they do much more poorly, even down to chance levels. If you think that is evidence from secondary tasks, is that because the frontal lobes are being asked to do two things at once?

Shimamura. Having control subjects perform in dual-task situations has been shown to be a useful way to simulate attentional deficits in patients with frontal lobe lesions. In many instances, findings from dual-task conditions do mimic patient data. However, you can't always make a perfect play between the two. For example, Juliana Baldo, a graduate student in my laboratory, and I have recently conducted a study comparing letter and category fluency in patients with frontal lobe lesions. In fluency tasks, subjects are asked to retrieve as many items as they can for a particular cue. In letter fluency the cues are letters (e.g., F, A, S), and in category fluency the cues are semantic categories (e.g., animals, occupations, fruits). In studies using dual-task conditions in normals, Morris Moscovitch has shown that letter fluency is affected by attention load but category fluency is not. In studies of patients with frontal lobe lesions, Juliana Baldo and I found that the patients are significantly impaired on both tasks, and the impairment is comparable in both fluency conditions. Thus, in this case, findings from dual-task conditions do not simulate the pattern of performance observed in patients with frontal lobe lesions.

Lindsay. There is some evidence of how stress can really narrow attention and one might think that really narrowing attention in certain conditions at least could lead to extremely good memory for perceptual aspects of the experience, but not very good integration of the features you are focusing on. I don't think the data are completely consistent on that. I wanted to ask you to speculate wildly about how we know the performance on direct or implicit memory tests are often hyperspecific, you see encoding specificity in a very big way. I think we are all thinking that fits with this notion that a trigger you might encounter is also hyperspecific and gives you a really good match, and might allow retrieval of decontextualized information. Could you comment on what that would mean for notions that people could be forgetting traumatic events that happen over and over again, every night and in the morning when they see their dad everything seems fine? That is to say, they are encountering very similar events. I had one case in which I consulted in which this woman allegedly every time she went to her therapist he was raping her, but that she kept making appointments because as soon as she walked out she didn't remember. I wonder if you think in encoding specificity terms if you can wildly speculate on that?

Shimamura. That's a tough one. I cannot make a convincing argument in support of that kind of really stark dissociation of consciousness. In terms of the implicit aspects of encoding, there is the notion that such forms of memory are not strongly bound to contextual information, such as source information, which is the term we use to describe memory for spatio-temporal context. If memory for an event is sparse in contextual information, then one can imagine that recollection of that information would be difficult to retrieve based on internal cues. However, one could imagine that certain external triggers could bring up the memory if the external cues closely fit the context of the prior event.

Briere. You are starting from lesion states and then talking about how those lesion states might produce the kind of mechanisms we've described here. I'm really curious if you have any ideas yourself about what psychologically non-lesion states might produce these difficulties to mimic lesion states. Can you front end us at all in terms of suggesting, for example, would the disorganising effects of high emotional states mimic the lesion states from which your data are based? Can you come up with any non-pathogenic or non-physiological lesion explanations that would mimic the kinds of processes you are showing?

Shimamura. I don't know of much research in terms of human work. There is some animal research on emotions and memory, but I don't think there has been much to link specifically frontal lobe dysfunction and memory disorders associated with highly emotional situations. Perhaps, in the future functional neuroimaging techniques may provide some clues concerning emotional states and brain function.

Briere. Can I push you a little bit more on this? It seems to me that what we have so far is that you are providing us with a structural and anatomic or neurostructural interpretation of how these mechanisms might show up later on. The problem we have with the model is that you got there through lesions. What is really fascinating, is that what we have to now replicate, if for instance you use tonic immobility as a biological model for catatonia, then what everyone is trying to work out is how would humans get to that biological state where suddenly the change matches what we know from a biological model? Can we or is anyone aware of any psychological phenomena with high stress, reduced attention processes, or whatever that would be environmental which would front-end us into this model somehow? It's probably not likely since the reports of recovered memories are from sexual as opposed to physical abuse, that I doubt that we are going to find that there were any lesions there. So the next question is how do we get there? This is valid because I suspect that there is stuff here that's valid and also in this model we have to do something different from what you have there if we don't assume there are neurological deficits, which is we have to say, what if someone had the equivalent to these lesion states, and then they didn't? Because they are now adults whatever those physiological phenomena that were going on we might presume they are not going on now. So now what they have are encoding difficulties that possibly cause all kind of problems, but now they have an active functional brain and they have to reconstruct the memory phenomenon. Is there any literature on what these kind of more psychological precursors might be?

Shimamura. That's the crux of the problem, in the case of reinstated memories, you could be dealing with normal functioning people at the time a psychologists see the client. What you need to do to is to assess their cognitive functioning at the time of the event, and of course we can't do that. If one is dealing with a situation in which there are lingering changes, then one can apply a neuropsychological perspective and determine if the changes are consistent with frontal lobe dysfunction or some other neurological dysfunction. Thus, one could obtain a neuropsychological profile of cognitive abilities in clients who report reinstated memories and see if there are any lingering effects.

Widom. I am not sure I can ask this clearly, but I think this is really fascinating. As you may know there's a whole theory about psychopathy which suggests that there are some problems with frontal lesions and certainly there is some experimental evidence which suggests that they perseverate. What if you have a group of children who, for example are physically abused and the physical abuse involved brain damage and the brain damage hits these areas. You would then see some of these behaviours which would provide the link for the people who are trying to explain the psychopathy, certainly the impulsivity, the clinical stuff you talked about at the very beginning with Phineas Gage's personality change that took place. What is interesting to me if you were to follow along the suggestions that you made and only take people who had reinstated memories, you might find a spurious relationship that you would miss because the physiological response which would affect memories would really be due to the childhood trauma and would have nothing to do with the reinstated memory, but you'd never see that because you never had that cell in your design.

Shimamura. That's absolutely right. One can imagine that clients who report reinstated memories are perfectly fine, because all the cognitive/emotional problems happened at the time of encoding and perhaps later when the memory was reported to be unavailable. You mentioned childhood injuries, and there's a slightly different picture when one incurs brain injury as a child. It is commonly reported that if you have a severe head injury before puberty, the array of cognitive deficits are often more widespread, but the amount of recovery is much more significant compared to having a comparable injury as an adult. It has been suggested that during childhood, the brain is more plastic and therefore has a better chance to recover.

Cameron. There is a tremendous complexity about this issue, that there is no all right or all wrong. From my study of women who were sexually abused as children, who said they had always remembered or forgotten, I find a tremendous amount of interest in this biological field and I think we are going to have methods of distinguishing them one day. By and large it's not going to matter that much, to pinpoint everything, but what I have found is that there are tremendous sensory and emotional memories which are very powerful, and what people get back are fragments, especially in the early stages, that eventually fill a picture puzzle and those fragments are intensively bright of what they were feeling, seeing or smelling. They come together so you do get a picture of something like your feelings and what someone else is doing. So a very powerful experience could replicate some of the things you are talking about physiologically.

Shimamura. I think there are cognitive techniques that could be used to study the idea that the act of reconstructing memories from fragments induces the "feeling" of a reinstated memory. I have a very agnostic way of looking at these things, because we don't know a lot about the clinical, biological, and cognitive factors that produce the kind of strong feelings that accompany a reinstated memory that was once unavailable and now is well remembered.

Wagaanar. What struck me about your model is that what you are saying is that these memories cannot be entirely correct and they also cannot be entirely wrong, and this mixture I find in many cases which are presented to us. It would be rather silly to argue that they are correct or wrong, but in the courts we have a line between what is true about these memories and what is not. What you are arguing is that indeed that is the case, the problem is not are they true or false, the problem is that a lot of it is true and a lot of it is false. Does your model tell us in any way how we could go about making a distinction or are we only saying yes that's what happens? Or is it also predicting what kind of aspects are likely true or not?

Shimamura. That is certainly the next step. If I had to speculate, there will be some aspects of an event that are particularly affected if one considered the possibility that the frontal lobes or the hippocampus were dysfunctional during a traumatic event. If there were frontal lobe dysfunction, the event would never have been adequately encoded, and, in particular, source or context memory would be severely affected. That is, the event would be poorly bounded to time and location information. In terms of hippocampal dysfunction, the findings would suggest again that the contextual information would be particularly affected, because the hippocampus appears to facilitate the long-term binding of poly-modal information and not information from specific sensory modalities. I think the main point I wanted to make is that at the time of recollection you have to put fragments together to reconstruct a memory, which is like remembering a story. This story is going to be rather unique for reinstated memories for two reasons: First, because of the high emotional content, the fragments may be charged and quite memorable. Second, frontal or hippocampal dysfunction during a traumatic event could make these fragments even less bound to contextual information than normal memories.

Wagenaar. Would you agree with the statement that if you find corroboration for parts of the story that it still doesn't mean that its all correct?

Shimamura. We have to assume that. Some of the examples of distorted memories where people introduce other events known to have occurred in a different context suggest that reconstructed memories can be mixtures of various past events or even fantasies. The real problem I think we have, particularly for clinicians, is in terms of the therapist's belief systems. To what extent should a clinician believe in the veridicality of a reinstated memory? One can go far and strongly believe in the report or one can be very skeptical and consider reports to be distorted until further corroboration is obtained. On the experimental side, there is something very interesting about the role of context on the retrieval of traumatic memories. Also, in terms of the frontal lobes, we know that this region has something to do with decision processes associated with metacognition, or knowing about what you know. For example, if you have problems in judgments or the "feeling of knowing," then you might feel like you know something when you don't and likewise not feel like you know something when you actually do.

11

ANOMALIES OF AUTOBIOGRAPHICAL MEMORY

Retrograde Amnesia, Confabulation, Delusional Memory, Psychogenic Amnesia, and False Memories

Michael D. Kopelman

United Medical and Dental Schools of Guy's and St. Thomas's Hospital
Lambeth Palace Road
London, United Kingdom

1. INTRODUCTION

Autobiographical memory, its deficits, and its relationship to other aspects of memory, has become a topic of burgeoning research interest during the past fifteen years (Rubin, 1982; Conway, 1990; Conway, Rubin, Spinnler & Waagenaar, 1992). In this chapter, I propose to review findings where autobiographical memory shows deficits or anomalies - in retrograde amnesia, confabulation, delusional memory, and psychogenic amnesia. I will then try to relate these observations to the debate concerning so-called false memories.

2. RETROGRADE AMNESIA

2.1. Autobiographical Memory Loss in Organic Amnesia

The first objective study of remote memory in amnesic patients employed a measure of famous faces (Sanders & Warrington, 1971). However, studies of autobiographical memory followed some time afterwards, including important studies by Zola-Morgan, Cohen and Squire (1983) and Butters and Cermak (1986).

Zola-Morgan et al. (1983) studied seven Korsakoff patients, patient NA (who has diencephalic pathology), post-ECT patients, and alcoholic (non-Korsakoff) and healthy controls. Ten stimulus words were presented to the subjects, who were asked to recall a specific autobiographical memory to each cue word, and then to try to date and to place the memory. The experimenter probed for the presence of a memory and for further details if necessary. Scoring was in terms of the number of memories recalled in the absence

Recollections of Trauma, edited by Read and Lindsay
Plenum Press, New York, 1997

of probing, and also in terms of the "specificity" of the response, whether or not probing had taken place. These authors found that, in the absence of probing, Korsakoff patients and patient NA produced significantly fewer personal memories than their respective controls, and that bilateral ECT patients showed a trend to perform worse within two hours of their convulsion than when retested four months later. On the other hand, Korsakoff patients and patient NA were able to produce autobiographical memories on prompting. Korsakoff patients did not differ significantly from their alcoholic controls in terms of the number of memories produced following prompting, and NA was capable of giving highly detailed responses to probes. Nevertheless, it was notable that the Korsakoff patients had to delve much further back into their remote past in order to retrieve autobiographical memories (mean = 30.4 years) than did comparison groups of non-Korsakoff alcoholics (mean = 20.1 years) or healthy controls (mean = 12.7 years).

Butters and Cermak (1986) studied patient PZ, an eminent scientist who had developed an alcoholic Korsakoff syndrome:

> These authors administered to PZ a series of standard anterograde tests, finding that PZ was unable to show any learning in four presentations of either a verbal or non-verbal paired associate learning task. They then administered the Albert, Butters and Levin (1979) Famous Faces test, finding that PZ's performance was, in general, more severely impaired than many Korsakoff patients, and that he manifested a relatively "flat" temporal gradient, i.e., he was more severely impaired than other Korsakoff patients for his earliest memories. The authors also constructed a test of "famous scientists", including names well known before or after 1965. PZ's results were compared with those of an academic of similar age and prominence: he was severely impaired for scientists prominent both before and after 1965, but particularly for the latter category. Finally, PZ was tested on information derived from his own published autobiography. He was asked about relatives, colleagues, collaborators, conferences, research assistants, research reports, and books mentioned prominently in the autobiography. The results indicated a clear temporal gradient with PZ recalling approximately 65% of items correctly for the period 1916–1930, 40% for 1940–1950, 25% for 1950–1960, and nothing for the period 1960–1980.

Taking all these findings together, Butters and Cermak (1986) concluded that PZ had a severe retrograde amnesia, encompassing autobiographical knowledge as well as public information, and that his autobiographical loss was characterised by a fairly prominent "temporal gradient". Other important case-studies were carried out by Cermak and O'Connor (1983) and Baddeley and Wilson (1986) (for review, see Kopelman, 1993).

Subsequent group studies confirm an extensive retrograde loss, going back many years or decades, in Korsakoff and Alzheimer patients, with a steep temporal gradient (relative sparing of early memories) in Korsakoff patients (Kopelman, 1989) and a gentler temporal gradient in Alzheimer patients (Sagar, Cohen, Sullivan, Corkin & Growdon, 1988; Kopelman, 1989; Greene & Hodges, 1996a, b). The steeper temporal gradient in Korsakoff than Alzheimer patients has been attributed to the relative sparing of early memories in "semantic" form by Korsakoff patients, as well as their severe loss of more "recent" memories because of their heavy drinking (Kopelman, 1989, 1993) (See Figures 1 and 2). Consistent with the view that semantic memory deficits may be contributing to the early remote memory losses of Alzheimer patients, Greene and Hodges (1996a) have attributed some of the remote memory deficits in Alzheimer patients to a loss of semantic knowledge.

It should also be noted that patients with frontal lobe lesions can show severe impairments in autobiographical and other aspects of remote memory. For example, Della Sala et al. (1993) found that 38% of a sample of patients with CT scan delineated lesions

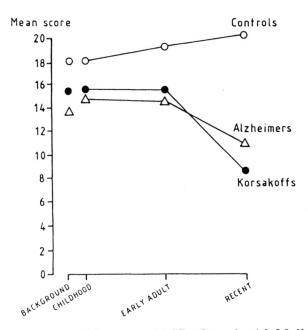

Personal semantic memory. Max. score = 21. SDs: Controls = 1.0–2.9; Korsakoffs = 2.0–4.7; Alzheimers = 3.6–4.25.

Figure 1. Personal semantic memory (facts) in Korsakoff and Alzheimer patients. Reproduced from *Neuropsychchologia*, *27*, 437–460, 1989.

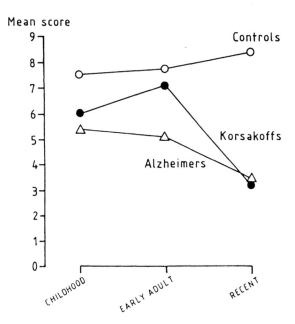

Autobiographical   memory.   SDs: Controls = 1.2–1.5;   Korsakoffs = 1.25–2.1; Alzheimers = 2.1–2.4.

Figure 2. Autobiographical memory (incidents) in Korsakoff and Alzheimer patients. Reproduced from *Neuropsychologia*, *27*, 437–460, 1989.

of the frontal lobes showed severe autobiographical memory loss, including all four patients in their sample who had bilateral lesions. Other studies demonstrating that patients with frontal lesions can show extensive retrograde memory loss include those by Baddeley and Wilson (1986), Mangels, Gershberg, Shimamura and Knight (1996), and Kopelman, Stanhope and Kingsley (1996), the last of whom also found that bilateral lesions produce the most severe impairment. This finding may have implications for understanding the nature of the retrieval deficit in other groups of patients with a remote memory loss, as substantial correlations between remote memory impairment and frontal/executive test performance are sometimes found (e.g., in Korsakoff and Alzheimer patients: Kopelman, 1991; 1992) and recent PET scan studies have emphasised the role of right frontal lesions in the retrieval of memories (Shallice, Fletcher, Frith, Grasby, Frackowiak & Dolan, 1994; Tulving, Kapur, Markowitsch, Craik, Habib & Houle, 1994).

2.2. Dissociations in Retrograde Amnesia

There is also evidence, both from group studies and single-case investigations, of dissociations within remote memory. Since greatest weight in this connection is often given to single-case studies, I will begin with group studies. Kopelman (1989) examined the pattern of intercorrelations amongst a number of remote memory tests in Korsakoff patients (Figure 3). It can be seen that several measures of the more "semantic" aspects of remote memory correlated significantly together (famous news events recall, famous news events recognition, a famous personalities test), and these also correlated significantly with current IQ. Likewise, measures of the recall of autobiographical incidents and of "personal semantic" facts correlated highly and significantly together. On the other hand, these two main clusters of tasks showed only low and non-significant correlations between one another - strong evidence that, at least in Korsakoff patients, these two aspects of remote memory may reflect the operation of independent brain systems. Likewise, Greene and Hodges (1996b) have suggested that differential patterns of decline in Alzheimer patients between autobiographical and the more semantic aspects of remote memory suggest

Test inter-correlations

	MQ	IQ	Famous personalities	News event: recog.	News event: recall	Personal semantic memory
Korsakoff patients *(n = 16)*						
Famous personalities	0.69*	0.54†				
News events: recognition	0.40	0.53†	0.53†			
News events: recall	0.37	0.45†	0.57*	0.78*		
Personal semantic memory	0.35	0.27	0.27	−0.06	0.26	
Autobiographical incidents	0.32	0.19	0.28	0.08	0.17	0.68*

*$P < 0.01$.
†$P < 0.05$.

Figure 3. Remote memory test inter-correlations in Korsakoff patients. Reproduced from *Neuropsychologia, 27,* 437–460, 1989.

independent components, although measures of relative decline are subject to artefacts such as scaling effects and floor effects.

Consistent with these findings is the contrast between a patient reported by De Renzi, Liotti and Nichelli (1987), on the one hand, and patients described by O'Connor, Butters, Miliotis, Eslinger and Cermak (1992) and Ogden (1993). De Renzi et al. (1987) reported the case of a 44-year-old woman who, following an episode of herpes encephalitis, displayed severe impairment of semantic knowledge, contrasting with normal memory for autobiographical events. In particular, she was impaired at any task demanding the retrieval of words or of their meaning, such as confrontation naming, a task requiring differentiation of correct sentences from those containing a semantic error, and a task requiring the classification of (e.g.) specific animal names to categories such as mammals, birds, fishes or insects. She was also impaired at knowledge for public information, e.g., she was unable to provide any information about World War II, the assassination of a recent Italian Prime Minister, or famous people, including Hitler, Mussolini and Stalin. Cueing helped her in some instances, but she was never able to achieve precise recollection. By contrast, O'Connor et al. (1992) have described a patient (LD) with extensive damage in right temporal lobe structures, resulting in a disproportionately severe impairment in the recall of autobiographical incidents, relative to remote semantic information. LD also exhibited severe visuo-perceptual deficits, and the authors argued that she might have a particular difficulty in conjuring up visual images necessary for the retrieval of past autobiographical experiences. Similarly, Ogden's (1993) patient showed damage to occipito-temporal pathways, also manifesting a severe and disproportionate impairment of autobiographical relative to semantic memory.

Consistent with these findings, Kopelman et al. (1996) in a group study of patients with herpes simplex encephalitis, predominantly affecting either the left or right temporal lobe, found that patients with predominantly right-sided lesions were severely impaired in the retrieval of autobiographical memories, whereas patients with unilateral left-sided lesions showed particular difficulty in "labelling" past famous people to word-completion cues. However, such findings should not be interpreted to suggest that the autobiographical and semantic components of remote memory are entirely separable from one another. First, examination of the distribution of the scores in a large series of patients administered remote memory tests does not indicate bimodality (Kopelman & Stanhope, 1996), and, indeed, there are very few outliers. Secondly, both the autobiographical and the more semantic components of remote memory may have retrieval systems in common: in particular, the correlation with frontal/executive tests occurs across a variety of different types of remote memory task (Kopelman, 1991, 1993), may indicate a common, underlying retrieval system.

In addition, a further dissociation has been postulated, in which there is focal or "isolated" retrograde amnesia, in the absence of anterograde memory loss. Whilst it does indeed appear that some degree of disproportion in remote memory impairment can occur (Kapur, Ellison, Smith, McLellan & Burrows, 1992), sometimes representing a differential pattern of recovery from initially severe anterograde and retrograde memory loss (Goldberg, Antin, Bilder, Gerstman, Hughes & Mattis, 1981), whether remote memory loss can ever be "isolated" is much more controversial (Kopelman, 1996). In many of the cases described in the literature, psychiatric factors have not properly been excluded: other cases do, in fact, show quite a severe anterograde memory loss or may reflect a primary semantic memory problem. Even in the remaining cases, it is not always clear that like has been compared with like, or that alternative explanations (such as a deficit in effortful or visual memory) have been excluded (for review, see Kopelman, 1996).

2.3. Summary

Autobiographical memory impairments are an important component of retrograde amnesia in patients with neurological lesions. There is evidence from both single-case and group studies that autobiographical memory may be dissociated from the more "semantic" aspects of remote memory, some patients (particularly those with right temporal lesions) showing a disproportionate impairment of autobiographical memory. On the other hand, frontal retrieval systems may be important in searching for and verifying both autobiographical memories and remote semantic memories. Cases of disproportionate retrograde memory loss have been described, although psychological factors may be important in some of these. To some degree, autobiographical memory loss in organic amnesia may provide a "template", against which to compare phenomena observed in psychologically based memory loss.

3. CONFABULATION

3.1. Characteristics of Confabulation

One of the most intriguing aspects of retrograde amnesia, of direct relevance to the present topic, is confabulation. The "spontaneous" form of confabulation, in which there is a persistent, unprovoked outpouring of erroneous memories, has usually been attributed to frontal lobe pathology (Luria, 1976; Stuss, Alexander, Liberman & Levine, 1978; Kapur & Coughlan, 1980; Baddeley & Wilson, 1986; Moscovitsch, 1989), although DeLuca and Ciccerone (1991) pointed out that it may also arise in transient, confusional states in various types of brain pathology. Baddeley and Wilson (1986) made the important distinction that, whereas some patients with frontal lobe pathology show confabulation, others show aspontaneous, non-fluent, inhibited retrieval of remote memories. Where confabulation arises, these authors commented that it is not limited to test situations: beliefs are held with a strong degree of conviction, and the patients will act on them; they show extreme resistance to argument or persuasion; and the beliefs are frequently preoccupying and bizarre. For example, Baddeley and Wilson described a patient, RJ, of whom they wrote:

> "One weekend while at home with his family, he sat up in bed and turned to his wife, asking her, "Why do you keep telling people we are married?" His wife explained that they were married and had children, to which he replied that children did not necessarily imply marriage. She then took out the wedding photographs and showed them to him. At this point, he admitted that the person marrying her looked like him but denied that it was he."

Johnson (1991) and Dalla Barba (1993a, b) have both argued that confabulation is, perhaps, best viewed as a deficit in reality-monitoring. The latter (Dalla Barba, 1993a, b) indicated that confabulation is usually confined to episodic memory and, where it affects semantic memory, he argued that this results from a deficit in general semantic processing. My colleagues and I (Kopelman, Ng & Van den Broucke, 1996) have recently described a 43-year-old woman who developed profuse confabulation, which extended across episodic, personal semantic, and general semantic memory. This lady's problems followed a Wernicke episode, which gave rise to a residual Korsakoff syndrome. However, shortly after her admission, a carcinoma of the cervix was diagnosed, which eventually resulted in metastases to the posterior part of the brain. The patient was severely impaired on frontal/executive tasks, and her confabulation showed remarkable consistency, despite various vicissitudes in her illness until her death eight months later. She was contrasted with a patient who had bilateral antero-medial frontal lesions, who showed confabulation only within personal semantic memory, and a patient with bilateral temporal lobe pathology, who did not show any confabulation despite severe anterograde amnesia.

Our patient, AB, confabulated spontaneously and floridly throughout her illness. For example, when she was first seen by our team, she told us that she was suffering from measles. On another occasion, she said that she had recently been home to the north of England with her parents, and that her father had suffered a stroke. In fact, her mother had been dead for 4 years and her father for 20 years. Twenty-four hours after being given the diagnosis of cancer, she could not remember this, but, interestingly, she did recall being upset by something the night before, which she attributed to "a commotion downstairs". Subsequently, she became preoccupied with the death of her grandmother which she said had occurred a few weeks earlier, although she got the date and the name of the hospital in which this had arisen wrong. She spent much of the time looking at the London skyline from her room, which she failed to recognise even though she had worked in London for the previous 20 years. She often believed she was in the hospital where she used to work, and when that hospital was pointed out to her from the current bedroom window, she would change her mind but state that she was in yet another hospital in London. She often confused who people were, mistaking doctors for family members or people she had never seen. When asked to describe a research psychologist who was 26 and brunette, she fluctuated in her descriptions from saying that this person was "a petite blonde" to a "rather over-weight, grey-haired 50-year-old woman"!

Within semantic memory, AB made errors about her own age, claiming that she was 30 when she was in fact 43. When administered Dalla Barba's (1993a) Confabulation Battery and asked what had happened in Kuwait in 1989, she claimed that the American army had occupied and taken over Kuwait and part of the Yemen territory, and that there was an uprising within the American army. She said that Robert Maxwell, the businessman who had died at sea, was shot "in an uproar" and that he continued to live quietly. She also perseverated about shootings, claiming that Princess Grace had been shot and survived, living quietly in Monaco. On one occasion, she described Stanley Baldwin as the current British Prime Minister.

We asked AB's brother to help us identify which of her confabulations represented "real memories" inappropriately retrieved, out of temporal context, and conflated together (compare Korsakoff, 1889; see Kopelman, 1995a). We were not able to put a precise figure on this, because there were instances where he was unsure, but there were many memories for which, either he knew that this was the case, or it seemed very possible that this had happened. Furthermore, perseveration seemed to be an important factor in AB's confabulation: for example, the reference to shootings (above) followed AB being asked about President Kennedy's death. Social context may also be an important contributor to the content of confabulations: because AB found herself in hospital, she assumed she was working there (she had indeed held a para-medical job).

This was also illustrated in another patient, who was the innocent victim of a bombing, during which he sustained a fairly severe head injury. This man was attended in hospital for the first 48 hours by very fierce-looking armed police officers but, by the time he came out of his confused state and post-traumatic amnesia (which was 72 hours approximately), the police had gone. During the course of the following week, the patient started to retrieve a few "fragments" of memory from within the amnesic gap, but he mentioned spontaneously that he was having difficulty determining when some of these memories had arisen: for example, he had a memory of looking up at a vehicle on a dark night, but he was unsure in what city this had occurred. However, some weeks later, he gave a graphic description of the police's response to him in hospital. Although this might conceivably have been a retrieved fragment of memory, I think that it is much more likely that this was a confabulation (he was very confused when the police were present) based on what his relatives and friends had told him about the admittedly very tense situation when he arrived in hospital.

Finally, it should also be mentioned that patients and healthy subjects can make fleeting intrusion errors or distortions on memory testing, which are sometimes known (particularly by clinicians) as momentary or "provoked" confabulations. It is important to note that these intrusion errors are made when healthy subjects remember something poorly, and that they resemble qualitatively some of the errors made by patients (Kopelman, 1987a; Hammersley & Read, 1986). For example, some years ago, I asked subjects to remember the logical memory passages from the Wechsler (1945) version of the Memory Scale, finding that healthy subjects tested at a one-week delay made almost as many intrusion errors/momentary confabulations as Korsakoff and Alzheimer patients did at immediate recall, and that they were of a qualitatively similar type. For example, asked about Anna Thompson who was robbed and reported this at a police station, the subjects would commonly say that she was a thief who had been arrested by the police (Kopelman, 1987a).

3.2. Summary

The spontaneous form of confabulation is thought to result from a deficit in reality-monitoring associated with frontal/executive dysfunction. The memories can be profuse, bizarre, preoccupying, and held with absolute conviction. Whilst resulting from underlying frontal pathology, the confabulations may reflect memories retrieved inappropriately and out of temporal context; they may result from perseveration of earlier responses; and they may reflect the social context. In much more moderate form, healthy subjects can produce fleeting distortions or intrusion errors when asked to retrieve something that they remember very poorly, in which case this is known as momentary confabulation. It is obviously of importance for the present debate that certain forms of brain damage can give rise to bizarrely erroneous memories, held with such strength, and that, because of the reconstructive character of memory (Bartlett, 1932), even healthy subjects may show fleeting intrusion errors.

4. DELUSIONAL MEMORIES

4.1. Characteristics of Delusional Memories

Superficially very similar are the delusional memories which can arise in certain forms of psychotic disorder, particularly schizophrenia. These delusional memories, which are rare, should be distinguished from the general run of delusions (common in schizophrenia), which often have a memory component. Strictly speaking, a delusional memory consists of either a true memory, which gives rise to a deluded interpretation, or (more commonly) a false memory arising in the context of psychosis. Many of its characteristics as a phenomenon resemble those of the spontaneous form of confabulation, as described by Baddeley and Wilson (1986). Commonly, it is only the context in which the phenomenon arises which distinguishes delusional memory from confabulation, i.e., psychosis rather than organic amnesia (Kopelman, 1987b; Buchanan, 1991).

Some years ago, I saw a 33-year-old man, who believed that he had been hired by Lord Lucan, a prominent English aristocrat, to kill his lordship's wife. He gave a graphic account of the meeting at which this hiring took place. He also recalled that he had indeed assaulted Lady Lucan and that he had killed both Lord Lucan and the couple's nanny, a reference to a notorious murder which had in fact occurred in London in 1973. His account was so convincing that I was just about to telephone the police when the patient told me about the "angels" on the bonnet of his car. This delusional memory did, in fact, occur in the context of other "first rank" symptoms of schizophrenia (the patient's first episode), and there was no evidence of any organic pathology. The delusional preoccupations were substantially ameliorated following treatment with thioridazine (a neuroleptic medication), although, as commonly occurs in such cases, the "memory" was never completely abolished.

More recently, my colleagues and I (Kopelman, Guinan & Lewis, 1995) have described a 47-year-old clerical worker, who had been studying for a PhD in English literature and is extremely articulate about Chaucerian and Shakespearean literature.

This patient (WM) claimed that, in 1970, she had been working on a fruit-picking farm during the summer in East Anglia, when she encountered an internationally famous orchestral conductor, who also happened to be fruit-picking there. No words were exchanged between them, but she claims that, subsequently, he traced her and followed her in London, and that her friends challenged him about this. She says that she retreated to a rural town, where her parents were then living, but the musician followed her there. She believes that he was in love with her, and she says that she was prepared "to meet him half way". She also claims that his parents had died around that time, that he had recently been divorced, and that he himself was psychologically unsettled at the time they met. Subsequently, he stopped pursuing her, and they have exchanged only a few words since, when she waited for him outside stage doors. However, she has written to him on a regular basis, although she does not receive any reply. On one occasion, he was sent a final demand by an expensive London store after she had purchased a wedding dress and arranged for the bill to be sent to him. On another occasion, she deposited her suitcases outside his flat, intending to move in.

It has to be emphasised that this lady is a very sober, apparently sensible lady, tidily dressed, somewhat anxious looking, and obviously intelligent. As already mentioned, she talks articulately about her PhD studies and about domestic problems in her life. However, her tone will switch immediately she is asked about the conductor, in which case a whole flow of detail about their recent interactions emerges (they communicate by "telepathy"). There is no evidence that the meeting on the fruit farm or any other meeting has ever taken place, and the patient describes a number of "first rank" symptoms of schizophrenia, which show little response to medication (she says that she takes this because "he" insists on it). It should be emphasised that all WM's abnormal beliefs appear to derive from her "memory" of meeting the conductor on a fruit farm.

In this latter case, my colleagues and I (Kopelman et al., 1995) carried out a number of cognitive tests and found that, unlike virtually all the patients with spontaneous confabulation described in the scientific literature, WM does not show any evidence of executive or frontal dysfunction. Somewhat similarly, David and Howard (1994) described four patients with delusional memories. A limited range of cognitive tests was carried out, but these included the cognitive estimates task (Shallice and Evans, 1978), on which none of their patients showed evidence of frontal or executive dysfunction. Their patients, like ours, were in general cognitively intact, although our patient and one of theirs showed impairment on a face recognition memory task. David and Howard (1994) argued that the perceptual characteristics of their patients' delusional memories were stronger than real memories, thereby misleading an "evaluation system" to accept the delusional memories as real, despite their inherent implausibility.

4.2. Summary

Delusional memories share many characteristics with "spontaneous" confabulation - they are held as absolute convictions, not amenable to argument, arising apparently spontaneously, and they are often bizarre and preoccupying. They differ in that they occur in the context of psychosis, rather than amnesia, and recent research suggests that frontal/executive dysfunction is not a necessary correlate of delusional memory (despite being almost universally found in spontaneous confabulation). In the present context, it is pertinent to note that psychiatric disorder (usually schizophrenia) as well as neurological disorder (organic amnesia) can give rise to false memories, held with absolute conviction.

5. PSYCHOGENIC AMNESIA

5.1. Fugue States

In recent years, my colleagues and I have seen a number of patients in an apparent fugue state, defined as a sudden loss of autobiographical memory and the sense of personal identity, usually associated with a period of wandering, and which resolves (most commonly in a few hours or days) to leave an amnesic gap for the period of the memory loss (Kopelman, 1995b).

Patient KG (Kopelman, Green, Guinan, Lewis & Stanhope, 1994) was a 55-year-old man, who had been charged with embezzlements from his work place that had taken place during the course of approximately one year. He claimed amnesia for the offences. In addition, he described two fugue episodes, when he went wandering for several hours and had no memory of what he had done during that time. The first of these occurred the day after he was charged with the offences, and, on that occasion, he went to buy a newspaper in South London at approximately 7.30 in the morning, and the next thing he could remember was "coming round" in the main railway station at Glasgow in Scotland. He asked a man where he was, and then was taken to a police station. It was approximately 5 pm. Glasgow had been Mr KG's home town, but he had not been there for approximately 30 years. He had no memories of the journey, but he possessed a valid ticket. He was admitted to the Royal Infirmary in Glasgow, where all investigations were normal. The second episode occurred three months later, the day after the police had searched his home. On this occasion, the patient apparently wandered through south-east and east London for several hours, being found by a vicar, at which point he was complaining of sore feet. Further investigations did not reveal anything. KG also complained of a progressive memory impairment which was, initially, of relatively mild severity, and which was also complicated by concomitant features of depression. Neuropsychological testing did not provide any evidence of fabrication, but it did indicate an impairment in anterograde memory, which slowly became worse through time. KG served a short prison sentence, during which he developed transient neurological signs, after which an MRI scan revealed multiple, small cortical and subcortical infarcts, including a large one involving the left hippocampus and parahippocampal gyrus. In brief, the circumstances of his disappearances (a severe precipitating stress and concomitant depression) seemed to indicate authentic fugue episodes, and the clinical and neuropsychological evidence confirmed a mild-to-moderate organic memory impairment of vascular aetiology.

Patient AT (Kopelman, Christensen, Puffett & Stanhope, 1994) "came round" on the London Underground unaware of who or where she was, and appearing rather perplexed. She carried a bag, containing some clothes and an envelope addressed to a name which (subsequently) turned out not to be hers. She was taken to the nearest hospital, before being transferred to the present author's unit. Detailed assessments were conducted at various time-points during the course of the following year. She performed normally on virtually all tests of anterograde memory, including recognition memory and word-completion priming tasks. However, she showed an extremely severe impairment of retrograde memory on both autobiographical and public information (news event) tasks with a prominent recency effect (Figure 4), which was quite different from the temporal gradient normally seen in patients with organic amnesia (although similar to some of those patients reported to have so-called "isolated" retrograde amnesia). She had an American accent, but it took us 15 months to find out who she was with the help of Scotland Yard's Missing Persons Bureau. After she had been identified, she failed to show normal word-completion priming for the names of people and places she had known before the onset of her amnesia, although word-completion priming for post-onset names was normal. Moreover, on a recognition version of this task, her "feelings-of-knowing" for pre-onset names and places were no greater than for "baseline" items (unknown to her), which was interpreted as evidence of some degree of simulation. Her memory largely recovered after we performed an Amytal abreaction with the patient now knowing that we knew all about her from her family.

After discovering the circumstances of AT's disappearance from the United States, and following further information from her family, it seemed to us likely that she had indeed experienced an authentic fugue state lasting approximately a week, but that, thereafter, she was at least partially simulating, despite her excellent performance on most laboratory-designed tests for simulation (Kopelman, Christensen, Puffett & Stanhope, 1994). Moreover, this does not mean that AT was deliberately malingering in the sense of being fully aware of what she was doing: AT very much gave the impression of being someone who had to come to believe her own "script" (Conway, 1990). From such behaviour, one can see how so-called "multiple personality" might evolve, if differing scripts

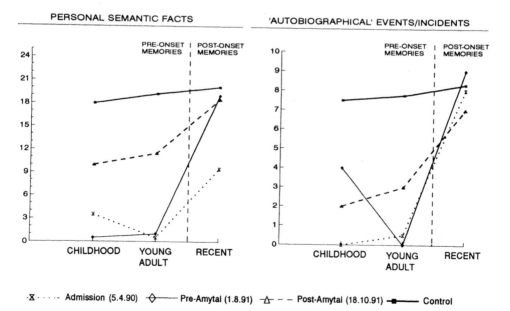

Figure 4. Personal semantic and autobiographical memory in patient AT. Reproduced from *Neuropsychologia, 32,* 675–691, 1994.

were encouraged and reinforced by doctors and psychologists as well as the outside world (Merskey, 1992, 1995). Interestingly, there were instances when AT was able to recognise something (such as the hotel she had initially stayed at in London) or "knew" something (for example, that pictures shown to her must be of her relatives) without being able to remember or consciously recollect anything else about them.

    Similar phenomena have been described by a patient recently under the care of the author. This man, who had had marital problems, disappeared from his home elsewhere in the country, shortly after finding his wife with a male friend at the family home. He had no memory for what happened in the ensuing seven days, but "came round" on a park bench with sore feet, still unable to remember his name or very much about his past. He was admitted to hospital, shortly after which he recovered his name, and he was identified by the Missing Persons Bureau. His memory impairment steadily resolved, and he was able to describe quite a lot about his past when administered the Autobiographical Memory Interview (Kopelman, Wilson & Baddeley, 1990), although significant gaps still remained. These gaps particularly concerned matters involving his wife and his work. Interestingly, he was able to describe a visit to London with his wife some months earlier,

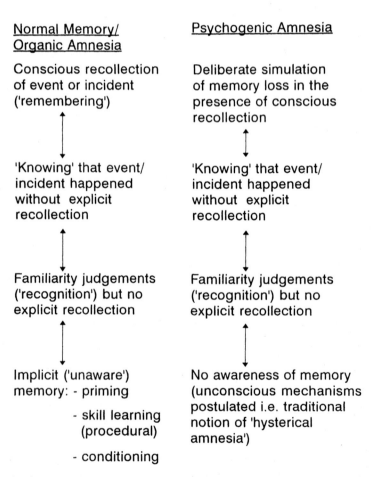

Figure 5. Levels of awareness in memory and amnesia. Reproduced from *Neuropsychologia*, *32*, 675–691, 1994.

and he "knew" of places he had visited, although the interconnecting memories, explicit recollection of what they had done, and any affective feeling for that period were absent - in Coriat's (1907) term, these memory fragments appeared "strange and unfamiliar". On the other hand, this patient was aware of emotional distress concerning his marital breakdown, despite the fact that he had very little "explicit" recollection of his wife. On the basis of these and similar observations, Kopelman (1995b) postulated that there can be a hierarchy of awareness in psychogenic amnesia (Figure 5), similar to that seen in normal memory or organic amnesia. In brief, there can be varying levels of awareness in memory, which may include "knowing" or recognition without full "conscious recollection" (compare Gardiner & Java, 1990).

Elsewhere, I have reviewed the factors which appear to predispose to fugue episodes (Kopelman, 1987b, 1995b). In brief, there is always a severe precipitating stress, such as marital or emotional discord, bereavement, financial problems, stress during wartime, or a charge of offending. Secondly, depressed mood is an extremely common antecedent, as was emphasised by Berrington, Liddell and Foulds (1956). (Both KG and our recent patient had been treated for depression by their general practitioners before their fugue episode occurred). Suicidal ideas just before or following a fugue are also common. Thirdly, there is commonly a past history of a transient, organic amnesia from head injury, epilepsy, or severe alcohol intoxication (so-called alcoholic blackouts). In brief, it appears that patients who have experienced a previous, transient organic amnesia, and who have become depressed and/or suicidal, are particularly likely to go into a fugue in the face of a severe, precipitating stress. Schacter (1996) has also emphasised how common is a past history of head injury or other organic pathology. Schacter (1996) drew attention to recent research indicating that glucocorticoid steroids, secreted in response to acute or chronic stress, may damage neurons (see also van der Kolk, 1994). In particular, there is evidence that patients on prednisolone for one year or more may show impaired explicit but not implicit memory (Keenan, Jacobson, Soleymani & Newcomer, 1995), although, unfortunately, that paper gave insufficient documentation concerning what clinical disorders required these patients to be on prednisolone in the first place. Furthermore, a careful study by Bremner et al. (1995) showed that veterans from the Vietnam War with posttraumatic stress disorder (PTSD) had a statistically significant 8 % smaller right hippocampal volume on MRI scan, compared with non-veteran control subjects, although there was no difference in any other volumetric measurement. The authors attempted to control for a history of substance abuse, and it is certainly intriguing to see whether this finding will be replicated. On the basis of these and other findings, Schacter (1996) speculated that reduced hippocampal volume, perhaps brought about by excessive exposure to glucocorticoids, may contribute to the memory problems of patients with dissociative identity disorder, given the frequent occurrence of head trauma in the past histories of these patients. Whilst these observations are certainly intriguing, my own suspicion is that the main relevance of a past history of organic amnesia is as a learning experience.

However, I am increasingly struck by how difficult it can be to separate out organic factors (including substance misuse) from psychological stresses in the aetiology of transient amnesias, and how the two may often interact to produce their effects.

Patient AH was a middle aged white male who arrived at our Central London Accident and Emergency Department at 2 o'clock one morning, claiming to have no memory for his name, his past, or where he came from. His last memory was of being in the home where he had been living for some weeks on the south coast. He had fragments of memory concerning being attacked by someone who had stolen his money from his wallet, and of going into a police station where he said that he had been sworn at. He then asked a passer-by about the nearest hospital, and he was brought to our Accident Department. He was a well-kempt, co-operative man, who looked a bit tense and anxious. By the time that he was examined on the ward, he was orientated in person as well as time and place. He was very preoccupied about his memory loss, and he wanted this investigated. Approximately 24 hours after admission, he started to show signs of alcohol withdrawal and he was put on medication to suppress the symptoms of this. He also began to appear increasingly distressed and depressed, especially as patchy memory of his past started to return, and treatment with an antidepressant was commenced. It later emerged that he had been depressed for some time since his third marriage had broken up; and he had been living very unhappily in a hostel on the south coast. We found out from other sources that there had been some kind of altercation in the hostel which immediately preceded his disappearance, although he had no memory for this. His memories gradually started to return, and we learned that he had had a long history of alcohol abuse. He disappeared from the ward on one occasion, returning intoxicated, and he subsequently discharged himself - we thought to resume drinking. Although his memory loss had many features of a fugue (loss of personal identity and of all his past autobiographical memories), it seems likely that it was precipitated by alcohol abuse.

More recently, I have been seeing patient SB, who has had a series of fugue-like episodes. In one of the first of these, she remembered leaving her home in her car to go shopping, and the next thing she recalled was finding herself at the admissions desk of a South London hospital (where she had previously worked, and where her former partner had died), not knowing how she had got there. Two hours had elapsed. She has had a series of these episodes, in the context of severe, and at times suicidal, depression following a series of adverse life events - bereavements involving a partner, child, and grandchild; two episodes of rape, one at knife point; and the experience of being stalked by her assailant. At the same time, SB has been a heavy drinker for some considerable time, and her intake has increased markedly in response to these traumas - it is quite common for her to consume a bottle of vodka, a bottle of brandy, or a bottle of wine in an evening. In these circumstances, it is very difficult to disentangle whether alcohol or severe stress and depression are the cause of her memory loss and, in view of the frequency of the attacks, I suspect that the two may interact in some way.

5.2. Amnesia for Offences

Many offenders claim amnesia for their offence. This is most common in homicide cases, but it also occurs in other violent crime and, occasionally, in shoplifting or fraud. Taylor and Kopelman (1984) found that 26% of homicide cases claimed amnesia, and 8% of other violent offenders. Other studies give figures between about 20% and 45% of those accused of homicide (Leitch, 1948; Guttmacher, 1955; O'Connell, 1960; Bradford & Smith, 1979; Parwatikar , Holcomb & Meninger, 1985).

Taylor and Kopelman (1984) found that these amnesic offenders fell into three main groups. First, there was a small group of patients whose psychosis interfered with encoding and/or retrieval, such that they gave a completely erroneous account of what had happened, sometimes amounting to a delusional memory.

A young man, who had a history of recurrent hospital admissions for schizophrenia, reported that he had gone into a fish and chip shop, that he had looked into the eyes of a Chinese serving woman, and that he had asked for cod roe. He then said the lights had become bright, and that he had fainted, and he could not remember anything else. In fact, there had been no loss of consciousness nor any report of an initial altercation - he had suddenly picked up a bar and started smashing the ovens. (Taylor & Kopelman, 1984)

In very occasional cases, such anomalous or even delusional memories may result in charges being brought inappropriately:

> A sailor claimed that he had killed an acquaintance at sea, following an angry dispute; and he gave a detailed and consistent account of the killing. He was charged with murder, but it emerged that he had been floridly psychotic at the time of his confession, and that he was referring to a voyage three years earlier, when nobody had been lost at sea. Eventually, he was acquitted, and his "confession" was attributed to a delusional memory, but by that stage, he had already served a lengthy period in prison on remand. (Taylor & Kopelman, 1984)

Secondly, a larger group of subjects had committed their offence in the context of heavy alcohol intoxication, and in all of these cases, there was a prolonged history of alcohol abuse. In short, the amnesia for the incident in these cases amounted to an alcoholic blackout. The third and most interesting group of amnesic offenders involved "crimes of passion". These were all homicide cases, all but one involving a lover, spouse, or close partner as victim, each episode being unplanned and unpremeditated, and occurring in a state of extreme emotional arousal, sometimes against a background of depression. It is easy to speculate that the offence was too painful to remember, and O'Connell (1960) gave examples of statements by offenders which did indeed suggest that this was the case.

The most obvious explanation for these amnesias is that the subjects are simulating in the hope that the charges against them might be reduced. For example, Schacter (1986, 1996; Schacter, Norman & Koutstaal, in press) has argued that "most experts agree that numerous alleged amnesias for violent crimes are feigned", although he did not specify who these experts were. Against the authenticity of such amnesias, he cited the case of Sirhan Sirhan who assassinated Robert Kennedy. On the other hand, he also described another patient, who killed his wife for suspected infidelity, was amnesic for this, and subsequently suicided. Schacter (1996) described this latter type of case as "exceedingly rare". But he has turned the matter on its head: the criminal justice system deals daily with the victims of domestic tragedy - people who kill their spouse or lover in states of extreme emotional arousal, which accounts for approximately 75% of homicides in the UK (Bluglass, 1979) of whom as many as 30% go on to suicide (West, 1967). It is the political assassins and terrorists who constitute a small minority. Hence, the Sirhan Sirhan example is very atypical.

The account of their amnesia that offenders give is strikingly consistent across different individuals and, elsewhere (Kopelman, 1987c, 1995b), I have put forward four main arguments, supporting the case that many of these amnesias are genuine. First, many amnesic subjects have been described in the literature who either reported their own crime or failed to take measures to avoid their capture. This makes an account of amnesia as simulation to avoid punishment seem less plausible.

> A 40-year-old Egyptian was married to an English woman with two young children. When he discovered that his wife was having an affair with a musician, he became depressed, and he was treated with an antidepressant as an outpatient at his local hospital. During the afternoon of the offence, he had a furious row with his wife, during which he threatened to kill the musician. Later, he could recall going to kiss his daughter good night, but he could not remember anything after that until the police arrived. However, he had in the meantime telephoned the police, and he was subsequently charged with the murder of his wife by stabbing. (Taylor & Kopelman, 1984, quoted by Kopelman, 1995b)

> A 67-year-old man had apparently battered his wife to death without any apparent motive, before telephoning the police and giving himself up. On their arrival, he reported that he had no memory of the actual attack, but that he recalled standing over the body realising that he had

been responsible for his wife's death. His memory had not cleared by the time of the Court hearing. (Gudjonsson & MacKeith, 1983)

Secondly, it should be noted that the factors which have been associated with amnesia in offenders overlap with those which have been implicated in cases of impaired recall by the victims or eyewitnesses of crime - notably violent crime, extreme emotional arousal, and alcohol intoxication (see e.g., Kuehn, 1974; Clifford & Scott, 1978; Loftus, 1979; Yuille & Cutshall, 1986; Yuille, 1987; Deffenbacher, 1988). Thirdly, in English law and in much of the United States, amnesia per se does not constitute either a barrier to trial or any defence. For amnesia to contribute to the question of responsibility, other issues have to be raised, such as epilepsy or other forms of organic brain disease. Most lawyers are aware of this, but this does not stop the clients continuing to claim amnesia, even in instances where recall of what actually happened would be helpful to their cause. (See the example of the sailor above). Finally, the demarcation between "conscious" malingering and "unconscious" forgetting may not be clear-cut. O'Connell (1960) quoted a non-amnesic offender describing how he let the memory " drift into the background ... like putting something into ... a safe and locking it away". By comparison, amnesic subjects described having "buried everything about (the) case" and feeling that recollection would be "so (horrifying) that I just can't remember anything" or that "there is something in my mind ... it seems to be forming a picture and then ... my head hurts ... it gets all jumbled up again". In terms of Figure 5 (above), such reports might be characterised as "knowing" without remembering, and similar phenomena could arise in amnesia for sexual abuse (below).

5.3. Summary

Examples have been given of psychogenic amnesia in fugue states, where it is global, and in offences, in which it is situation-specific. In all these cases, the question of possible organic aetiology or of simulation always arises. Unequivocal organic causes (such as in epilepsy or hypoglycaemia) must, of course, be identified, and various methods are available for detecting simulation (Kopelman, 1995b). However, these various factors can also interact. Patients in fugue have often had a past history of organic amnesia, which probably served as a learning experience, and it does appear that some patients may come to adopt their own "scripts" as they emerge from an "authentic" amnesia. Alcohol and depression seem to be common precursors to both fugue episodes and to amnesia for crime and, in the latter case, the "obviousness" of the possible motive does not necessarily undermine the genuineness of the experience. Given the extensive literature on memory failure in the eyewitnesses and victims of crime, it should hardly be surprising that recall can fail in offenders. Indeed, this is an important point in the present context - both the alleged perpetrators and the alleged victims of an offence may be liable to omissions, distortions, or frank intrusion errors in their recall of an event.

6. THE NOTION OF REPRESSION

6.1. Definitions and Empirical Research

These observations lead straight to repression, but this turns out to be a very fickle notion indeed. Schacter (1996) pointed out how Freud moved from arguing that repression was an "intentional" process (see Freud & Breuer, 1895) to its becoming an unconscious defence. Ceci and Loftus (1994) have pointed to a distinction between complete and partial repression, and between that associated with early Oedipal conflicts versus that associated with later trauma. They argued that, for empirical researchers, such distinctions amount to trying to hit a moving target because common terms are used to convey different meanings by different writers. Fonagy and Target (1996) have identified three stages at which Freud employed the term "repression" in differing ways, in the last of which primary and secondary repression were distinguished. These various distinctions are not exhaustive, or even the most important as far as empirical research is concerned. When he wrote the *Introductory Lectures*, Freud (1915/1917) considered that the outcome of repression was anxiety, whereas by the time he wrote the *New Introductory Lectures* (Freud, 1933), the outcome of repression was the alleviation of anxiety. Even within the same book, Freud used repression in different ways, such that in the *Introductory Lectures*, he employed the term to mean both a general tendency to recall pleasant rather than unpleasant memories, as well as to refer to the specific outcome of an unconscious conflict between the reality and pleasure principles.

There has been a long history of empirical investigations into the notion of repression, although the first phase of these investigations petered out precisely because of these problems in definition (e.g., Pear, 1914; Wolf, 1914; Meltzer, 1930; Thomson, 1930; Fisher & Marrow, 1933; Gilbert, 1938; Edwards, 1942). Whilst it has clearly been established that pleasant memories are more speedily and more readily retrieved than unpleasant memories in healthy subjects (Lishman, 1974; Master, Lishman & Smith, 1983) and, more interestingly, that this trend is reversed in depression (Lloyd & Lishman, 1975), such findings appear to corroborate Freud's more general remarks about pleasant and unpleasant memories, but say nothing about the role of unconscious conflict. On the other hand, attempts to introduce conflict into the experimental situation (e.g., Edwards, 1942) are vulnerable to the psychoanalysts' saying that the "right" sort of conflict has not been measured - Ceci and Loftus's (1994) moving target.

Many of the recent empirical studies have been stimulated by the false memory debate. Findings have been reviewed in a number of publications (Loftus, 1993; Pope & Hudson, 1995; Schacter, 1996; Schacter et al., in press). In particular, Pope and Hudson (1995) sought studies which attempted to test whether memories of childhood sexual abuse had been repressed. Omitting single-case studies, the authors found only four investigations bearing on this issue - Herman and Schatzow (1987); Briere and Conte (1993); Loftus, Polonsky and Fullilove (1994); and Williams (1994). They criticised these studies on the basis that *either* the original abuse had not been corroborated, *or* the findings were heavily dependent on self-report, in which case a report of past forgetting needed to be corroborated. Moreover, the reasons for failure to report a past abuse can be various and need to be explored. On the basis of these observations, the authors concluded that "present evidence is insufficient to permit the conclusion that individuals can "repress" memories of childhood sexual abuse". On the other hand, given the difficulty of corroborating past abuse or past forgetting, there was suggestive evidence within the cited studies that subsamples of the subjects involved might have experienced forgetting at some time (19% in the Loftus et al. (1994) study).

For what it is worth, my own clinical experience is that complaints of memory loss for child abuse tend to be rather different from the memory loss seen in fugue states or reported by offenders. In fugue states, there is a global loss of memory while the fugue lasts. In amnesia for offences, there is also a severe loss of memory, which encompasses a discrete period, usually a matter of a few minutes up to about one hour (longer if alcohol is implicated). In both cases, cueing seldom brings back the memories. On the other hand, I have quite frequently seen patients who have been described by psychotherapists or others as having memory loss for a period of child abuse, but when one talks through the experience with the subject, there is usually a vagueness or "cloudiness" in their memory, without there being complete forgetting. In one particular example, patient DV developed late-onset epilepsy and apparently focal retrograde amnesia following what he considered a toxic exposure to chemicals at his place of work. On the Autobiographical Memory Interview (Kopelman et al., 1990), he did indeed show a severe and disproportionate memory loss, such that he performed far worse than the mean scores of Alzheimer and Korsakoff patients for childhood and early adult memories, but he was performing entirely normally for "recent" memories. On the other hand, when he was not challenged with a memory "test", but I took him through his past life in an informal manner (somewhat akin to the so-called "cognitive interview"), I found that he could recall a lot about his past life, including an episode of homosexual rape at puberty, which he said had been very traumatising. In brief, it may be that such distressing memories are put to the back of the subject's mind, in a manner analogous to what O'Connell (1960) described in some offenders; they are not thought about or rehearsed; and then they are forgotten until the appropriate context or retrieval cues are provided. Alternatively, in some patients, the memories may never be actually forgotten, but they are retained in a vague, unelaborated form, because they have never been rehearsed (compare Schacter, 1996; Schacter et al., in press).

Should fugue states and amnesia for offences be taken as evidence of repression? Alternatively, do they arise from "dissociation" in abnormal states of arousal? In my writings, I have usually tried to avoid the use of either of these terms, partly because of the theoretical baggage with which they come (and conflicting baggage at that), and partly because these notions in fact explain very little, if you strip that baggage aside. I would favour that we start to examine whether we can provide an explanation of these phenomena in terms more akin to the general memory literature and studies of organic amnesia: for example, in terms of faulty encoding in states of high emotional arousal, the context of retrieval, encoding-retrieval interactions and/or state-dependency, the interaction of affect and memory processes, or the interaction between frontal control mechanisms and retrieval cues.

6.2. Summary

There has been a long history of empirical investigations into repression. The early studies were fraught by the conflicting definitions of the term, and consequently petered out in a stalemate. The more recent studies have concentrated upon child sexual abuse. Given the sheer difficulty of carrying out studies to the standard which Pope and Hudson (1995) would require, the findings can be regarded as, at best, equivocal and, at worst, unconvincing. It may be more appropriate to examine instances of memory loss employing concepts derived from cognitive psychology.

7. SEXUAL ABUSE AND FALSE MEMORIES

7.1. Prevalence and Issues

There can be little doubt that (remembered) sexual abuse is widely prevalent. Mullen, Martin, Anderson, Romans and Herbison (1993) conducted a postal survey of 2,250 women in Dunedin, New Zealand, of whom 61% replied (71% of those under 65).

All those reporting some form of child sexual abuse were interviewed, as well as a comparison group not reporting a history of abuse, and current and past psychiatric symptoms were recorded using standardised methods. Thirty-two percent of the sample reported some form of sexual abuse before the age of sixteen, 20% describing genital contact, and 6% reporting actual or attempted intercourse. There was a raised prevalence of subsequent depression, anxiety disorder, drug dependence, alcohol abuse, eating disorders, and suicide attempts, with the prevalence of many of these complaints being related to the severity of the original abuse. However, the authors pointed out that these complaints were very varied, and that they were not necessarily present in abuse victims; and consequently, other factors must have interacted with the history of abuse in producing them. A subsequent paper examined these other factors (Romans, Martin, Anderson, O'Shea & Mullen, 1995). Obviously this study investigated those who, by definition, remembered the abuse, and the data were entirely dependent upon self-reports. Oliver (1993) has emphasised the need to obtain information from a wide variety of sources, bringing to attention cases of documented abuse (not necessarily sexual), which were not reported in self-report surveys, some of which Oliver attributed to "memory blockages".

On the other hand, it is, of course, equally devastating to be accused of an offence which was not committed. Citing the Loftus (1993) shopping mall experiment amongst many others, Lindsay and Read (1994) concluded their extensive review by stating:

"One of the most unnerving implications of the cognitive psychological research reviewed in this paper is that people can be very confident in their memories and beliefs and, at the same time, very wrong. People can believe they are remembering events in their own lives when those events never happened. Experts can believe they are observing powerful correlations when none actually exist. It is difficult to confront this evidence of our fallibility, but that evidence is overwhelmingly clear. We take this cautionary message to heart. Perhaps we are wrong. Perhaps psychotherapy clients receiving memory recovery therapy are very rarely led to create illusory memories. But we believe that our concern about the possibility of illusory memories of childhood sexual abuse is better grounded in reality than the beliefs of people who deny the fallibility of memory and argue for the unqualified acceptance of all reports of recovered memories of childhood events."

One reads and listens to the stories of parents who have been devastated by such accusations, and they are heart-wrenching: in some respects, they are reminiscent of those whose children were drawn into quasi-religious cults involving parental rejection (e.g., Sargant, 1957). One then reads the accounts given by their accusers in *Accuracy About Abuse* and they are equally tragic and sickening. How does one make sense of these conflicting accounts and understand how they have come about? Can false memories simply be blamed on the practices of bad therapists, or did false beliefs arise in seed-beds of dispute, misunderstanding, sexual ambiguity and misinterpreted cues? Unfortunately, the answers are not to be found, as yet, in the pages of academic journals; and they will certainly not be discovered in the law courts.

There is no doubt that this issue raises massive questions for psychotherapists, and one suspects that this is why some participants to the debate have jumped on board (e.g., Webster, 1995). Bad therapy certainly exists. My wife (a psychotherapist herself) was asked to be an expert witness in a case in which a totally unqualified therapist had lain on top of a number of female patients, and had inserted his finger into their mouths to help "recover" their memories of childhood abuse. My wife was asked by a barrister (attorney) whether this is regular practice in psychotherapy. It is not! But it is not only bad therapy that is challenged. Many people have long been concerned by therapists' over-interpretations and antiquated theoretical systems, couched in language which Orwell (1946) would deplore. Accusations of implanting memories of sexual abuse are potentially explosive to the whole psychotherapy infrastructure, in a way that empirical studies of repression or of therapeutic efficacy were not. Relatively few therapists seem to have taken this on board as yet, although some are struggling with the issue (Fonagy & Target, 1996), and Boakes (1995) has taken an admirably bold stand.

Ultimately, the solution to this matter probably lies in rather mundane matters, such as the registration of therapists, and in tighter regulation and scrutiny by their professional bodies. It does not lie in naive gestures. At the *Practical Aspects of Memory Conference* two years ago, it was suggested that every time a patient reports sexual abuse to a therapist, independent corroboration by another therapist should be obtained. This would mean that, if a patient had plucked up courage after two years in an unforced environment to tell a therapist about sexual abuse (it does happen), the appropriate response would be: "Well. I'm glad you've told me about that - now we must go and tell somebody else!"

However, I am also very concerned that the notion of "false memory" can itself be abused. I know of one case, which attracted some publicity and where false memory was used as a defence, in which it had been clearly documented that the accused had said to his victim "Well, it didn't do you any harm, did it?". When challenged in private about this, the accused gave a very unsatisfactory reply, but the case collapsed, mainly because of the way it was handled by the prosecution's side. In another case, false memory was raised as the defence, where a pre-pubescent child was the accuser: although there are undoubtedly problems in obtaining evidence from children, this is a long way from the context in which false memory debate has previously been conducted. Likewise, false memory has been raised in sexual assault cases between adults. In one of these, I was asked by the accused to use information about the other party to argue for a false memory. When I explained that in a heated, fraught, emotional situation, both parties would be liable to memory errors - omissions, distortions, and intrusion errors - the client said to me: "Are you, Dr Kopelman, putting my memory on the same level as his/hers?" The answer was an unequivocal "yes".

7.2. Summary

Whilst sexual abuse of children is undoubtedly widespread, and its consequences varied and complex, precise prevalence figures are difficult to obtain, and multiple sources of information need to be used. There is no doubt that the false memory dispute offers a major challenge to much psychotherapeutic practice and, as yet, relatively few therapists seem to have taken this on board. The polarisation of the debate, exacerbated in legal cases, prevents what is most required - namely, research studies of how seed-beds of misunderstanding are sown. Moreover, there is a real danger that the notion of false memories will itself become abused as alleged offenders use such a defence in all sorts of cases. As the study of other types of offenders shows, it is not only the victims, but also the alleged perpetrators of offences who are liable to manifest memory omissions, distortions or intrusions.

8. CONCLUDING COMMENTS

Studies of retrograde amnesia in patients with neurological brain disease show that disproportionate impairments in autobiographical memory can arise, associated with particular lesions. Whether they ever arise independent of any degree of anterograde amnesia in neurological disorders remains controversial. However, both group studies and individual case-studies clearly indicate a structure within memory, in which the recollection of autobiographical incidents and personal facts can show damage independently of any impairment in remote memory for public information. At the same time, there are control systems, based partly (perhaps wholly) in the frontal lobes, which operate upon both components of memory.

False memories undoubtedly occur in a number of different contexts. Patients with organic amnesia (particularly if the medial aspects of the frontal lobes are also implicated) can show confabulation which is spontaneous, florid, preoccupying and often bizarre. These patients may act upon their beliefs, and they are not amenable to argument. Secondly, occasional patients with psychiatric disorder may display delusional memories, which have many clinical features in common with the spontaneous form of confabulation - also being bizarre, preoccupying, and absolute convictions which determine the patients' behaviour. These delusional memories sometimes arise in patients who continue their day-to-day life apparently normally, and the "madness" only manifests itself when one asks questions about topics relating to the delusional memory. Thirdly, healthy subjects may show distorted memories or intrusion errors, when they remember something badly. These errors can be quite striking, and the subjects may be very confident that they are accurate. Such errors have been demonstrated in a large number of studies. All these factors make it highly plausible that false memories for sexual abuse could arise in an appropriate context, which might be a seed-bed of dispute and misunderstanding, fanned by over-interpretative therapist interventions.

It also follows from what I have written that psychogenic amnesia can and does occur, even if this has been difficult to demonstrate unequivocally in cases of sexual abuse (Pope & Hudson, 1995). Some reductionists may prefer a pseudo-physiological explanation (e.g., Webster, 1995), and others may want to attribute some of the cases to simulation. However, fugue states and amnesia for offences are widely reported, and the "obviousness" of the motive in some cases does not necessarily undermine the reality of the experience, which is one reason why attributions of "secondary gain" are often unhelpful. Also unhelpful are "explanations" in terms of repression or dissociation, both terms having been used in so many different senses that they have become virtually empty of meaning. My own preference would be for us to develop explanations derived from cognitive concepts employed elsewhere, looking at the role of (for example) frontal control and inhibitory systems and how they interact with particular types of affect and retrieval cues (compare Shimamura, 1996). Having said this, I must add that the amnesia often claimed for sexual abuse appears to me different in certain respects from that seen in fugue states and offences. In both of the latter cases, there is a clearly demarcated and virtually total loss of recall; whereas in child sexual abuse, the subject often appears to have a "clouded memory" in the back of her (or his) mind: "clouded memory" being a phrase previously used by Baddeley and Wilson (1986) to describe a subgroup of patients with frontal lobe lesions. This hypothesised distinction between complete amnesia and "clouded memory" should be entirely amenable to empirical investigation by students of autobiographical memory. Likewise, why certain things are remembered and others forgotten, and why subjects differ in their response to trauma, are intriguing questions also amenable to empirical investigation.

It remains an open question what has happened in any given case in which the issue of false memory has arisen. Social and family psychologists and psychiatrists might have been able to resolve such matters by interviewing the various parties involved, individually and together, if the situation had not now become so fraught with political and legal considerations. While memory theory and amnesia investigations clearly find that false memories are entirely plausible, and are almost to be expected, the term itself has already become subject to abuse. Those of us involved in medico-legal cases need to be very much on our guard against the misuse of this defence.

Footnote: some details of the patients mentioned have been changed to preserve confidentiality.

REFERENCES

Albert, M.S., Butters, N., Levin, J. (1979). Temporal gradients in the retrograde amnesia of patients with alcoholic Korsakoff's disease. *Archives of Neurology, 36*, 211–216.

Baddeley, A.D. & Wilson, B. (1986). Amnesia, autobiographical memory, and confabulation. In D.C. Rubin (Ed.), *Autobiographical memory*. Cambridge: Cambridge University Press.

Bartlett, F.C. (1932). *Remembering: a study in experimental and social psychology*. Cambridge: Cambridge University Press.

Berrington, W.P., Liddell, D.W. & Foulds, G.A. (1956). A reevaluation of the fugue. *Journal of Mental Science, 102*, 281–286.

Bluglass, R. (1979). The psychiatric assessment of homicide. *British Journal of Hospital Medicine, 22*, 366–377.

Boakes, J. (1995). False memory syndrome. *Lancet, 346*, 1048–1049.

Bradford, J. & Smith, S.M. (1979). Amnesia and homicide: the Podola case and a study of thirty cases. *Bulletin of the American Academy of Psychiatry and the Law, 7*, 219–31.

Bremner, J.D., Randall, P., Scott, T.M., Bronen, R.A., Seibyl, J.P., Southwick, S.M., Delaney, R.C., McCarthy,G., Charney, D.S. & Innis, R.B. (1995). MRI-based measurement of hippocampal volume in patients with combat-related posttraumatic stress disorder. *American Journal of Psychiatry, 152*, 973–981

Briere, J. & Conte, J. (1993). Self reported amnesia for abuse in adults molested as children. *Journal of Traumatic Stress, 6*, 21–31.

Buchanan, A. (1991). Delusional memories: first-rank symptoms? *British Journal of Psychiatry, 159*, 472–474.

Butters, N. & Cermak, L.S. (1986). A case study of the forgetting of autobiographical knowledge: implications for the study of retrograde amnesia. In D.C. Rubin (Ed.), *Autobiographical memory*. Cambridge: Cambridge University Press.

Ceci, S.J. & Loftus, E.F. (1994). "Memory work': a royal road to false memories? *Applied Cognitive Psychology, 8*, 351–364.

Cermak, L.S. & O'Connor, M. (1983). The anterograde and retrograde retrieval ability of a patient with amnesia due to encephalitis. *Neuropsychologia, 21*, 213–234.

Clifford, B.R. & Scott, J. (1978). Individual and situational factors in eyewitness testimony. *Journal of Applied Psychology, 63*, 852–9.

Conway, M.A. (1990). *Autobiographical memory: an introduction*. Buckingham, Uk: Open University Press.

Conway, M.A., Rubin, D.C., Spinnler, H. & Waagenaar, W.A. (1992). *Theoretical perspectives on autobiographical memory*. Dordrecht and London: Kluwer Academic Publishers.

Coriat, I.H. (1907). The Lowell case of amnesia. *Journal of Abnormal Psychology. 2*, 93–111.

Dalla Barba, G. (1993a). Confabulation: knowledge and recollective experience. *Cognitive Neuropsyschology, 10*, 1–20.

Dalla Barba, G. (1993b). Different patterns of confabulation. *Cortex, 29*, 567–581.

David, A.S. & Howard, R. (1994). An experimental phenomenological approach to delusional memory in schizophrenia and late paraphrenia. *Psychological Medicine, 24*, 515–524

De Renzi, E., Liotti, M. & Nichelli, P. (1987). Semantic amnesia with presevation of autobiographical memory. *Cortex,, 23*, 575–597.

DeLuca, J. & Cicerone, K.D. (1991). Confabulation folllowing aneurysm of the anterior communicating artery. *Cortex, 27*, 417–423.

Deffenbacher, K. (1988). Eyewitness research: the next ten years. In M. Gruneberg, P. Morris & R. Sykes (Eds.), *Practical aspects of memory* (Vol 1). Chichester: Wiley.

Della Sala, S., Laiacona, M., Spinnler, H. and Trivelli, C. (1993). Impaired autobiographical recollection in some frontal patients. *Neuropsychologia, 31*, 823–840.

Edwards, A.L. (1942). The retention of affective experiences - a criticism and re-statement of the problem. *Psychological Review*, *49*, 43–53.

Fisher, V.E. & Marrow, A.J. (1933). Experimental study of moods. *Character and Personality*, *2*, 201–208.

Fonagy, P. & Target, M. (1996). The recovered memory debate: an empirical and psychoanalytic perspective. *Journal of American Psychoanalytic Assocation*. Submitted.

Freud, S, (1915–1917).*Introductory lctures on pychoanalysis* (Trans. J. Strachey, 1974). Harmondsworth: Penguin.

Freud, S. (1933). *New introductory lectures on psychoanalysis* (Trans. J. Strachey, 1974). Harmondsworth: Penguin.

Freud,S. & Breuer, J. (1895). *Studies on hysteria*. (Trans. J. Strachey, 1966). New York: Avon Books.

Gilbert, G.M. (1938). The new status of experimental studies on the relation of feeling to memory. *Psychological Bulletin,*, *35*, 26–35.

Goldberg, E., Antin, S.P., Bilder, R.M., Gerstman, L.J., Hughes, J.E.O. & Mattis, S. (1981). Retrograde amnesia: possible role of mesencephalic reticular activation in long-term memory. *Science*, *213*, 1392–1394.

Greene, J.D.W. & Hodges, J.R. (1996a). Identification of famous faces and famous names in early Alzheimer's disease. Relationship to anterograde episodic and general semantic memory. *Brain*, *119*, 111–128.

Green, J.D.W. & Hodges, J.R. (1996b). The fractionation of remote memory. Evidence from a longitudinal study of dementia of Alzheimer type. *Brain*, *119*, 129–142.

Gudjonsson, G.H. & MacKeith, J. (1983). A specific recognition deficit in a case of homicide. *Medicine, Science and the Law*, *23*, 37–40.

Guttmacher, M.S. (1955). *Psychiatry and the law*. New York: Grune and Stratton.

Hammersley, R. & Read, J.D. (1986). What is integration? Remembering a story and remembering false implications about the story. *British Journal of Psychology*, *77*, 329–41.

Herman, J.L. & Schatzow, E. (1987). Recovery and verification of memories of childhood sexual trauma. *Psychoanalytic Psychology*, *4*, 1–14.

Johnson, M.K. (1991). Reality monitoring: evidence from confabulation in organic brain disease patients. In G.P. Prigatano & D.L. Schacter, (Eds.) *Awareness deficit after brain injury: clinical and theoretical issues*. New York: Oxford University Press.

Kapur, N. & Coughlan, A.K. (1980). Confabulation and frontal lobe dysfunction. *Journal of Neurology, Neurosurgery and Psychiatry*, *43*, 461–463.

Kapur, N., Ellison, D., Smith, M., McLellan, L. & Burrows, E.H. (1992). Focal retrograde amnesia following bilateral temporal lobe pathology: a neuropsychological and magnetic resonance study. *Brain*, *116*, 73–86.

Keenan, P.A., Jacobson, M.W., Soleymani, R.M. & Newcomer, J.W. (1995). Commonly used therapeutic doses of glucocorticoids impair explicit memory. *Annals of New York Academy of Sciences*, 400–402

Kopelman, M.D. (1987a). Two types of confabulation. *Journal of Neurology, Neurosurgery and Psychiatry*, *50*, 1482–1487.

Kopelman, M.D. (1987b). Amnesia: organic and psychogenic. *British Journal of Psychiatry*, *150*, 428–442.

Kopelman, M.D. (1987c). Crime and amnesia: a review. *Behavioural Sciences and the Law*, *5*, 323–342.

Kopelman, M.D. (1989). Remote and autobiographical memory, temporal context memory, and frontal atrophy in Korsakoff and Alzheimer patients. *Neuropsychologia*, *27*, 437–460.

Kopelman, M.D. (1991). Frontal lobe dysfunction and memory deficits in the alcoholic Korsakoff syndrome and Alzheimer-type dementia. *Brain*, *114*, 117–137.

Kopelman, M.D. (1992). The 'new' and the "old': components of the anterograde and retrograde memory loss in Korsakoff and Alzheimer patients. In L.R. Squire and N. Butters (Eds.), *The neuropsychology of memory* (2nd ed.). New York: Guilford.

Kopelman, M.D. (1993). The neuropsychology of remote memory. In F. Boller & H. Spinnler (Eds.), *Handbook of neuropsychology* (Vol 8). Amsterdam: Elsevier Science Publishers.

Kopelman, M.D. (1995a). The Korsakoff syndrome: a clinical and neuropsychological review. *British Journal of Psychiatry*, *166*, 154–173.

Kopelman, M.D. (1995b). The assessment of psychogenic amnesia. In A. Baddeley, B.Wilson, & F. Watts (Eds.). In *Handbook of memory disorders*. Chichister: John Wiley and Sons.

Kopelman, M.D. (1996). Isolated retrograde amnesia - an exceptionally critical review - in preparation.

Kopelman, M.D., Christensen, H., Puffett, A. & Stanhope, N. (1994). The Great Escape: a neuropsychological study of psychogenic amnesia. *Neuropsychologia*, *32*, 675–691.

Kopelman, M.D., Green, R.E.A., Guinan, E.M., Lewis, P.D.R. & Stanhope, N. (1994). The case of the amnesic intelligence officer. *Psychological Medicine*, *24*, 1037–1045.

Kopelman, M.D., Guinan, E.M., & Lewis, P.D.R. (1995). Delusional memory, confabulation, and frontal lobe dysfunction: a case study in de Clérambault's syndrome. *Neurocase*, *1*, 71–77.

Kopelman, M.D. Ng, N. & Van Den Broucke, O. (1996). Confabulation extending across episodic, personal semantic, and semantic memory: a case-study. About to be submitted.

Kopelman, M.D. & Stanhope, N. (1996). Correlates of retrograde memory loss in 72 patients with organic amnesia. In preparation.

Kopelman, M.D., Stanhope, N. & Kingsley, D. (1996). The nature of retrograde amnesia in patients with focal diencephalic, temporal lobe or frontal lesions. Submitted for publication

Kopelman, M.D., Wilson, B.A. & Baddeley, A.D: (1990). *The autobiographical memory interview.* Bury St Edmunds: Thames Valley Test Company.

Korsakoff, S. S. (1889). Psychic disorder in conjunction with peripheral neuritis (trans. M. Victor & P.I.Yakovlev, 1955). *Neurology, 5,* 394 - 406.

Kuehn, L.L. (1974). Looking down a gun barrel: person perception and violent crime. *Perceptual and Motor Skills, 39,* 1159–64.

Leitch, A. (1948). Notes on amnesia in crime for the general practitioner. *Medical Press, 219,* 459–63.

Lindsay, D.S. & Read, J.D. (1994). Psychotherapy and memories of childhood sexual abuse: a cognitive perspective. *Applied Cognitive Psychology, 8,* 281–338.

Lishman, W.A. (1974). The speed of recall of pleasant and unpleasant experiences. *Psychological Medicine, 4,* 212–218.

Lloyd, G.G. & Lishman, W.A. (1975). Effect of depression on the speed of recall of pleasant and unpleasant experiences. *Psychological Medicine, 5,* 173–180.

Loftus, E.F. (1979). *Eyewitness testimony.* Cambridge, Mass: Harvard University Press.

Loftus, E.F. (1993). The reality of repressed memories. *American Psychologist, 48,* 518–537.

Loftus, E.F. Polonsky, S. & Fullilove, M.T. (1994). Memories of childhood sexual abuse: remembering and repressing. *Psychology of Women, 18,* 67–84.

Luria, A.R. (1976). *The Neuropsychology of memory.* New York: John Wiley.

Mangels, J.A., Gershberg, F.B., Shimamura, A.P. & Knight, R.T. (1996). Impaired retrieval from remote memory in patients with frontal lobe damage. *Neuropsychology,* in press.

Master, D. Lishman, W.A. & Smith, A. (1983). Speed of recall in relation to affective tone and intensity of experience. *Psychological Medicine, 13,* 325–331.

Meltzer, H. (1930). Individual differences in forgetting pleasant and unpleasant experiences. *Journal of Educational Psychology, 21,* 399–409.

Merskey, H. (1992). The manufacture of personalities. The production of multiple personality disorder. *British Journal of Psychiatry, 160,* 327–340.

Merskey, H. (1995). Multiple personality disorder and false memory syndrome. *British Journal of Psychiatry, 166,* 281–283

Moscovitch, M. (1989). Confabulation and the frontal system: Strategic vs. associative retrieval in neuropsychological theories of memory. In H.L. Roediger & F.I.M. Craik (Eds.), *Varieties of Memory and Consciousness: Essays in Honour of Endel Tulving.* Hillsdale, NJ: Erlbaum.

Mullen, P.E., Martin, J.L. Anderson, J.C., Romans, S.E. & Herbison, G.P. (1993). Childhood sexual abuse and mental health in adult life. *British Journal of Psychiatry, 163,* 721–732.

O'Connell, B.A. (1960). Amnesia and homicide. *British Journal of Delinquency, 10,* 262–276.

O'Connor, M., Butters, N., Miliotis, P., Eslinger, P. & Cermak, L.S. (1992). The dissociation of anterograde and retrograde amnesia in a patient with herpes encephalitis. *Journal of Clinical and Experimental Neuropsychology, 14,* 159–178.

Ogden, J.A. (1993). Visual object agnosia, prosopagnosia, achromatopsia, loss of visual imagery, and autobiographical amnesia following recovery from cortical blindness: case MH. *Neuropsychologia, 31,* 571–589.

Oliver, J.E. (1993). Intergenerational transmission of child abuse: rates, research, and clinical implications. *American Journal of Psychiatry, 150,* 1315–1324.

Orwell, G. (1946). Politics and the English language. Reprinted (1962). in *Inside the Whale and Other Essays.* (pp 143–158). Harmondsworth, Penguin Press.

Parwatikar, S.D., Holcomb, W.R. & Meninger, K.A. (1985). The detection of malingered amnesia in accused murderers. *Bulletin of the American Academy of Psychiatry and the Law, 13,* 97–103.

Pear, T.H. (1914). The role of repression in forgetting (1). *British Journal of Psychology, 7,* 139–146.

Pope, H.G. Jr. & Hudson, J.I. (1995). Can memories of childhood sexual abuse be repressed? *Psychological Medicine, 25,* 121–126

Romans, S.E., Martin, J.L., Anderson, J.C., O'Shea, M.L. & Mullen, P.E. (1995). Factors that mediate between child sexual abuse and adult psychological outcome. *Psychological Medicine, 25,* 127–142.

Rubin, D.C. (1982). On the retention function for autobiographical memory. *Journal of Verbal Learning and Verbal Behavior, 21,* 21–38.

Sagar, H.J., Cohen, N.J., Sullivan, E.V., Corkin, S. & Growdon, J.H. (1988). Remote memory function in Alzheimer's disease and Parkinson's disease. *Brain, 111,* 185–206.

Sanders, H and Warrington, E. (1971). Memory for remote events in amnesic patients. *Brain, 94,* 661–668.

Sargant, W. (1957). *Battle for the mind.* London: Heinemann.

Schacter, D.L. (1986). Amnesia and crime: how much do we really know. *American Psychologist*, *41*, 286–295.

Schacter, D.L. (1996). *Searching for memory: the brain, the mind and the past.* New York: HarperCollins.

Schacter, D.L., Norman, K.A., & Koutstaal, W. (1997). The recovered memory debate: a cognitive perspective. In (M.A. Conway, ed.) *False and recovered memories*, Oxford, Oxford University Press (in press).

Shallice, T., Fletcher, P., Frith, C.D., Grasby, P.M., Frackowiak, R.S.J. & Dolan, R.J. (1994). Brain regions associated with acquisition and retrieval of verbal episodic memory. *Nature, 368*, 633–5.

Shallice, T. & Evans, M.E. (1978). The involvement of the frontal lobes in cognitive estimates. *Cortex, 14*, 294–303.

Shimamura, A.P. (this volume). Neuropsychological factors associated with memory recollection: what can science tell us about reinstated memories? In J.D. Read, & D.S. Lindsay (Eds.). *Recollections of Trauma: Scientific Research and Clinical Practice.* New York and London: Plenum Press. (This volume).

Stuss, D.T., Alexander, M.P., Liberman, A. & Levine, H. (1978). An extraordinary form of confabulation. *Neurology, 28*, 1166–1172.

Taylor, P.J. & Kopelman, M. (1984). Amnesia for criminal offences. *Psychological Medicine, 14*, 581–8.

Thomson, R.H. (1930). An experimental study of memory as influenced by feeling tone. *Journal of Experimental Psychology, 26*, 462–468.

Tulving, E., Kapur, S., Markowitsch, H.J., Craik, F.I.M., Habib, R. & Houle, S. (1994). Neuroanatomical correlates of retrieval in episodic memory: auditory sentence recognition. *Proceedings of the National Academy of Science, USA, 96*, 2012–2015.

van der Kolk, B.A. (1994). The body keeps score: memory and the evolving psychobiology of posttraumatic sstress. *Harvard Review of Psychiatry, 1*, 253–265.

Webster, R. (1995). *Why Freud was wrong: sin, science and psychoanalysis.* Harper Collins: London.

Wechsler, D. (1945). A standard memory scale for clinical use. *Journal of Psychology, 19*, 87–95.

West, D.J. (1967). *Murder followed by suicide*, London: Heinemann

Williams, L.M. (1994). Recall of childhood trauma. A prospective study of women's memories of child sexual abuse. *Journal of Consulting and Clinical Psychology, 62*, 1167–1176.

Wolff, A. (1914). The role of repression in forgetting (2). *British Journal of Psychology, 7*, 147–153.

Yuille, J.C. (1987) *The effects of alcohol and marijuana on eyewitness recall.* Paper presented at Conference on Practical Aspects of Memory, Swansea: UK (unpublished)

Yuille, J.C. & Cutshall, J.L. (1986). A case study of eye-witness memory of a crime. *Journal of Applied Psychology, 71*, 291–301.

Zola-Morgan, S. Cohen, N.J. & Squire, L.R. (1983). Recall of remote episodic memory in amnesia. *Neuropsychologia, 21*, 487–500.

COMMENTARY ON ANOMALIES OF AUTOBIOGRAPHICAL MEMORY: RETROGRADE AMNESIA, CONFABULATION, DELUSIONAL MEMORY, PSYCHOGENIC AMNESIA, AND FALSE MEMORIES

Elizabeth F. Loftus

1. INTRODUCTION

Kopelman (this volume) describes a variety of patients who have had devastating experiences - injuries, strokes, and other mishaps - that created problems of autobiographical memory. Virtually all of these patients have had organic injuries of one sort or another, and so their ability to inform our discussion of remembering and forgetting after psychological trauma is unclear. Nonetheless, to facilitate this endeavor it may be useful to classify the brain-damaged patients according to the type of memory impairment that they show. The simplest dichotomy for characterizing these cases is the two-by-two table, where an individual could in reality have not experienced some critical event or, alternatively, may have had a critical experience. And within these two possibilities, individuals might be in one of two recall states - not recalling the event, or, alternatively, recalling the event.

2. FALSE NEGATIVES AND FALSE POSITIVES

One type of memory deficit shown by these patients is a "false negative" - the failure to remember events that actually did occur. The eminent scientist PZ, who developed an alcoholic Korsakoff syndrome, provides one example. PZ was asked about professional experiences (colleagues, conferences, research mentioned prominently in his autobiography), but could remember few of these experiences if they had occurred around the onset of his disease. The frontal lobe patients also show severe impairments of autobiographical memory - especially those with bilateral lesions. And many offenders, especially in homicide cases, appear to have amnesia for known past acts - with alcohol intoxication playing a role in many cases.

Another type of memory deficit shown by many of Kopelman's patients is a "false positive" - the explicit recall of events that did not occur. The schizophrenic patients with delusional memories of experiences that they never had provide one example. Another class are the confabulating patients with frontal lobe lesions who sometimes report detailed personal memories for things that could not have happened. Patient AB, for example, remembered that she had recently visited her parents, a memory that could be proven to be false. (In point of fact, her mother had been dead for four years and her father had been dead for 20). WM was positively convinced that a certain man was in love with her. These patients show that frontal patients sometimes show beliefs that are held with a strong degree of conviction, that patients will act on these convictions, and that they sometimes show extreme resistance to arguments or persuasion. Often the beliefs are quite bizarre. (For more examples of the types of errors that confabulators make, see Burgess & Shallice, 1996). The false recollections of confabulators bring to mind a poem by Hughes Mearns (1875–1965), that reads like it could have been written by one of these patients:

"As I was going up the stair
I met a man who wasn't there
He wasn't there again today;
I wish, I wish he'd stay away."

3. NO RECALL FOLLOWED BY RECALL

The 2 × 2 classification of patients does not provide an ready place for one important group - those who have, for a period of time, no recall of an experience, but later they regain their memory. Kopelman's patient descriptions reveal that some do indeed have this experience. The Korsakoff patients for example, have been shown to recall fewer personal memories spontaneously, but when prompted with cue words they do remember more - a kind of "forgetting" and later "remembering."

More dramatically, there are the fugue cases, where in the apparent absence of any organic injury, patients lose their personal identity and large sectors of their memory for personal past. Later they regain these memories. Typically the amnesia is precipitated by severe emotional or psychological trauma. Patient KG, the 55 year old man who had been charged with embezzlement from the workplace, claimed complete amnesia for the offenses, and also lost memory of his entire personal history. Neurological testing suggested that organic causes may have played a role. The patient AT was found wandering around the London underground with loss of identity, and later regained her memory after an amytal abreaction. Other evidence suggested that this might be a case of deliberate simulation.

Fugue cases can be found sprinkled throughout the literature (see Goldenberg, 1995; Kopelman 1995; Schacter, Wang, Tulving & Freedman, 1982). Generally after some traumatic episode, there is first a fugue state in which individuals wander around for variable periods of time, ranging from minutes to months and are unaware of their memory loss. Next individuals may be asked questions about their past that they cannot answer, and they become aware of their memory loss, although they may still be experiencing amnesia. This stage typically lasts several days, but might last longer (e.g., for weeks) on occasion. The final stage is the clearing of the amnesia, which sometimes occurs spontaneously and sometimes in response to a cue, or to some intervention such as sodium amytal treatment. In numerous fugue cases, investigators have reported a prior history of brain damage, which has led some investigators to suggest that some preexisting neurological dysfunction may interact with the emotional trauma to produce the fugue experience (Schacter & Kihlstrom, 1989). In this same vein, Kopelman (this volume) discusses the fact that suicidal ideas just before or after the fugue are common, as is a past history of transient organic amnesia from head injury, epilepsy, or severe alcoholic intoxication. We might keep in mind, then, that these may be experiences that predispose someone to have an experience of extraordinary lack of recall, followed by fairly complete recollection.

The fugue cases reveal that memories can be quite dramatically "lost" and then recovered. While many cases contain facts that make it unknown whether there is some organic involvement, it does appear to be the case that some truly functional amnesia can occur. Schacter and Kihlstrom have defined this as "memory loss that is attributable to an instigating event or process that does not result in damage or injury to the brain, and produces more forgetting than would normally occur in the absence of the instigating event or process" (1989, p. 209). While many theories have been offered to account for the peculiar behaviors that fugue patients display (including "dissociation", and "selective failure of episodic memory"), there are no strong empirical grounds for distinguishing amongst them, and, according to Schacter and Kihlstrom (1989) a critical challenge for future research is to construct and implement empirical tests to discriminate between the different theories.

It should be kept in mind that there are other situations, besides the fugue cases, where true memories appear to be lost and then regained, but were not discussed by Kopelman. For example, consider the survivors of one of the world's most devastating marine disasters, the sinking of the car ferry Estonia (Taiminen & Tuominen, 1996). On September 28, 1994 the Estonia was sailing to Stockholm when it suddenly tilted and began sinking. Approximately 900 passengers and crew members died by drowning or freezing, but 128 were rescued from life boats, life rafts, or directly from the sea by helicopters or ships that had come to the disaster area. Thirty-eight of these survivors were taken to a hospital in Finland, and the investigators who studied them noted that severe dissociative amnesia or paramnesia was present in four cases. These patients remembered everything except the last few hours before being rescued. In all four cases, the patients had lost a relative in the disaster and they regained their memories within two days.

Is there any connection between the memory loss and recovery in fugue patients and the memory loss that is claimed in some cases of child sexual abuse? Kopelman thought the connection was tenuous, noting that in the fugue patients the memory loss is demarcated and virtually total. In the child sex abuse cases he claimed that the memory loss was characterized by a cloudiness without complete forgetting. Or course, some of the more dramatic and controversial cases of alleged child sexual abuse do indeed claim complete banishment of memories from conscious awareness and subsequent recovery of those memories. Thus, this subset cannot be distinguished from the fugue cases on the basis of the cloudiness criterion.

Kopelman did not go as far as some would like in explicitly extracting from his vast experience with these patients some useful elements that might help us understand the claims of forgetting and remembering of childhood abuse. He might have spent more time discussing the duration of amnesia in patients. In the fugue cases the amnesia is resolved typically in a matter of days. In the Estonia survivors, the dissociative amnesia disappeared in two days. In contrast, in many cases of reported massive repression, the memories of abuse are sometimes claimed to be lost for decades. Kopelman might have also spent more time discussing the false memories of confabulators. In the frontal patients, the confabulators sometimes produce bizarre recollections, and they stick to them in the face of contrary evidence. In at least some cases of reported massive repression, the memories are modified by individuals when they are confronted with contradictory facts. If the possessor of a repressed memory later finds out that her sister could not have been present at the time of the murder, the sister is conveniently removed from the memory. These are but a few of the ways in which the losses and gains of memory experienced by these patients are sometimes quite different from the losses and gains reported by some more extreme cases of recovered memory clients.

Kopelman's chapter, taken as a whole, provides a very nice contribution to the literature on anomalies of autobiographical memory. He engagingly describes the maladies of memory that have inflicted his unfortunate patients. Their provocative behaviors and dissociations of memory help us appreciate the wonder of a memory that is working properly, and might potentially help us understand the forgetting and remembering of psychological traumas. And he does one more thing quite well: he reminds us repeatedly, lest we forget, that alleged perpetrators and alleged victims are both liable to memory errors - to omissions, distortions, and frank intrusions.

REFERENCES

Burgess, P. W. & Shallice, T. (1996). Confabulation and the control of recollection. *Memory*, 4, 359–411.

Goldenberg, G. (1995). Transient Global Amnesia. In A.D. Baddeley, B.A. Wilson, & F.N. Watts (Eds). *Handbook of memory disorders*. London: John Wiley & Sons Ltd., (p. 109-133.)

Kopelman, M. D. (1995). The assessment of psychogenic amnesia. In A.D. Baddeley, B.A. Wilson, & F.N. Watts (Eds). *Handbook of memory disorders*. London: John Wiley & Sons Ltd. (p 427–448.)

Schacter, D. L. & Kihlstrom, J. F. (1989). Functional amnesia. In F. Boller & J. Grafman (Eds) *Handbook of neuropsychology, Vol 3*. Amsterdam: Elsevier Science Publishers, (p 209–231.)

Schacter, D.L., Wang, P.L., Tulving, E. & Freedman, M. (1982). Functional retrograde amnesia: a quantitative case study. *Neuropsychologia*, 20, 523–532.

Taiminen, T. J. & Tuominen, T. (1996). Psychological responses to a marine disaster during a recoil phase: Experiences from the Estonia shipwreck. *British Journal of Medical Psychology*, 69, 147–153.

QUESTION AND ANSWER SESSION

Schooler. That was a very enlightening talk. I think the point about the shades of grey of forgetting was an important insight. One thing that I had trouble getting a handle on is the woman with the fugue state. You claim that, on the one hand, she was so successful on many these memory techniques that are shown to catch simulators and yet, at the same time there is speculation that the true fugue lasted only for a week and that she wrote to one of her children three months later. I wonder if you could help us get a better intuition about how she could beat these simulation tests and at the same time write to her children.

Kopelman. My impression is that beating tests of simulation is not hard. I've seldom seen a patient who scores below chance on the recognition tests and yet these are taken as the hallmark of a test to detect simulation. The various other tests which are proposed are not very good, they may catch a few, but not very many. Again, one can't prove that she didn't plan it all over a period of time. All I can say is that a period of a week of complete amnesia is much more consistent with the literature. The fact that she has never been able to recall what took place during that week seems to be consistent with her having had an initial fugue. After that, three months later she wrote back to her child, but I just want to put the idea again that it is not black or white. I have a feeling that what happened to her was that she came round and she created for herself a whole new lifestyle and she came to believe her own script. One suspects that if she's successful in this and you gave her a lot of reinforcement, when she gets into another problem she might develop another role and start to believe in that script. My understanding of multiple personality, if it exists, is that this could be how it arises. However, I can't disprove it to the people who will want to interpret this as her having simulated all along.

Shimamura. I found lots of things very fascinating, one of which was this idea that some kind of organic event could actually trigger or act as a learning experience for a psychiatric memory disorder. I think that's a very interesting aspect and one that hasn't really been covered very much. What I really wanted to ask you about though is this notion of the right hemisphere and its role in many of these things. It's interesting that some of the data point to the frontal lobes and some of the data point to the right hemisphere, not necessarily the frontal lobes, and I'm wondering if it's just the right hemisphere, in its capacity to do these global and imaginal and visual types of things that may be very important for autobiographical memory, maybe more than semantic memory. It may be some kind of marker. I noticed that one of the cases, which might have been a delusional case, had a very bad face recognition performance on the Warrington recognition test, whereas the words were just fine, and again it suggests that it's some kind of visual memory problem associated with that. It reminded me of one thing that Steve Lynn (this volume) said about some of the victims of child sexual abuse where they are high in fantasy proneness and one might imagine that might have an imagery component as well. What are your thoughts on the specific role of the right hemisphere in this situation ?

Kopelman. Well I didn't present all the data we've recently got on autobiographical memory and organic brain disorders because I was really just trying to set the scene for discussing other issues. But there does seem to be in the recent data we've collected a right/left difference for patients with temporal lobe lesions so that right damage is worse for autobiographical memory, whereas left damage might affect the linguistic labelling of remote memories. But in the frontal lobe group we've also got patients with unilateral left and unilateral right and bilateral damage and there you don't get the right/left difference or at the most, it's only trends. In the frontal group it's the bilateral patients who do worst on remote memory tasks. As to the second part of your question, the patient with delusional memories, yes, it is actually noticeable that she has a disproportionate deficit on face recognition memories. When I've presented her before to people like Andy Young, they've picked up on this, and of course he is finding that a lot of patients with Capgras syndrome are also down on face recognition memory. In fact it crops up so often in deluded patients that I'm not quite sure what to do with it because I'm not sure whether it's very specific. Also, although on the Warrington recognition memory test she was very down on face memory, but she was down on verbal memory on the revised Weschler scale.

Eth. I read the clinical experiences somewhat differently than you do. It seems as if you are suggesting that there are very neat discrete categories much like Beth Loftus" 2x2 diagram in which we can place patients so that there are factitious patients who are intentionally lying to us; that there are patients with delusional memories and confabulation who are sincere but who are telling us falsehoods and then there are patients who genuinely forget either for organic or psychological reasons. It seems to me that there is considerable overlap and that it is not always clear which category a patient falls within. The patients may move among the categories, that a delusional patient may have had a real event around which there is a delusional elaboration. We heard earlier that the PTSD combat veteran may have seen a movie and incorporated some of the movie scenes into his own autobiographical memory and that it's not always a task that an expert or psychiatrist can make in deciding which of these discrete categories patients fall into; therefore, we are obligated to treat them and to accept the accounts that they tell us in an effort to assist them in relief of their symptoms.

Kopelman. Two points - first of all I was trying to make the point a propos the psychogenic, that I didn't regard the issue as black or white, that they must be either faking or totally genuine, but I was trying to postulate a continuum. Secondly, I make a distinction between content and form, and I would certainly agree that within the content of what the delusional memory patients described and also within the content of what the organic confabulating patient would say, there was stuff that a psychodynamic oriented therapist could write books about as to why these particular delusions or confabulated ideas concerned this particular content in this particular patient. On the other hand, looking at the circumstances of the patient, there is no doubt that the patient AB who I presented had severe organic brain disease which had precipitated the confabulated ideas, whatever their particular content, and that was a consequence of her poor frontal lobe and executive function. Likewise in the two patients with deluded memories, there were a lot of other features which I didn't talk about, which suggested that they had a psychotic disorder. So although the content of any particular patient's abnormal memories could be interpreted in a dynamic way if you like, the fact that they got them arises from distinguishable circumstances and actually has implications for treatment, because the confabulator was not treatable as such (although she had of course received high doses of thiamine and cytotoxic drugs), whereas the deluded patients did respond to medication and the psychogenic patients also wouldn't have responded to medication.

Briere. I think it becomes a bit of a red herring to make childhood sexual abuse the archetypal or classic case of trauma motivating avoidance of memory. I think it's much bigger than that. This field started in sexual abuse, but for instance much of my work over the last years has been on adult trauma, gang rapes, torture, etcetera, and yet you hear about the sexual abuse because that's where we were before, but the danger is if we marginalize it, and sexual abuse has its own whole series of problems, then we get cross interference because problems associated with sexual abuse, which are very complex, can reach over to the broader issue which is how trauma relates. I think we're all making that mistake of making that primary equation. The other question was that I too was very interested in your idea that if someone had some kind of neurological insult or constitutional difficulty, that they could learn from that and that might increase the likelihood that they might engage in some kind of psychogenic process later. My sense of that, and on this I come out more conservative than you do, is usually if I hear there was a preexisting brain event, I'm likely to assume that later events that I saw also had a neurological basis but were subtle. In PTSD we have what we call a priming effect, where you've been traumatised then later smaller amounts of trauma can produce a post-traumatic stress event. I'm not saying that it's the same here, I just wonder if we can rule out whether a stressor later in life might exceed some threshold more easily because there is a neurological difficulty. So how do you think people could learn from those neurological events such as they become psychological events later? If that's true then that's a very interesting notion.

Kopelman. I think the fact that organic damage often precedes what I've chosen to call psychological amnesia is fairly well established. A paper by Berrington found a high rate of head injuries in their patients and a paper by Stengel emphasised a past history of epilepsy. It's one of the factors which I've extracted from my review of the literature and other people, such as Dan Schachter, make exactly the same point about there being high rates of previous transient organic amnesia. The second point I'd make is that in these patients, KG and AT, they did of course have very full physical investigations, and in KG there was subsequently reason to believe that there was a vascular problem that accounted for his everyday and progressive learning difficulties but that still doesn't convince me that his two episodes of going wandering and becoming amnesic the day after being confronted with his offence and the day after the police had come to his home should be regarded as organic. Dan Schachter interprets these higher rates of past organic amnesia as perhaps something a previous head trauma has done to your gluco-corticoids and has somehow had an effect on neuronal functioning in the medial temporal lobes, which somehow makes you more vulnerable to an episode of transient amnesia later. That's a plausible hypothesis, but I take the much simpler view that it actually involves a learning episode so that when you become suicidally depressed and you're confronted with a severe precipitating stress, you somehow become amnesic.

Wagenaar. Clearly there are two states, first she really believed she was amnesic and was confused and later on when she started to write to her children she started prolonging the illusion because there was some value in it for her. Would it be possible that there is some sort of trance like state that could be easily elicited by a situation so that she would go back to this state and not simulate anything at all and shift from one state to the other when she needed to do that - is that possible ?

Kopelman. I think that the period of the first week which I am interpreting as a genuine fugue could be very like what you're describing as a trance-like state, but I don't think that the state she was then in and maintained for a year was like that. I don't think one could say she was in a trance-like state for this period.

REFERENCES

Berrington, W.P., Liddell, D.W., & Foulds, G.A. (1956) A reevaluation of the fugue. *Journal of Mental Science,* *102,* 281–286.

Schacter, D.L., (1996). *Searching for memory: the brain, the mind and the past.* New York: Harper Collins.

Stengel, E. (1941). On the aetiology of the fugue states. *Journal of Mental Science, 87,* 572–599.

12

HYPNOSIS, PSEUDOMEMORIES, AND CLINICAL GUIDELINES

A Sociocognitive Perspective

Steven Jay Lynn,[1] Bryan Myers,[1] and Peter Malinoski[2]

[1]State University of New York at Binghamton
Binghamton, New York 13902
[2]Ohio University
Athens, Ohio 45701

1. INTRODUCTION

Hypnosis has never been far from the center of controversy. Indeed, hypnosis has been intimately associated with historical debates concerning the nature of hysteria, dissociation, repression, and now, memory (see Lynn, Rhue, & Spanos, 1994). While hypnosis is currently riding an unprecedented wave of popularity among clinicians, and while researchers are moving hypnosis forward into the mainstream of psychology, debate rages in the hypnosis and broader psychological community about the role and potential usefulness of hypnosis in memory retrieval (Loftus & Ketcham, 1994; Lindsay & Read, 1995; Lynn & Nash, 1994).

If hypnosis were not viewed as something "special," then it is unlikely there would be much debate about whether hypnosis can improve memory, nor much concern about whether hypnosis can create false memories in psychotherapy. The idea that there is something special about hypnosis is a vestige of 18th-century mesmerism and later hypnosis which associated hypnosis with the idea of unusual and even supernatural capabilities. Mesmer and Puysegur claimed that hypnotic phenomena depend on the special prowess or supernatural skills of the hypnotist. Other 18th-century and 19th-century investigators argued that magnetized (and later hypnotized) subjects could see without the use of their eyes, travel mentally to distant planets and report back accurately about the inhabitants, spot disease by seeing through the skin to the internal organs of sick individuals, and communicate with the dead. The belief that hypnosis had a special power to retrieve lost memories was shared by luminaries such as Janet, Breuer, and Freud (see Lynn et al., 1994).

Whereas many of these beliefs are now regarded as outlandish, the belief that hypnosis is a special state or condition that enhances memory continues to beguile modern

Recollections of Trauma, edited by Read and Lindsay
Plenum Press, New York, 1997

workers in the field. For instance, Hayward and Ashworth (1980) purport that hypnosis can, "induce a mental state which facilitates recall and enables the subject to produce more information than he would be able to provide in the so-called waking state" (p. 471). However, in the last decade or so, the tide of scientific opinion has turned to the point that it is widely acknowledged that memory is reconstructive and that hypnosis either has no effect on memory (Erdelyi, 1994) or that it can seriously impair and even distort recall (Orne et al., 1996; Perry, in press). Nevertheless, the lay public, certain clinically oriented scholars (Hammond et al., 1995), and many practicing clinicians continue to believe that hypnosis can have a useful role in recovering memories of trauma and abuse.

Since Loftus and Loftus (1980) found that 84% of psychologists and 69% of nonpsychologists endorsed the statement that "memory is permanently stored in the mind and that "... with hypnosis, or other specialized techniques, these inaccessible details could eventually be recovered," survey research has documented the pervasiveness of the idea that hypnosis improves memory. Six years later, McConkey and Jupp (1986) found that 94.6 % of Australian students (N = 203) agreed with the statement that hypnosis "can make responsive subjects remember things that they could not normally remember," and McConkey (1986) replicated this high rate of endorsement with University of Pennsylvania and Temple University subjects (N = 173). More recently, Whitehouse and his colleagues (1991) found that 93% of college age subjects reported that hypnosis enhances memory retrieval.

Of course, hypnosis is a reciprocal process that depends on the therapist's beliefs and expectancies, as well as the participant's. Yapko (1994) recently surveyed over 850 psychotherapists in private practice and found that they endorsed the following items with high frequency:

1. 75%: "Hypnosis enables people to accurately remember things they otherwise could not".
2. 47%: "Therapists can have greater faith in details of a traumatic event when obtained hypnotically than otherwise".
3. 31%: "When someone has a memory of a trauma while in hypnosis, it objectively must actually have occurred".
4. 54%: "Hypnosis can be used to recover memories of actual events as far back as birth".
5. 19%: "Hypnotically obtained memories are more accurate than simply just remembering".
6. 27%: Disagreed with statement that there was a "legitimate basis for believing that hypnosis can be used in such a way as to create false memories".

Survey research also documents the fact that a sizable minority of psychologists in the United States report that they use hypnosis to help clients recall memories of sexual abuse. Poole, Lindsay, Memon, and Bull (1995) surveyed 145 licensed U.S. doctoral level psychotherapists who were randomly sampled from the National Register of Health Service Providers in Psychology in two studies (N = 145), and 57 British psychologists who were sampled from the Register of Chartered Clinical Psychologists. Twenty-nine percent and 34% of U.S. psychologists in the two surveys, respectively, reported that they used hypnosis to help clients recall memories of sexual abuse. Five percent of the British therapists responded accordingly.

Given the apparent investment of many clinicians in the use of hypnotic procedures, it is not surprising that the American Society of Clinical Hypnosis (ASCH) recently issued guidelines for clinical hypnosis aimed at memory improvement or recovery (Hammond et al., 1995). These guidelines legitimize this practice among psychotherapists and are fast becoming the standard of care in the field. Hence, there is a pressing need to examine the literature in this area and to evaluate pertinent justifications or contraindications for the use of hypnosis in improving memories.

Our chapter responds to these needs by presenting a socio-cognitive model of hypnosis and memory, and by addressing the following questions: 1.) Does hypnosis improve memory? 2.) Are hypnotized participants particularly vulnerable to the effects of misleading information? 3.) Do hypnotic procedures enhance unwarranted confidence in remembered events? 4.) Can hypnotic age regression enhance memory of events in the distant past? and 5.) What are the determinants of hypnotic pseudomemories? We conclude our chapter with an examinaiton of certain guidelines proffered by the American Society of Clinical Hypnosis in light of the extant literature on hypnosis and memory. We argue that although the guidelines represent an important and ambitious initiative to educate clinicians about the potential limitations of hypnosis, and although the guidlines contain valuable information that could well limit risky practices in psychotherapy, they, nevertheless, have notable limitations and do not provide adequate justification for the use of hypnosis as a memory recovery tool in psychotherapy.

2. A SOCIO-COGNITIVE MODEL OF HYPNOSIS AND MEMORY

Before we address the questions listed above, we advance a socio-cognitive model of hypnosis and memory that constitutes the framework for our discussion. This model can be traced to attacks by Sarbin and Coe and Barber on the concept of hypnosis as an altered state of consciousness (see Lynn et al., 1994). These authors argued that despite external appearances, hypnotic responses were not particularly unusual and therefore did not require the positing of unusual states of consciousness. There now exists a virtual consensus among researchers that the effects of hypnosis are not due to the induction of a special state with particular causal or defining features associated with it (Kirsch & Lynn, 1995).

This convergence of opinion is, at least in part, the byproduct of the following research findings which have accrued over the past two decades. People can respond to suggestions for alterations in sensation, perception, thought, feeling, and action without prior induction of hypnosis. This is typically referred to as "waking" suggestibility. The term "waking" is often placed in quotes because the idea that hypnosis is in any way akin to sleep has been widely rejected, and the term nonhypnotic might be preferable. Nonhypnotic suggestions are administered with brief instructions about the task (e.g., "I'd like to see how well you can experience a series of suggestions that I will make") replacing the more elaborate induction procedures, in which people are led to understand that they are entering hypnosis. It has been established that people can respond to the full range of hypnotic suggestions without a prior induction and that the effect of the induction is merely to increase responsiveness to suggestion (Barber, 1969; Hilgard, 1977). For most people, the increase is very small. For example, a person who, when hypnotized, responds successfully to 7 suggestions on a 12-suggestion suggestibility scale might respond to 6 of them without a hypnotic induction. Furthermore, correlations between waking and hypnotic suggestibility range between .63 and .85 (Barber & Glass, 1962; Hilgard & Tart, 1966). Given this much common variance, it seems likely that the causes of the response are the same in both situations, which is one reason for the widespread rejection of the altered state hypothesis. Another reason for the rejection of this hypothesis is that decades of research have failed to show that hypnotized and nonhypnotized participants reliably differ

on markers of physiological responding, particularly when adequate experimental control
are imposed (see Dixon & Laurence, 1992; Kirsch & Lynn, 1995).

In summary, the function of an hypnotic induction is merely to increase suggestibil
ity to a minor degree. This increase in suggestibility can also be achieved with nonhypno
tic procedures when subjects have positive response expectancies, attitudes, motivation
and information regarding how to respond to suggestions. In fact, social cognitive theo
rists including Barber, Sarbin, Spanos, Coe, Chaves, Kirsch and Lynn have identified
these and other social and cognitive variables, including rapport with the hypnotist, situ
ational demands, response biases, and performance standards, as influential determinants
of hypnotic responses, including memories elicited during hypnosis (see Lynn & Rhue
1991).

According to this perspective, hypnotized subjects strive to fulfill role demands and
behave in a manner consistent with their expectancies (e.g., Kirsch & Lynn, 1995; Shee
han & McConkey, 1982; Spanos, 1986). As far as memory goes, prehypnotic attitudes an
beliefs that hypnosis facilitates recall, as well as the hypnotic proceedings them
selves—including suggestions that hypnosis involves an altered state—generate expectan
cies that posthypnotic recall will be improved. Hence, it is not surprising that hypnotize
subjects frequently recall more information in hypnotic than in nonhypnotic contexts tha
do not generate such expectancies. By encouraging imagination, relaxation, and the com
plete experience of suggestions, hypnotic situations discourage critical evaluation of sug
gested events and memories and lower the threshold for reporting an imagined event as
"memory". Combined, these factors raise levels of confidence in inaccurate as well as ac
curate memories, although as we shall see later, the false confidence effect is not invari
ably large.

Social-cognitive theorists do not deny that certain abilities—including imaginative
and fantasy abilities—play a role in hypnotic responding. However, a consistent finding i
that the relation between measures of imaginative traits and dissociation and hypnotic re
sponsiveness is quite small (see Kirsch & Lynn, 1995). Patterns of imaginative activit
may, however, increase the distinctiveness and life-like quality of memories and lead to
increased and unwarranted confidence in their accuracy. This, however, would be posite
to occur in any situation that encourages imagination and discourages critical evaluation
of memory. Indeed, a social-cognitive account of memory and hypnosis assumes tha
memory distortions are not unique to hypnosis, and that when research controls for atti
tudes, expectancies, suggestive influences, and motivation to report memories, difference
between hypnotic and nonhypnotic conditions should be minimal or nonexistent. Never
theless, hypnotic procedures can and do increase pseudomemory risk, above and beyon
nonsuggestive procedures, as we will document below.

3. HYPNOSIS AND PSEUDOMEMORIES

3.1. Does Hypnosis Improve Memory?

We now turn to the first question we posed at the outset: Does hypnosis improv
memory? In a recent review of the literature, Erdelyi (1994) classified laboratory studie
according to the type of stimulus and memory tests employed in an attempt to bring a de
gree of order to what he regarded as a chaotic literature. Classifying 34 studies published
before 1988 in this manner, Erdelyi concluded that recall tests for high sense stimuli such
as poetry and meaningful pictures almost always produces hypermnesia or enhancemen

of memory. However, recognition tests for high sense and recognition and recall tests for low-sense stimuli such as nonsense syllables or word lists failed to show evidence of hypnotic hypermnesia. Erdelyi argued that a problem in interpreting these results is that even when hypnosis results in greater recall, there is an attendant increase in incorrect information. Hence, without controlling for response criteria, it is not possible to evaluate recall levels.

In two recent studies (Dinges, Whitehouse, Orne, Powell, Orne, & Erdelyi, 1992; Whitehouse, Dinges, Dinges, & Orne, 1988) that evaluated hypermnesia with response productivity controlled by means of a forced choice recall procedure, hypnosis did not produce enhanced recall beyond nonhypnotic hypermnesia. In fact, in one of the studies (Dinges et al. 1992), hypnosis not only failed to enhance retrieval of correct items, but it also increased the production of incorrect information. Relatedly, a study by Dywan and Bowers (1983) found that subjects who were hypnotized reported twice as many items and three times as many errors as nonhypnotic controls.

Hypnosis does not always evoke more information or increased error rates (Sanders & Simmons, 1983; Sheehan, 1988a; Sheehan & Tilden, 1983). In many studies, hypnotized and nonhypnotized subjects cannot be distinguished when careful controls are imposed, buttressing Erdelyi's (1994) conclusion that "no hypnosis-specific effect on memory has been observed" (p. 383). In short, the available evidence provides no warrant for the use of hypnosis as a memory aid, a conclusion entirely consistent with the socio-cognitive model.

3.1.1. Hypnosis and Emotional Stimuli. The guidelines for the use of clinical hypnosis advanced by the American Society of Clinical Hypnosis take exception to this conclusion with regard to meaningful, emotionally arousing stimuli, so it is important to carefully evaluate this contention. The authors of the guidelines state that "...with emotion-laden memories for meaningful material, we believe it likely that hypnosis has the potential to clearly prove helpful with some individuals". (p. 15)

It is claimed that in such instances emotional trauma has created a block to memory because of the state-dependent nature of some memories and the manner in which the encoding context and mood may be reinstated through hypnosis. The report thus endorses a "robust repression" model in which memories are blocked or locked away, and hypnosis can provide a key to the door of memory. This model has come under critical fire lately, and is far from universally accepted in the scientific community (see Ofshe & Singer, 1994). Moreover, state-dependent learning effects are often nonexistent and unreliable. When such effects do occur, they tend to be manifested in only a limited range of circumstances such as when participants experience strong, stable moods; when they play an active part in generating target events; and when they take responsibility for producing cues required to retrieve the events (Eich, 1995, p. 74). Hence, state-dependent learning effects fail to constitute a sufficient rationale for using hypnosis to reinstate context and mood. In closing, the reinstatement of context and mood in no way guarantees that information recalled will be accurate or protected against the usual vagaries of memory and suggestive influences.

The ASCH report justifies the use of hypnosis to enhance recall of early trauma by maintaining that early traumatic memories are encoded in visual images more than in verbal form, and that hypnosis enhances the vividness of imagery in hypnotizable persons. However, the idea that early traumatic memories are specifically encoded in visual images that can be accurately retrieved in adulthood lacks an empirical foundation and is not widely accepted scientifically (see Spanos, 1996).

Perhaps more problematic, encouraging persons to imagine during hypnosis, pa ticularly when recall is hazy or absent, constitutes a license to confabulate, a proble compounded by the fact that vivid imagery can increase the compelling quality of mem ries, independent of accuracy (e.g., Johnson, Hashtroudi, & Lindsay, 1993; Johnson Raye, 1981). For instance, Johnson, Raye, Wang, and Taylor (1979) showed that peop who scored high on a standard test of imagery tended to perform more poorly on a reali monitoring test, in which they were to distinguish between items they had previously se versus items they had previously imagined seeing. Indeed, later in the chapter we will r view studies which demonstrate hypnotizability is a risk factor for the production pseudomemories.

The ASCH report further contends that "Since hypnosis is believed by many peop in the field to be a controlled dissociation... and because of the evidence that many traum and abuse victims enter trance-like, dissociative states during and after trauma ... recrea ing an emotional and dissociative context through hypnosis integrated within psychothe apy may facilitate both the recovery and working through of traumatic memories". (p. 1. It is not altogether evident what is meant by the phrase "recreating an emotional and di sociative context through hypnosis," and the term "trance-like dissociative states" equally obscure. However, in our opinion, using dissociative recall techniques to establis a "dissociative context" is very risky, if dissociative techniques include such procedur as inviting clients to watch split screen television images or having them leave their bod to watch a traumatic scene unfold. These techniques are highly suggestive in nature. I deed, the report appears to be contradictory in the sense that it advocates establishing dissociative context while it cautions the reader that dissociative techniques may carry degree of risk to the client.

Finally, the argument that hypnosis and dissociation can be equated is not supporte by the available evidence. Across many studies, measures of dissociation are, on averag correlated with hypnotizability at .14 (see Green & Lynn, 1995). With appropriate co trols for context effects, the correlation vanishes to near zero. If the authors of the repo mean by dissociation something different than what dissociation scales measure, then it necessary to specify what is meant in this regard.

In their defense of hypnosis as a potentially valuable memory recovery tool, th authors of the guidelines argue that laboratory research has limited ecological validit and that it is possible to overgeneralize experimental findings to real-world trauma vic tims. This point is beyond dispute. After all, many laboratory studies involved bystande or witnesses of events rather than trauma victims. Furthermore, there are ethical cor straints attached to the treatment of experimental subjects in the laboratory that unde standably make researchers chary of exposing subjects to high levels of negativel arousing stimuli.

Nevertheless, a number of experimental studies, the majority of which were n cited in the ASCH report, have been conducted that compare hypnotic versus nonhypnoti memory in the face of relatively emotionally arousing stimuli. Many of these studies hav used stressor films, some with demonstrable physiological and subjective manipulatio checks (De Piano & Salzberg, 1981), which have involved depictions of fatal stabbing (Grabowski, Roese, & Thomas, 1991); an actual murder that was videotaped serendipi tously (Sheehan, Garnett, & Robertson, 1993); a transorbital lobotomy (DePiano & Salzberg, 1981); shop accidents and mutilations (DePiano & Salzberg, 1981); sexual inte course (DePiano & Salzberg, 1981); and an event either described as the aftermath of a accident, a shoplifting incident, or a violent robbery (Kaltenbach & Lynn, 1996). Other re searchers have had subjects read a gory story (Wagstaff & Sykes, 1984), or have expose subjects to an emotionally arousing news announcement (Baker & Patrick, 1987) or a mock assassination (Timm, 1981). In all, seven laboratory studies have failed to confirm the hypothesis that hypnosis is effective in enhancing memory in emotionally arousing situations when appropriate controls are used. These studies yield a clear and consistent conclusion: Hypnosis neither improves recall in emotionally arousing situations nor does arousal level mediate hypnotic recall.

Erdelyi (1994) has suggested that the findings from Sloane's (1981) doctoral dissertation with the Los Angeles Police Department counters the argument that the results of "contrived" laboratory studies are totally irrelevant to true-life traumas. Sloane found that hypnosis did not augment recognition memory for victims of violent crimes such as rapes and shootings. Although clinical situations may well differ from more sterile laboratory situations, and traumatic memories may differ in certain respects from emotional yet non-traumatic memories, there is no empirical ground for concluding that hypnosis has a role in the recovery of emotional or traumatic memories and, hence, no justification for the use of hypnosis to recover such memories.

3.2. Are Hypnotized Participants Particularly Vulnerable to Misleading Information?

Hypnosis may not only fail to improve memory, but introducing subtle leading questions and misinformation can impair recall. Putnam (1979), Zelig and Beidelman (1981), and Sanders and Simmons (1983) found that hypnotized subjects made more memory errors in response to leading questions than did subjects in waking control groups, although Rainer (1984) and Sheehan et al. (1993) found no such differences in responses to leading questions across hypnotic and nonhypnotic groups. Misinformation effects are thus not limited to hypnosis.

As far as hypnotizability goes, Register and Kihlstrom (1988) failed to find that high versus low hypnotizable subjects responded differently to leading questions. Although Sheehan et al. (1993) found that high hypnotizable subjects accepted more false suggestions than did low hypnotizable subjects, they failed to confirm their prediction that high hypnotizable subjects during hypnotic instruction would show most evidence of accepting false information in response to strongly cued leading questions.

In conclusion, hypnotic subjects are at least as likely as nonhypnotic subjects to be misled in their recall by leading questions and sometimes are more prone to the biasing effects of leading questions. There also are indications that high hypnotizable persons are particularly vulnerable to memory distortion in response to misleading information. None of the research, however, indicates that hypnosis produces more accurate recall than waking conditions or somehow immunizes against the effects of misinformation (see Spanos, 1996).

3.3. Do Hypnotic Procedures Enhance Unwarranted Confidence in Remembered Events?

Studies indicate that although hypnosis does not always increase confidence for memories, hypnotized individuals often express a level of confidence in memories that is higher than the accuracy of the memories warrant. This effect is apparent in both recognition and recall memory tests (Sheehan & Tilden, 1983, 1984, 1986) and in situations in which deliberate attempts are made to mislead subjects by way of leading questions (see

Sheehan, 1988a,b's program of research) and in which no such attempts are made (e.g., Dywan & Bowers, 1983).

Why might this be so? The survey research reviewed earlier implies that merely defining the situation as "hypnotic" generates demands for recall. Unfortunately, there are no countervailing demands for accuracy. Buckhout, Eugenio, Licitra, Oliver, and Kramer (1981) found that when subjects exhibited little or no memory for critical details, 90% of the hypnotized subjects versus only 20% of the nonhypnotized controls reported motivation to guess the correct response. In short, hypnosis sanctions guessing within the expectational context that whatever is remembered is accurate.

Research indicates that hypnotizability level plays a role in the degree of confidence expressed, with high hypnotizable subjects evidencing more confidence in recall than low hypnotizable subjects (Dywan & Bowers, 1983; Sheehan & Tilden, 1983). Ability may be important insofar as relatively imaginative subjects' vivid representations of suggested events render them prone to confuse imaginings with memories. However, another possibility is that relatively high hypnotizable subjects are particularly sensitive to situational demands that contribute to confidence effects.

This latter point is underscored by research with simulating subjects—that is, low hypnotizable subjects who are instructed to role play the responses of excellent hypnotic subjects, as a control for situational demand characteristics. Nonhypnotized simulating subjects generally display high levels of confidence in the memories they report during simulated hypnosis (Sheehan, 1988a,b)—sometimes in excess of that displayed by high hypnotizable subjects (Redston & Knox, 1983; Sheehan & Tilden, 1984) and sometimes equivalent to that of hypnotizable subjects. In the one study in which hypnotizable subjects exhibited greater confidence than simulators, Sheehan (Study 4, 1988a) suggested that the hypnotizable subjects might have scrutinized the misinformation less critically than did simulators.

Gwynn and Spanos (1996) have argued that confidence effects and the relation between confidence and hypnotizability is mediated by context-based expectancies. In many studies, subjects are tested for memory or pseudomemory as part of the same experiment in which their hypnotizability is assessed. When high hypnotizable subjects are aware of their hypnotizability scores, they are likely to act in terms of how they believe a high hypnotizable subject should respond. Increased confidence, then, is thought to reflect a carryover of expectancies across hypnotizability and memory test situations. Spanos, Quigley et al. (1991) tested high and low hypnotizable subjects' abilities to identify mug shots of an offender in a videotaped mock murder following either hypnosis or alert test conditions. Care was taken to not inform the nonhypnotic subjects that they had been selected on the basis of their hypnotizability scores. The investigators found that neither hypnotizability nor the administration of an hypnotic induction influenced the nonhypnotized subjects' accuracy of mug shot identifications. In contrast, hypnotizability and confidence were correlated in terms of incorrect identifications on the part of the hypnotic subjects. Hypnotizability and confidence were not correlated in nonhypnotic subjects. These results support the hypothesis that the relationship between hypnotizability and confidence is mediated by context-based expectancies.

The sensitivity of confidence ratings to contextual variations might be one explanation for why increased and/or unwarranted confidence in hypnotic recollections is neither uniformly present nor inevitably strong. For instance, in some studies the effect was not found at all (Mingay, 1977; Putnam, 1979; Reston & Knox, 1983; Sheehan et al., 1993; Zelig & Beidelman, 1981); in a number of other studies, when the effect was found, it was not very impressive in magnitude. For example, in Whitehouse et al. (1988), the confidence of hypnotized participants in inaccurate recollections increased from "just guessing" to "much doubt". Nogrady, McConkey, and Perry (1985) and Spanos et al. (1989) reported similarly small effects. Sanders and Simmons (1983) reported that hypnotized subjects did not report significantly higher confidence ratings than nonhypnotized controls when the measure used was "willingness to testify in court".

Some influential workers in the field (Orne, 1979) have argued that unwarranted confidence in hypnotically augmented memories is so strong that effective cross-examined is precluded. Only one study exists on this subject, but the research by Spanos et al. (1989) and his associates indicates this is not the case. In a paradigm designed to induce misinformation effects in high and low hypnotizable subjects, Spanos et al. found that hypnotic subjects were just as likely as nonhypnotic subjects to break down under cross examination by disavowing their earlier false recollections. Hence, hypnotic testimony was no more resistant to cross-examination than nonhypnotic testimony. Additionally, after cross-examination, marked by clear demands for disavowing earlier testimony, the pseudomemory reports (i.e., misattributions) of high and low hypnotizables converged because the high hypnotizables showed a greater drop in misattributions.

Our conclusions are in keeping with those of Spanos (1996): "Both hypnotic and nonhypnotic subjects are frequently overconfident about the accuracy of what they recall. Although the evidence is mixed, some studies suggest that hypnotic subjects exhibit even larger overconfidence effects than nonhypnotic subjects". (p. 93–94) Whereas confidence effects are, at times, sizable (see McConkey, 1992; Wagstaff, 1989), they are neither invariably large nor do they necessarily preclude cross examination. Nevertheless, given the small data base on the effects of hypnosis on the ability to withstand cross examination, it seems premature to draw definitive conclusions at this time. It is, however, appropriate to conclude that the literature does not support the idea that hypnosis selectively increases confidence in accurate memories.

3.4. Does Hypnotic Age Regression Facilitate Recall of Distant Past Events?

We have so far considered memories of events in the recent past. However, earlier we referred to survey data indicating that many clinicians use hypnosis to recover very early memories of child sexual abuse. It is therefore important to examine the impact of hypnosis on memories of events in the distant past. After all, if hypnosis is not a viable way of recovering memories of the recent past, there is no reason to believe it would be any more effective in recovering events in the distant past. A corpus of experimental evidence on hypnotic age regression supports this conclusion.

The compelling and potentially persuasive nature of hypnotized subjects' memory reports is no better illustrated than in the case of age regression. This point can be highlighted by an anecdote based on the senior author's (SJL) clinical work. His client missed a therapy session. Because she had a history of suicide attempts and was depressed at the time, he decided to contact her the next day. She was puzzled by his concern and stated, "Are you kidding me, I was there". But as it turned out, she had no memory for what was discussed during the session. Nevertheless, it was difficult to convince her that she missed her appointment. At the next session, SJL age regressed her to the time of the previous session in order to explore her memory lapse. During hypnosis, she stated that she was angry with her 7-year-old son, left her house crying, and drove to a nearby cemetery. With much emotion, she related how she went to an open grave, got in the grave, and became terrified when she could not get out of the grave. After several frantic attempts, she finally succeeded in extricating herself from the grave. She then drove home and reported that she went to sleep. After hypnosis, she was extremely upset by the thought that she would do this.

SJL, however, had his doubts. The next night they visited the grave together. There was no such grave at the site that matched her description. When he interviewed her son, he informed him that his mother had slept through our session! Her vivid experience was, perhaps, a dream or a fantasy generated during hypnosis. His mother, a classic fantasy prone person, had, over the years, confused fantasy and reality on a number of occasions. If no effort were made to ascertain the validity of the client's claims, it would have been very easy to accept her dramatic and seemingly convincing narrative.

Many studies of hypnotic age regression indicate that age regression narratives can be dramatic and compelling yet fail to correspond to historical events. In his exhaustive review of over 100 years of hypnosis research on temporal regression, Nash (1987) failed to find any special correspondence between the behavior and experience of hypnotized adults and that of actual children. The conclusion at which he arrived is that whereas the products of hypnotic age regression are often clinically useful, the client's responses, which often reflect their beliefs and assumptions about childhood characteristics and experiences at certain ages, cannot be accepted as face value. In fact, Nash (1992) argued that a literal reliving of an historical event is not humanly possible and that a client's report may have little or nothing to do with an actual event. No matter how dramatic, no matter how subjectively compelling to the client, and no matter how clinically useful, clients are not able to literally return to a state of childhood functioning (Nash & Lynn, 1994).

To provide relevant examples, we will summarize several studies conducted in our laboratory. The first study (Hamel & Lynn, 1996), used Naglieri's (1986) Draw A Person test, which provides a valid measure of developmental level based on figure drawings. The investigators age-regressed hypnotized and simulating subjects to the second grade and asked them to draw pictures of a man, a woman, and of themselves. Hypnotized subjects gave their age during age regression as 7.1 years, and simulators gave their age as 7.2 years. Furthermore, the subjects spelled words in a childlike manner, showing clear changes between their adult and child handwritings. However, the age regressed hypnotized and the simulating subjects did not perform in a manner consistent with their stated ages on the figure drawing tasks. In fact, the hypnotized subjects performed in a manner consistent with children who were nearly 9 years old (8.97 years) and the simulating subjects performed in a manner consistent with children who were nearly 8 years old (7.98 years). In short, despite their compelling role enactments, subjects apparently fused or intermingled more recent memories with old memories, impairing their ability to perform in a childlike manner on the figure drawing test.

The second age regression study underlined the fact that what may be remembered during hypnosis is not an exact replay of an historical event. Nash, Drake, Wiley, Khalsa, and Lynn (1986) attempted to corroborate the memories of subjects who participated in an earlier age regression experiment. This experiment involved age regressing hypnotized and simulating subjects to age 3 years to a scene in which they were in the soothing presence of their mothers. During the experiment, subjects reported the identity of their transitional objects (e.g., blankets, teddy bears). Third-party verification (parent report) of the accuracy of recall was obtained for the two groups: 14 hypnotized subjects and 10 simulation control subjects. Despite the similarity to children in their way of relating to transitional objects, hypnotic subjects were less able than control subjects to correctly identify the specific transitional objects actually used. Hypnotic subjects' hypnotic recollections, for example, matched their parent's report only 21% of the time, whereas simulators' reports after hypnosis were corroborated by their parents 70% of the time. Furthermore, all recollections obtained during hypnosis were incorporated into posthypnotic recollections, regardless of accuracy. These finding imply that clinicians should not assume the veridicality of specific content reported during or after hypnosis.

In the next study, Sivec and Lynn (1996a) compared hypnotized versus alert imagining subjects' performance when it was suggested that a person experience a meaningful event at an age that it was possible to verify that the event did not occur. Sivec and Lynn age regressed subjects to the age of 5 and suggested that they played with a Cabbage Patch Doll if they were a girl or a He-Man toy if they were a boy. These were the most popular toys released by Mattel Toy Company for a 5-year period. Half of the subjects received hypnotic age regression instructions and half of the subjects received suggestions to age regress that were not administered in a hypnotic context. However, the toy was not released until two or three years after the target time of the age regression suggestion. Interestingly, none of the nonhypnotized persons were clearly influenced by the suggestion. They did not rate the memory of the experience as real, nor were they confident that the event occurred at the age they were regressed to. However, 20% of the hypnotized subjects rated the memory of the experience as real and were confident that the event occurred at the age to which they were regressed. Hence, the pseudomemory effect was specific to the hypnosis condition. The data are consistent with the idea that hypnosis can increase false confidence in remembered events.

Whereas it is not ethical to study the malleability of abuse reports in the laboratory, it is possible to examine the effects of social influence on early memories that cross the two-year threshold of infantile amnesia. Researchers converge in their opinion that memories before age two are not likely to be veridical descriptions of actual historical events (see Malinoski, Lynn, & Sivec, in press). In one such study, Sivec and Lynn (1996b) asked hypnotized and nonhypnotized subjects about their earliest memories. Only 3% of the 40 subjects in the alert condition recalled a memory earlier than two years the first time they were asked to report their earliest memory. However, 23% of the 40 hypnotized subjects reported a memory earlier than age 2, 20% reported a memory earlier than 18 months, 18% reported a memory earlier than a year, and 8% reported a memory of earlier than 6 months. The second time they were asked for an early memory, only 8% of the nonhypnotized subjects reported a memory earlier than two years, and only 3% reported memories of 6 months or earlier, statistics consistent with large surveys we have done with college students. In contrast, 35% of hypnotized subjects reported memories earlier than 18 months, 30% of subjects reported memories earlier than a year, and fully 13% of subjects reported a memory before six months.

Before leaving the topic of hypnotic age regression, it is important to describe a study done in Spanos's laboratory that illustrates the importance of expectancies transmitted prior to actual age regression procedures. In a series of studies Spanos, Menary et al. (1991) showed that prehypnotic expectancies affected the characteristics that subjects attributed to "past-life identities" and the extent to which past-life identities described themselves as having been abused during childhood. Spanos, Burgess, and Burgess (1994) stated that, "When constructing their past lives, subject shape the attributes and biographies attributed to these identities to correspond to their understandings of what significant others believe these characteristics to be" (p. 435). These findings are consistent with many studies inspired by the social-cognitive model showing that prehypnotic expectancies affect a variety of responses including amnesia, pain perception, and the experience of involuntariness.

Of course, pseudomemories are not restricted to hypnotic contexts. In a recent study that Malinoski and Lynn (1966) conducted, interviewers asked subjects to report their earliest memory, and questioned subjects until they denied any earlier memories for two sequential probes. Interviewers then asked subjects to close their eyes, see themselves "in their mind's eye" as a toddler or infant, and "get in touch" with memories of long ago. Interviewers also informed subjects that most young adults can retrieve memories of very early events—including their second birthday—if they "let themselves go" and try hard to visualize, focus, and concentrate. Interviewers then asked for subjects' memories of their second birthday, after which they received additional instructions to visualize, concentrate, and focus on even earlier memories and were complimented and reinforced for reporting increasingly early memories.

The mean age of the initial reported memory was 3.70 years, with only 11.3% of subjects reporting initial earliest memories at or before age 24 months. Furthermore, the more fantasy prone and open to experience a person was, the more likely they were to report an earlier initial memory. The mean age of the earliest memory report elicited prior to the visualization procedure was 3.16 years, with 15% of subjects reporting memories at or before 24 months. However, after receiving the visualization instructions, 59.4% of the subjects reported a memory of their second birthday. After the birthday memory was solicited, interviewers pressed subjects for even earlier memories. The mean age of the earliest memory reported was 1.60 years, fully two years less than their initial memory report.

One of the most interesting findings was that 78.2% of the sample reported at least one memory that occurred at 24 months of age or earlier. Furthermore, 56% of the subjects reported a memory between birth and 18 months of life, a third of the subjects reported a memory that occurred at age 12 months or younger, and 18.0% reported at least one memory of an event that occurred at six months or younger. Finally, 4% of the sample provided memory reports from the first week of life.

Interestingly, measures of compliance, fantasy proneness, interrogative suggestibility, and hypnotizability correlated significantly with either memories of the second birthday or at least one memory from 24 months of age or earlier. Perceived clarity of earliest memory report emerged as a strong predictor of confidence in the accuracy of the very earliest memory ($r = .58$, $p < .001$). In a final questionnaire, subjects indicated moderate-to-high levels of confidence in the accuracy of their memory reports. Further, subjects believed their memories were, overall, quite accurate, and reported they did not feel much pressure to report increasingly early memories and that they did not "make up things to please the experimenter". It is noteworthy that this questionnaire was completed anonymously, minimizing the effects of demand characteristics on subjects' responses.

This study indicates that very early memory reports are sensitive to social pressure and suggestions to report early memories. The veridicality of early memories was not assessed. However, the age of many of the memory reports make it unlikely that they were actual memories of events at the claimed age of occurrence. In conclusion, hypnotic enactments and memories can be very compelling yet inaccurate. Moreover, with sufficient pressure, even nonhypnotic early memory reports are malleable and, although implausible, embraced with confidence.

3.5. Hypnotic Pseudomemories: What Are Their Determinants?

With the exception of age regression studies, we have so far reviewed studies that use relatively subtle questions or information designed to mislead subjects. We have not considered studies in which unsubtle, explicit leading suggestions are administered with the expressed goal of creating so-called pseudomemories. Early figures in the history of hypnosis including Bernheim, Janet and Forel were aware of the fact that hypnotic suggestions were capable of permanently altering memories.

The phenomenon of hypnotically-induced pseudomemory is exemplified in Bernheim's dramatic case of "Marie, G".: "where is the case of a somnambulist, Marie G...., an intelligent woman... I hypnotize her into a deep sleep and say, "you got up in the night?" She replies, "Oh, no." "I insist upon it; you got up four times to go to the water closet, and the fourth time you fell on your nose. This is a fact, and when you wake up no one will be able to make you believe the contrary." When she wakes I ask, "How are you now?" "Very well," she answers, "but last night I had an attack of diarrhea. I had to get up four times. I fell, too, and hurt my nose." I say, "You dreamed that. You said nothing to me about it right now. Not one of the patients saw you." She persists in her statement, saying that she had not been dreaming, that she was perfectly conscious of getting up, that all the patients were asleep; - and she remains convinced that the occurrence was genuine" (pp. 164–165).

More recently, Orne (1979) developed a procedure for demonstrating pseudomemory which, interestingly, bears a certain resemblance to the procedures used by Bernheim in the case of Marie. Orne's description of the procedure follows: "First, I carefully establish and verify that a particular subject had in fact gone to bed at midnight on say February 17, and had arisen at 8 a.m. the following morning. After inducing deep hypnosis, it is suggested that the subject relive the night of February 17 - getting ready for bed, turning out the light, and going to sleep at midnight. As the subject relives being asleep, he is told that it is now 4 a.m. and then is asked whether he has heard the two loud noises. Following this question (which is in fact a suggestion), a good subject typically responds that the noises awakened him. Now instructed to look around and check the time, he may say it is exactly 4:06 a.m. If then asked what he is doing, he may describe some activity such as going to the window to see what happened or wondering about the noises, forgetting about them, and going back to sleep.

Still hypnotized, he may relive waking up at 8 a.m. and describe his subsequent day. If, prior to being awakened, he is told he will be able to remember the events of February 17 as well as all the other things that happened to him in hypnosis, he readily confounds his hypnotic experience with actual memory on awakening. If asked about the night of February 17, he will describe going to sleep, and being awakened by two loud noises. If one inquires at what time these occurred, he will say, "Oh, yes, I looked at my watch beside my bed. It has a radium dial. It was exactly 4:06 a.m...." The subject will be convinced that his description about February 17 is accurately reflecting his original memories" (pp. 322–323; see also Barnes, 1982).

Adapting Orne's (1979) pseudomemory creation procedure, Laurence and Perry (1983) provided the first quantitative investigation of pseudomemory. Highly hypnotizable subjects were asked to select a night of the previous week during which they reported no specific memories of awakening or dreaming. After being hypnotically age-regressed to the night in question, subjects were administered a suggestion to hear "Some loud noises that may sound like back-firings of a car, or door slammings...some loud noises". (p. 524). After hypnosis, 76.5% of the subjects who previously accepted the noise suggestion (13/17), or 48% of the total sample, demonstrated pseudomemory by maintaining that the sounds had actually occurred or reported that they were uncertain about whether or not the noises were real.

Replications of the pseudomemory effect using the above design, which has come to be termed the "nocturnal events" paradigm, have been obtained from different laboratories with rates ranging between 39–81% for high hypnotizable subjects (Labelle, et al., 1990; Labelle & Perry, 1986; Laurence et al., 1986; Lynn, et al., 1992; McCann & Sheehan, 1988, Study 1; Spanos & McLean, 1986;Weekes, et al., 1992). In the process of addressing increasingly sophisticated questions, researchers have gone beyond merely demonstrating the pliability of memory reports in response to suggestion, to specifying the aptitudinal, interpersonal, and situational variables that affect such reports. In the next section, we consider a number of determinants of pseudomemories.

3.5.1. Hypnotizability. According to a socio-cognitive perspective, hypnotically suggested memories resemble other suggested responses in key respects. Not surprisingly, studies have demonstrated a relation between hypnotizability and responsiveness to pseudomemory suggestions. In general, high and medium hypnotizable subjects report more pseudomemories than do lows (see Lynn & Nash, 1994). In some studies, medium hypnotizables perform comparably to highs (Sheehan, Statham, & Jamieson, 1991b), and in other studies, medium hypnotizables display less pseudomemory than highs, but more than lows (Sheehan, Statham, & Jamieson, 1991a). The fact that many medium hypnotizable persons, who represent the modal subjects in the population, report pseudomemories indicates that the effect may be much more pervasive than certain writers have contended (e.g., Brown, 1995).

Interestingly, high hypnotizable subjects exhibit pseudomemories to a greater extent than low hypnotizables in nonhypnotized as well as hypnotized conditions (McConkey, Labelle, Bibb, & Bryant, 1990; Sheehan, Statham, Jamieson, & Ferguson, 1991; Spanos, Gwynn, Comer, Baltruweit, & DeGroh, 1989). This suggests that pseudomemory responding is associated with a general suggestibility or compliance factor that transcends the hypnotic situation. However, a recent retrospective analysis (E.C. Orne, Whitehouse, Dinges, & M. T. Orne, 1996) of results from several studies of hypnotically influenced memories indicate that even low hypnotizable subjects can be vulnerable to false memories in hypnotic conditions.

It is necessary to include nonhypnotic control groups in order to evaluate the extent to which pseudomemory is specific to hypnosis. Studies comparing pseudomemory rates among hypnotized and nonhypnotized "waking" conditions have produced mixed results. Research by Sheehan and his associates (Sheehan, 1991, Studies 1 & 2; Sheehan et al., 1991 a, b) consistently demonstrated higher rates of pseudomemory among hypnotized subjects compared to waking controls given questionnaire filler tasks to equate for the time required to deliver hypnotic inductions. In contrast, studies by Barnier and McConkey (1992) and McConkey et al. (1990) found that hypnotic and nonhypnotic controls reported equivalent levels of pseudomemory in response to suggested items (see also Spanos et al., 1989).

A socio-cognitive account of hypnosis emphasizes participants' motivations, expectancies, and demand characteristics inherent in the testing situation. Differences in pseudomemory between hypnotic and nonhypnotic treatments such as responding to filler tasks may be due to differential motivation and demand characteristics across these two situations. Weekes, Lynn, Green, and Brentar (1992) compared the pseudomemory rates of hypnotized and awake task motivated subjects (Barber, 1969; see also Sheehan & Perry, 1976) using the nocturnal events paradigm. Task motivation is operationally similar to hypnosis insofar as subjects are told that the experimenter is interested in subjective experience and they are also told that the experiment is designed to test their ability to imagine and visualize events in tests of imagination. The researchers found that subjects in both conditions exhibited equivalent levels of pseudomemory (69%).

In a related experiment, Lynn, Rhue, Myers, and Weekes (1994) again used the nocturnal events paradigm and administered the pseudomemory suggestion to high hypnotizable hypnotized subjects and low hypnotizables instructed to simulate or "fake" hypnosis (Orne, 1959). Both treatments produced equivalent levels of pseudomemory. In two other studies in our laboratory, to which we refer later, the finding that hypnotized and simulating subjects report pseudomemories at the same rate was replicated. Taken together, these findings suggest that pseudomemory reports are neither unique nor specific to hypnosis and further suggest that false memory reports are influenced by the situational demands inherent within the experimental context.

3.5.2. Social and Contextual Factors. According to the social cognitive model of hypnosis, a variety of situational and interpersonal factors influence hypnotic responses, with memory being no exception. Consistent with this emphasis on contextual factors, in two studies, Sheehan, Green, and Truesdale (1992) found that rapport between hypnotist and subject affected the rate of pseudomemory, with reduced rapport appreciably lowering the pseudomemory rate. McCann and Sheehan (1988, Study 1), in a replication of Laurence and Perry's original (1983) study, found that varying the instructions provided to subjects in the hypnotic context greatly influenced subjects' pseudomemory reports. When subjects were informed that the hypnotic effects (including the pseudomemory suggestion) would be carried over or persist following the termination of the hypnotic procedures, the pseudomemory rate was 70%. However, when the hypnosis and waking treatments were clearly differentiated, the pseudomemory rate dropped to 20%.

Relatedly, McConkey et al. (1990) found that the experimental context strongly affected the rate of pseudomemory. Upon immediate testing, approximately 50% of hypnotizable subjects reported pseudomemory. However, when contacted by telephone at home 4–24 hours later by an experimenter who was not part of the earlier session, the rate decreased dramatically to 2.5%. Barnier and McConkey (1992) replicated the finding that the overall pseudomemory rate declined from 60% for a false suggestion that a thief depicted in a series of slides was wearing a scarf, to 10% when the experimental context shifted to imply to subjects that the experiment had ended. Similarly, pseudomemory rate for a false suggestion that he had been carrying a bouquet of flowers dropped from 27%-3%. McCann and Sheehan (1987) were also successful in "breaching" pseudomemory. When subjects were presented with incontrovertible evidence relating to the original memories, by giving them a recognition test involving the videotape of a robbery they observed, pseudomemory rates decreased substantially.

In an attempt to reduce pseudomemory reports by varying the demands of the experimental testing situation, Murrey, Cross, and Whipple (1992) offered a monetary award to subjects able to distinguish real memories and suggested false memories. Subjects given monetary incentives to report accurately were less likely to report pseudomemories than subjects not given monetary incentives. A study by Spanos and McLean (1986) showed that false memories could be breached by providing subjects with information during hypnosis that affected their expectancies about appropriate responding during hypnosis. The researchers incorporated the "hidden observer" technique (e.g., Hilgard, 1977) into an adaptation of the nocturnal events paradigm to "breach" or reverse subjects' initial pseudomemory reports. Initially, almost 82% (9/11) of subjects who accepted the false memory suggestion reported pseudomemories. Subjects were then administered the following hidden observer instructions: "During deep hypnosis people often confuse reality with things that were only imagined. The hypnotized part of a person's mind accepts suggestions so completely that what was suggested actually seems to have been happening...Yet at the same time that you are experiencing suggestions, there is some other part of your mind, a hidden part, that knows what is really going on...The hidden part can always distinguish what was suggested from what really happened (p. 157)". With this instructional set, all but 2 subjects reversed their responding and reported that the noises had only been suggested to them. When the experimenter instructed subjects that she wished to shift from the "hidden part" back to the hypnotized part, subjects again reported pseudomemories.

Two studies by Weekes, Lynn, Brentar, Myers, and Green (Lynn et al., 1994 & Weekes et al., 1992), to which we referred previously, employed a nonhypnotic manipulation which informed subjects that they can successfully distinguish between fantasy and reality through the use of "deep concentration". Unlike Spanos and McLean's (1986) hidden observer manipulation, the deep concentration manipulation failed to reverse subjects' pseudomemory reports. Unlike the deep concentration instructions, the hidden observer instructions provided clear demands for subjects to reverse their earlier pseudomemory reports, while simultaneously permitting them to remain in the role of a responsive hypnotized subject, without contradicting themselves.

In a third study, Green, Lynn, and Malinoski (1996) attempted a close replication of Spanos and McLean's (1986) procedures by using their instructions and assessing hidden observer responses during hypnosis, as they did. Even though Green et al. followed Spanos and McLean's procedures, the former investigators were once again unable to show that the majority of persons who report pseudomemories reverse them in the face of shifting demand characteristics. That is, only 22% of persons who initially showed pseudomemories reversed their reports under hidden observer instructions. The reasons for the failure to replicate Spanos and his colleagues' findings are unclear. However, it appears that pseudomemory reports can be obdurate and recalcitrant to modification. In summary, there is a growing body of evidence that implicates contextual factors in the genesis of pseudomemories. However, it is also clear that once pseudomemories are instated, they may be difficult to reverse.

3.5.3. Confidence in Pseudomemory Reports. In Laurence and Perry's initial investigation, subjects were classified as demonstrating pseudomemory if they reported that the suggested events occurred or reported that they were uncertain whether the events actually took place. The majority of pseudomemory studies do not indicate what criterion of certainty, if any, was used when calculating pseudomemory. Nor do the majority of pseudomemory studies (two exceptions being Lynn, Weekes, & Milano, 1989; Lynn, Milano, & Weekes, 1991) assess the degree to which the subject was able to experience age regression, the pseudomemory suggestion, or even hypnosis. However, studies conducted in three laboratories (Barnier & McConkey, 1992; Lynn et al. 1991; Sheehan, et al. 1991a, b; Weekes, Lynn, & Myers, 1996) have shown that subjects who report pseudomemories are frequently unsure about the accuracy of their memories. Hence, it is not surprising that such subjects have been found to be less confident of the accuracy of their recall than subjects who do not report pseudomemories (Sheehan et al. 1991a, b). The fact that subjects are not confident about their recall suggests that original memory traces may still be available to some degree and that pseudomemories may be more fragile than is generally acknowledged. At the same time, as noted above, research in our laboratory has shown that pseudomemories, once instated, may be difficult to reverse.

3.5.4. Memory as a Decision Process: Event Base Rates and Distinctiveness. According to the socio-cognitive perspective, hypnotic responses and experiences are the byproduct not only of expectancies but also of decision making processes based on performance standards. Lynn, Green, and Jaquith (1996) have shown that performance standards can have an appreciable effect on hypnotic responses. Contrary to how most subjects actually perform, one group of subjects was informed prehypnotically that subjects who respond to more than a few suggestions imagine suggested events as lifelike and "as real as real (events)" and respond immediately and involuntarily to suggestions. In comparison to subjects who received standard prehypnotic instructions that accompany standardized hypnotizability scales, subjects who received the instructions that established a stringent or difficult response criterion believed they responded to only two and a half suggestions, passed nearly three fewer suggestions, and reported far less suggestion related involuntariness than subjects in the standard instruction condition. Hence, hypnotized persons use information at their disposal to make decisions about their responses.

Memory is also the endproduct of decision and inferential processes: Pseudomemories result when participants mistakenly decide that a suggested event occurred when in fact it did not. In situations in which there is a vivid memory of an event, it is plausible that the event occurred, and the event is highly distinctive, the decision about whether the memory occurred is an easy one. Under these circumstances, most individuals would say that the event occurred. However, it is not always that easy to decide whether an event occurred or did not occur. Often we are unsure about what occurred or when it occurred, and our memories are not all that vivid and lack life-like qualities. Hence, the criteria adopted and the inferences generated to evaluate whether a memory occurred or not can play a role in distinguishing fantasy and reality and pseudomemory formation (see Johnson & Raye, 1981; Johnson et al., 1993).

Strack and Bless (1994) contended that if a person is certain they would have recalled an event had they witnessed it, they would have a basis for inferring the nonoccurrence of the event, even if they could not recall the specific event. The example the authors give is of a student who is asked whether a professor was wearing a sombrero during a lecture. The student is able to deny this occurrence with confidence because metacognitive knowledge (about one's own mental functioning) can be applied to the conclude that the event should be remembered if it in fact occurred. That is, in the case of an event that "is conceptually or categorically distinct" (p. 205), the lack of a memory provides a powerful cue that the event did not occur. On the other hand, with less salient events, such as asking whether the professor was wearing eye glasses during the lecture, Strack and Bless maintain that the absence of a memory would not lead to a confident denial of the occurrence in that the event would not have been thought to be memorable.

Decision making processes are relevant to suggested events and the influence of misleading information. The principle of discrepancy detection (Hall, Loftus, & Tousignant, 1984) states that misleading information is most likely to bias participants when they do not detect discrepancies between post-event information and memory for an original event (p. 135). Tousignant, Hall, and Loftus (1986) found a relation between participants' degree of scrutiny of information designed to mislead them (i.e., reading a postevent narrative containing misleading information slowly) and the degree to which misinformation was resisted. Furthermore, when there is substantial forgetting of items associated with long retention intervals, or subjects are uncertain about whether an event actually took place, they may be vulnerable to misleading suggestions (e.g., Belli, 1989; Belli, Windschitl, McCarthy, & Winfrey, 1992; Brainerd & Reyna, 1988; Lindsay, 1990). As an extension of the principle of discrepancy detection, when the contents of hypnotic suggestions conflict with the memory for events that participants are certain did not take place, such suggestions are unlikely to elicit pseudomemory reports.

Our discussion implies that whether a person reports that a suggested event occurred may well vary with respect to the nature of the event and the attendant certainty or lack of it regarding its actual occurrence. In keeping with this idea, McCann and Sheehan (l988) and Lynn, Weekes, and Milano, 1989) have argued that events that are publicly verifiable and in the person's direct field of experience are associated with relatively low pseudomemory rates. In contrast, hazy or uncertain memories of current or childhood events may be prone to distortion by deliberate or inadvertent suggestion (Lynn & Nash, 1994; Loftus, 1993).

In research inspired by Orne's original (1979) pseudomemory demonstration, the target event was a loud noise such as a door slamming or a car backfiring (e.g., Labelle & Perry, 1986; Labelle, et al., 1990; Laurence & Perry, 1983; Lynn, et al., 1994; McCann & Sheehan, 1988, Study 1; Weekes, Lynn, Green, & Brentar, 1992) that occurred while participants were asleep. Presumably, these events have a high base rate of occurrence in everyday life and are not particularly distinctive. Thus, participants might not believe that they would remember whether an event of this nature occurred, and might be uncertain of whether the event occurred on a particular occasion. Under these circumstances, it would be expected that participants would adopt a lax pseudomemory report criterion (i.e., say the event occurred when in doubt or when prompted by task demands to report pseudomemory or had a vivid imaginal representation of the event), and be vulnerable to the effects of leading questions that promote pseudomemory responding by implying that the event actually occurred (e.g., "Tell me when you hear the noise;" see also Spanos & McLean, 1986). Indeed, research using everyday stimuli or events with a relatively high base rate of occurrence has documented pseudomemory rates ranging from 39–81%.

In another line of pseudomemory research, Lynn, Weekes, and Milano (1989) used a very different pseudomemory suggestion. The target event involved participants' hearing a telephone ringing and a conversation with the experimenter that occurred during the actual experiment, which was conducted in a classroom. Because classrooms are not ordinarily equipped with telephones, and telephones do not typically ring during experiments, this highly distinctive event had a low base rate of occurrence in the test setting. In sharp contrast to the rates secured with Orne's paradigm, Lynn, et al. (1989) demonstrated that the pseudomemory rate did not exceed 11.5% (on open-ended reports) when a telephone ring was used as the target event. With such a blatant stimulus, participants appeared to adopt a much more stringent criterion for reporting that the suggested event occurred in reality. In several other studies using this stimulus, we found comparably low base rates of responding to the pseudomemory suggestion, which parallel low pseudomemory rates obtained by others (Barnier and McConkey, 1992; McCann & Sheehan, 1987, 1988) with publicly verifiable events with a low base rate of occurrence.

In a recent study, Weekes, Lynn, and Myers (1996) directly compared two publicly verifiable events that varied in terms of their distinctiveness and perceived base rates of occurrence. Consistent with predictions, the researchers found that pseudomemory rates were higher with respect to a nondistinctive event with a high perceived base-rate of occurrence. That is, subjects had a much higher pseudomemory rate (63%) in response to a suggestion that a door slammed in the hallway the previous week, than in response to a suggestion that a telephone rang in the room the previous week (25%).

This research implies that base rate information and the distinctiveness or perceived likelihood of an events' occurrence play a role in pseudomemory formation. One possibility is that if therapists convey to their clients that a history of sexual abuse is a high base rate event that could account for the symptomatology manifested (e.g., depression, relationship problems), and that the event could well have been repressed (low perceived likelihood of remembering the event), an increased pseudomemory risk may eventuate.

Another implication of the idea that memory is a decision making process related to event likelihood has to do with the age at which suggested memories occur. For example, if a suggested event happened later in life, the person would likely infer that if it indeed occurred, it would be remembered. Therefore, the fact that it was not remembered would constitute evidence that the event did not, in fact, occur, as suggested. However, with early life events, even if they were distinctive, a person might be less likely to say, "I would have remembered it," and therefore more likely to be influenced by suggestions or by expectancies about what might have occurred at the target age.

On the other hand, if a person were able to visualize early life events or suggested events with particular vividness or intensity, the imagined events may well assume "realistic" characteristics (see Belli & Loftus, 1993; Zaragoza & Lane, 1994) and lead to an attribution that the event did occur, when the person was in doubt. Consistent with this possibility, in a recent study on autobiographical memories, Lynn, Malinoski, Aronoff, and Zelikovsky (1966) found that subjects who reported memories in the first year of life were more fantasy prone and had more vivid and detailed memories than subjects who reported later memories.

Returning to our experiment on base rates and event distinctiveness (Weekes et al., 1996), we also tested the hypothesis that participants who report pseudomemories adopt a relatively lax criterion for reporting that events that did not take place did, in fact, occur in reality. That is, we predicted that participants who reported hypnotic pseudomemories would also indicate that more (nonsuggested) events (e.g., small tiles falling from the ceiling) occurred during the screening session of the previous week than participants who were not misled by the pseudomemory suggestion. Our results supported this hypothesis and implied that, when in doubt, participants who report pseudomemories exhibit a bias toward reporting that events occurred, regardless of whether they occur in actuality.

Our findings imply that such a bias is consistent with the characteristics of high hypnotizable individuals, and speak to the possible broad relevance of hypnotizability as an individual difference variable in this context. The general relevance of hypnotizability and individual differences can also be seen in the autobiographical memory study we conducted (Lynn et al., 1996) which found that hypnotizability and the tendency to report early memories was correlated at .26, even when context effects were controlled.

At this point it is worth noting that the issue of whether pseudomemory reports merely reflect responses biases, in the absence of subjective conviction in the reality of suggested events, is not settled. The response bias explanation implies that subjects are able to distinguish the original information and the false, suggested information. According to this view, subjects' reports that they were awakened by a noise, for example, occur in response to demand characteristics, not because their memories were truly altered. However, hypnosis studies have not given adequate attention to subjects' ability to distinguish the original and suggested information and to subjects' belief in the reality of the suggested event's occurrence in the face of shifting demand characteristics (see McConkey, 1991).

One of the primary if not overriding demands of the hypnotic situation is to fully experience suggested events. Very few hypnosis researchers believe that most hypnotic subjects merely comply with demands absent some degree of subjective experience. Thus, some subjects or clients may experience genuine memory alterations in the sense that they come to believe that they experienced the suggested events, even though they may initially question whether the memories were imagined versus accurate representations of life experiences. Indeed, subjects' reports, if we take them at face value, imply that this is the case (see Lindsay & Read, 1995). Moreover, hypnosis pseudomemory researchers would do well to examine more fully sophisticated research questions such as "Are real and suggested memories integrated? Do they coexist?" and to exploit the creative experimental designs (e.g., McCloskey & Zaragoza, 1985) of the broader literature on misinformation effects in memory.

Yet even with these pieces of unfinished business, a reasonable question is whether we have enough information about hypnosis and memory to dispense with hypnosis as a memory recovery tool. As a clinician, it is wise to embrace the physician's dictum, "First do no harm". It must be acknowledged that pseudomemory studies have not been done in strictly clinical conditions, so questions about generalization can be raised. However, it must also be acknowledged that a great deal of evidence converges on the conclusion that hypnosis does not increase recall of accurate information and can, in certain instances, impair recall. As clinicians, if we are to err, and err we shall, it must be on the side of safety, of protecting the client.

Many of the variables that increase pseudomemory risk in experimental situations are arguably just as relevant, if not moreso, in clinical and forensic interview situations. For example, in these latter situations, every effort is made to establish rapport with the client, no attempt is made to confront or cross-examine the client about recovered memories, repeated attempts at recall are often made, and the memories or events exhumed are rarely verifiable. We simply cannot wait for definitive evidence from more clinically oriented research and ignore the available evidence that sends a clarion message: Do not use hypnosis for the purpose of memory recovery, particularly when accuracy of recall is at a premium or inaccurate information can prove harmful or destructive.

4. WHITHER GUIDELINES FOR CLINICAL HYPNOSIS?

Where does this leave us with respect to guidelines for using clinical hypnosis for memory improvement? In our opinion, the guidelines proffered by the American Society for Clinical Hypnosis (ASCH) provide a good deal of valuable information about hypnosis and represent an important, ambitious, and well-intended initiative to educate clinicians about the pitfalls of human memory, and about the risks of certain psychotherapeutic procedures. For instance, the ASCH report acknowledges that memory is reconstructive and that leading and suggestive procedures can engender pseudomemories. The guidelines underscore the importance of providing clients with informed consent, of avoiding blatantly suggestive interventions and providing clients with the alternative "I don't know" in answering questions, and of avoiding potentially harmful metaphors such as "the mind is like a tape recorder" that can remember repressed events. If widely implemented, the guidelines could serve to deter many therapists from engaging in a number of risky and potentially destructive psychotherapeutic practices.

The ASCH guidelines clearly indicate that all memories, whether hypnotically derived or otherwise, need to be corroborated. However, we are concerned that clinicians will interpret the guidelines to imply that if the practices suggested are adhered to, false memory risk will be completely eliminated. It would be unfortunate if clinicians did not fully appreciate that whatever advantage in accurate recall hypnosis provides, it is accompanied by a tradeoff in recall errors. Furthermore, contrary to the implication in the ASCH guidelines, as we argued earlier, the available evidence indicates that hypnosis provides no special recall benefit in terms of improving memories associated with relatively arousing situations. Before implying that hypnosis might be of particular benefit in helping trauma victims recall information, it would be prudent to await convincing experimental data that supported this contention. Although the ASCH report may be correct that hypnosis improves so-called emotional or traumatic memories, this still remains a speculative proposition.

The model advanced in the ASCH report implies that memories must be recovered and worked through before true or complete healing can be achieved. However, age regression and memory recovery procedures are fraught with potential problems, and evidence is lacking that any uncovering approach, hypnotic or otherwise, provides benefits that outweigh inherent risks. Although the report is no doubt correct in noting that "hypnosis has the potential to clearly prove helpful with some individuals," (p. 15) hypnosis and, any other suggestive technique for that matter, has the potential to evoke possibly damaging false recollections in other individuals.

The ASCH guidelines also specify the conditions under which "exploratory techniques...used to encourage insight into...the contribution of feelings or earlier life experiences to current problems" should be used in the following terms: "When patients present with long-standing and complex symptoms that have generalized to a larger number of life areas, where the initial assessment suggests adaptive functions and conflicts may be associated with patient problems, and where the patient's present life stressors and relationships do not seem to adequately account for symptomatic complaints..". (p. 26) The ASCH guidelines also recommend that "Hypnotic uncovering also seems most compatible with patients...who enter treatment with the expectation that insight will be curative and who wish to pursue a therapeutic goal of self-awareness". (p. 26) Our concern is that it is just this sort of client, who is searching for answers and for whom present-day stressors and relationships do not seem to provide satisfactory explanations of symptoms, who would be prone to believe that repressed traumatic events provide a viable account of current difficulties. The fact is there is no empirical justification for favoring uncovering procedures with this or any type of client, relative to more present-oriented, mastery-based treatments.

The ASCH report maintains that increased confidence in memories in hypnosis is "most likely due to the use of suggestions that create expectations on the part of the patient for accurate recall" (p. 26). This assertion is problematic in that the sources of increased confidence in hypnosis are certainly not limited to direct suggestions conveyed during hypnosis. The report further avers that "...such contaminating effects may be controlled considerably with neutral expectations created prior to hypnosis and during hypnotic induction and age regression" (p. 26). There is some support for the idea that providing warnings about the possibility of misinformation can reduce suggestibility effects (Greene, Flynn, & Loftus, 1982; Warren, Hulse-Trotter, & Tubbs, 1991). But there is no guarantee that warning by conveying "neutral expectations" will counteract well-ingrained beliefs about hypnosis as well as unrealistic wishes, hopes, and fantasies about the salutary effects of hypnosis in psychotherapy.

Green and Lynn (1996) recently completed a warning study using Orne's nocturnal events paradigm, which has a high base rate of persons reporting pseudomemories, often exceeding 50%. In one condition, an experimental assistant informed participants about myths regarding hypnosis, including the idea that hypnosis can make participants remember things they cannot normally remember. We took the following sentences directly from the ASCH guidelines: "Memory is imperfect, whether or not hypnosis is used. Memory is not like a tape recorder, and rarely will all the details of any recollection be fully accurate. People have been shown to be capable of filling in gaps in memory, of distorting information, and of being influenced in what is "remembered" by leading questions or suggestions (p. 50). Participants were further informed that: "Hypnosis does not improve memory. If a person is unable to recall something before hypnosis, it is unlikely that they will accurately recall it during or after hypnosis. Hypnotized participants may confuse what they imagine with what really occurred. This can lead to false memories". In the unwarned group, participants received information about other myths regarding hypnosis, but none pertaining to memory.

Our findings indicated that subjects in the warned condition were less likely to report that they heard a suggested noise during hypnosis: 38% of the warned participants indicated they heard the noise versus 75% of the unwarned participants. Hence, there appears to be justification for using warnings to reduce the effects of suggestive procedures in hypnosis. However, we also found that warnings were a far from a fail-safe means of preventing pseudomemories. That is, when we examined pseudomemories among the individuals who indicated they heard the noise, a very different picture emerged: the warning had no effect on the pseudomemory rate in those participants who were influenced by suggestions to report that they heard the suggested noise. In fact, fully 75% of those persons in the warned condition believed the noise occurred in reality, versus 58% of the unwarned persons. Furthermore, the warned participants were just as confident in their false memories as were the unwarned participants.

The limited warnings that were made in this study did not reduce false confidence. The ASCH recommendations have mandated that clinicians expend far more extensive efforts to structure neutral expectations on the part of patients before, during, and after hypnosis. ASCH has also offered guidelines mandating that therapists do not provide suggestions to clients that may increase confidence artificially. We do not yet have research on the degree to which full compliance with these recommendations will reduce recall confidence, but the available evidence indicates that warnings will not fully eliminate pseudomemories or reduce confidence in false memories once they are instated. We also believe it is important to provide clients with informed consent documents that contain information concerning the possible risks of using suggestive procedures for recall enhancement. Clearly much remains to be learned about the effects of warnings and informed consent procedures on memory.

The ASCH guidelines also provide suggestions for interviewing clients. The report advises that, "Patients should be instructed that questions will be asked that should not be interpreted as suggestions, but as inquiries for information" (p. 30). However, this warning is of questionable value. Why would the therapist ask particular questions if they were not relevant? Do not most, if not all, questions contain an implicit suggestion? Indeed, the pseudomemory literature reveals that subtle questions such as, "Did you hear a noise that awakened you at night?" function as suggestions that alter memory reports after hypnosis.

One of the most serious problems with the ASCH guidelines is that they do not caution therapists against the use of ideomotor signaling methods. The report states that "The hypnotic technique of ideomotor signaling, while not a truth serum nor a direct line to the unconscious, may be useful in both clinical and investigative hypnosis in providing another source of information to be balanced with material already in conscious awareness" (p. 30). In ideomotor signaling, the person is invited to respond to questions with a finger movement, which is to occur automatically rather than intentionally. The implication is that the finger movement is directly activated by the unconscious or by a special or altered state of hypnosis. Unfortunately, there is no evidence to support either of these possibilities. The danger is that if the therapist or client believe these responses tap into some truly wise, knowing, or ordinarily inaccessible recess of the mind, they might give answers to ideomotor questions more credibility than warranted and engender pseudomemories. Whether these sorts of questions place pressures to respond beyond ordinary inquiry methods is unknown.

5. CONCLUSIONS

In conclusion, hypnosis is not a reliable means of helping clients recall either traumatic or nontraumatic memories. Hence, hypnosis should not be used to recover memories in psychotherapy. Nevertheless, hypnosis does have a role in the treatment of persons with continuously available memories, preferably in the context of a present-centered, mastery-based treatment. In these instances, hypnotic procedures can be readily combined with behavioral and psychophysiological approaches of proven benefit (Kirsch, Montgomery, & Sapirstein, 1995). Yet even in these instances, great care should be taken to avoid leading procedures, and the therapist should have an appreciation for the difficulty, if not impossibility, of completely eliminating inappropriate and counter-therapeutic suggestive influences.

It would be unfortunate if hypnosis comes to be singled out as a particularly risky procedure, somehow more "dangerous" than many other interventions. This could eventuate because of the tendency to view hypnosis as something "special" noted at the outset; because pseudomemory risk has been most intensively studied and well-documented in hypnotic contexts, and because there is, perhaps, a natural tendency to defend one's own preferred mode of treatment by way of invidious comparisons with other approaches. If hypnosis were to be scapegoated in this fashion, and we can see some indications that it has already begun to occur, it would be most unfortunate. Whether geared to memory recovery or not, no psychotherapy or treatment technique protects against pseudomemory formation. All therapies contain many of the elements that our review indicates are associated with false memories in the hypnotic context. Clinicians would do well to evaluate their practice of psychotherapy in light of the proposition that there is no such thing as risk-free therapy.

6. REFERENCES

Baker, R.A., & Patrick, B.S. (1987). Hypnosis and memory: The effects of emotional arousal. *American Journal of Clinical Hypnosis, 29*, 177–184.

Barber, T.X. (1969). *Hypnosis: A scientific approach.* New York: Van Nostrand.

Barber, T. X., & Glass, L. B. (1962). Significant factors in hypnotic behavior. *Journal of Abnormal and Social Psychology, 64*, 222–228.

Barnier, A. J., & McConkey, K, M. (1992). Reports of real and false memories: The relevance of hypnosis, hypnotizability, and the context of memory test. *Journal of Abnormal Psychology, 101*, 521–527.

Belli, R. F. (1989). Influences of misleading postevent information: Misinformation interference and acceptance. *Journal of Experimental Psychology: General, 118*, 72–85.

Belli, R.F., & Loftus, E. (1993). Recovered memories of childhood abuse: A source monitoring perspective. In S.J. Lynn & J.W. Rhue (Eds.). *Dissociation: Theoretical and clinical perspectives.* New York: Guilford. (pp. 415–434).

Belli, R.F., Windschitl, P.D., McCarthey, T.T., & Winfrey, S.E. (1992). Detecting memory impairment with a modified test procedure: Manipulating retention interval with centrally presented event items. *Journal of Experimental Psychology: Learning, Memory, and Cognition, 18*, 356–367.

Brainerd, C.J., & Reyna, V.F. (1988). Memory loci of suggestibility development: Comment on Ceci, Ross, and Toglia (1987). *Journal of Experimental Psychology: General, 117*, 197–200.

Brown, D. (1995). Pseudomemories: The standard of science and the standard of care in trauma treatment. *American Journal of Clinical Hypnosis, 37*, 1–24.

Buckhout, R., Eugenio, P., Licitra, T., Oliver, L., & Kramer, T. H. (1981). Memory, hypnosis and evidence: Research on eyewitnesses. *Social Action and the Law, 7*, 67–72.

DePiano, F. A. & Salzberg, H. C. (1981). Hypnosis as an aid to recall of meaningful information presented under three types of arousal. *International Journal Of Clinical and Experimental Hypnosis, 29*, 383–400.

Dinges, D. F., Whitehouse, W. G., Orne, E. C., Powell, J. W., Orne, M. T., & Erdelyi, M. H. (1992). Evaluating hypnotic memory enhancement (hypermnesia and reminiscence) using multitrial forced recall. *Journal of Experimental psychology: Learning, Memory, and Cognition, 18*, 1139–1147.

Dixon, M. & Laurence, J. R. (1992). Hypnotic susceptibility and verbal automaticity: Automatic and strategic processing differences in the Stroop color naming task. *Journal of Abnormal Psychology, 101*, 344–347.

Dywan, J. & Bowers, K. S. (1983). The use of hypnosis to enhance recall. *Science, 222*, 184–185.

Eich, E. (1995). Searching for mood dependent memory. *Psychological Science, 6*, 67–75.

Erdelyi, M. (1994). Hypnotic hypermnesia: The empty set of hypermnesia. *International Journal of Clinical and Experimental Hypnosis, 42*, 379–390.

Grabowski, K. L., Roese, N. J., & Thomas, M. R. (1991). The role of expectancy in hypnotic hypermnesia: A brief communication. *International Journal of Clinical and Experimental Hypnosis, 34*, 193–197.

Greene, E., Flynn, M. S., & Loftus, E. F. (1982). Inducing resistance to misleadng information. *Journal of Verbal Learning and Verbal Behavior, 21*, 207–219.

Green, J.P., & Lynn, S.J. (1995). Hypnosis, dissociation, and simultaneous task performance. *Journal of Personality and Social Psychology, 61*, 728–735.

Green, J.P., Lynn, S.J., & Malinoski, P. (1996). *Hypnotic pseudomemories: The effects of warnings and hidden observer instructions.* Manuscript submitted for publication.

Gwynn, M. I. & Spanos, N. P. (1996). Hypnotic responsiveness, Nonhypnotic suggestibility, and responsiveness to social influence. In R. G. Kunzendorf, N. P. Spanos, & B. Wallace (Eds.), *Hypnosis and Imagination* (pp. 147–175). New York: Baywood.

Hall, D.F., Loftus, E.F., & Tousignant, J.P. (1984). Postevent information and changes in recognition for a natural event. In G. Wells and E.Loftus (eds), *Eyewitness testimony: Psychological perspectives.* Cambridge: Cambridge University Press.

Hamel, J., & Lynn, S.J. (1996). *Figure drawings: A new look at trance logic.* Unpublished manuscript, Ohio University.

Hammond, D.C., Garver, R.B., Mutter, C.B., Crasilneck, H.B., Frischholz, E., Gravitz, M.A., Hibler, N.S., Olson, J., Scheflin, A., Spiegel, H., & Wester, W. (1995). *Clinical hypnosis and memory: Guidelines for clinicians and for forensic hypnosis.* Des Plaines, IL: American Society of Clinical Hypnosis Press.

Hayward, L., & Ashworth, A. (1980). Some problems of evidence obtained by hypnosis. *Criminal Law Review*, 469–485.

Hilgard, E. R. (1977). *Divided consciousness: Multiple controls in human thought and action.* New York: Wiley.

Hilgard, E. R., & Tart, C. T. (1966). Responsiveness to suggestions following waking and imagination instructions and following induciton of hypnosis. *Journal of Abnormal Psychology, 71*, 196–208.

Johnson, M.K., Hashtroudi, S., & Lindsay, D.S. (1993). Source monitoring. *Psychological Bulletin, 114*, 3–28.

Johnson, M.K., & Raye, C.L. (1981). Reality monitoring. *Psychological Review, 88*, 67–85.

Johnson, M.K., Raye, C.L., Wang, A.Y., & Taylor, T.H. (1979). Fact and fantasy: The roles of accuracy and variability in confusing imaginations with perceptual experiences. *Journal of Experimental Psychology: Human Learning and Memory, 5*, 229–240.

Kaltenbach, P., & Lynn, S.J. (1996). *Contextual reinstatement as an aid to recall of the eyewitness.* Unpublished manuscript, Ohio University.

Kirsch, I., & Lynn, S.J. (1995). The altered state of hypnosis: Changes in the theoretical landscape. *American Psychologist, 50*, 846–858.

Kirsch, I., Montgomery, G., & Sapirstein, G. (1995). Hypnosis as an adjunct to cognitive bheavioral psychotherapy: A meta-analysis. *Journal of Consulting and Clinical Psychology, 63*, 214–220.

Labelle, L., Laurence, J. R., Nadon, R., & Perry, C. (1990). Hypnotizability, preference for an imagic cognitive style, and memory creation in hypnosis. *Journal of Abnormal Psychology, 99*, 222–228.

Labelle, L., & Perry, C. (1986). *Pseudomemory creation in hypnosis.* Paper presented at the 94th annual convention of the American Psychological Association, Washington, DC.

Laurence, J.-R., Nadon, R., Nogrady, H., & Perry, C. (1986). Duality, dissociation, and memory creation in highly hypnotizable participants. *International Journal Of Clinical and Experimental Hypnosis, 34*, 295–310.

Laurence, J.-R., & Perry, C. (1983). Hypnotically created memory among highly hypnotizable participants. *Science, 222*, 523–524.

Lindsay, D.S. (1990). Misleading suggestions can impair eyewitnesses' ability to remember event details. *Journal of Experimental Psychology: Learning, Memory, and Cognition, 16,* 1077–1083).

Lindsay, D.S., & Read, J.D. (1995). "Memory work" and recovered memories of childhood sexual abuse: Scientific evidence and public, professional, and personal issues. *Psychology, Public Policy, and Law, 1,* 846–908.

Loftus, E. F. (1993). The reality of repressed memories. *American Psychologist, 48,* 518–537.

Loftus, E.F., & Ketcham (1994). *The myth of repressed memories.* New York: St. Martins Press.

Loftus, E.f., & Loftus, G.R. (1980). On the permanence of stored information in the brain. *American Psychologist, 35,* 409–420.

Lynn, S.J., Green, J., & Jaquith, L. (1996). *Hypnosis and performance standards.* Unpublished manuscript, Ohio University.

Lynn, S.J., Malinoski, P., Arnoff, J., & Zelikovsky, N. (1996). *Early memory reports, fantasy proneness, and hypnotizability.* Unpublished manuscript.

Lynn, S. J., Milano, M. J., & Weekes, J. R. (1991). Hypnosis and pseudomemories: The effects of prehypnotic expectancies. *Journal of Personality and Social Psychology, 60,* 318–326.

Lynn, S. J., Milano, M. J., & Weekes, J. R. (1992). Pseudomemory and age regression: An exploratory study. *American Journal of Clinical Hypnosis, 35,* 129–137.

Lynn, S.J., & Nash, M.R. (1994). Truth in memory: Ramifications for psychotherapy and hypnotherapy. *American Journal of Clincial Hypnosis, 36,* 194–208.

Lynn, S.J., & Rhue, J.W. (1991). An integrative model of hypnosis. In S.J. Lynn & J.W. Rhue (Eds.). *Theories of hypnosis: Models and perspectives.* New York: Guildord.

Lynn, S.J., Rhue, J.W., Myers, B., & Weekes, J.W. (1994). Pseudomemory and hypnosis: Real versus simulating subjects. *International Journal of Clinical and Experimental Hypnosis, 52,* 118–129.

Lynn, S.J., Rhue, J.W., & Spanos, N.P. (1994). Hypnosis. In K. Ramachadran (Ed.), *Encyclopedia of human behavior,* Volume 2. New York: Academic Press.

Lynn, S.J., Weekes, J.R., & Milano, M. (1989). Reality versus suggestion: Pseudomemory in hypnotizable and simulating subjects. *Journal of Abnormal Psychology, 98,* 75–79.

Malinoski, P., Lynn, S.J., & Sivec, H. (in press). The pliability of early memory reports: Vulnerability to social influence. In S.J. Lynn, K.M. McConkey, & N.P. Spanos (Eds.), *Truth in memory.* New York: Guilford Press.

McCann, T., & Sheehan, P. W. (1987). The breaching of pseudomemory under hypnotic instruction: Implications for original memory retrieval. *British Journal of Experimental and Clinical Hypnosis, 4,* 101–108.

McCann, T., Sheehan, P. W. (1988). Hypnotically created pseudomemories: Sampling their conditions among hypnotizable participants. *Journal of Personality and Social Psychology, 54,* 339–346.

McCloskey, M., & Zaragoza, M. (1985). Misleading postevent information and memory for events: Evidence against memory impairment hypotheses. *Journal of Experimental Psychology: General, 114,* 1–16.

McConkey, K.M. (1986). Opinions about hypnosis and self-hypnosis. *International Journal Of Clinical and Experimental Hypnosis, 34,* 311–319.

McConkey, K.M. (1991). The construction and resolution of experience and behavior in hypnosis. In S.J. Lynn, & J.W. Rhue (Eds.), *Theories of hypnosis: Current models and perspectives.* New York: Guilford.

McConkey, K.M., & Jupp, J.J. (1986). A survey of opinions about hypnosis. *British Journal of Experimental and Clinical Hypnosis, 3,* 162–166.

McConkey, K. M., Labelle, L., Bibb, B. C., & Bryant, R. A. (1990). Hypnosis and suggested pseudomemory: The relevance of test context. *Australian Journal of Psychology, 42,* 197–206.

Mingay, D. J. (1987). Hypnosis and memory for incidentally learned scenes. *British Journal of Experimental and Clinical Hypnosis, 3,* 173–183.

Murrey, G.J., Cross, H. J., & Whipple, J. (1992). Hypnotically created pseudomemories: Further investigation into the "memory distortion or response bias" question. *Journal of Abnormal Psychology, 101,* 75–77.

Naglieri, J.A. (1986). Draw a person: A quantitative scoring system. San diego, CA: The Psychological Corporation, Harcourt Brace Jovanovich, Inc.

Nash, M. R. (1987). What, if anything, is age regressed about hypnotic age regression? A review of the empirical literature. *Psychological Bulletin, 102,* 42–52.

Nash, M. R. (1992). *Retrieval of childhood memories in psychotherapy: Clinical utility and historical veridicality are not the same thing.* Paper presented at the annual convention of the American Psychological Association, Washington, D.C.

Nash, M.R., Drake, M., Wiley, R., Khalsa, S., & Lynn, S.J. (1986). The accuracy of recall of hypnotically age regressed subjects. *Journal of Abnormal Psychology, 95,* 298–300.

Nogrady, H., McConkey, K. M., & Perry, C. (1985). Enhancing visual memory: Trying hypnosis, trying imagination, and trying again. *Journal of Abnormal Psychology, 94,* 195–204.

Ofshe, R.J., & Singer, M.T. (1994). Recovered-memory therapy and robust repression: Influence and pseudomemories. *International Journal of Clinical and Experimental Hypnosis, 42,* 391–410.

Orne, M. T. (1959). The nature of hypnosis: Artifact and essence. *Journal of Abnormal and Social Psychology, 58,* 277–299.

Orne, M. T. (1979). The use and misuse of hypnosis in court. *International Journal Of Clinical and Experimental Hypnosis, 27,* 311–341.

Orne, E.C., Whitehouse, W.G., Dinges, D.F., & Orne, M.T. (1996). Memory liabilities associated with hypnosis: Does low hypnotizability confer immunity? *International Journal of Clinical and Experimental Hypnosis, 44,* 354–369.

Perry, C. (1996). *The accuracy of traumatic and untraumatic memories elicited by hypnosis and other procedures.* Unpublished manuscript, Concordia University, Montreal, Canada.

Poole, D.A., Lindsay, D.S., Memon, A., & Bull, R. (1995). Psychotherapy and the recovery of memories of childhood sexual abuse: U.S. and British practitioners' opinions, practices, and experiences. *Journal of Consulting and Clinical Psychology, 68,* 426–437.

Putnam, W. H. (1979). Hypnosis and distortions in eyewitness memory. *International Journal Of Clinical and Experimental Hypnosis, 28,* 437–488.

Rainer, D.D. (1984). *Eyewitness testimony: Does hypnosis enhance accuracy, distortion and confidence?* Unpublished doctoral dissertation, University of Wyoming, Laramie.

Register, P. A. & Kihlstrom, J. F. (1988). Hypnosis and interrogative suggestibility. *Personality and Individual Differences, 9,* 549–558.

Redston, M. T. & Knox, J. (1983, October). *Is the recognition of faces enhanced by hypnosis?* Paper presented at the 35th Annual Meeting of the Society of Clinical and Experimental Hypnosis, Boston.

Sanders, G. S., & Simmons, W. L. (1983). Use of hypnosis to enhance eyewitnes accuracy: Does it work? *Jounal of Applied Psychology, 68,* 70–77.

Sheehan, P. (1988a). Confidence and memory in hypnosis. In H. M. Pettinati (Ed.), *Hypnosis and memory* (pp. 95–127). New York: Guilford.

Sheehan, P. (1988b). Memory distortion in hypnosis. *International Journal Of Clinical and Experimental Hypnosis, 36,* 296–311.

Sheehan, P. W. (1991). Hypnosis, context, and commitment. In S. J. Lynn & J. W. Rhue (Eds.), *Theories of hypnosis: Current models and perspectives* (pp. 520–541). New York: Guilford Press.

Sheehan, P.W., Garnett, M., & Robertson, R. (1993). The effects of cue level, hypnotizability, and state instruction on responses to leading questions. *International Journal of Clinical and Experimental Hypnosis, 41,* 287–304.

Sheehan, P.W., Green, V, & Truesdale, P. (1992). Influence of rapport on hypnotically induced pseudomemory. *Journal of Abnormal Psychology,* 101, 690–700.

Sheehan, P.W., & McConkey, K.M. (1982). *Hypnosis and experience: The exploration of phenomena and process.* Hillsdale, NJ: Erlbaum.

Sheehan, P.W., & Perry, C.W. (1976). *Methodologies of hypnosis.* New Jersey: Erlbaum.

Sheehan, P. W., Statham, D., & Jamieson, G. A. (1991a). Pseudomemory effects and their relationship to level of susceptibility to hypnosis and state instruction. *Journal of Personality and Social Psychology, 60,* 130–137.

Sheehan, P. W., Statham, D., & Jamieson, G. A. (1991b). Pseudomemory effects of time in the hypnotic setting. *Journal of Abnormal Psychology, 100,* 39–44.

Sheehan, P. W., Statham, D., Jamieson, G. A., & Ferguson, S. R. (1991). Ambiguity in suggestion and the occurrence of pseudomemory in the hypnotic setting. *Australian Journal of clinical and Experimental Hypnosis, 19,* 1–18.

Sheehan, P. W. &Tilden, J. (1983). Effects of suggestibility and hypnosis on accurate and distorted retrieval from memory. *Journal of Experimental Psychology: Learning, Memory, and Cognition, 9,* 293–293.

Sheehan, P. W. &Tilden, J. (1984). Real and simulated occurrences of memory distoriton in hypnosis. *Journal of Abnormal Psychology, 93,* 47–57.

Sheehan, P. W. &Tilden, J. (1986). The consistency of occurrences of memory distortion following hypnotic induction. *International Journal of Clinical and Experimental Hypnosis, 34,* 122–137.

Sivec, H., & Lynn, S.J. (1996a). *Hypnotic age regression from the cabbage patch: Hypnotic vs. nonhypnotic pseudomemories with a verifiable event.* Unpublished manuscript, Ohio University.

Sivec, H., & Lynn, S.J. (1996b). *Early life events: Hypnotic vs. nonhypnotic age regression.* Unpublished manuscript, Ohio University.

Sloane, M. C. (1981). *A comparison of hypnosis vs. waking state and visual vs. non-visual recall instructions for witness/victim memory retrieval in actual crimes.* Doctoral dissertation, Florida State University. (Dissertation Abstracts International; University Microfilms No. 81–25, 873.)

Spanos, N. P. (1983). Hypnotic Behavior: A social psychological interpretation of amnesia, analgesia, and "trance logic". *Behavioral and Brain Sciences, 9,* 449–467.

Spanos, N.P. (1996). *Multiple identities and false memories.* Washington, DC: American Psychological Association.

Spanos, N. P., Gwynn, M. I., Comer, S. L., Baltruweit, W. J., & deGroh, M. (1989). Are hypnotically induced pseudomemories resistant to cross-examination? *Law and Human Behavior, 13,* 271–289.

Spanos, N. P., Menary, E., Gabora, N. J., DuBreuil, S. C., & Dewhirst, B. (1991). Secondary identity enactments suring hypnotic past-life regression: A sociocognitive perspective. *Journal of Personality and Social Psychology, 61,* 308–320.

Spanos, N. P., Quigley, C. A., Gwynn, R. I., Glatt, R. L., & Perlini, A. H. (1991). Hypnotic interrogation, pretrial preparation, and witness testimony during direct and cross-examination, *Law and Human Behavior, 15,* 639–653.

Spanos, N.P., & McLean, J. (l986). Hypnotically created pseudomemories: Memory distortions or reporting biases? *British Journal of Experimental and Clinical Hypnosis, 3,* 155–159.

Spanos, N.P., Burgess, C.A., & Burgess, M.F. (1994). Past life identities, UFO abductions, and satanic ritual abuse: The social construction of "memories". *International Journal of Experimental and Clinical Hypnosis, 42,* 433–446.

Strack, F., & Bless, H. (1994). Memory for nonoccurrences: Metacognitive and presuppositional strategies. *Journal of Memory and Language, 33,* 203–217.

Timm, H. W. (1981). The effect of forensic hypnosis techniques on eyewitness recall and recognition. *Journal of Police Science and Administration, 9,* 188–194.

Tousignant, J.P., Hall, D., & Loftus, E.F. (1986). Discrepancy, detection and vulnerability to misleading postevent information. *Memory & Cognition, 14,* 329–338.

Wagstaff, G.F. (1989). Forensic aspcts of hypnosis. In N.P. Spanos & J. F. Chaves (Eds.), *Hypnosis: The cognitive-behavioral perspective* (pp. 430–357). Buffalo, NY: Prometheus.

Wagstaff, G. F. & Sykes, C. T. (1984). Hypnosis and the recall of emotionally-toned material. I*RGS Medical Science, 12,* 137–138.

Weekes, J. R., Lynn, S. J., Green, J. P., & Brentar, J. T. (1992). Pseudomemory in hypnotized and task-motivated participants. *Journal of Abnormal Psychology, 101,* 356–360.

Weekes, J.R., Lynn, S.J., & Myers, B. (1996). *Pseudomemories and hypnosis: The effects of base-rates and event distincitiveness.* Manuscript submitted for publication.

Whitehouse, W.G., Dinges, D.f., Orne, E.C., & Orne, M.T. (l988). Hypnotic hypermnesia: Enhanced memory accessibility or report bias? *Journal of Abnormal Psychology, 97,* 289-295.

Yapko, M.D. (1994). Suggestibility and repressed memories of abuse: A survey of psychotherapists' beliefs. *American Journal of Clinical Hypnosis, 36,* 194–208.

Zaragoza, M.S., & Lane, S.M. (1994). Source misattributions and the suggestibility of eyewitness memory. *Journal of Experimental Psychology: Learning, Memory, and Cognition, 20,* 934–945.

Zelig, M. & Beidleman, W. B. (1981). The investigative use of hypnosis: A word of caution. *International Journal Of Clinical and Experimental Hypnosis, 29,* 401–412.

COMMENTARY ON HYPNOSIS, PSEUDOMEMORIES, AND CLINICAL GUIDELINES: A SOCIOCOGNITIVE APPROACH

Willem A. Wagenaar, Leiden University, The Netherlands

This is a clear and complete review of what we know about hypnosis and memory, which needs no commentary at all. Therefore I will limit my comments to a few side remarks.

1. OVERVIEW

Let me first attempt to summarise the paper in six questions plus answers.

a. Does hypnosis improve memory? No.

b. Are hypnotised subjects more receptive to misleading information? No

c. Does hypnosis increase unwarranted confidence? No

d. Can hypnotic age regression enhance memory? No

e. Can hypnosis induce pseudo memories? Yes

f. Are the guidelines offered by the American Society of Clinical Hypnosis adequate? No.

Taken together, to me these answers suggest that hypnosis is not an advisable tool for the reinstatement of memories assumed to be lost.

2. MEMORY METAPHORS

Many memory models make in one way or another use of the library metaphor. This metaphor has two parts: a store of information, like books on the shelves; and a set of procedures, used for the storage and retrieval of information. Sometimes it is claimed that the store is permanent, and that all memory problems are caused by storage and retrieval processes. Others claim that the stored information can be changed, for instance through interference with more recently stored information. The idea that hypnosis may improve memory is clearly based upon a notion of a permanent store, made inaccessible through retrieval problems. Hypnosis is supposed to restore the access to a previously inaccessible store. Lynn's paper demonstrates that hypnosis does not have such an effect. I want to stress that this finding does not logically lead to the rejection of the library model with a permanent store and fallible storage/retrieval procedures. On the contrary, if it is assumed that the access problem can be overcome only by presenting other and more effective retrieval cues, the prediction is that hypnosis will not help.

3. UNANCHORED CASE HISTORIES

I cannot resist the temptation to give some comments on the case of the missed therapy session discussed by Lynn. In my own contribution I have argued that case histories may only help if they are firmly anchored by means of extensive information, on to a body of beliefs shared by us all. This case is not anchored in such a way. It is supposed to illustrate the compelling nature of false memories produced in a condition of hypnotic age regression. But why should we accept this as an example of age regression? The client only went back a few days! Why should we accept that the client really believed her own story? Could it not be that she generated an acceptable excuse for not showing up in a therapy session? Did she get around paying for the missed session in this way? If, as stated, she was a classic fantasy-prone person, why was hypnosis needed to let her come up with this story? How do we know that hypnosis contributed anything at all? Was this memory, produced in a hypnotic state, more clear than her other fantasies? Why is the story presented as compelling? Is it compelling because she was in a hypnotic state, so that the therapist did not expect any fantasies? Would others have believed her? In what way has hypnosis helped this client to become a normal person, instead of an "interesting case", walking around graveyards with her therapist? The anecdote makes good reading, but it did not help me at all, apart from suggesting that some therapists are compelled by poorly anchored narratives.

4. ASCH GUIDELINES

To many of us the problem of recovered memories is a very practical one. We would be helped by clear and practical answers. The quote from the ASCH guidelines illustrates the unpractical and wishy-washy nature of many compromise-type statements that I have come across recently.

> ".... with emotion-laden memories for meaningful material, we believe it likely that hypnosis has the potential to clearly prove helpful with some individuals."

Imagine that you want to know whether there will be a bus, to take us all back to the airport at the end of these weeks. The message from the organisation is:

> ".... with respect to the bus to the airport, we believe it likely that there may be a bus that clearly has the designed capacity to be helpful to transport perhaps some individuals."

I would not rely on it.

QUESTION AND ANSWER SESSION

Elliott. I had a comment and a suggestion. Sometimes we polarise this as a debate between cognitive scientists and clinicians: I think to see both you and Willem Wagenaar talk points out it is clear that it's not just about cognitive scientists and clinicians, but that within clinicians we have differences of opinions. I wondered if you have any idea about how the use of hypnotism in the treatment of CSA has any specific implication apart from memory based on the research you have and even given that this is not a conference about CSA and hypnosis and that obviously you use it to treat a wider range of trauma in general, could you comment about whether you would be more cautious in other uses of hypnosis knowing what you know about the suggestibility of memory? Would you still use it with sexual abuse survivors, would you stop using it in ways other than just about the recovery of memory?

Lynn. Actually, hypnotic techniques can be very useful with a wide variety of clientele. Just because someone has been sexually abused, would I shy away from using hypnosis? Definitely not. In fact, I hate to think of people in terms of categories, such as a "sexual abuse survivor." Instead, I would consider the therapeutic agenda, the conflicts, issues, and behaviours that needed to be addressed and modified on a very individual basis before I intervened with any procedure. Just how hypnosis would fit into the overall treatment scheme would depend on my assessment of the person. With persons with a history of sexual abuse, I tend to focus my hypnotic interventions on developing present-centered coping and mastery strategies for containing affect and feeling strong. I might use imaginative or cognitive-behavioral rehearsal techniques for coping with future situations. There are many, many applications for positive suggestions that are soothing, ego-strengthening, and that can have a beneficial influence on perceptions, and how people view their bodies and frame their experiences, for example. With hypnosis, clients can come to appreciate how malleable their cognitions and feelings are, and better appreciate the control they have over their experiences. Self-hypnotic techniques and posthypnotic suggestions can also be used to generalise treatment gains. But let me underscore the point that hypnosis and other therapeutic procedures should not, in my opinion, be used for memory recovery. At the same time, let's not make hypnosis a scapegoat. Any therapy can and does have potentially negative effects, so safeguards against suggestive influences should be employed in any treatment. I would be no more or less careful with hypnosis than I would with any other procedure. I would be careful in all cases, regardless of whether I was treating a person with a traumatic past or not.

Donovan. It seems to me that if you think about the trauma field over the last ten or fifteen years, especially dissociative disorders, some approaches have been very highly ritualistic. Hypnosis has been very much at the core of the trauma field over the last 10 years, and it's very highly ritualistic. One of the problems that I think this has created is the notion in many people's minds we have to have a highly ritualistic, structured approach to solve a problem. Then if life throws you a curve that doesn't fit into that particular situation, you have a big problem. Let me give you an example of the other side of that coin. We had a 40-year old, 300-lb individual who had spent four years in the Harvard system, and was diagnosed as MPD, moved to Florida and decided to go into treatment. They were warned that it wouldn't be MPD systems treatment and that I do not have hospitalised patients, so she had to be prepared not to go into hospital and not to hurt herself. One of my patients did get himself hospitalised, a 36 year old very handicapped person. So I took two $300 per hour attorneys to the psychiatric hospital to get him released, which we did. While I was at the hospital this woman called. She was on thirty medications, because she had very complex, life threatening medical problems as well and was decompensating and didn't know what to do. She wanted to know if she could increase her medication. I told her in any case you'll still have your problems when it's over. She was in a house she'd just moved into, all full of boxes that hadn't been emptied, I said that the antidote to chaos is order, pick a box and put it away. That's what we have done that for the last year and a half, and this woman who has been on psychiatric disability for five years is getting ready to go back to work. No hypnosis, no ritualised structured treatment, and every problem that came up we just had to deal with. So how do you feel about the ritualistic aspects of hypnosis as opposed to the spontaneous aspects of just dealing with problems that arise?

Lynn. That question defies a short answer. I view hypnosis as a cultural ritual, with many of the classical hypnotic phenomena or effects such as hypnotic involuntariness, the feeling that your hand is lifting up automatically, for example, as based on the specific wording of the suggestions and culturally-based expectations about hypnosis. I think that much of what occurs in a hypnotic context is people respond in terms of their expectancies and do their best to experience the suggested event. I don't think that most people fake their responses. Just like responses in non-ritualized, less structured situations, hypnotic responses are complexly determined. It is not altogether clear what mediates or optimises treatment effects in any therapeutic situation, whether it is ritualised or not, hypnotic or non hypnotic in nature. Expectancies seem to be important across therapies, but so are other non-specific factors like the therapeutic alliance, as well as the specific techniques used in relation to the problem treated. It is also important to keep in mind that there are suggestive and ritualised elements in many therapies, and drawing a line between hypnosis and other therapies that are much less direct or ritualised can be very difficult. Yet even within situations defined as hypnotic, there are differences in how ritualised, authoritative, and direct the procedures are versus more free-flowing, spontaneous, permissive, and indirect. In fact, we reviewed the literature on so-called direct versus indirect suggestions in hypnotic and non hypnotic contexts in a 1993 article in the *International Journal of Clinical and Experimental Hypnosis*. In the case of direct suggestions, the suggestions are administered in an authoritative manner and it is very clear how the hypnotist, for example, wants the person to respond. In the case of indirect suggestions, the suggestions are generally less ritualised, more permissive, metaphoric, less authoritative, and the relation between the suggestion and the response is less clear or direct. When you examine this literature, what is striking is the lack of differences between the direct and indirect procedures. The ritual, the hocus pocus, seems to be less important than the fact that the person is able to discern what is required to respond successfully—that is that the therapeutic demand is clear and the person has the willingness and ability to conform to that demand.

Bill Matthews and his colleagues conducted an interesting study where they shared creative metaphors with individuals in a non-ritualized situation and people were able to discern the meaning of the metaphor. Contrary to what some therapists have suggested, the metaphor did not operate "unconsciously." In general, although certain people like to be talked to in a metaphoric way, they are able to tell you what the point of the metaphor is, so attempting to disguise a directive or suggestion in terms of a metaphor with a child, by way of a story, for example, can be, in actuality, no different than telling a child, for example, to "brush your teeth, go to sleep on time, or listen to your mom or dad." So, as I said earlier, this is a complex and fascinating area for clinicians and researchers to develop and explore more fully.

Shuman. Given your review of literature, are there circumstances you would approve the use of hypnotic techniques for memories to be refreshed?

Lynn. I am not sure that I approve of using hypnosis for refreshing memory in any situation. But in certain forensic situations, it is conceivable that it could be useful, so I would be hesitant to rule out its use entirely. Let me say, I am still undecided. But I think the verdict is out regarding situations where you have basically little or nothing to risk by using hypnosis, such as a desperate situation (e.g., a kidnapping) and few or no leads and restrict the use of hypnosis to looking for information that can be potentially corroborated. In the event that hypnosis is used, the procedures would have to be "very clean" and absolutely non-suggestive, and any information obtained would need to be independently corroborated. Of course, depending on the jurisdiction, the courts could throw this information out and may even strike non hypnotic testimony from the record in the event hypnosis was used, so this possibility must be considered before hypnosis is implemented. Each situation must be carefully evaluated on a case-by-case basis, and hypnosis should only be used—if it is used at all—as a very last resort. In general, though, my opinion is that hypnosis should not be used to refresh memory—although there may be some room for flexibility in certain rare instances. It is important to keep in mind that forensic and clinical situations are typically very different. In forensic situations, memories are recorded and certain safeguards are put in place. Suggestive elements of the procedures can be carefully examined and evaluated on a videotaped record. But I am hoping that the tide will turn in the clinical area in that clinicians will be equally cautious and conscientiously record their use of hypnosis in clinical situations.

Hyman. Mine is a question about analogue studies such as being awakened by the phone ringing, experiences we have all had. Are they pseudomemories or is it just that you got them confused about the time it happened?

Lynn. Your question is a legitimate one. Confusion about when something happened is a possibility, although recall that participants earlier denied, in the case of Orne's paradigm, that the event occurred at the indicated time. We are taking our research one step at a time, and using different kinds of suggestions in the context of different paradigms. There may be problems with individual paradigms, but we are gaining converging information that memories are malleable, and learning more about the circumstances in which memories are pliable. I think we need to move on to more real life analogue situations, but we have learned a lot from paradigmatic laboratory investigations.

REFERENCES

Lynn, S.J., Neufeld, V., & Mare, C. (1993). Direct versus indirect suggestions; A conceptual and methodological review. *International Journal of Clinical And Experimental Hypnosis, 41*, 124–152.

Matthews, W., & Langdell, S. (1989). What do clients think about the metaphors they receive? *American Journal of Clinical Hypnosis, 31*, 242–251.

13

INFORMED CLINICAL PRACTICE AND THE STANDARD OF CARE

Proposed Guidelines for the Treatment of Adults Who Report Delayed Memories of Childhood Trauma

Christine A. Courtois

The Center: Posttraumatic Disorders Program
The Psychiatric Institute of Washington
Washington, D. C. 20037

1. INTRODUCTION

The impetus for this paper comes from two different but related professional initiatives: 1) the development of guidelines and scientifically validated standards of practice and 2) the treatment of adults who report delayed memory for past trauma, especially child sexual abuse. The purpose of the paper is the articulation of guidelines for the informed treatment of adults who report childhood trauma. Special attention is devoted to clinical issues that arise when the patient reports new (delayed, recovered, re-instated) memories of abuse during the course of therapy; suspects past trauma/abuse on the basis of recovered or delayed memories that occur within or outside of therapy; or suspects past trauma/abuse in the absence of specific recollections.

In recent years, a number of professional organizations have empaneled working groups and task forces to study the issue of delayed memory for child abuse trauma and to make recommendations for research, clinical, and forensic practice. The pertinent findings and recommendations of these various working groups are incorporated in the guidelines discussed in this paper and form the basis of the evolving standard of care for this treatment population.

This paper is organized as follows: the first half consists of two sections, the first devoted to a discussion of the scientifically based standards of practice and the standard of care, and the second providing a brief review of major developments in the knowledge base relevant to treatment of the long-term effects of child sexual abuse. The second half of the paper presents proposed guidelines for post-traumatic therapy with specific attention to reports of abuse that are the result of recovered/delayed memories and to suspicions of abuse (when clear recall is lacking). It includes attention to ethical principles of

Recollections of Trauma, edited by Read and Lindsay
Plenum Press, New York, 1997

practice, the knowledge, competency and training needs of practitioners, and the general organization and main areas of intervention of this proposed treatment approach.

2. DEFINING STANDARDS OF PRACTICE AND THE STANDARD OF CARE

This section begins with a brief discussion of what is meant by standards of practice and the standard of care (See Chambless, 1995; Hayes, Follette, Dawes, & Grady, 1995, for broader discussions of these issues). We then narrow the focus to consider the applicability of standards of practice and the standard of care to the treatment of post-traumatic conditions in general and delayed memory for past trauma in particular. These efforts form the backdrop of the more specific focus of this paper. It is explicitly acknowledged that the development of empirically supported standards for the treatment of past trauma (including attention to delayed memory) and the evolving standard of care must occur within the context of and be coordinated with profession-wide initiatives. Additionally, until more data are available and a specific standard of care established, clinicians who work with traumatized (or possibly traumatized) populations must practice within the currently available codes of ethics and generic standards promulgated by the various mental health professions.

2.1. Standards of Practice

Standards of psychological practice refer to general bounds set on practice that are consistent with current scientific evidence and knowledge. They encompass hortatory or prescriptive standards describing what a practitioner "ought to do" as well as minatory or proscriptive standards describing what "not to do" (Dawes, 1995). Efforts to demonstrate the efficacy of psychological treatments are increasingly important to the working clinician due to a number of factors including but not limited to the growth and developing sophistication of the behavioral and mental health fields, changes that are occurring in the health care delivery system where greater accountability is being demanded, and, as noted above, the demands of consumers and interested or affected third parties (e.g., insurance companies, the courts).

Developing a scientific basis for specific practice interventions is a complex and multidetermined endeavor. It is at once an eminently practical and rational process (as well as an aspirational one) but is very difficult to operationalize in terms of developing and implementing evaluation criteria (Chambless, in press; Chambless et al., 1996). Typically, the task is undertaken by working groups of recognized experts in a topic area who review the available authoritative literature to determine the "state of the data". The findings of a review of this sort then form the basis for recommended assessment and intervention efforts and suggest areas in which additional research is needed (Hayes, 1995). At present, preliminary efforts are being made within the American Psychological Association to develop criteria for evaluating the efficacy of assessment and intervention efforts and the American Psychiatric Association has recently published guidelines for the treatment of a variety of psychiatric disorders (American Psychiatric Association, 1996; Chambless et al., 1996). These efforts are not without critics, however, particularly concerning such important issues as what criteria to establish, what validation level to meet, how many studies are needed, and whether these efforts will result in a restriction of practice (Garfield, 1996; Kovacs, 1996).

2.2. The Standard of Care

The choice and efficacy of interventions and of the overall treatment strategy are increasingly salient issues in the forensic setting, especially in determining the standard of care in malpractice cases. "Standard of care" is a legal term applied in those cases in which the burden is on the plaintiff to prove that treatment was below standard and was the proximate cause of harm. In a general sense, the standard of care refers to professional peer and expert opinion and testimony, authoritative research, and applied clinical literature, developed within applicable regulatory statutes as well as professional practice standards and ethical codes (Brown, 1995).

Brown (1995) suggested that the standard of care for trauma treatment "is defined by the evolving literature on diagnosis, as defined by *DSM-IV*, and on trauma treatment written by trauma experts" (p. 16). This encompasses a review of the available literature on the "state of the science" and "state of applied science and practice" in the field of traumatic stress studies. In terms of delayed memory issues, it also takes into consideration the recommendations and cautions of cognitive memory experts.

3. DEVELOPMENT OF THE CONTEMPORARY TREATMENT MODEL FOR ADULTS SEXUALLY ABUSED AS CHILDREN: AN OVERVIEW OF MAJOR CONTRIBUTIONS

The treatment of adults abused as children is a relatively recent specialty in clinical practice. Three distinct but interrelated lines of research (all undertaken beginning in the early 1970s) have made independent and collective theoretical contributions to understanding the initial and long-term effects of child abuse and furthermore have been seminal in the development of the treatment strategy under discussion in this chapter. These are: 1) the study of child abuse/child sexual abuse; 2) the study of posttraumatic responses and Posttraumatic Stress Disorder; and, 3) the study of psychological dissociation and its relation to trauma.

3.1. The Study of Child Abuse/Child Sexual Abuse

The context for the contemporary study of child abuse and child sexual abuse was initially the identification of and publicity surrounding the "battered child syndrome" (Kempe et al., 1962) and the study of violence against women. These two areas cross-referenced each other in several significant ways. Studies of battered children resulted in the identification of other forms of family violence that often occurred concurrently—wife abuse and the sexual abuse of children. Studies of violence against women found sexual assault to be quite prevalent and perpetrated more often by acquaintances (including family members) than strangers.

As these various forms of abuse were investigated in more depth, they were identified as traumatic stressors and their initial and long-term effects as fitting a posttraumatic conceptualization (Burgess & Holmstrom, 1974; Peters, 1976; Sgroi, 1982). Initial attempts at intervention and treatment were undertaken as the widespread prevalence of abuse and the seriousness of its aftereffects (both personal and societal) became more evident. A preliminary professional literature emerged on the treatment of child victims of ongoing physical and sexual abuse/incest (Burgess et al., 1978; Sgroi, 1982) and adult victims of past abuse (Butler, 1978; Courtois & Watts, 1982; Herman, 1981; Meiselman, 1978) and current battering (Walker, 1988).

3.2. The Study of War Trauma/Posttraumatic Stress Disorder

During the same time period, the study of war trauma accelerated in response to the needs of Vietnam veterans. Findings from these studies brought renewed attention to the traumatic consequences of war and resulted in the development and inclusion of formalized diagnostic nomenclature and criteria for severe posttraumatic reactions, Posttraumatic Stress Disorder (PTSD), in the *Diagnostic and Statistical Manual III* (*DSM*, American Psychiatric Association, 1980). Criteria included bi-phasic reactions of intrusion and numbing of the trauma along with physiological hyperarousal and startle response, often accompanied by anxiety and depression. The reaction was usually experienced acutely in the immediate aftermath of the trauma but could emerge in delayed fashion and/or could become chronic. This new diagnosis was instrumental in challenging the traditional view of psychopathology as predominantly intrapsychic—researchers and clinicians began to identify the unacknowledged etiological role external trauma could play in the development of psychological distress and mental illness.

Throughout the 1980s, as other types of trauma and traumatized populations were studied, the cumulative data suggested that the human trauma response—like the human stress response identified by Selye (1976)—has a rather common pattern of occurrence irrespective of the type of traumatic stressor (Figley, 1985; McCann & Pearlman, 1990; McCann, Pearlman, Sakheim & Abrahamson, 1988; van der Kolk, 1984, 1987) and that PTSD could be applied to the reactions of other types of trauma victims besides war veterans. Over time, however, researchers argued for a spectrum of trauma responses by type of trauma (Herman, 1992b). In particular, they noted more complex reactions in individuals subjected during childhood to trauma involving conditions of secrecy, entrapment, helplessness, and powerlessness and chronic and escalating violation perpetrated by someone on whom the victim is dependent and/or has an ongoing relationship. This type of trauma is prototypic of child abuse/child sexual abuse. These reactions often lead to severe developmental damage to the personality structure and to personal and interpersonal functioning that is above and beyond reactions associated with standard PTSD. A new diagnosis based on this formulation, Complex PTSD or Disorders of Extreme Stress Not Otherwise Specified (DESNOS), was proposed and field tested but, to date, is not included in the *DSM* (Herman, 1992a, 1992b).

3.3. The Study of Psychological Dissociation

The study of psychological dissociation by both cognitive scientists and clinical researchers resumed during the same time period, spurred on in part by the new investigations of child abuse, domestic violence, and war trauma. As a clinical phenomenon, and following the original formulation of Janet (1889), dissociation is viewed as a normal psychophysiological response that often (but not always) occurs following severe traumatization allowing the individual to detach from emotionally difficult material and from noxious physical responses and sensations.

A specific category of dissociative disorders was first included in the *DSM-III* in 1980, the same year the diagnosis of PTSD was introduced (American Psychiatric Association, 1980). As currently defined, "The essential feature of the Dissociative Disorders is a disruption of the normally integrated functions of consciousness, *memory*, identity, or perception of the environment. The disturbance may be sudden or gradual, transient or chronic" (American Psychiatric Association, 1994, p. 477; emphasis added) (consistent with different onset and durations patterns associated with PTSD as noted above). Dissociative amnesia, one of the five identified dissociative disorders "is characterized by an *inability to recall important personal information, usually of a traumatic or stressful nature*, that is too extensive to be explained by ordinary forgetfulness" (p. 477; emphasis added). The memory disturbance aspect is highlighted here because it provides an explanatory mechanism for the fragmented and delayed/recovered memory found to be associated with different types of trauma (Elliott & Briere, 1995; van der Kolk & Fisler, 1995). Although more research is needed, a growing body of data now indicates a connection between a history of trauma, especially chronic severe trauma beginning in early childhood, and dissociative disorders in adulthood (Putnam, 1989; Ross, 1989). Many researchers and clinicians consider the alternating posttraumatic phases of intrusion and numbing/denial as inherently dissociative. Highly symptomatic and severely traumatized clients often carry dual diagnoses of PTSD and a dissociative disorder.

3.4. The Development of Treatment Models

The research from these three areas (i.e., child abuse, war trauma, and dissociation) spawned the development of theoretical formulations and treatment approaches. A general treatment paradigm for posttraumatic conditions and disorders was developed using the newly available research on traumatic stress reactions as its foundation (Brown & Fromm, 1988; Figley, 1985; McCann & Pearlman, 1990; Ochberg, 1988; van der Kolk, 1984, 1987). More specific to the topic of this paper, preliminary models were developed for the treatment of the long-term effects of child sexual abuse (Briere, 1989, 1991; Butler, 1978; Courtois, 1988; Dolan, 1990; Gil, 1988; Herman, 1981; Jehu, 1988; Kluft, 1990; Meiselman, 1978, 1990) and/or dissociative post-traumatic conditions (i.e., Dissociative Identity Disorder/Multiple Personality Disorder and the other Dissociative Disorders) (Braun, 1986; Kluft, 1985; Putnam, 1989; Ross, 1989). Although these treatment models developed rather independently of one another, inspection of them reveals that each relied on reviews of the scientific literature available at the time and on original research and theoretical formulations produced by each author. These models shared many commonalities and, in a sense, cross-referenced and cross-validated each other. They also all followed a posttraumatic approach, largely to counterbalance the neglect of trauma found in almost all previous psychotherapeutic approaches.

In 1991, a National Institute for Mental Health (NIMH) consensus panel of trauma and sexual abuse experts was organized with a mandate to review the scientific and clinical data pertaining to the treatment of adults sexually abused as children. Following review of the available research and clinical literature, recommendations were made regarding the need for additional study and continued theoretical and treatment refinement. In particular, the need for outcome research on the efficacy of treatment models and specific strategies was recommended (Beutler & Hill, 1993; Hill & Beutler, 1993). Methodological problems were also identified and recommendations made for more rigorous research specifications (Briere, 1993). It is an interesting footnote in light of the later emergence of the memory controversy that issues of memory and memory retrieval were not given much consideration in the recommendations. This omission was not because memory issues were viewed as unimportant but because they were not emphasized; work on memory and memory retrieval were viewed as inherent to the treatment of post-traumatic conditions and as only one focus of treatment, among many. The recommendations made by this group of experts continue to be relevant and point the way for a more scientifically based treatment, but now new recommendations must specifically encompass and emphasize issues of memory.

More recently, a "second generation" of treatment models has been published that builds on and extends the earlier work, integrating posttraumatic approaches with other models of psychotherapy (e.g., cognitive-behavioral, ego psychology, object relations, psychoanalytic) and attending more to issues of memory. Some address the generic treatment of posttraumatic reactions (Everly & Lating, 1995; Flannery, 1992; Herman, 1992b; Meichenbaum, 1994; van der Kolk, McFarland & Weisaeth, 1996; Williams & Sommer, 1994; Wilson & Lindy, 1994; Wilson & Raphael, 1993), some the long-term effects of child sexual abuse/incest (Briere, 1992, 1996; Davies & Frawley, 1993; Draucker, 1992; Herman, 1992b; Kepner, 1995; Pearlman & Saakvitne, 1995; Pope & Brown, 1996; Salter, 1995; Scharff & Scharff, 1994; Waites, 1993), and some are specific to the dissociative disorders (Cohen, Birzoff, & Elin, 1995; Kluft & Fine, 1993; Spira, 1996; Speigel, 1994). This entire body of work provides a preliminary consensus regarding the treatment of posttraumatic conditions and, more particularly, the treatment of adults sexually abused as children. It also serves as a strong foundation for informed practice and the evolving standard of care.

4. THE CONTROVERSY REGARDING POST-ABUSE THERAPY

Controversy regarding the focus and methods of the new post-abuse therapy first erupted in 1992. Here we review some of the events that led to the controversy and some of the main critiques and rejoinders.

4.1. The Impact of the Self-Help Literature and the Media

A number of lay and self-help books were published in tandem with the publication of the professional literature (Bass & Davis, 1988; Blume, 1990; Davis, 1991; Engel, 1989; Littauer, 1990; Poston & Liston, 1989). These books presented an overview of the effects of incest/child sexual abuse and the healing/recovery process that was generally consistent with the professional literature but overgeneralized beyond the available data. Some of the statements made about abuse prevalence and the ubiquity of absent memory and about symptoms and aftereffects as conclusive of an abuse history (especially in the absence of *any* memory of abuse) were especially problematic.

Both the professional and self-help literature received extensive media coverage that was so pervasive that, within the span of a decade, incest and other family problems (e.g., alcoholism, physical violence) went from being the most taboo and shameful of personal and family experiences to ones that were highly sensationalized. The media coverage was cataclysmic in its impact. It created a social context and made it more acceptable for many adults to report and remember past experiences of abuse and to question whether, in fact, abuse could account for some of their past and present difficulties. As a result, a huge influx of adults sought therapeutic assistance specifically for abuse-related memories and issues. Many sought formal psychotherapy with mainstream licensed professionals while others engaged in "alternative therapies" provided by a wide range of providers, many of whom had little or no mental health training or certification but who advertised as "therapists" or "sexual abuse experts" nevertheless.

4.2. Challenges in the Clinical Setting

The clinical setting underwent major challenges as a result of this groundswell. Since most therapists had received no training in either their graduate courses or clinical placements in the identification or treatment of any type of traumatic stress (much less such complicated forms as incest or other family violence), they were hard-pressed to know how to respond to the needs of the individuals seeking their assistance for abuse-related issues. As a consequence, many learned to treat this population "on the job and in the trenches" by attending continuing education workshops and reading the newly available "first generation" clinical writings on the treatment of incest and sexual abuse. Much of this literature discussed reluctant disclosure and delayed/recovered memory as common patterns among abuse survivors but, by and large, did not discuss the reconstructive nature of memory nor the clinical complexities of working with these issues. Additionally, although this literature did address some of the personal and professional challenges in treating traumatized/relationally damaged clients, many therapists experienced these issues and dilemmas firsthand without adequate training or supervisory assistance.

Since that time, it has become clear that these various issues contributed to some of the clinical excesses and errors that have come under criticism. It has also become clear that the psychological treatment of adults reporting past abuse is complex. A consensus has developed that treatment of this population should not be undertaken by the novice therapist without prior training and supervision nor should it be undertaken at all by a lay person. It is also abundantly clear that a significant clinical population of formerly abused individuals is in need of treatment and that more sophisticated approaches and strategies are needed. The "second generation" literature is a start toward addressing these issues and in providing proposed guidelines of competent treatment leading to a more defined standard of practice.

4.3. The Impact of Legislative Changes

During this same time period, virtually all state legislatures changed statutes of limitation and delayed discovery requirements to allow adults to bring civil actions for childhood abuse against alleged perpetrators, including parents. It was in the forensic setting with its burden of proof standard that the current controversy first emerged. As these cases developed, clinicians were called as experts for the plaintiffs to explain posttraumatic stress disorder, the long-term damages resulting from childhood sexual abuse, and delayed reactions and recovered memory. Cognitive psychologists specializing in memory research were hired as defense experts and challenged the concept of repressed/delayed memory for repeated abuse as inconsistent with the available literature on the workings of human memory. They called into question some of the techniques that therapists described using to help their clients retrieve memories. They further criticized as naive and in error therapists who believed their patients' delayed memory productions as the veridical representation of historical truth rather than as narrative reconstruction.

4.4. The False Memory Critique

The memory critique reached the public domain in the spring of 1992 mainly due to the establishment of the False Memory Syndrome Foundation and the media coverage it received. This organization, whose membership includes individuals who claim to be falsely accused of abuse and whose professional advisory board consists of eminent memory researchers (some of whom had served as defense experts in the aforementioned civil cases) charged that the U.S. was in the midst of an epidemic of false memories of abuse and false accusations. The epidemic was directly attributed to a course of therapy labeled "Recovered Memory Therapy" in which therapists used problematic memory enhancement techniques with clients who had suspicions but no clear cognitive memory of having been abused. The most problematic of these techniques were identified as hypnosis (with or without age regression), guided imagery, some forms of "journalling", interpreting current physical symptoms as "body memories" of childhood events, and interpreting dreams as accurate memories of childhood events, along with several ancillary approaches used to promote the recovery of memories, i.e., recommending that clients read self-help books on abuse effects and memory retrieval, suggesting that they join sexual abuse survivor groups, and countering their doubts about the accuracy of their abuse memories (See Lindsay & Read, 1994, for a detailed discussion).

Clients were said to develop "false memory syndrome" (or false memories of abuse that never occurred) due to the systematic and indiscriminate application of these problematic techniques by therapists holding seriously flawed beliefs about the workings of human memory and about repressed memories in particular. These same therapists tended to overattribute many common symptoms of psychological distress to past sexual abuse. Moreover, many of these therapists tended to believe in the reality of any and all memory productions, no matter how improbable or without tangible evidence (e.g., past life abuse, alien abduction abuse, Satanic abuse). Even more seriously, the repercussions were felt outside of the therapy setting as adults, on the basis of their newly recovered memories, accused their parents and others of past abuse, limited or stopped contact with family members and, in some cases, initiated civil lawsuits.

Trauma therapists and researchers as well as adult survivors and their advocates were alarmed by the scope and the tone of the critique. They charged that the false memory advocates took a sensationalized and adversarial stance that unnecessarily polarized the issues and that they virtually dismissed the possibility of repressed/delayed memory for any type of trauma, despite clinical and research evidence to the contrary. Professionals representing the trauma perspective further raised concerns that the scope of the problem was misrepresented. They argued that the critics did not have adequate data to substantiate their claim that large numbers of therapists were either routinely using or misusing the suspected techniques, nor was there a formalized course of posttrauma treatment labeled "Recovered Memory Therapy" oriented only towards retrieval of abuse memories. Furthermore, no data from clinical studies were available to substantiate the claim that false memories were *created* by therapists using certain techniques. Brown (1995) decried the non-differentiation of professional and self-help approaches as follows:

> The problem with some recent articles speculating about false-memory production in therapy...is their failure to address the standard of care in the authoritative literature on trauma treatment. Instead they make a general indictment of the entire profession of psychotherapy by confounding the expert professional literature on trauma treatment with anecdotal accounts of sub-standard care drawn largely from the self-help trauma literature" (p. 16).

4.5. The Need for Common Ground

As the controversy has matured and some of the polemic has diminished, the legitimacy of concerns raised by both camps has been acknowledged and the need for increased communication and common ground is ever more evident (Courtois, 1995; Lindsay, this volume). False memory critics have tempered their position somewhat as clinicians have made clear that they have changed some of the ways they practice in response to a number of their cautions. The remainder of this paper is devoted to the exposition of the clinicians' perspectives on what constitutes the current (and evolving) standard in post-trauma treatment, including its rationale, strategy, and course.

5. PROPOSED GUIDELINES FOR TREATING ADULTS WHO REPORT PAST TRAUMA

These guidelines have as their basis the currently available research and literature on trauma, abuse, and memory, the consensus among experts regarding treatment approaches and strategies, and the cautions and recommendations of cognitive scientists, practitioners, and professional working groups (American Medical Association, 1993; American Psychological Association, 1994, 1996; American Psychiatric Association, 1993; Barach, 1994; British Psychological Association 1995; Canadian Psychiatric Association, 1995; Courtois, 1996; Hammond et al., 1995; Lindsay, 1994; Lindsay & Read, 1994; Loftus, 1993; Yapko, 1993. See also Grunberg & Ney, this volume).

Despite the considerable body of literature now available on this treatment, a recently published caution must be noted. Van der Kolk, McFarland, and van der Hart (1996) in their review chapter of treatment approaches to posttraumatic stress disorder wrote that: "...systematic investigation of what constitutes effective treatment is still in its infancy" (p. 417) and "Until more comprehensive treatment outcome studies are available, we continue to be critically dependent on clinical wisdom in treating these patients. Thus, we must remain aware of the caveat that there can be significant gaps between clinical impressions and scientific data" (p. 418). This situation is not much different than is found in other areas of psychological practice and the movement towards scientifically validated treatment approaches, as discussed in the early part of this paper; nonetheless, the efficacy of treatment must be studied and demonstrated systematically and the standard discussed here will evolve with continued development of the knowledge base.

The aim of these practice guidelines is to provide clinicians from all mental health professions with guidance (both hortatory and minatory) for conducting psychotherapy with adults who disclose abuse histories at the outset of psychotherapy, who report new or delayed abuse memories during the course of therapy, or who, on the basis of no clear memory and/or sketchy recall, question whether they have been abused. Several assumptions underlie them: (a) the majority of individuals who seek treatment for abuse-related issues have retained some memory for the abuse; (b) some clients may recall additional details or experiences of abuse during the course of therapy because research has shown that accessibility to trauma memories can be quite variable, and psychotherapy is conducive to self-exploration and self-revelation; (c) memory for past trauma may return after a period of total lack of recall (but that these situations are the exception rather than the norm); (d) some memories reflect narrative versus historical truth; and (e) absent evidence, witnesses, or other corroboration, the therapist has no way of knowing whether delayed recollections represent real events, hence whether such memories are true or false.

5.1. Professional Standards of Practice and Codes of Ethics

Therapists who work with abused or possibly abused individuals must practice within currently available professional standards and codes of ethics. According to London (1994), the issue of repressed memories has been "Balkanized" from the mainstream practice of psychotherapy, a practice that must be reversed. General practice guidelines and standards apply, as do professional ethics. Therapists must stay in their assigned roles and guard against any personal or extra-therapeutic agenda influencing the therapy. Quoting London:

> The education, training, and experience of the psychologist [or other mental health professional] does prepare one to be an objective, neutral, professional who can integrate the art and science to help patients empower themselves. There is nothing in the skill-base that qualifies one to be an advocate, clinical detective, diviner of truth, judge, jury, or prosecutor. Therapists are not direct observers of past events, nor are they extensions of the client. Conversely, patients are not extensions of the therapist...This is an issue that requires a competent, scientifically based, professional approach. The professional must provide an objective assessment, a full informed consent, and comprehensive treatment. The therapist must consider the implications of one's work. The professional must consider the patient, the family, the professional, and public policy (p. 64).

Ethics codes provide a framework for ethical professional practice and are designed to protect the practitioner and the patient; however, they are inherently ambiguous and, at times, may contradict each other, legal requirements, or other mandates in the client's best interest. Abuse, trauma and memory issues can further complicate the picture (see Adshead, this volume; American Psychological Association, 1996b, 1996c; Daniluk & Haverkamp, 1993; and Hotelling, 1995, for additional discussion). It is the professional's job to be aware of these issues and to take them into consideration from the outset of treatment. Competing requirements must be evaluated as they arise, always with a focus on the patient's best interest. Consultation and peer review are advisable when major ethical dilemmas or contradictions present themselves.

5.2. Competence and Training Issues

High levels of experience and competence are needed to work with the complex issues presented by traumatized individuals, including adults abused as children. General agreement exists among experts that this treatment should not be left to the trainee or novice. Unfortunately, information on human traumatization, the traumatic stress response, and its treatment has not been systematically included in either the core curriculum or in clinical placements of the mental health professions (Alpert, Brown, & Courtois, 1996; Hoteling, 1995; Payne, 1995). As noted earlier, this has placed a heavy professional burden on many practitioners who have needed to develop knowledge as well as competence on the job and through extra-curricular education and training. Clinicians treating these patients have a responsibility to seek specific education and to keep abreast of newly emerging information in a number of areas, as the following authors suggest:

> In addition to the general areas of competence required of all psychologists who practice psychotherapy, the psychologist [or other mental health professional] should have working knowledge of areas of particular relevance to abuse and memory issues such as: basic memory principles, autobiographical memory, infantile amnesia, implicit and explicit memory, traumatic memory research, research on the prevalence and impact of abuse, strengths and limitations of techniques designed to gain greater access to memory, forms of dissociation and the similarities and differences between repression and dissociation, and the manifestations of post-traumatic stress disorders (Campbell, Courtois, Enns, Gottlieb & Wells, 1995, p. 2)

Supervision and consultation are recommended as essential for all therapists working with the population of abused or possibly abused individuals (not only the novice or trainee) for many reasons, not the least of which are the complexity and co-morbidity of these patients, the many high-risk situations that emerge in their treatment, and the intense relational demands made by many traumatized patients. Practitioners have an obligation to monitor continuously their level of competence, choice of treatment approach, countertransference issues, caseload intensity and balance, vicarious traumatization, burn-out, and self-care. This is especially the case during periods of intense stress or personal crisis in a therapist's life. Additionally, therapists with a personal history of abuse and trauma should optimally have dealt with these issues in their own treatment, should maintain vigilance about over- or under-identification with the patient, and have additional sources of consultation/supervision (Briere, 1989; Pearlman & Saakvitne, 1995). It should further be understood that not all therapists are interested in or able to provide this form of treatment. When this is the case, patients with abuse issues should be referred to therapists willing and competent to treat them.

5.3. The Treatment Frame and the Therapeutic Relationship

The foundation of post-trauma treatment is relative safety and predictability within an ongoing relationship; yet, the therapeutic relationship with PTSD patients (and Complex PTSD and Dissociative Disorder patients in particular) is notoriously demanding and intricate due to the re-play of interpersonal aspects of the trauma such as mistrust, betrayal, dependency, love, hate, sexualization, and aggression (Briere, 1989; Courtois, 1988; Davies & Frawley, 1993; Pearlman & Saakvitne, 1995). The therapist should provide a great deal of information and obtain informed consent at the start of treatment. Informed consent is not a one-time event, and should be considered an ongoing process to be revised and updated according to the needs of the patient as they change over the course of treatment. Special informed consent forms are recommended for use with any specialized, experimental, or controversial technique such as hypnosis (Hammond et al., 1995; Scheflin & Shapiro, 1989) or Eye Movement Desensitization and Reprocessing (EMDR) (Shapiro, 1996) so the patient is made aware of the implications and the risks/benefits of its use.

The use of a "Rights and Responsibility" statement at the outset of treatment is advisable as a general informed consent statement (APA, 199 ; Courtois, 1996). In a document of this sort, the practitioner outlines a number of issues, including but not limited to the following: his/her therapeutic orientation and usual ways of working; mutual rights and responsibilities; confidentiality and its limitations including state reporting laws regarding patient reports of ongoing or past abuse (state laws vary considerably so the clinician must be aware of local statutes) and actions needed in the case of clear and present danger to self or others; fees, billing, insurance and payment issues; assessment, goal-setting with attention to available resources (e.g., personal, familial, financial), and treatment planning; therapist availability outside of session and back-up coverage during absences and vacations; cancellation and therapy termination policies; issues of non-compliance with treatment; adjunctive evaluations and treatment; collateral assessments and releases of information; the use of contracts and plans for specific issues (e.g., self-harm and suicide); safety issues; and how and when hospitalization or psychopharmacological evaluation might be considered. Of necessity, documents of this sort vary by the therapist's orientation and style—what is most important is that the method of practice is conveyed clearly to the prospective patient.

Records should be kept in sufficient detail to document major communications with the patient and to keep ongoing documentation of the assessment and treatment, per routine professional standards. Every effort should be made to maintain records that are neutral in perspective and tone and that record any disclosures as "reported by" the patient rather than as documented historical events.

A collaborative approach that is empowering to the patient is recommended for all trauma treatments to counter the lack of control and powerlessness inherent in victimization (Ochberg, 1988). This approach diffuses somewhat the patient's tendency to view the therapist as the "authority on high" to be feared, deferred to, etc., and establishes an expectation that the patient play an active role in his/her treatment. Furthermore, such an egalitarian permissive approach does not establish conditions most likely to result in memory confabulation such as a highly powerful and persuasive authority figure in a closed relationship (Brown, 1995). Although this approach is deliberately fostered and the therapist adheres to the basic therapy principles of empathy, respect, and genuineness, s/he retains ultimate responsibility and control for the course of treatment.

Another critical issue is the maintenance of personal and professional boundaries between therapist and patient. Practitioners working with this population must be especially scrupulous about maintaining their professional authority and avoiding dual relationships. Abused individuals have had their personal boundaries violated and have been enjoined in dual role relationships repeatedly; they may attempt to replicate these relationship patterns with the therapist, a circumstance that the therapist should anticipate and work with but not reenact. The therapist must gain an awareness of the many ways that abuse dynamics might come into play in the therapy relationship and work to interpret and change them for optimal healing to occur (Pearlman & Saakvitne, 1995; Wilson & Lindy, 1994).

5.4. Pre-Treatment Assessment

The therapist begins the treatment process by conducting a comprehensive and objective psychosocial assessment that follows normal intake procedures. The assessment should include questions about the patient's family, social, medical, developmental, and occupational history as well as the severity and course of any previous symptoms and mental health difficulties (e.g., anxiety, depression, mood swings, psychosis, substance abuse, self-harm, suicidality, and post-traumatic and dissociative symptoms). Past treatment history including previous diagnoses should also be assessed. Questions about problematic childhood and family experiences and a history relevant to violence and all forms of trauma (including family violence, sexual abuse, physical abuse, medical trauma, accidents, devastating personal and family losses, and natural disasters) should be included among other questions in the initial history-taking to provide a baseline and to indicate to the patient that these issues are relevant and open to discussion. All questions should asked in as neutral and open-ended way as possible.

Some abused individuals readily report an abuse/trauma history, some will not disclose even upon direct inquiry (sometimes deliberately and sometimes because they genuinely do not know). Other patients have nothing of this sort to disclose because they were not abused. As a general matter, the therapist should not make assumptions regarding the meaning of a lack of disclosure—at its most simple, it means that the individual does not have an abuse/trauma history; however, when the individual's symptom picture is acute and/or consists of a number of posttraumatic symptoms or symptoms of the type most correlated with an abuse history (Neumann, Houskamp, Pollack, & Briere, 1996), the possibility of undisclosed or unrecognized abuse or other trauma should be given consideration.

5.4.1. When Abuse Is Disclosed. When abuse is disclosed during the assessment, the therapist should record the information factually and objectively as reported by the patient. A description of the abuse should be obtained in as much detail as possible including the nature and particulars of its occurrence; the identity and relationship to the perpetrator; the individual's role in the experience; the subjective thoughts and feelings about the experience and any action taken or not taken; the effect of the trauma on the individual's life and on perceptions of self and others; the individual's coping style, ego strength, and level of cognitive functioning (Courtois, 1988; Scurfield, 1985; van der Kolk, McFarlane & Weisaeth, 1996) and how long the patient has known the history and whether there have ever been memory gaps or lack of memory accessibility. The therapist must take care to ask questions in an open-ended, objective yet sensitive and supportive manner. Some patients will respond readily and others will be overwhelmed and will need to answer these questions over time.

In the case of disclosed abuse, the practitioner further assesses for symptoms associated with posttraumatic reactions including intrusive reexperiencing, autonomic hyperarousal, numbing of responsiveness and affect (with attention to substance abuse and other addictive/compulsive difficulties), intense emotional reactions, learning difficulties, memory disturbances and dissociation, medical problems and psychosomatic reactions, interpersonal difficulties (such as problems with personal boundaries, aggression against self or others and ongoing abuse), and any criminal justice/legal difficulties. The therapist should ask in detail about the individual's current level of safety in terms of self-harm and violence to and from others. Individuals with a trauma history—especially involving incest/child sexual abuse—often have high degrees of revictimization and reenactment experiences in adulthood, including self-injury and suicidality. Therapy must begin with attention to the possibility that these issues are current. Finally, another important area of inquiry concerns whether the patient has taken any legal action regarding the abuse or is contemplating any in the future.

The clinician should anticipate a range of symptomatology and severity and should not assume that all abused individuals respond the same way. Some may have few, if any, serious reactions and concerns but the majority in a clinical setting are likely have moderate to serious aftereffects and symptoms (Courtois, 1988). The assessment is further complicated by some of the characteristics of the posttraumatic response as discussed by Campbell, Courtois, Enns, Gottlieb, and Wells (1995, p. 3):

> In cases of long term trauma, the client may not have experienced the necessary conditions for acquiring a coherent, consolidated sense of self or may have encountered ongoing abuse in adulthood that resulted in significant disruptions of the client's self structure. The consequences of long-term abuse may be manifested through a wide range of problems in defining and integrating aspects of the self, including identity confusion or fragmentation, the tendency to experience normally integrated process as separate aspects of the self, and distortions of body image or personal esteem. Furthermore, the client may exhibit behaviors such as either-or thinking, affective instability, impulsivity, rapid shifts in emotional or cognitive states, or self-injurious behavior. Careful assessment regarding the strength and nature of the client's self-structure is necessary for planning optimal interventions and establishing whether the client is prepared to deal with traumatic memories.

Many issues such as these and other post-traumatic symptoms do not show up on standard psychological assessment instruments (Briere, 1995). When personality testing is undertaken, the practitioner should include one or more of the newly available instruments designed specifically to assess post-traumatic and dissociative symptoms (Carlson, 1996; Steinberg, 1995).

5.4.2. When Abuse Is Suspected But Not Remembered. If an individual enters treatment suspecting but not explicitly remembering abuse and has unrealistic expectations of therapy and/or memory retrieval, the therapist should begin by finding out what has led to such suspicions or expectations. These might include previous therapy involving the use of problematic techniques or a specific and closed perspective; participation in previous therapies where abuse was directly suggested or implied; previous involvement in a self-help or therapy group for abuse survivors; reading and personal interpretations of specific self-help literature; and, social compliance issues. Any misunderstanding about abuse and memory processes should be corrected (and noted explicitly in the patient's chart) and the patient urged to take a more open-ended, exploratory stance over a period of time. Also, the practitioner should consider additional evaluation for other risk factors associated with possible false-memory production (Brown, 1995). Standardized instruments for the assessment of hypnotizability (Speigel & Speigel, 1978) and interrogatory suggestibility (Gudjohnsson, 1984, 1992) are available.

When specific memory is absent, it is crucially important that the therapist not "fill-in" or "confirm" reported suspicions of a non-remembered abuse history—the patient needs to come to his or her own understanding and may need to tolerate considerable uncertainty, especially when corroboration is lacking. The therapist must be able to tolerate ambiguity and uncertainty and must also be aware that, in some highly traumatized individuals, the story will only emerge in a disguised and fragmented manner that requires patience and careful attention. The practitioner must honestly monitor personal assumptions and biases and take care to avoid leading questions, suggestions of abuse, premature closure of exploration or, alternatively, a premature focus on sexual abuse as the only possible explanation of a patient's distress, and/or an overacceptance of the patient's circumstances as evidence of the historical truth of abuse. The therapist must also be prepared to correct misinformation and, at times, confront improbable and unwarranted conclusions. When the patient's beliefs or conclusions have a frankly paranoid, delusional and/or psychotic quality, additional assessment is called for. It is necessary to underscore, however, that these symptoms might be posttraumatic adaptations rather than frank psychosis. Obviously, differential diagnosis can be quite difficult in these cases and standard personality assessment instruments supplemented with those that specifically assess posttraumatic and dissociative symptoms should be considered.

When abuse is suspected but not explicitly remembered or corroborated and when posttraumatic reactions and symptoms are not in evidence, the general treatment orientation follows a generic rather than a posttraumatic model.

Since an assumption of past trauma should not be automatically made, treatment under this circumstance should resemble therapy of a more generic sort and all but the most general of post-traumatic education and emphasis be deleted. This strategy can be shifted in the event that memory returns and/or other evidence emerges to support the occurrence of trauma.

5.4.3. Additional Areas of Pre-Treatment Assessment. Inquiry about the individual's personal and financial resources is also warranted. A preliminary assessment of the individual's ego strength, personal resilience, health status (including any areas of disability, compromise, or disease) is done at this time along with discussion of reasons for seeking therapy and preliminary goals. Information about the impact of the individual's culture, social class, ethnicity, sexual orientation, disability/limitation also require assessment attention. These factors may impact the patient's perspective in a number of ways and need to be taken into account in assessing resilience and areas of difficulty and in determining goals. Inquiry regarding financial resources includes attention to living expenses and arrangements, financial stability and difficulties, job security, health care resources and interpersonal support network. These need to be on par with the individual's capacity to do the work; otherwise, they may need to be negotiated for a better fit.

Finally, adjunctive consultation (medical, psychiatric, neurological, vocational/occupational) might be considered and a second opinion sought regarding diagnosis and treatment. Previous therapy experience is also of interest. With written consent, records of previous therapists should be requested for review and comprehensive treatment planning.

5.5. Diagnosis

The therapist considers and assimilates all of the information gained during assessment in making a diagnosis and developing a treatment strategy. It is useful to complete all five axes of the *DSM* (American Psychiatric Association, 1994) to include attention to characterological issues, medical illness, past and current stressors, and level of functioning. Adults with a past trauma history often have had a number of previous therapies and diagnoses. The practitioner thus may have to sort through a range of diagnoses to determine which, if any, apply in the present circumstance. Further complicating the picture is the fact that the population of trauma survivors has been found to have a high degree of co-morbidity. Multiple diagnoses may therefore be appropriate and can be listed in order of severity and/or order of treatment priority.

PTSD is often considered a superordinate diagnosis but it should only be given when a trauma history is reported (not just suspected). Criterion A of the diagnosis is the experiencing or witnessing of a traumatic stressor, something that is not always a certainty when clear recollection is absent. Although this situation is of the "chicken and egg" variety in truly traumatized individuals who do not recall the trauma due to their posttraumatic response, the therapist errs on the side of caution by not assigning the diagnosis (or assigning it provisionally) until all of the criteria are met. Critics have charged that PTSD diagnosis has been applied without appropriate attention to whether previous trauma was specifically remembered rather than suspected.

Similarly, the diagnosis of a dissociative disorder needs to be undertaken with care. When a patient exhibits dissociative behavior and symptoms, practitioners need to consider all of the dissociative disorders, not only Dissociative Identity Disorder, and may benefit from consultation with colleagues experienced in the diagnosis of these conditions.

5.6. The Structure of Post-Trauma Treatment

Experts in the treatment of trauma are in agreement that the therapy process is progressive. As noted earlier, although a collaborative working relationship is the model of choice, the therapy is not laissez-faire and the therapist is in charge of its general structure, organization, emphasis, pace, and tone. This even includes attention to the structure of the individual session and closing each session in a way that insures that the patient is not left in a vulnerable and open emotional state.

Most often, psychodynamically informed individual psychotherapy is the treatment of choice, supplemented by group therapy at different points in the course of treatment, if feasible. Nevertheless, some individuals will only have access to group therapy due to financial and insurance limitations and/or due to the philosophy of various mental health agencies. Whether treatment involves individual, group, or some combination of both, it should be organized according to the following sequenced model consisting of three phases each with a variety of tasks and objectives. In this model, issues of memory make up only one aspect of the treatment and are generally not the major focus; rather, memories are addressed according to the patient's symptoms and level of distress but within the broader treatment model.

5.6.1. Early Phase: Alliance-Building, Safety, and Stabilization. This phase is measured in terms of the mastery of skills, not time. In fact, a great deal of time may be needed to accomplish the tasks and skills of this phase before undertaking any work in the next. When and if the trauma is addressed directly, it is only when the patient has achieved enough stability, skills, and ego strength to be able to manage and tolerate the strong emotions likely to be generated. McCann and Pearlman (1990) labeled this progressive process "self work before trauma/memory work". In this phase (and in the model in general) the patient is continuously focused on the need for safety, symptom stabilization and management, and the maintenance of functioning. Any work with traumatic or abuse material in this phase is cognitive and educational in format, directed toward actively teaching the patient about the process and aftermath of traumatization and about the management of posttraumatic symptoms. This structure works against an ambiguous and open-ended treatment that creates conditions of dependence, retraumatization and decompensation due to premature work on trauma without adequate safeguards in place, or against those conditions that are suggestive or conducive to memory elaboration (described in more detail below).

The development of the therapeutic relationship, the establishment of the parameters of treatment and the maintenance of safety and relative life stability are critical foundation tasks. In many ways, the work of this phase resembles that of non-trauma therapy; yet it differs quite substantially when compounded by posttraumatic influence. For example, the development of the therapeutic alliance, a more or less straightforward process with a nontraumatized patient, is often a daunting challenge with one who has been seriously abused. The therapist may be perceived as a stand-in for other untrustworthy and abusive authority figures to be feared, mistrusted, challenged, tested, distanced from, raged against, deferred to, clung to, sexualized, etc. A relationship of trust and mutual respect often takes an enormous amount of time, energy, and patience.

The establishment of a treatment frame and a collaborative contract for the therapy helps with relationship development and safety. The contract includes attention to such issues as a commitment to sequenced work and progressive skill building, the establishment of healthy boundaries between self and others (modeled by the therapist), the development of a safety plan, the preservation of functioning in all life spheres to the degree possible, the maintenance and/or development of a support network apart from the therapist, neutrality concerning memories, and a commitment to not engage in any impulsive and unplanned disclosures, confrontations, family cut-offs and/or legal action.

Although these issues are discussed and agreed at the outset of treatment, a degree of non-compliance and avoidance should be anticipated. Some seriously traumatized individuals are notoriously difficult to engage as they seek (consciously or unconsciously) to continue to avoid painful material. This problem requires that the therapist spell out and adhere to the parameters of the therapeutic contract while maintaining flexibility and sensitivity. The capacity of the patient to do the work must be constantly assessed and titrated accordingly in order for the patient to stay in treatment. Even when the patient choses to stop treatment, it is advisable to leave the door open for future contact and possible resumption of the treatment (McFarlane, 1994; van der Kolk, 1996).

The therapeutic issues encompassed in this phase are many, some of which emerge only after the resolution of others (Jehu, 1988). The treatment plan is collaboratively determined to whatever degree possible. Each plan is different, tailored to the patient's unique concerns, symptoms, and resources. The tolerance and modulation of affect, the undoing of cognitive errors and distortions, and the teaching of grounding and stabilization skills for use with posttraumatic symptoms are all essential to this phase. Typical therapeutic issues include education regarding trauma and posttraumatic reactions/adaptations, the verbalization of feelings and somatic states, and the development of personal stabilization mechanisms, coping skills, ego defenses and ego strengths, safety and self-protection strategies, life skills, and self-care capacities (Briere, 1989; Courtois, 1988, 1991; Herman, 1992b; Kepner, 1995; McCann & Pearlman, 1990; van der Kolk et al., 1996). Critical to this phase and related to the ability to make progress on these issues is the stabilization of mood disturbances, personality issues, and posttraumatic and dissociative symptoms through cognitive-behavioral and psychopharmacologic approaches.

Depending on the range and severity of the patient's symptoms and needs, this phase may take a great deal of time and effort. Some relatively intact patients can progress rather quickly but the norm is for the work to go slowly. The time-intensive nature of this work is comparable to what has previously been described in the clinical literature on the treatment of the borderline personality patient (who quite often has had a history of abuse and neglect) (Gabbard & Wilkinson, 1995; Linehan, 199). Once mastery of the tasks of this phase has been achieved, some patients choose to stop treatment. Others discontinue because they lack the personal, motivational, family or financial resources to proceed. In either case, the patient is ideally healthier and has more personal and interpersonal resources and stability than when treatment began.

5.6.2. Middle Phase: Trauma Work—De-Conditioning, Mourning, and Resolution. This phase involves systematic attention to the traumatic material, titrated according to the capacities and defenses of the patient. The primary goal is for the patient to gradually face and make sense of the trauma material along with its associated emotions at a pace that is safe and manageable. Most often, this involves facing the material in small, manageable increments with attention to not overshooting or undershooting the "therapeutic window" (Briere, 1994). It does not mean high-intensity reexperiencing or "re-living" that re-traumatizes patients and results in their decompensation nor does it mean actively digging for memories. Patients are not encouraged to do this work to foster regressive dependency or to get stuck in a morass of more and more serious trauma, and certainly not to create traumatic memories; rather, the purpose is to allow for a deconditioning of the traumatic material and a re-structuring of trauma-related cognitions and a personal narrative in the interest of resolution. Van der Kolk et al. (1996) is most eloquent on the critical purpose and nature of this phase:

When patients have gained stability, control, and perspective, treatment can be terminated. There is no intrinsic value in dredging up past trauma if a patient's current life provides gratification, and the present is not invaded by emotional, perceptual, or behavioral intrusions from the past. However, if such involuntary emotional perceptual, or behavioral intrusions continue to interfere with people's current functioning, controlled and predictable exposure to the traumatic memories can help with regaining mastery...

A therapist's natural proclivity is to help a patient avoid experiencing undue pain; however, learning to tolerate the memories of intense emotional experiences is a critical part of recovery. The psychotherapist who understands the nature of trauma can aid the process of integration by staying with the patient through his or her suffering; by providing a perspective that the suffering is meaningful and bearable; and by helping in the mastery of trauma through putting the experience into symbolic, communicable form (i.e., through putting perception and sensations into words). (p. 428).

In this phase, the patient directly faces both the occurrence of the abuse and its consequences. This phase usually involves the experiencing of intense emotional pain and anguish and a process of mourning the losses associated with abuse. It is in this phase that "things get worse before they get better" (something the patient should be informed of and give consent to ahead of time), but getting worse for a period of time is clearly in the interest of getting better, not in getting mired in the past or in deepening levels of dysfunction.

5.6.3. The Late Phase: Self and Relational Development. This phase involves continued work on self-development, a self apart from the trauma and less encumbered by traumatic intrusions and cognitions. A major focus is the reestablishment of secure social connections and an accumulation of restitutive emotional experiences with the therapist and with others (van der Kolk et al., 1996). Attention continues to be directed to personality issues and emotional development, mood stability, personal safety, self-care, and personal boundary management. Optimally, the patient has achieved a new level of personal development and maturity beyond the limitations imposed by post-traumatic responses and adaptations. These, in turn, lead to other changes. Relationships often require reassessment, rebalancing, direct therapeutic intervention, or termination. Relationship work occurs in the context of family of origin, work relationships, friendships, intimate relationships, sexual functioning, and childrearing. Patients may be further freed up to develop aspects of their lives that were previously untended or constricted, including educational and occupational endeavors, recreational activities and hobbies, physical activities and pursuits, etc.

Termination of treatment can be exhilarating, difficult, and poignant. The decision to end treatment is most efficacious when it is arrived at mutually when the patient's treatment goals have been accomplished. As in other therapies, termination often causes a resurgence of feelings about previous losses and abandonments, particularly difficult issues for abuse/trauma survivors. Adequate time should therefore be planned to address the issues and feelings that surface. It is generally recommended that treatment end with something of a safety net in place: that the patient can occasionally return for "check-ups" or "check-ins" or can return to treatment if s/he experiences a resurgence of symptoms or issues (which may occur as the result of developmental changes, such significant issues as the death of the alleged abuser, or other life crises). Even after a treatment ends, the therapist should guard against the development of a dual relationship since it would complicate and preclude a return to treatment.

5.7. Therapy Issues Pertaining to Memory

Brown (1995) summarized this treatment strategy as follows:

Most trauma experts agree that classic abreaction and the use of memory recovery techniques as a *main* focus of treatment are contraindicated. This is not to say that memory recovery doesn't have a proper place within phase-oriented treatment, but only after stabilization. Uncovering is usually conducted primarily with free-recall uncovering strategies along with coping-enhancement and affect-regulatory methods that help establish the emotional state through which memories come forth in a way that minimizes leading. While memory recovery is not always indicated, it is often indicated. Outcome research has shown that exposure to traumatic memories is associated with treatment gain in behavioral treatment of PTSD...and in the psychodynamic treatment of severe dissociative disorders. (p. 16).

Throughout the course of the treatment, the therapist must "walk a fine line" to be neutrally supportive of the patient, especially in those cases when the patient is confused and when clear memory of trauma/abuse is not available. Patients must be supported as they struggle with their ambivalence because true victims of abuse often doubt their perceptions and memories. The practitioner must however steer between suggestion or dismissal of abuse in the patient's background and must carefully manage risk factors that would encourage the production of false beliefs or reports during the course of treatment (American Psychiatric Association, 1993; American Psychological Association, 1994, 1996; Courtois, 1995a; Hammond et al., 1994). The results of numerous laboratory studies indicate that the production of false beliefs is lowest with a free-recall or free-narrative retrieval strategy in contrast to structured, leading, or repetitive questioning. The therapist must therefore adopt a style closest to free-recall strategy (Geiselman et al., 1993), adopt a scientific attitude of openness and hypothesis-testing over time, avoid an authoritarian approach or role, avoid closed-ended or suggestive inquiry, and must take the patient's level of suggestibility and hypnotizability into consideration (Brown, 1995).

As the quote from Brown (1995) implies, memory exploration is warranted in a number of circumstances for resolution and the cessation of the most intractable symptoms. Memory exploration, when it occurs, should only be undertaken in the context of ongoing therapy and not be farmed out to self-styled "memory recovery experts," split off to other therapeutic formats such as short-term group therapy, self-help groups, or weekend "intensives" or undertaken with special techniques or medications such as hypnosis or sodium amytal (the latter might be warranted in exceptional circumstances but the therapist would be well advised to work with a panel of expert consultants to make this determination).

In any event, when the patient is struggling with the possibility of abuse when memory is absent or spotty, the therapist makes efforts to educate him/her about the malleability, limitations and suggestibility of memory, about infantile and childhood amnesia, about possible post-event influence on memory, and the possible condensation of different memories across time. This information must be counterbalanced, however, with information about memory for emotional events and the somatosensory and fragmented nature of post-traumatic recall. It is important that cautions about memory not be interpreted as denial of the possibility of abuse or other trauma.

Hypnosis for memory retrieval, guided imagery, expressive therapies (artwork, journalling, storytelling), reading of self-help books and membership in self-help abuse groups have all been identified as especially problematic in the possible production of false memories. If and when any of these techniques and strategies are considered for use, appropriate cautions must be in place and their limitations must be explicitly discussed with the patient. For example, hypnosis should not be used for memory retrieval per se but can be very useful in symptom management and resolution. Before its use, the patient should be educated about its benefits and limitations and the possible inaccuracy of trauma images and memories (as well as personal beliefs) that may emerge in trance. It is particularly recommended that therapists have training in whatever technique they use and further that they have familiarity with materials they might recommend (e.g., self-help reading, particular groups).

Some patients seek outside sources of information and possible corroboration. Patients should be encouraged to consider the potential risks and benefits of such a search especially if it involves the alleged abuser (and/or other family members in the case of incest) and a range of possible responses and outcomes. Ironically, a lack of evidence or corroboration may pose as much a crisis for some patients as the gaining of evidence does for others. Because of this, patients should identify clear goals, anticipate disappointment as well as success, and enlist the help of their support network. The therapist should not undertake corroboration as a therapeutic task or mandate nor should they pressure patients to seek out corroboration. It should be kept in mind that denial by alleged perpetrators does not mean that abuse did not occur and that certain evidence (medical and school records, family pictures, diaries kept in childhood and adolescence) may suggest abuse but may not be definitive absent direct admission by the perpetrator or witnessing by others.

As implied above in the discussion of phase one issues and approaches, the patient is continuously returned to issues of safety, stability, functioning and life quality and not to the uncovering of more and more horrific abuses and trauma. Although the exploration of trauma and new memories is important, it is necessary for the therapist to assist the patient to achieve closure at some point regarding the past and to shift focus to present-day concerns. As with other aspects of this therapy, this closure occurs on an individual basis. As noted by Enns et al. (1995, p. 233):

> Efforts to remember the past must always be framed as a method for creating greater meaning in the present. Childhood sexual abuse [as well as other types of trauma] is always associated with the shattering of the client's self and the client's assumptive world. Thus, working through memories may be necessary to help the survivor discontinue the reenactment of behaviors that are rooted in the traumatic experience, transform memories, reconstruct the self, provide a new perspective about the past, view oneself as a survivor rather than as a victim [or as worthy of abuse], and refocus energy from protecting the self from old pain to deal effectively with new developmental tasks.

5.8. Transference and Countertransference

Discussion of post-trauma treatment is incomplete without mention of transference and countertransference as it affects the therapeutic relationship and supports or interferes with the ultimate success of the treatment. Traumatized patients can be very difficult to treat and present significant challenges to the therapist who, without specialized knowledge and attention to transference and countertransference issues, can end up inadvertently reenacting aspect of the abuse to the detriment of the patient and him/herself. The post-traumatic symptomatology (including self-harm, suicidality, revictimization, and risk-taking), the content of the traumatic material itself, and the patient's relational style and needs tend to be offsetting and anxiety-provoking for the therapist (especially the novice and/or anyone untrained in or unaware of these issues). Additionally, "These therapies are uniquely challenging because of the inevitability that sexual abuse survivors will engage in unconscious or dissociated reenactment of traumatic interpersonal experiences that invite therapists to respond in complementary ways" (Pearlman & Saakvitne, 1995, p. 4).

Although particulars are beyond the scope of the present chapter, attention to these relational reenactments and to the therapist's responses is crucial. It is the author's belief that countertransference errors have, in part, resulted in some of the therapeutic excesses pointed out by the critics. A number of substantive books have recently been published on transference and countertransference issues in the treatment of trauma and are to be recommended (Davies & Frawley, 1994; Figley, 1995; Lindy & Wilson, 1995; Pearlman & Saakvitne, 1995). Therapists need more training in these relational dimensions to avoid some of the most common errors, including overidentification with and rescuing, avoidance, and abandonment of and anger toward the patient that may lead to exploitation or disengagement. And all of these can lead to errors having to do with the patient's memories. As a means of avoiding these problems, consultation and supervision around issues of transference and countertransference can be invaluable.

6. CONCLUSION

Informed treatment and the evolving standard of care for abused and possibly abused individuals posits a therapy that is sequenced, paced and titrated, and directed toward stabilization and the resolution of major symptomatology, which is sometimes achieved through direct work with the traumatic content. The therapist who works within the parameters of this standard, and who recognizes that delayed memories and false memories of past abuse are both possible, is best able to provide a rational and balanced therapeutic approach to these issues. The model presented in this paper is derived from the currently available clinical literature on the treatment of post-traumatic conditions and is responsive to the critiques of cognitive memory scientists. It is further presented within the context of other efforts across mental health fields to develop a scientifically informed therapeutic strategy and standard of care.

REFERENCES

American Medical Association Council on Scientific Affairs (1994). *Memories of childhood abuse, CSA Report 5-A-94.* Chicago: Author.

American Psychiatric Association. (1980). *Diagnostic and statistical manual of mental disorders.* (3rd ed.). Washington, DC: Author.

American Psychiatric Association. (1994). *Diagnostic and statistical manual of mental disorders.* (4th ed.). Washington, DC: Author.

American Psychiatric Association. (1996). *Practice guidelines.* Washington, DC: Author.

American Psychiatric Association Board of Directors. (1993). *Statement on Memories of Sexual Abuse.* Washington, DC: Author.

American Psychological Association (1994). *Interim report of the Working Group on Investigation of Memories of Childhood Abuse.* Washington, DC: Author.

American Psychological Association (1996). *Final report of the Working Group on Investigation of Memories of Childhood Abuse.* Washington, DC: Author.

American Psychological Association ad hoc Committee on Legal and Ethical Issues in the Treatment of Interpersonal Violence. (1996a). *Potential problems for psychologists working with the area of interpersonal violence.* [Brochure]. Washington, DC: Author.

American Psychological Association ad hoc Committee on Legal and Ethical Issues in the Treatment of Interpersonal Violence. (1996b). *Professional, ethical, and legal issues concerning interpersonal violence, maltreatment and related trauma.* [Brochure]. Washington, DC: Author.

Barach, P. M. (1994). *ISSD guidelines for treating dissociative identity disorder (multiple personality disorder in adults.* Skokie, IL: The International Society for the Study of Dissociation.

Bass, E., & Davis, L. (1988). *The courage to heal: A guide for women survivors of child sexual abuse.* New York: Harper & Row.

Beutler, L., & Hill, C. (1992). Process and outcome research in the treatment of adult victims of childhood sexual abuse: Methodological issues. *Journal of Consulting and Clinical Psychology, 60,* 204–212.

Blume, E. S. (1990). *Secret survivors: Uncovering incest and its aftereffects in women.* New York: John Wiley & Sons.

Braun, B. G. (Ed.). (1986). *Treatment of multiple personality disorder.* Washington, D.C.: American Psychiatric Press, Inc.

Briere, J. (1989). *Therapy for adults molested as children:Beyond survival.* New York: Springer Publishing Co.

Briere, J. (Ed.). (1991). *Treating victims of child sexual abuse.* San Francisco: Jossey-Bass, Inc.

Briere, J. (1992). *Child abuse trauma: Theory and treatment of the lasting effects.* Newbury Park, CA: Sage.

Briere, J. (1993). Methodological issues in the study of sexual abuse side effects. *Journal of Consulting and Clinical Psychology, 60,* 196–203.

Briere, J. (1995). *Trauma Symptom Inventory (TSI) Professional Manual.* Odessa, FL: Psychological Assessment Resources, Inc.

Briere, J. (1996a). A self-trauma model for treating adult survivors of severe child abuse. In J. Briere, L. Berliner, J. A. Bulkley, C. Jenny, & T. Reid (Eds.). *The APSAC Handbook on Child Maltreatment* (pp. 140–157). Thousand Oaks, CA: Sage.

Briere, J. (1996b). *Therapy for adults molested as children: Beyond survival.* (2nd Ed.). New York: Springer Publishing Co.

Briere, J., Berliner, L., Bulkley, J. A., Jenny, C., & Reid, T. (Eds.). (1996). *The APSAC Handbook on Child Maltreatment.* Thousand Oaks, CA: Sage.

British Psychological Association (1995). *Recovered memories: The Report of the Working Party of the British Psychological Society.* London: Author.

Brown, D. (1995). Pseudomemories: The standard of science and the standard of care in trauma treatment. *American Journal of Clinical Hypnosis, 37,* 1–24.

Brown, D., & Fromm, E. (1986). *Hypnotherapy and hypnoanalysis.* Hillsdale, NJ: Lawrence Earlbaum Associates.

Burgess, A. W., Groth, A. N., Holmstrom, L. L., & Sgroi, S. M. (1978). *Sexual assault of children and adolescents.* Lexington, MA: Lexington Books.

Burgess, A. W., & Holmstrom, L. L. (1974). Sexual trauma of children and adolescents: Pressure, sex and secrecy. *Nursing Clinics of North America,10,* 554–563.

Butler, S. (1978). *Conspiracy of silence: The trauma of incest.* New York: Bantam Books.

Campbell, J., Courtois, C. A., Enns, C., Gottlieb, M., & Wells, M. (1995). *Psychotherapy guidelines for working with clients who may have an abuse or trauma history.* American Psychological Association Division 17 (Counseling Psychology) Committee on Women.

Carlson, E. B. (1996). *Trauma research methodology.* Lutherville, MD: Sidran Press.

Chambless, D. L. (in press). In defense of dissemination of empirically supported psychological interventions. *Clinical Psychology: Science & Practice.*

Chambless, D. L. et al. (1996) An update on empirically validated therapies. *The Clinical Psychologist, 49,* 3–18.

Cohen, L., Berzoff, J., & Elin, M. (Eds.). (1995). *Dissociative identity disorder.* Northvale, NJ: Jason Aaronson.

Courtois, C. A. (1988). *Healing the incest wound: Adult survivors in therapy.* New York: W.W. Norton & Co.

Courtois, C. A. (1991). Theory, sequencing, and strategy in treating adult survivors. In J. Briere (Ed.)., *Treating victims of child sexual abuse.* San Francisco: Jossey-Bass.

Courtois, C. A. (1995). Scientist-practitioners and the delayed memory controversy: Scientific standards and the need for collaboration. *The Counseling Psychologist, 23,* 290–293.

Courtois, C. A. (1996). *Practice guidelines for the treatment of adult clients possibly abuse as children (those who initially report no memories of abuse or who do not disclose at the outset of therapy).* Unpublished manuscript.

Courtois, C. A., & Watts, D. L. (1982). Counseling adult women who experienced incest in childhood or adolescence. *Personnel and Guidance Journal, 60,* 275–279.

Daniluk, J. C., & Haverkamp, B. E. (1993). Ethical issues in counseling adult survivors of incest. *Journal of Counseling & Development, 72,* 16–22.

Davies, J., & Frawley, M. G. (1994). *Treating the adult survivor of childhood sexual abuse: A psychoanalytic perspective.* New York: Basic Books.

Davis, L. (1991). *Allies in healing: When the person you love was sexually abused as a child.* New York: Harper Perennial.

Dawes, R. M. (1995). Standards of practice. In S. C. Hayes, V. M. Follette, R. M. Dawes, & K. E. Grady. *Scientific standards of psychological practice: Issues and recommendations.* Reno, NV: Context Press.

Dolan, Y. M. (1990). *Resolving sexual abuse: Solution-focused therapy and Ericksonian hypnosis for adult survivors.* New York: W.W. Norton & Co.

Draucker, C. (1992). *Counseling survivors of childhood sexual abuse.* Newbury Park, CA: Sage.

Elliott, D., & Briere, J. (1995). Posttraumatic stress associated with delayed recall of sexual abuse: A general population study. *Journal of Traumatic Stress, 8,* 629–648.

Engel, B. (1989). *The right to innocence: Healing the trauma of childhood sexual abuse.* Los Angeles: Jeremy P. Tarcher, Inc.

Enns, C. Z., McNeilly, C. L., Corkery, J. M., & Gilbert, M. S. (1995). The debate about delayed memories of child sexual abuse: A feminist perspective. *The Counseling Psychologist, 23,* 181–279.

Everly, G. S., & Lating, J. M. (Eds.). (1995). *Psychotraumatology: Key papers and core concepts in post-traumatic stress.* New York: Plenum.

Figley, C. R. (Ed.). (1985). *Trauma and its wake: The study and treatment of post-traumatic stress disorder*. New York: Brunner/Mazel.

Figley, C. R. (Ed.). (1995). *Compassion fatigue: Coping with secondary traumatic stress disorder in those who treat the traumatized*. New York: Brunner/Mazel.

Flannery, R. B. (1992). *Post-traumatic stress disorder: The victim's guide to healing and recovery*. New York: Crossroad.

Gabbard, G., & Wilkinson, S. (1994). *Management of countertransference with borderline patients*. Washington, D.C.: American Psychiatric Press, Inc.

Garfield, S. L. (in press). Some problems associated with "validated" forms of psychotherapy. *Clinical Psychology: Science and Practice*.

Geiselman, R. E., Fisher, R. P., MacKinnon, D. P., & Holland, H. L. (1993). Eyewitness memory enhancement in the police interview: Cognitive retrieval mnemonics versus hypnosis. *Journal of Applied Psychology, 70*, 401–412.

Gil, E. (1988). *Treatment of adult survivors of childhood abuse*. Walnut Creek, CA: Launch Press.

Gudjonsson, G. (1992). *The psychology of interrogations, confessions, and testimony*. Chichester, England: John Wiley & Sons.

Hammond, D. C. et al. (1994). *Clinical hypnosis and memory: Guidelines for clinicians and for forensic hypnosis*. Chicago: American Society for Clinical Hypnosis Press.

Hayes, S. C. (1995). What do we want from standards of psychological practice? In S. C. Hayes, V. M. Follette, R. M. Dawes, & K. E. Grady. *Scientific standards of practice: Issues and recommendations*. Reno, NV: Context Press.

Hayes, S. C., Follette, V. M., Dawes, R. M., & Grady, K. E. (1995). *Scientific standards of practice: Issues and recommendations*. Reno, NV: Context Press.

Herman, J. L. (1981). *Father-daughter incest*. Cambridge, MA: Harvard University Press.

Herman, J. L. (1992a). Complex PTSD: A syndrome in survivors of prolonged and repeated trauma. *Journal of Traumatic Stress, 3*, 377–391.

Herman, J. L. (1992b). *Trauma and recovery: The aftermath of violence-from domestic to political terror*. New York: Basic Books.

Herman, J. L., & van der Kolk, B. (1987). Traumatic antecedents of borderline personality disorder. In B. van der Kolk (Ed.). *Psychological trauma* (pp. 111–126). Washington, DC: American Psychiatric Press, Inc.

Hill, C., & Alexander, P. (1993). Process research in the treatment of adult victims of childhood sexual abuse. *Journal of Interpersonal Violence, 8*, 415–427.

Hotelling, K. (1995, August). *Ethical issues in the recovery of sexual abuse memories*. Paper presented at the annual meeting of the American Psychological Association, New York City.

Janet, P. (1889). *L'automatisme psychologique*. Paris: Alcan.

Jehu, D. (1988). *Beyond Sexual Abuse: Therapy with women who were childhood victims*. New York: John Wiley & Sons.

Kempe, C. H., Silverman, F. N., Steele, B. F., Droegemueller, W., & Silver, H. K. (1962). The battered child syndrome. *Journal of the American Medical Association, 181*, 17–24.

Kepner, J. I. (1995). *Healing tasks: Psychotherapy with adult survivors of childhood abuse*. San Francisco: Jossey-Bass.

Kluft, R. P. (Ed.). (1985). *Childhood antecedents of multiple personality*. Washington, DC: American Psychiatric Press, Inc.

Kluft, R. P. (Ed.). (1990). *Incest-related syndromes of adult psychopathology*. Washington, DC: American Psychiatric Press, Inc.

Kluft, R. P., & Fine, C. G. (Eds.). (1993). *Clinical perspectives on multiple personality disorder*. Washington, DC: American Psychiatric Press, Inc.

Kovacs, A. A. (1995). We have met the enemy and he is us! *The Independent Practitioner, 15*, 135–137.

Lindsay, D. S. (1996, June). *Increasing sensitivity*. Paper presented at the NATO Advanced Study Institute, Port de Bourgenay, France.

Lindsay, D. S., & Read, J. D. (1994). Psychotherapy and memories of childhood sexual abuse: a cognitive perspective. *Applied Cognitive Psychology, 8*, 281–338.

Linehan, M. (1993). *Cognitive-behavioral treatment of borderline personality disorder*. New York: Guilford.

Littauer, F., & Littauer, F. (1990). *Freeing your mind from memories that bind: How to heal hurts from the past*. San Bernadino, CA: Here's Life Publishers.

Loftus, E. (1993). The reality of repressed memories. *American Psychologist, 48*, 518–537.

London, R. (1994). Therapeutic treatment of patients with repressed memories. *The Independent Practitioner*, 64–67.

McCann, I. L., & Pearlman, L. A. (1990). *Psychological trauma and the adult survivor: Theory, therapy, and transformation.* New York: Brunner/Mazel.

McCann, I. L., Pearlman, L. A., Sakheim, D. C., & Abrahamson, D. J. (1988). Trauma and victimization: A model of psychological adaptation. *The Counseling Psychologist, 16*, 531–594.

Meichenbaum, D. (1994). *A clinical handbook/practical therapist manual for assessing and treating adults with post-traumatic stress disorder (PTSD).* Waterloo, Ontario, Canada: Institute Press.

Meiselman, K. C. (1978). *Incest: A psychological study of causes and effects with treatment recommendations.* San Francisco: Jossey-Bass.

Meiselman, K. C. (1990). *Resolving the trauma of incest:* Reintegration therapy with survivors. San Francisco: Jossey-Bass.

National Institute of Mental Health, Division of Biometry and Applied Sciences, Antisocial and Violent Behavior Branch. (1990). *Research workshop on Treatment of Adult Victims of Childhood Sexual Abuse,* Washington, DC.

Neumann, D. A., Houskamp, B. M., Pollock, V. E., & Briere, J. (1996). The long-term sequelae of childhood sexual abuse in women: A meta-analytic review. *Child Maltreatment, 1*, 6–17.

Ochberg, F. M. (Ed.). (1988). *Post-traumatic therapy and victims of violence.* New York: Brunner/Mazel.

Payne, A. B. (1995, August). *Training and supervision issues regarding trauma and recovery of memories.* Paper presented at the annual meeting of the American Psychological Association, New York City.

Pearlman, L. A., & Saakvitne, K. W. (1995). *Trauma and the therapist: Countertransference and vicarious traumatization in psychotherapy with incest survivors.* New York: W. W. Norton.

Peters, J. J. (1976). Children who are victims of sexual assault and the psychology of offenders. *American Journal of Psychotherapy, 30*, 398–421.

Pope, K., & Brown, L. (1996). *Recovered memories of abuse: Assessment, therapy, forensics.* Washington, DC: American Psychological Association.

Poston, C., & Lison, K. (1989). *Reclaiming our lives: Hope for adult survivors of incest.* New York: Little, Brown.

Putnam, F. W. (1985). Dissociation as a response to extreme trauma. In Kluft, R. (Ed.). *Childhood antecedents of multiple personality* (pp. 65–98). Washington, DC: American Psychiatric Association Press, Inc.

Putnam, F. W. (1989). *Diagnosis and treatment of multiple personality disorder.* New York: Guilford Press

Ross, C. A. (1989). *Multiple personality disorder: Diagnosis, clinical features, and treatment.* New York: John Wiley & Sons.

Russell, D. E. H. (1986). *The secret trauma: Incest in the lives of girls and women.* New York: Basic Books.

Salter, A. C. (1995). *Transforming trauma: A guide to understanding and treating adult survivors of child sexual abuse.* Newbury Park, CA: Sage.

Scharff, J. S., & Scharff, D. (1994). *Object relations therapy of physical and sexual trauma.* Northvale, NJ: Jason Aaronson Inc.

Scheflin, A. W., & Shapiro, J. L. (1989). *Trance on Trial.* New York: Guilford.

Scurfield, R. M. (1985). Post-trauma stress assessment and treatment: Overview and formulations. In C. R. Figley, (Ed.). *Trauma and its wake: The study and treatment of post-traumatic stress disorder* (pp. 219–256). New York: Brunner/Mazel.

Selye, H. (1976). *Stress in health and disease.* Boston: Butterworth.

Sgroi, S. M. (1982). *Handbook of clinical intervention in child sexual abuse.* Lexington, MA: Lexington Books.

Shapiro, F. (1995). *Eye movement desensitization and reprocessing: Basic principles, protocols, and procedures.* New York: Guilford.

Spiegel, D. (Ed.). (1994). *Dissociation: Culture, mind, and body.* Washington, DC: American Psychiatric Press, Inc.

Spiegel, H., & Spiegel, D. (1978). *Trance and treatment: Clinical uses of hypnosis.* New York: Basic Books.

Spira, J. L. (Ed.). (1996). *Treating dissociative identity disorder.* San Francisco: Jossey-Bass.

Steinberg, M. (1995). *Handbook for the assessment of dissociation: A clinical guide.* Washington, DC: American Psychiatric Press, Inc.

van der Kolk, B. (Ed.). (1984). *Post-traumatic stress disorder: Psychological and biological sequelae.* Washington, DC: American Psychiatric Press, Inc.

van der Kolk, B. (1987). *Psychological trauma.* Washington, DC: American Psychiatric Press, Inc.

van der Kolk, B., & Fisler, R. (1995). Dissociation and the fragmentary nature of traumatic memories: Overview and exploratory study. *Journal of Traumatic Stress, 8*, 505–525.

van der Kolk, B., McFarland, A., & van der Hart, O. (1996). A general approach to treatment of posttraumatic stress disorder. In B. van der Kolk, A. McFarland, & L. Weisaeth (Eds.). *Traumatic stress: The effects of overwhelming experience on mind, body, and society* (p. 417–440). New York: Guilford.

van der Kolk, B., McFarland, A., & Weisaeth, L. (Eds.). (1996). *Traumatic stress: The effects of overwhelming experience on mind, body, and society.* New York: Guilford.

Waites, E. A., (1993). *Trauma and survival: Post-traumatic and dissociative disorders in women.* New York: W.W. Norton & Co.

Walker, L. E. (1984). *The battered woman syndrome.* New York: Springer.

Williams, M. B., & Sommer, J. F. (Eds.). (1994) *Handbook of post-traumatic therapy.* Westport, CT: Greenwood Press.

Wilson, J. (1989). *Trauma transformation and healing: An integrative approach to theory, research, and post-traumatic therapy.* New York: Brunner/Mazel.

Wilson, J., & Lindy, J. (Eds.). (1994). *Countertransference in the treatment of PTSD.* New York: Guilford.

Wilson, J., & Raphael, B. (Eds.). (1993). *International handbook of traumatic stress syndromes.* New York: Plenum.

Yapko, M. D. (1994). *Suggestions of abuse: True and false memories of childhood sexual trauma.* New York: Simon & Schuster.

COMMENTARY ON INFORMED CLINICAL PRACTICE AND THE STANDARD OF CARE: PROPOSED GUIDELINES FOR THE TREATMENT OF ADULTS WHO REPORT DELAYED MEMORIES OF CHILDHOOD TRAUMA

D. Stephen Lindsay, University of Wales—Bangor, U.K., University of Victoria, Canada

1. PRAISE

I greatly admire Christine Courtois, not only as someone who undertakes the tremendously difficult task of working with trauma survivors, but also as someone who has responded to the controversy about memory work in a constructive way. Courtois has emerged as the leading figure among trauma-oriented psychologists working to develop and communicate sensible guidelines for trauma-oriented psychotherapy designed simultaneously to maximize support for incest survivors and minimize risks of inadvertent suggestive influences. I would not be surprised to learn that her efforts in this direction have provoked criticism from some fellow traumatologists. Courtois had already been a target of critics of memory work because of her publications arguing that abuse survivors may not remember their abuse, that working through abuse memories may be important for such clients, and that clinicians should therefore create conditions that foster remembering of childhood trauma. Courtois did not promote high-pressure searches for suspected hidden memories in clients who disavow abuse histories, but nonetheless she has taken flak from critics of memory work (e.g., Lindsay & Read, 1994). Thus I suspect she now finds herself in a position to which I too aspire, in which one is sometimes a target of criticism from both sides of this controversy.

I first encountered Courtois's efforts toward developing guidelines for trauma-oriented therapy at the 1994 Midwestern Conference on Child Sexual Abuse and Incest. I was impressed with these tentative guidelines, and heartened to see them, but of course I had some criticisms and suggestions, and I wrote to her expressing these opinions. As one index of the constructive stance Courtois has taken, I received a cordial reply and the news that some of my suggestions had been incorporated into ongoing revisions of the guidelines.

I agree with much of what Courtois has said in her lecture, and salute her for it. I particularly welcome her acknowledgment that the media indulged in extensive sensationalization of uncritical accounts of recovered memories of bizarre abuse in the late 1980s and early 1990's, and that such media shows interacted with pop-psychology sources such as the Bradshaw television series and the popularization and generalization of 12-step programs and self-help literatures. I also appreciate Courtois's comments about the necessity of a high level of training and skill for practitioners working with childhood abuse, and her observation that some therapists with little or no formal training were greatly influenced by the media and popular press presentations. Even more important is her acknowledgment that some highly trained professionals, too, were unduly influenced by such material—in part because of the paucity of better material and in part because of the shocking extent to which professional psychotherapists rely on popular books as a source of information (Beutler, Williams, & Wakefield, 1993). Most important, I appreciate Courtois's statements regarding the necessity of avoiding highly suggestive techniques and approaches. I note particularly her statement that, because Criterion A of the PTSD diagnosis is the occurrence of a trauma, this diagnosis should not be given unless a trauma history is established, and her recommendation that clinicians should obtain full informed consent before embarking on a course of treatment that is expected to make the client get worse before getting better. These arguments, by a traumatologist of Courtois's stature, are bound to have a tremendous positive impact, reducing use of suggestive techniques without undercutting support for victims of abuse.

The approach Courtois advocates would, if adopted, eliminate the most extreme suggestive searches for hidden memories. But I am not entirely confident that it would restrict practice to approaches that have minimal risk. My concerns regarding Courtois's approach to therapy are more tentative and harder to articulate than my alarm about the most aggressive archeological digs for suspected hidden memories, and I hope that my discussion of these concerns does not overshadow the fact that I greatly admire and appreciate the contribution Courtois has made by developing these guidelines.

2. CONCERNS

2.1. Minimization of the Problem of Risky Memory Work

In some parts of her lecture, Courtois appeared to me to minimize bases for concern about suggestive searches for suspected hidden memories. One example is her statement that evidence does not support the contention that large numbers of therapists conduct archaeological digs for lost memories. I think that this statement echoes a common point of confusion that arises when people fail to keep in mind the very large number of therapists. Suppose, for example, that during the 5-year period from 1987 to 1992, 5% of North Americans who provide insight therapies used powerfully suggestive approaches to memory work. That would mean, of course, that 95% did not use such approaches. Five percent sounds very small, but how many clients, during that 5-year period, would have been exposed to highly suggestive forms of memory work? I do not think it is possible to give a precise estimate, but consider the order of magnitude. What number would one achieve if one added up the PhD, PsyD, MA, MD, MSW, clergy, and people without formal training who provide insight therapies in North America? The answer is on the order of several hundred thousand, most of whom work with dozens of clients per year. Thus a small percentage of therapists translates into a substantial number of therapists and an even larger number of clients.

2.2. The Target Population

One of my concerns has to do with the population of clients for whom these guidelines are advocated (for related concerns, see Don Read's comment on John Briere's lecture). In her title and several times in her lecture, Courtois defined the target population as "clients who report delayed memories of abuse." This implies that the guidelines are to apply to work with clients who have already reported abuse histories. As guidelines for working with clients who seek assistance in dealing with past trauma, I think Courtois's recommendations are thoughtful, thorough, meticulously detailed, and that they cleave to a very high standard of professional care and accountability while admirably emphasizing appropriate and sensitive empathic support for the client. The recommended approach makes ample room for clients to work with their trauma issues, but does not rush them into doing so.

Unfortunately, the definition of the target population of clients for whom the guidelines are recommended becomes less clear as one reads through the guidelines. For one thing, the dividing line between clients who enter therapy with accessible memories of childhood trauma and those who do not is not so obvious as one might think. For example, some clients remember certain instances of abuse when they enter therapy but later experience recovery of memories of other, qualitatively different sorts of events. Given the vagueness of the definition of terms such as "trauma" and "abuse," it may be that virtually all clients enter therapy with memories of experiences that might be viewed as traumas. Furthermore, elsewhere Courtois indicated that the guidelines also apply to work with clients who present with suspicions but no clear memories of abuse. Finally, Courtois indicated that the target population also includes clients who seek help for "problems associated with childhood sexual abuse," but it is not clear whether this is meant to refer only to clients who themselves view their problems as being associated with childhood sexual abuse, or also to clients whose symptoms are interpreted as being associated with childhood sexual abuse.[*]

Despite the title, it appears that Courtois's traumatological approach to therapy has been and is being advocated for and used with clients who initially do not remember or suspect any history of childhood sexual abuse. Much to her credit, she stated quite plainly that failure to "disclose" should not automatically be taken as denial, argued that the diagnosis of PTSD should not be made unless the client reports some trauma that satisfies Criteria A, and counseled caution in the use of memory recovery techniques with clients who do not report abuse. Indeed, she explicitly said that when an abuse history is merely suspected, treatment should follow a generic, rather than a posttraumatic, model. And yet the pervasive undercurrent of the approach seems to be that childhood trauma (and, particularly, childhood sexual abuse) is quite likely to lie at the root of adulthood psychological problems, and that working through such trauma is an important part of therapy. For example, consider the following quotation: "When the individual's symptom picture is acute

---

[*] It is worth noting that although Courtois claimed that critics of memory work focused on cases in which clients sought help for abuse or for suspicions of abuse, the fact is that critics have focused primarily on cases in which clients sought help for common psychological problems (e.g., anxiety, depression, relationship difficulties, sleep disturbance, sexual dysfunction, eating disorders, substance-abuse problems) and did not remember childhood abuse but were told that their symptoms were consistent with an abuse history, that many people with abuse histories do not remember them, that psychological healing in such cases depends on and is evidenced by recovering trauma memories, and that various exercises may be helpful in exploring the possibility of a hidden history of abuse.

and/or consists of a number of post-traumatic symptoms or symptoms of the type most correlated to an abuse history . . . the possibility of undisclosed or unrecognized abuse or other trauma should be given consideration." I do not know why an "acute" symptom picture indicates undisclosed trauma, I am not convinced that there is any known constellation of symptoms that can be taken as likely indicators of a hidden history of childhood sexual abuse, and I am troubled at what Courtois seems to have in mind when she says that the possibility of undisclosed abuse should be "considered" in such cases.

2.3. Hypothesis-Confirming Approach

Courtois advocated a hypothesis-confirming approach when there are perceived grounds for considering the possibility of undisclosed trauma. For example, she suggested that given such suspicions clinicians should look for autonomic hyperarousal, numbing of responsiveness and affect, intense emotional reactions, learning difficulties, memory disturbances and dissociations, aggression against self and others, interpersonal difficulties, psychosomatic reactions, substance abuse and other addictive/compulsive difficulties, impulsivity, and problems with body image or self-esteem. Presumably, finding such symptoms would add to one's suspicions of non-remembered childhood trauma. This is deeply worrying to me. For one thing, oftentimes multiple symptoms should not add incrementally to confidence in a hypothesis regarding a hidden history of abuse, because oftentimes symptom clusters are not independent but rather are highly correlated aspects of a condition (Ceci & Loftus, 1994). For another thing, it seems to me that most people seeking psychotherapy have at least a few of the symptoms Courtois listed, and the probability that such symptoms indicate non-remembered abuse is relatively low. Finally, looking for particular symptoms—especially if they are not well-defined—may well increase the likelihood of noting (and perhaps even creating) their presence due to various cognitive and social-psychological processes (e.g., expectancy effects, demand characteristics, self-fulfilling prophecies, etc.).

2.4. Probability That Symptoms Indicate Non-Remembered Abuse

The recommendation that clinicians should suspect non-reported abuse given certain symptoms and therefore seek confirming evidence for that suspicion rests on the belief that a substantial percentage of clients with such symptoms are suffering the after-effects of non-reported abuse. Courtois stated that adult survivors of childhood sexual abuse who suffer after-effects serious enough to require clinical services make up a high percentage of all adults in both in- and out-patient populations. The meaning of the term "high" was not specified. I would like to learn what sort of figure she had in mind and how much of the evidence for it comes from studies of representative samples as opposed to samples of clients receiving therapy from traumatologists or MPD specialists. My impression is that studies vary dramatically in their estimates of the base rate of abuse histories among people seeking therapy (see Read & Lindsay, 1994, p. 423). More to the point, numerous lines of evidence suggest that only a very small percentage of psychotherapy clients have problems that are caused by non-remembered histories of abuse.

Consider, for example, evidence on the base rate of various kinds of childhood sexual abuse. Finkelhor's (1994) review of retrospective self-report studies of the prevalence of childhood sexual abuse indicates that, as a conservative estimate, approximately 20% of U.S. women report having experienced some form of sexual abuse during childhood. Finkelhor noted that many reports are of extra-familial abuse, that many are of one-time instances, and that a third of the perpetrators of reported abuse are said to have been under age 18 years when the abuse occurred. Finkelhor's review indicated that something on the order of 5% report childhood abuse involving penetration or oral-genital contact. Compared to the beliefs of just a few decades ago (e.g., that only 1 in a million North Americans, or .0001%, experience incest) these prevalence estimates are shockingly high. But, taken together, retrospective self-report studies suggest that the kinds of abuse emphasized by traumatologists (e.g., traumatic, chronic, and escalating violation perpetrated by a loved adult) are reported by a small percentage of respondents in large-scale retrospective self-report studies. (A large number of victims, but a small percentage of people.)

Of course, retrospective self-report studies likely underestimate prevalence, for a variety of reasons, and it may be that the base rate of abuse survivors is somewhat higher among psychotherapy clients than among the general population. But first consider the fact that only some victims of severe CSA demonstrate lasting harm, and then consider the myriad insults to mental health that confront North Americans: neglect, poverty, violence, the disintegration of the extended family and, more recently, of the nuclear family, drugs, crime, bereavement, ever increasing demands and ever decreasing social support to meet those demands, etc. Think of reasons your own children might someday seek psychological help; I suspect that most people can imagine that their own children might someday seek psychotherapy for the kinds of problems Courtois listed as indicators of non-reported abuse, even if their children were not sexually abused. Childhood sexual abuse is an important social problem and a psychopathogen, but I think it is a mistake to return to Freud's early belief that it lies at the root of all, most, or even a large minority of psychological problems.

I also believe that most survivors of traumatic abuse beyond infancy do not forget that it happened. Courtois claimed that "The memory disturbance aspect [of dissociative disorders diagnoses] . . . provides an explanatory mechanism for the fragmented and delayed/recovered memory found to be associated with different types of trauma" (p. 10), but in my opinion (a) claims about Dissociative Amnesia do not amount to an "explanatory mechanism" and (b) the claim that fragmented and delayed/recovered memory is associated with trauma goes far beyond the data. I am not saying that all trauma survivors remember the trauma, nor am I saying that it is impossible for trauma survivors to not remember the trauma for decades and then later remember it. On the contrary, I think there is compelling evidence that people can and do forget traumas and later remember them. What I am saying is that such people make up a small percentage of the small percentage of people with histories of genuine trauma.

When all of these arguments are put together (evidence regarding the prevalence of extreme forms of abuse, evidence that some abuse survivors are asymptomatic, evidence that most abuse survivors remember their abuse, and consideration of the myriad insults to psychological health that confront members of our society), I think the belief that a large percentage of people seeking psychotherapy for help with common psychological problems are suffering the after-effects of non-remembered trauma is severely challenged. This argument undermines the rationale for hypothesizing that clients with particular symptoms have hidden histories of abuse, and suggests that practitioners should be at least as open to considering other possibilities. Indeed, given that other factors with higher base rates may be equally strongly related to particular symptoms, it may be that practitioners should be biased toward entertaining other hypotheses. I acknowledge that Courtois stated that practitioners should keep an open mind, and that childhood sexual abuse is not the only factor that may underlie psychological problems; but to my ear such statements come across as caveats, a brake applied to the project of looking for hidden trauma memories. Far better to have such a brake than none, but I am not sure it sufficiently slows the momentum toward suggestive searches for suspected hidden memories of childhood sexual abuse.

2.5. Efficacy of Memory Work

Another rationale for the statement that practitioners should suspect non-reported abuse in clients with certain symptoms is the belief that for such clients working through issues related to abuse is an important part of therapy. Courtois cited Brown (1995) as stating that "exposure to traumatic memories is associated with treatment gain in behavioral treatment of PTSD . . . and in the psychodynamic treatment of severe dissociative disorders." I am aware of two carefully done controlled studies supporting the hypothesis that detailed recounting of the rape can be more helpful for rape victims than other treatments, but these studies did not include women who did not know that they had been raped. I know of one conference presentation reporting a study evaluating trauma-oriented therapy, but my understanding is that it did not lead to better results than the comparison treatment (Spiegel, 1994, cited in Ceci & Loftus, 1994). There are, of course, many case studies in the traumatology and MPD literatures, but in my view interpretation of these reports is quite problematic. I am not saying that working through trauma is unimportant for trauma survivors; I am merely saying that to the best of my knowledge we lack solid evidence for the belief that best practice when working with psychotherapy clients with the symptoms Courtois enumerated includes exploring for hidden memories of traumatic childhood sexual abuse.

In support of the claim that clinicians should consider the possibility that clients with certain symptoms have hidden histories of CSA, Courtois argued that "Suppressing true memories of past abuse is as potentially serious and damaging as suggesting (false) memories of abuse that never occurred." First, I am not quite sure of the relevance of the first half of the statement: To the best of my knowledge, no one has suggested that therapists should suppress true memories of abuse. Second, if the claim is that failing to work at eliciting true reports of abuse is as damaging as suggesting false abuse, then I challenge that claim. Imagine we do a study, in which some clients receive highly suggestive memory work and others receive, say, behavioral interventions targeted to helping them respond effectively to their current psychological problems. Courtois's claim implies that both treatments would be damaging (the former because it suggests false memories, the latter because it does not encourage clients to explore true ones), but I suspect that the suggestive treatment would be damaging and the behavioral intervention would be helpful. If the claim is merely that practitioners should not deny or trivialize clients' reports of abuse, then I agree with it but think it should have been more clearly articulated. As stated it seemed to be a rationale for working (however gently) at eliciting reports of suspected abuse.

In a similar vein, Courtois said that sodium amytal might be warranted in exceptional circumstances as a way of exploring for memories of abuse in order to resolve the most intractable symptoms. I would be interested in learning more about the circumstances that warrant use of sodium amytal as a memory-recovery technique (see Piper, 1993). Finally, Courtois suggested that clients should be informed about the "somatosensory" nature of posttraumatic recall. I would also like to learn more about this phenomenon.

2.6. The Voice of Authority and Consensus

Courtois speaks with considerable authority and, at times, in a voice that suggests that she represents a broad if preliminary consensus among psychologists who work with trauma survivors. For example, she several times used terms such as "The contemporary treatment strategy," and made statements such as "Most often, psychodynamically informed individual psychotherapy is the treatment of choice, supplemented by group therapy at different points in the course of treatment if feasible" (p. 35). I noted that clinicians who are best known as MPD specialists (e.g., Braum, Kluft, Putnam, Ross) figured prominently in Courtois's list of those who contributed to the development of "the" general treatment strategy. As Mulhern points out in her Commentary in this volume, there are close links between the MPD phenomenon and the recovered memories phenomenon. In any case, I suspect that there may not be so broad a consensus across clinical psychologists regarding treatment of trauma survivors as Courtois's comments sometimes seem to imply.

3. CONCLUSION

I argued in my lecture that we should grapple with the difficult issues that lie between extreme positions. It is relatively easy to make firm and clear statements about the extremes. For example, I think most would agree that it is inappropriate to tell clients who report abuse histories that their memories are likely fantasies; similarly, most would agree that it is inappropriate to encourage clients who report no abuse history to undertake searches for hidden memories of such a history. But between these extremes lie gray areas in which statements are more open to debate. Courtois's lecture puts us somewhere in the midst of two important gray areas: that between clients who have always remembered childhood trauma versus clients who had no inkling of trauma until memories were recovered, and that between approaches to therapy that pose no risk of iatrogenic illusory memories or false beliefs and approaches to therapy that pose substantial risk.

In closing, I want to make it clear that I believe that even when childhood sexual abuse is restricted to relatively extreme forms of contact abuse, there are millions of survivors of such abuse. I also believe that such abuse is profoundly wrong and that it can cause long-lasting harm. Thus I have no doubt that childhood trauma is an important issue for very large numbers of people in the general population, and I applaud the work of the many psychologists, social workers, and other professionals who help such people to improve their psychological health and well-being. I entirely agree that practitioners should be open to their clients' reports of past trauma, and I agree that asking clients about trauma histories is a sensible procedure in many therapy situations. I salute Courtois for stating quite clearly that her approach does not focus on exploring trauma for its own sake, but rather only as a means of enhancing well-being, and applaud her for the many very reasonable and helpful statements she made about reducing the suggestiveness of trauma-oriented psychotherapy. Although, as indicated above, I have some lingering concerns, in general I think that her proposed guidelines are a major and very admirable accomplishment.

REFERENCES

Beutler, L. E., Williams, R. E., & Wakefield, P. J. (1993). Obstacles to disseminating applied psychological science. *Applied and Preventative Psychology, 2*, 53–58.

Brown, D. (1995). Pseudomemories, the standard of science and the standard of care in trauma treatment. *American Journal of Clinical Hypnosis, 37*, 3–29.

Ceci, S. J., & Loftus, E. F. (1994). "Memory work:" A royal road to false memories? *Applied Cognitive Psychology, 8*, 351–364.

Finkelhor, D. (1994). Current information on the scope and nature of child sexual abuse. *The Future of Children,* 4, 31–53.

Lindsay, D. S., & Read, J. D. (1994). Psychotherapy and memories of childhood sexual abuse: A cognitive perspective. *Applied Cognitive Psychology, 8,* 281–338.

Piper, A., Jr. (1993). "Truth serum" and "recovered memories" of sexual abuse: A review of the evidence. *Journal of Psychiatry and Law, Winter,* 447–471.

Read, J. D., & Lindsay, D. S. (1994). Moving toward a middle ground on the "false memory debate:" Reply to commentaries on Lindsay and Read. *Applied Cognitive Psychology, 8,* 407–435.

QUESTION AND ANSWER SESSION

Widom. I consider myself right in the middle. One of the things that troubles me, and I hope I come from a neutral stance, is that in the same way that we've asked Chris to talk about guidelines for clinicians and how can we monitor and get more responsible behaviour on the part of clinicians and not leading, misrepresenting, or engaging in expertise beyond our expertise, I really think as researchers we need to consider the APA guidelines on professional behaviour. I'm increasingly concerned that we ought to devote the same attention to very explicit guidelines about when our scientific expertise is appropriate to use in a courtroom. I think we really need to monitor ourselves and seriously think about this and not point the arrow only towards the clinicians.

Shuman. I want to discuss how we deal with this as a system, how do we prevent this? You talked about standards of care and obviously the wave of litigation is facing in the direction of therapists because they have malpractice insurance and the courts in the US have been limiting the homeowners' policies for these kinds of claims. The problem is that as courts look for standards so that they don't decide each of these cases differently, they look in part to the professional organisation. What they get from them, as we've talked about it, are politically acceptable agreements that provide a consensual level of generalisation which essentially say nothing useful in looking at individual cases. I think what's lovely about the guidelines you've provided is that they move down from Mount Olympus and actually talk specifically about what ought to be done in individual cases. The beauty of them, of course, is that they do provide guidance so that this isn't partisan experts in individual cases sorting this out, but rather a set of neutral guidelines that exist independent of that, and I want to commend you for that.

Schooler. Your talk was really encouraging to see the care and thought given to these issues. If one could know that these are the types of techniques that are being used out there I think everyone would feel much more assured. How can we have it happen that the types of techniques that your suggesting get used out there? It's really alarming to think that people can go through a 16-hour training class, (as you described in your oral presentation), put a notice up, and actually treat trauma. As long as they can do that, they're going to do that and, while I hear that many therapists are changing, I guess I don't have entire confidence in the trickle down view of that. It seems like real policy changes have to happen to ensure that it's the enlightened types of therapy that you're suggesting that are actually being used.

Courtois. It is a very complicated matter and I think some of it has to do with policing our own, but some of it begins by adopting different regulations that don't allow people to use terms such as "psychotherapist" without a specific training. I know there's controversy about that, but at least it's a preliminary step to guarding some boundaries and making sure there are some competent standards and some training standards that are in place. I also think the information is being disseminated among many therapists, but certainly not all. I'm doing a lot of workshops and therapists are lining up to get this information: they are not unaware. They may not know what to do and they may not know the parameters of the problem per se, but they know there's a problem and they know that they need to really watch how they are practising.

Creamer. I wanted to ask about treatment outcome studies and how we might go about assessing the efficacy of this kind of intervention. It struck me that one of the really difficult problems is the actual diagnosis because if one of my clients has a diagnosis of PTSD I might work quite differently compared to someone who's got a diagnosis of borderline personality disorder. I just wondered if you could comment quite generally on how we could go about looking at treatment outcome and perhaps with reference to particular diagnostic groups. I suppose the issue really was that we're presenting it as a treatment for adult survivors of childhood sexual abuse and yet that's different from the way we would normally set up our studies, which is looking at the diagnostic category. I wonder how we can match the two? We're presenting a treatment for an etiological cause, whereas normally we design our studies based on a diagnosis at the time and I'm having difficulties reconciling the two in terms of how we might do our treatment efficacy studies. Rather than saying is this an effective treatment for adult survivors of childhood abuse is this sufficient or do we have to say more about the presenting pathology?

Courtois. I think we need to say something more specific and I think some of the new instruments such as John Briere's trauma symptom inventory, as an example, provide us with instruments that could be used to look at some of those presenting symptoms that are characteristic of this population, or some of the PTSD screens could be used to do pre/post testing at least initially.

Browne. I wanted to pick up on the point that the false positive, false negative, debate is just as applicable to the offender as it is to the victim and yet we seem to have concentrated this debate on the victim. Therefore I'd like you to comment on why we've done that and whether you feel that the suggestion that society was ready to accept physical abuse and neglect and is less shocked by that, even though it kills two children a week in Britain and two children a day in the States, and yet we're more shocked about child sexual abuse. It was said twenty years ago that society's first reaction to this is denial, and I wonder how much you see our concentration on the false positive, false negative, debate as us still being in a process of denial. I also have a second question that relates to that, which is that I'm puzzled, especially as I come initially from the discipline of ethology and the biological bases of behaviour, why have we spent so much time looking at cognitive processes and the spoken word. Surely in false allegations and true allegation, non-verbal communication and the socio-emotional behaviour of the child is just as important. Sixty percent of communication is non-verbal and forty percent is verbal. So to the experimentalists and the researchers here, I plead that you put non-verbal behaviour into your experiments to look at the reactions of some of these children when they are attempting to relate a memory as true or false. I think that's where there is some really useful material that we can explore that could tease apart true and false allegations.

Courtois. I think that I was trying to convey some of this at the start. The issue of sexual abuse and most particularly incest, is still something that we have a difficult time looking at. We also have a very difficult time acknowledging that incest occurs across demographic categories and that is still very hard to accept and that is part of the socio-political context of what has sparked this controversy. As Florence Rush said, it is one of the "best kept secrets". There has been a very asymmetrical handling of the material, because we have not looked at the issue of false memory in perpetrators as much as we have in people who say they've been victimised. I would suggest that we really need to shift that focus and be more even-handed about it, especially as criminology studies have documented pretty conclusively that offenders have denial and honesty difficulties and may have problems with forgetting as well. Many perpetrators have substance abuse problems which might lead to black-outs and associated memory deficits.

14

GENDER AND RECALL OF CHILD SEXUAL ABUSE

A Prospective Study

Linda M. Williams[1*] and Victoria L. Banyard[2]

[1]The Stone Center, Wellesley College
106 Central Street
Wellesley, Massachusetts 02181-8268
[2]Department of Psychology
University of New Hampshire
Durham, New Hampshire 03824

1. INTRODUCTION

One critical question at the heart of the debate on recovered memory is "how common is it to have no memory of sexual abuse that occurred in one's childhood?" An increasingly large number of studies have documented that traumatic events from childhood may be forgotten (see Williams & Banyard, in press). Much of this research has specifically focused on adults' experiences with forgetting child sexual abuse and is based on naturalistic studies of clinical samples of men and women in treatment for the consequences of sexual abuse. This research reveals that many adults who now recall sexual abuse that occurred during childhood report that there were prior periods when they did not remember the abuse. For example, Herman and Schatzow (1987) found that over half of the women participating in an outpatient group for incest survivors reported some degree of prior forgetting of the sexual abuse they had experienced and that 28% of the women reported prior severe memory deficits. Prior studies have not focused on memories of sexual abuse among males or on possible differences in memory status for men and women who have experienced sexual abuse in childhood.

Two studies (Briere & Conte, 1993; Elliott & Briere, 1995) have offered some comparison of prior periods of forgetting child sexual abuse for males and females. Although

* This research was supported by the US Department of Health and Social Services, National Center for Child Abuse and Neglect Grants #90-CA-1495 to the Joseph J. Peters Institute and #90-CA-1406 and #1552 to the University of New Hampshire (Linda M. Williams, principal investigator). The authors gratefully acknowledge the assistance of Jane Siegel, Project Director.

Recollections of Trauma, edited by Read and Lindsay
Plenum Press, New York, 1997

this was not the focus of their work, Briere and Conte (1993) reported that in a clinical sample of 420 women and 30 men in treatment for sexual abuse there were no statistically significant gender differences in the frequency of reports of such forgetting. Data presented in tabular form in that article permit us to calculate that 59% of the women and 63% of the men reported prior periods of forgetting. Consistent with this, Elliott and Briere (1995) reported that in a community sample in which retrospective recollection of prior memory problems were studied there were no differences in abuse memory status based on gender of the respondent. While these studies contribute to our understanding of memories for child sexual abuse, they are retrospective in nature. That is, they rely on current reports of victimization in childhood. This is problematic in that both the sexual abuse history as well as the forgetting may be uncorroborated. Furthermore, retrospective designs are unable to examine those cases in which the sexual abuse experienced in childhood continues to be forgotten. Prospective studies of cases of child sexual abuse such as the one described in this chapter, can address some of these problems.

Based on previous research, one would not expect to find a gender difference in rates of actual forgetting of sexual abuse experienced in childhood, although it has been suggested that men may be less willing than women to *report* experiences to interviewers due to social pressure, embarrassment or shame (Widom & Morris, 1996). In this study we examine forgetting of abuse in a community sample of men with documented histories of child sexual abuse and compare the rates of forgetting for these men with previously reported rates of forgetting among a similar sample of women (Williams, 1994; 1995).

2. METHOD

Men and women were interviewed in 1990–1994 as part of a study of the long-term consequences of child sexual abuse. One hundred and forty-seven men and 206 women comprised the original sample of boys and girls with documented histories of child sexual abuse. These children had been seen 17 to 20 years earlier (in the early 1970s) when the sexual abuse was reported and they were examined and treated in a hospital emergency room where all sexual abuse victims in that jurisdiction were routinely taken. Details of the sexual assault were documented in the hospital records contemporaneous to the report of the abuse. At the time of the report of the abuse the girls and their caregivers also participated in research interviews for a study of the immediate consequences of sexual assault (McCahill, Meyer, & Fischman, 1979). The male victims seen at the hospital did not participate in the research in the 1970s.

In 1990 - 1994 the women and men were located and asked to participate in a follow-up study of adults who during childhood had received medical care at the identified hospital. The 47 men and 129 women who were interviewed are representative of the original sample of boys and girls seen at the hospital for sexual abuse. Informed consent following human subjects' guidelines was obtained. As was specified by the protocol, the men and women were not informed of their victimization histories. During a private face-to-face interview that averaged 3 hours in length, the men and women were asked questions about their childhood and adult life experiences. Their current social and psychological functioning was assessed using a variety of measures. To assess their recall of child sexual abuse a series of fourteen separate, detailed screening questions about sexual experiences in childhood and other unwanted sexual contact were asked following the approach of Russell (1986). The interviewers were blind to the circumstances of the sexual abuse reported in the 1970s and, in the case of the interviews with the men, the interviewers (two White women and one African-American woman) were blind to the men's membership in the victim or comparison group of males (i.e., whether the man had been seen at the hospital in the 1970s for child sexual abuse or for strictly other reasons.) Table 1 shows the demographics and the characteristics of the index child sexual abuse for the females and males interviewed in the 1990s.

The interview data were recorded and coded. Two raters reviewed each interview and the data from the archived files to assess whether the men and women had recalled the index abuse (the abuse reported in the 1970s). Taking an approach that would result in a conservative estimate of the proportion who did not recall the abuse, the raters used information in the case records from the 1970s to decide if the abuse (if any) that was recalled in the 1990s even remotely resembled the previously documented index abuse. (See Williams, 1994, for additional details on the methodology used for assessing recall of the index abuse.)

For purposes of our examination of gender and memory, data analysis proceeded in several steps. The first was to examine whether there were differences between men and women in recall of the sexual abuse documented in the 1970s. The second was to examine whether gender and/ or differences in the characteristics of the abuse experience were associated with current recall status.

3. RESULTS

Upon interview in the 1990s, 38% of the 129 women (Williams, 1994) and 55% of the 47 men did not appear to recall the sexual abuse documented in their hospital records. Statistical analyses reveal that this difference is statistically significant ($F(1, 174)=4.23$, $p<.05$) with the men less likely than the women to recall the sexual abuse they experienced in childhood. Although many men did not report the index abuse, most of the men showed no reluctance to talk about other sexual victimization in childhood. Half of the men who did not recall the index abuse told our interviewers about other, clearly different child sexual abuse experiences. In the total sample of male victims 28% recalled no history of sexual victimization in childhood. Among the women we have previously reported that 12% recalled no sexual abuse from childhood (Williams, 1994).

Analyses were conducted to determine if differences in the sexual abuse experiences of the boys and girls were responsible for the observed differences in recall status for the

Table 1. Characteristics of female and male samples

Variable	Female	Male
Demographics		
Current age	M=26 (3.37)	M=27 (3.36)
African-American	86%	89%
High school graduate	36%	55%
Currently employed	16%	36%
Currently married	34%	19%
Abuse characteristics		
Age at time of abuse	M=8.25 (3.37)	M=7.53 (3.12)
Penetration	69%	98%
Genital trauma	29%	53%
Family member perpetrator	36%	12%

men and women, and to explore the direct contribution of these abuse characteristics to abuse memory status. Previous analyses of the characteristics of abuse associated with forgetting in the sample of women (Williams, 1994) revealed that young age at time of abuse was a predictor of forgetting. Figure 1 shows the proportion of male and female survivors in each of two age groups (0–6 years old and 7–13 years old at the time of abuse) with no recall of abuse. Analyses of variance indicate main effects for age and an effect for gender that approaches significance, but no significant interaction between to two. This suggests that age does not operate differently for men and women. For both samples, younger age at time of abuse was related to higher rates of no recall.

Other abuse characteristics were then examined. Williams' (1994) previous analyses based on the sample of 129 women revealed that, in multivariate analyses, younger age at time of abuse and close relationship to the perpetrator both contributed to a decreased likelihood that the index abuse would be recalled. The present analyses examined the role of these variables in the combined sample of men and women. However, the analyses with male subjects involve some different variables and are, therefore, not directly comparable to reported results with the sample of women (Williams 1994). Because the boys had not been interviewed by researchers immediately following the abuse, information on the characteristics of their index abuse was based only on the data contained in the medical records from the hospital where they were seen in the 1970s. The data on the boys, therefore, is less complete and is not based on multiple measures from two or more sources as is the information on the girls' index abuse. Furthermore, there is no consistently recorded information from the boys records on the degree of force used in the assault. Thus, we examined the contribution of age at time of the abuse, genital trauma, family perpetrator and gender to abuse memory status (recall) at time of interview in the 1990s.

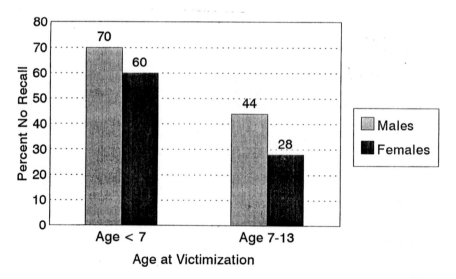

N=176; Main Effects:
Gender F=3.14, p=.078   Age F=16.17, p<.001
2-way Interaction: Gender & Age F=0.149, p=.70

Figure 1. Age at time of victimization and proportion with no recall of index abuse: Comparison of males and females.

Table 2 presents the results of the logistic regression of gender and abuse characteristics on recall. When all these variables (gender, age at time of abuse, genital trauma and family perpetrator) are entered, only age at the time of abuse makes a significant contribution to recall of the index abuse.

4. DISCUSSION

This brief report has provided an examination of the combined results of a prospective study of male and female survivors of child sexual abuse with regard to rates of recall of a documented experience of child sexual abuse. Contrary to prior research (Briere & Conte, 1993; Elliott & Briere, 1995) the present study, using bivariate analyses, did find gender differences in rates of no recall for child sexual abuse. The gender differences, however, did not remain significant in multivariate analyses in which age at the time of abuse emerged as an important explanatory variable. The boy victims were somewhat younger than the girls at the time of victimization. And, when taken as a proportion of the entire sample, there were more very young victims in the male sample. Once these age variations were taken into account the associations between gender and recall disappeared. As has been suggested by research on early autobiographical memory and "infantile amnesia," it is not surprising that survivors who were very young at the time of the abuse were also likely to have no recall of the incident in adulthood.

A number of interesting findings emerge from this study. The first is the fact that for both women and men there were survivors who were as old as 12 or 13 at the time of abuse who did not appear to recall this abuse upon reinterview in adulthood. Such findings raise a number of important questions. The first is whether these individuals represent true cases of forgetting or whether the study participants who did not report the index abuse were simply reluctant to disclose their experiences to an interviewer. Williams (1994) found that most of the women told interviewers about other personal information such as other experiences with child sexual abuse, substance abuse, and details of their sexual functioning. Preliminary analyses with the male sample have revealed a similar pattern, with those who did not report the index sexual abuse just as likely as those who did not recall the abuse to reveal other personal information about themselves during the interview. Of course, it is impossible to know the extent to which failure to report the abuse is attributable to a desire to keep the abuse private due, for example, to embarrassment or shame, or to actual forgetting of the abuse. Furthermore, the exact mechanism for any forgetting (e.g., infantile amnesia, simple forgetting due to lack of salience, problems with encoding or retrieval of the memory, dissociation, or repression) is unknown and undoubtedly varies across the sample (see Williams & Banyard, in press).

There are some limitations to the current study. The first is that we had to rely only on official hospital reports for details of the boys' index sexual abuse experiences. There-

Table 2. Logistic regression of gender and abuse characteristics on recall

Variable	B	SEB	p
Age at time of abuse	.17	.05	.001
Genital trauma	-.32	.37	N.S.
Family perpetrator	-.01	.39	N.S.
Gender	-.34	.49	N.S.

fore, the descriptions of the abuse characteristics for the male sample is much more limited than for the female sample (for further discussion of the impact of different measures of abuse characteristics on findings with this sample see Banyard & Williams, 1996). It may be that a lack of association between recall status and such variables as genital trauma, penetration, and closeness of the relationship to the perpetrator has to do with limits on the validity of the data used to create these variables. Furthermore, there was less variation in the types of abuse experienced by the men [e.g., nearly all of the men (98%) experienced child sexual assault involving penetration—either oral or anal sexual intercourse], thus hampering analyses of the contribution of this variable to recall status. Future research with larger and more diverse samples of survivors may be able to examine these questions more conclusively.

Future studies of memory for child sexual abuse should continue to examine gender as a variable. Research and clinical work with male survivors of child sexual abuse has revealed that males and females differ in the types of sexual abuse they are likely to experience (Finkelhor, 1993) and also in the responses they receive from their families and from society. Less attention has been focused on male survivors, perhaps contributing to greater silencing of their experiences. Men may find sexual assault by a male to be even more shameful and stigmatizing than women, perhaps making it less likely that they will readily disclose their experiences to interviewers. These factors are likely to affect willingness to report child sexual abuse (Widom & Morris, 1996) and may also affect memory of abuse. The findings from the multivariate analyses reported here suggest, however, that there are no gender differences in rates of forgetting child sexual abuse. In our interviews in which sufficient rapport was established with the men and women survivors and in which 14 detailed, behaviorally specific questions were asked about sexual experiences in childhood, we found no gender differences in rates of reporting of sexual abuse documented in childhood. It may be that in this study we were able to break through many of the barriers that can prevent men from reporting abuse experiences. This may be one reason why, contrary to Widom and Morris (1996)[†] but consistent with studies based on clinical samples, we found no difference in the rate of recall of child sexual abuse by males and females when controlling for age at time of abuse.

These findings do offer further support to those concerned that large, community-based retrospective studies of child sexual abuse may misclassify as non-abused a significant number of adults who were, indeed, abused in childhood. For the combined sample (n=176) of women and men who were victimized in childhood, one-sixth (16%) recall no child sexual abuse upon reinterview in adulthood. This poses a significant problem to be overcome in conducting retrospective studies (Banyard & Williams, 1996). In this sample, over one-half of men sexually abused in childhood did not recall the abuse documented in their hospital records. Although many of these did disclose to the interviewer the details of some other child sexual abuse experience, a full 28% of the sample with documented histories of child sexual abuse denied any history of sexual victimization in childhood. These findings suggest that abuse committed against younger boys, particularly abuse of boys younger than age 7, may be likely to go undetected in retrospective studies in which adults are asked about victimization histories. These findings have implications for estimation of the incidence and prevalence of child sexual abuse, as well as for studies of its consequences.

---

† Widom and Morris (1996) conducted a similar prospective study but with a smaller sample of male victims of sexual abuse (n=19) who were asked fewer questions about sexual abuse experiences. Widom and Morris also did not match the abuse reported to the index sexual abuse. This means that some of those who reported that they had been abused were referring to different sexual abuse experiences and may not have recalled the index abuse.

In summary, the high rates of no recall of child sexual abuse found in this study of male survivors suggest that memory problems related to child sexual abuse are not limited to female survivors. This is an important area for future inquiry.

REFERENCES

Banyard, V.L., & Williams, L.M. (1996). Characteristics of child sexual abuse as correlates of women's adjustment: A prospective study. *Journal of Marriage and the Family*,*58*, 853–865.

Briere, J., & Conte, J. (1993). Self-reported amnesia for abuse in adults molested as children. *Journal of Traumatic Stress, 6*, (1), 21–31.

Elliott, D.M., & Briere, J. (1995). Posttraumatic stress associated with delayed recall of sexual abuse: A general population study. *Journal of Traumatic Stress, 8* (4), 629–648.

Finkelhor, D. (1993). Answers to important questions about the scope and nature of child sexual abuse. *The future of children*. Los Altos: CA: David and Lucille Packard Foundation.

Herman, J.L., & Schatzow, E. (1987). Recovery and verification of memories of childhood sexual trauma. *Psychoanalytic Psychology*, *4*(1), 1–14.

McCahill, T., Meyer, L.C., & Fischman, A. (1979). *The aftermath of rape*. Lexington, MA: Lexington Books.

Russell, D.E.H. (1986). *The secret trauma: Incest in the lives of girls and women*. New York: Basic Books.

Widom, C.S., & Morris, S. (1996). *Accuracy of adult recollections of childhood victimization*. Unpublished paper: University at Albany.

Williams, L.M. (1994). Recall of childhood trauma: A prospective study of women's memories of child sexual abuse. *Journal of Consulting and Clinical Psychology*, *62*(6), 1167–1176.

Williams, L.M. (1995). Recovered memories of abuse in women with documented child sexual victimization histories. *Journal of Traumatic Stress*, *8*(4), 649–673.

Williams, L.M. & Banyard, V.L. (in press). Perspectives on adult memories of childhood sexual abuse: A research review. *American Psychiatric Press Review of Psychiatry*. Washington, D.C. : American Psychiatric Press.

15

A COGNITIVE CORROBORATIVE CASE STUDY APPROACH FOR INVESTIGATING DISCOVERED MEMORIES OF SEXUAL ABUSE

Jonathan W. Schooler,[1] Zara Ambadar,[1] and Miriam Bendiksen[2]

[1]University of Pittsburgh
635 LRDC
Pittsburgh, Pennsylvania 15260
[2]Bendiksen and Bendiksen
Virikveien 17
3212 Sandefjord
Norway

1. INTRODUCTION

In recent years, memory researchers have convincingly illustrated the dangerous role that suggestion may play in inducing fabricated memories of childhood trauma. Although post-event suggestion had long been known to alter the recollection of details of events (e.g., Loftus, Miller, & Burns, 1978; Schooler, Gerhard, & Loftus, 1986), recent research has demonstrated that experimenter suggestions can cause the vivid recollection of events that never occurred (Ceci, Loftus, Leichtman, & Bruck, 1994; Hyman, 1995; Loftus & Ketcham, 1994). Suggestions can even cause individuals to falsely recall being repeatedly exposed to negative situations that are unlikely to have ever happened (see Lindsay, this volume). The documented power of suggestion to induce memories of experiences that never occurred is especially alarming in light of the suggestive techniques that a minority of therapists are known to use with their clients in pursuit of forgotten memories of abuse (e.g., Polusny & Follette, 1996; Poole, Lindsay, Memon, & Bull, 1995; Yapko, 1994). If individuals can be induced to recall false memories under the modest persuasive pressures used in the laboratory, one can only imagine the dangers of therapy settings in which potentially unwarranted suggestions of abuse are made: 1) by a trusted authoritative figure; 2) over potentially years of sessions, and; 3) with a patient who may be particularly suggestible either due to hypnosis (cf. Lynn, this volume) or as a natural consequence of their dissociative tendencies (cf. Hyman & Billings, 1995) which are commonly associated with patients "diagnosed" as likely victims of abuse.

The alarming dangers of suggestion-induced memories of trauma have caused many memory researchers to sound the alarm, alerting the field and, in particular, clinicians of the potential risks of certain therapeutic practices (e.g., Ceci, Loftus, Leichtman, & Bruck, 1994; Lindsay & Read, 1994, 1995; Loftus, 1993). Such warnings are gravely needed, and indeed, of such priority that it is understandable that memory researchers have focused their efforts on further illuminating the risks of suggestion. Nevertheless, we believe that the time has come for basic memory researchers to also begin to investigate the other side of the issue; namely, how individuals may sometimes discover memories corresponding to actual trauma. As we have noted in the past (Schooler, 1994; Schooler, Bendiksen, & Ambadar, in press), such an endeavor will necessarily require the adoption of methodologies and sources of data that lack the rigor we have grown accustomed to in the laboratory. However, although perfectly suited for certain memory questions, the laboratory also has its costs, sacrificing ecological validity for control (cf. Neisser, 1978). Recollections of seemingly forgotten memories of sexual abuse are, for a host of pragmatic, ethical, and possibly scientific reasons, unlikely to ever be fully reproducible in the laboratory. As a result, examination of these types of memories requires that we investigate actual cases in which recollections of allegedly forgotten trauma have been reported. This chapter reviews our recent efforts to examine such cases. Our approach draws on cognitive principles and uses as much methodological rigor as possible, but, it ultimately relies on the imperfect sources of data that cases afford.

1.1. Discovered Memories

Before discussing our cases, it is important to clearly define the phenomenon under investigation. Our goal has been to characterize and corroborate recollective experiences in which individuals discover memories of seemingly forgotten abuse. Much confusion has arisen over the name for this alleged phenomenon. Such recollections have been characterized as recovered (e.g., Pezdek & Banks, 1996), repressed (e.g., Loftus, 1993), delayed (e.g., Harvey & Herman, 1994), exhumed (e.g., Kihlstrom, 1996), and re-instated (Shimamura, this volume). However, in our opinion none of these terms are entirely adequate. The term repressed implies a highly questionable set of mechanisms by which the memories were forgotten and later remembered. The terms recovered, delayed, and re-instated all imply that the memories were lost and then found, a claim which is problematic if the actual authenticity of the experience and the extent of forgetting is unknown. Exhumed, besides possessing an inherently negative connotation, presumes that the memories were retrieved through some extensive digging rather then spontaneously, as is often reported. Although we recognize that any new name will undoubtedly also be vulnerable to criticism, we nevertheless suggest that the term "discovered memories" (and variants such as "memory discoveries" and "discovered memory experiences") may have real merit. First and foremost, the term discovery focuses us on what we believe to be the defining characteristic of these experiences, namely that *the individual has the strong sense of discovering something important in their memory that was not appreciated before.* Second, it does not imply any specific mechanism of forgetting or conditions of recollection. Finally, it encourages patients, clinicians, and indeed the field as a whole to treat such recollections with both the gravity and caution appropriate to all major discovery claims. A memory discovery may be as accurate as that of the double helix or as groundless as the discovery of cold fusion. It may also may be, like Columbus' discovery of America, very significant but not at all what it first seemed to be—Columbus, after all, thought he had found India!

1.2. Authenticating the Components of Discovered Memories

In investigating the reality of discovered memories three distinct issues arise, each deserving of separate consideration. First there is the *reality of the event*, that is, whether the discovery corresponds, in at least a general sense, to an actual event or set of events. Second, there is *the reality of the forgetting*, that is whether the individual was in fact unaware of the existence of the memory prior to its discovery. Third, there is *the reality of the discovery experience*, that is, whether the individual actually had an experience of discovering memories of which they believe they were previously unaware. In short, memory discovery experiences should not be considered as black and white cases, either factual or false. Rather, each component of each case must be assessed on its own merit.

2. A CORROBORATIVE INVESTIGATION OF FOUR CASES

In the last few years, we became acquainted with several cases of discovered memories of sexual abuse for which corroborative evidence was available. Our approach to assessing these cases has been relatively straightforward. We first queried the individuals regarding: 1) the discovery experience; 2) their perceptions regarding the prior extant of forgetting; 3) the existence of any sources of corroboration for the event, and; 4) the existence of any sources of corroboration of the forgetting. Following our interviews, we attempted to contact other individuals who could corroborate the event and/or the extent of prior forgetting. These cases are described in greater detail in Schooler, Bendiksen, and Ambadar (in press). In the following discussion we briefly review the characteristics and corroboration of the cases (see Schooler, Bendiksen, & Ambadar, in press, for a more detailed description).

Case 1. The first case was brought to our attention by a colleague of the first author. It involved JR, a 39-year-old male who, at the age of 30 remembered being fondled by a parish priest when he was 12 years old. Subsequent to this initial recollection, JR recalled additional episodes of abuse spanning several years.

Case 2. The second case came to the attention of the second author (a practicing clinician) as a result of a referral from a patient. It involved WB, a 40-year-old female, who at the age of 37 recalled being raped while hitchhiking at age 16.

Case 3. The third case was brought to our attention through a colleague of the first author. It involved TW, a 51-year-old woman, who at the age of 34 recalled being fondled by a family friend while on vacation in Jamaica at age 9.

Case 4. The fourth case involved DN, who brought her case to the attention of the first author following a colloquium presentation that he gave on this topic. DN was a 41-year-old female, who at the age of 35 recalled having been raped and successfully convicting her attacker at age 22.

2.1. Characterization of the Memory Discovery Experiences

Two striking features emerge when we compare the memory discovery experience in each of these four cases. First, in each case the memory "trigger" had some significant correspondence to the original experience. Second, in each case the discovery was accompanied by marked shock and surprise.

Case 1. JR's experience of discovering a memory of having been abused by a priest occurred after he watched a movie in which the main character grapples with sexual abuse. He reported great shock at the discovery of the memory which occurred "fairly suddenly" with great vividness. As JR described it "I was stunned, I was somewhat confused you know, the memory was very vivid and yet... I didn't know one word about repressed memory."

Case 2. WB's experience of discovering a memory of being raped while hitchhiking occurred the morning after a male friend made an off-hand remark about the virginity of a young woman (WB had been a virgin when she was raped). She also reported great shock at the recollection of this memory noting "complete chaos in my emotions." As she put it "I awoke the next morning with a sudden and clear picture: "My God... I had been raped!! I was 16, just a kid! I couldn't defend myself."

Case 3. TW's experience of discovering a memory of being molested at age 9 occurred after she was invited to see a talk on sex abuse. TW characterized her reaction to the discovery experience as follows, "When I first remembered it, I was surprised. Completely taken back by it. Then I.. I don't even remember speaking... I was completely out of it."

Case 4. DN's experience of discovering a memory of being raped and going to court occurred while driving home thinking about her group therapist's remark that survivors of childhood sex abuse are often also abused as adults (DN had always been aware of her childhood abuse). As with the others, DN was completely taken aback by the memory. As she recounted it: "I had to just sit there for a while because it was just this extreme emotion of fear and total disbelief. Disbelief that it happened, disbelief that I could have forgotten something that traumatic."

2.2. Characterization of the Prior Forgetting

In each case, the individuals were asked several questions regarding their beliefs about their knowledge of the trauma prior to their memory discovery experiences. Three of the four individuals were quite confident that they would not have recalled the experiences even if they had been asked about them directly. However, one individual (WB) was less confident on this question.

Case 1. JR was completely unambiguous in his account of his perceived awareness of the memory prior to discovery, observing

"If you had done a survey of people walking into the movie theater when I saw the movie...asking people about child and sexual abuse "have you ever been, or do you know anybody who has ever been", I would have absolutely, flatly, unhesitatingly, said no!"

Case 2. In response to the question of whether she would have denied the experience even if asked about it directly, WB was a bit more uncertain, noting

"I actually think this is the case. When I wrote my story about rape [WB is a novelist] I can honestly say I had absolutely no connection to the fact that it had been a personal experience. I was writing it "on behalf of others," I thought this is what it must be like for those who experienced rape. I am really uncertain how I would have responded if someone had asked me directly."

Case 3. As with JR, TW also believed that she had no knowledge whatsoever about the existence of the memory prior to its discovery. As she put it, "the state of my memory in that period was none.. non-existent."

Case 4. DN also characterized herself as being completely unaware of the existence of the memory prior to her memory discovery experience, stating

"It's like how could I forget this. As horrible as it was having to go to court ...and having to tell what happened and everything, how could I forget that? I had no idea when I did forget it but I really feel that it had been totally forgotten until that night."

2.3. Corroboration of the Abuse

In each case, efforts were made to identify independent corroborative evidence supporting the individuals' claims regarding their abuse. Although in no case was it possible to find absolutely incontrovertible evidence that documented the precise details of the abuse (e.g., pornographic photos) in each case we were able to find at least reasonably compelling independent sources of support that some type of abuse did occur.

Case 1. In addition to JR's report that he confronted the priest who admitted the abuse, we also independently acquired corroborative evidence in the form of an interview with another individual. This individual reported that he had also been the victim of sexual advances by the priest (a memory which he reported he had never forgotten).

Case 2. We interviewed WB's ex-husband who had talked with WB the day after the alleged rape occurred. He indicated that she initially reported having had a "bad experience" in which she had sex "involuntarily" but had not protested and that a few days later she had described it as "something like rape".

Case 3. As with WB, TW also discussed her experience with her former husband prior to her memory discovery experience. In an separate interview, TW's husband reported that she had mentioned the abuse incident several times over the course of their marriage (which ended prior to the discovery).

Case 4. Because DN's case was actually taken to trial, corroboration was relatively straightforward. In a telephone interview, her lawyer at the time (who is now a judge) verified that the case did in fact go to court, and that the accused was found guilty of rape.

2.4. Corroboration of the Forgetting

All aspects of discovered memories are inherently difficult to substantiate, but, the actual extent of prior forgetting is perhaps the most difficult of all. Indeed, even scientifically speaking it is not always entirely clear what is meant by the construct of complete forgetting. Does it mean not recalled for an extended period of time, or not recalled even under conditions that might be expected to cue it (whatever those might be), or actually lost from memory, that is, unavailable under any circumstances? As Tulving and Pearlstone (1966) noted years ago, a memory can be available (i.e., in principle retrievable given the appropriate cuing conditions) even if it is not currently accessed (i.e., recalled under the present cuing conditions). These subtleties illustrate that the notion of complete forgetting is a hypothetical construct which is really quite difficult to define and even more difficult to demonstrate. Nevertheless, in two of our cases we do have suggestive evidence that the memories of the experiences may have been less accessible at certain points in their lives. For example, a former therapist of JR's indicated that JR had discussed many other embarrassing experiences but had never mentioned being abused by a priest (note the issue of sexual abuse was never mentioned during therapy). Similarly, when DN entered therapy for victims of sexual abuse, she was given an initial interview to assess her history of abuse. During this interview (as revealed in hospital records made available to the first author), DN described, in detail, her abuse as a child, but did not mention her rape experience.

Although some degree of forgetting is suggested in two of our cases in two other cases, we have rather compelling evidence suggesting that the prior forgetting was not as great as our cases believed. Both WB and TW discussed their abuse experiences with their husbands during a time in which they believed that they had forgotten about the events. They both reported being shocked to learn that they had talked about their abuse experiences with their ex-husbands. In recounting her reaction to learning that she had told her ex-husband about it, DN said she "felt like falling over. Absolutely shocked and floored that it [telling her husband] happened. And I still am. .. I can't remember telling him, I can't think of anything about the memory before [the discovery], and it's very disturbing, actually."

3. WHAT CAN WE EXTRACT FROM THESE CASES?

As we have noted in the past (Schooler et al., in press), the precise conclusions that one draws from the above cases is likely to be influenced by one's a priori beliefs about the phenomenon. If one believes that discovered memories might, at least sometimes, correspond to actual events, then the above cases may seem quite compelling. Alternatively, if one is skeptical that memory discovery experiences ever correspond to actual traumas, then there are certainly ways of dismissing the above cases. We respect the differences in opinion that such a priori beliefs will, and indeed, should cause. We note, however, that a priori beliefs might also lead to skepticism regarding the applicability of laboratory research to this issue. If one is highly doubtful that memories of abuse could be suggested, they might reasonably question the generalizability of suggested memory experiments which, for obvious reasons of ethicality, cannot involve experiences as severe as those mentioned here. We, as noted at the outset, are deeply committed to the view that experimental evidence does have important implications for this issue. Our point is simply that applying laboratory findings to discovered memories of trauma also requires a step between data and conclusion. Although this step is of a different nature (and perhaps magnitude) then that involved in the case studies reported here, it nevertheless illustrates that inferences can be warranted even with imperfect mappings between data and conclusions. In this context, we suggest that the above cases provide reasonably compelling evidence that discovered memories of sexual abuse may sometimes correspond to actual events. In addition, they may offer some useful clues into the nature of discovered memories, in particular: the conditions under which they occur, their phenomenological quality, and the manner in which they may distort estimations of prior forgetting. We briefly review these three issues.

3.1. The Conditions of Recollection

One notable characteristic of the above cases is the cues that elicited the discovered memories all had some significant correspondence to the original experience: a movie about sexual abuse, an off-hand remark about the virginity of a young woman, the prospect of seeing a talk on sexual abuse, and the observation that survivors of childhood abuse are often abused as adults. This correspondence between retrieval conditions and the original experience suggests the possible involvement of the *encoding specificity principle* (Tulving & Thompson, 1973) which suggests that the probability of retrieval is maximized when the retrieval conditions correspond to encoding conditions. Accordingly, memory discovery experiences may be most likely to be prompted by cues that have some correspondence to the original trauma.

3.2. The Phenomenology of the Discovery Experience

A second striking quality of the above cases is the sudden unpacking and affective on-rush associated with the discovery experience. As WB put it "like a flood, the locks were opened." TW characterized this experience as "like a.. a package of some sort... something there that's completely unwound instantly." In this context, the term memory discovery seems particularly applicable because it highlights the parallels between discovering memories of trauma and other types of cognitive discoveries. A well known correlate of cognitive discoveries in the context of problem solving is the "aha" or insight experience in which individuals have a sudden realization followed by an emotional on-rush (Gick & Lockhart, 1995; Schooler, Fallshore, & Fiore, 1995). Although the affective valence of discovering a traumatic memory is obviously quite different from that of discovering a solution to a problem, there still may be important parallels between the surprise and affective on-rush of problem solving and memory discoveries. If so, then the insight processes associated with problem solving discoveries (cf. Sternberg & Davidson, 1995) might have some important relevance to discovered memories.

3.3. Misconstruing Prior Forgetting

A third noteworthy quality of at least two of the cases described here is that they suggest one can forget about a period in which a memory had been remembered. Both WB and TW appeared to be astounded to discover that they had told their husbands about the incidents at a time in which they thought the memory had been forgotten. Such underestimation of prior knowledge has not been well documented before, however the overestimation of prior knowledge certainly has. Research on hindsight biases such as the "knew-it-all-along effect" (e.g., Fischoff, 1982) has demonstrated that receiving new information on a topic influences individuals' assessments of their prior knowledge such that they overestimate what they previously knew. It seems quite possible that a process analogous to the knew-it-all-along effect, which we have termed the "*forgot-it-all-along-effect*" (Schooler et al., in press), may occur in the context of some memory discovery experiences. Accordingly, if individuals assess their prior degree of forgetting on the basis of their current state, then the emotional agitation at the time of retrieval may cause them to underestimate their prior knowledge about the event in question. They may reason on the basis of their implicit theories regarding the consistency of psychological attributes (cf. Ross, 1989) "If I am this shocked and surprised now, then I must have previously completely forgotten about the experience." While the memory might be perceived to have been recalled for the first time in years, in reality it may have been recalled previously but without as much emotional punch, perhaps with a less negative interpretation. Indeed, both WB and TW's husbands reported that their wives earlier discussions of their experiences had been "emotionally flat". Of course, it is not clear that this forgot-it-all-along effect is involved in all memory discovery cases, and indeed, it does not seem to fit well with some of the cases described here. However, it does seem at least partially applicable to two of our cases in which the abuse was found to have been remembered at a time in which it was believed to have been forgotten.

4. SUMMARY

Although fraught with challenges, the cognitive corroborative case study approach to investigating discovered memories of abuse has proven to be a useful endeavor. Through such investigations we have found further evidence that memory discovery experiences can correspond to actual incidents of abuse. We have also been able to identify several characteristics of the cases that hint at possible mechanisms. The striking matches between the abuse experiences and the retrieval conditions indicates a possible role of encoding specificity. The "aha" like quality of the memory discovery experience suggests the possible involvement of insight like processes. And the misconstrual of prior forgetting suggests a new type of hindsight bias, termed the "forgot-it-all-along effect," whereby, in the context of emotional recollective experiences, individuals may underestimate their prior knowledge of the memory. We must emphasize that these cases should not be construed as countering the serious risks of suggestive therapy techniques, and more importantly, none of these cases occurred in the context of aggressive recovered memory therapy. Moreover these cases simply do not speak to the relative frequency with which discovered memories are apt to be authentic, fabricated, or some combination of the two. Despite these important limitations, at least one strong conclusion is warranted at this time: A corroborative case study approach, grounded in an understanding of basic cognitive mechanisms, is likely to provide an important tool for furthering our understanding of how individuals can have the shocking experience of discovering memories of seemingly unknown trauma.

REFERENCES

Ceci, S. J., Loftus, E. F., Leichtman, M. D., & Bruck, M. (1994). The possible role of source misattributions in the creation of false beliefs among preschoolers. *International Journal of Clinical and Experimental Hypnosis*, *42*, 304–320.

Fischoff, B. (1982). For those condemned to study the past: Heuristic and biases in hindsight. In D. Kahneman, P. Slovic, & A. Tversky (Eds.), *Judgment under uncertainty: Heuristic and biases* (pp. 335–351). New York: Cambridge Univ. Press.

Gick, M. L., & Lockhart, R. S. (1995). Cognitive and affective components of insight. In R.J. Sternberg, & J. E. Davidson (Eds.), *The nature of insight* (pp. 197–228). Cambridge, MA: The MIT Press.

Harvey, M. R., & Herman, J. L. (1994). Amnesia, partial amnesia and delayed recall among adult survivors of childhood trauma. *Consciousness and Cognition*, *3*, 295–306.

Hyman, I. E. (1995). False memories of childhood experiences. *Applied Cognitive Psychology*, *9(3)*, 181–197.

Hyman, I. E. & Billings, F. J. (1995). *Individual differences and the creation of false childhood memories*. Submitted for publication.

Kihlstorm, J. F. (1996). The trauma-memory argument and recovered memory therapy. In K. Pezdek, & W. P. Banks (Eds). *The recovered memory/false memory debate*, (pp. 297–311), San Diego, CA: Academic Press.

Lindsay, D. S., & Read, J. D. (1994). Psychotherapy and memories of child sexual abuse: A cognitive perspective. *Applied Cognitive Psychology, 8*, 281–338.

Lindsay, D. S., & Read, J. D. (1995). "Memory work" and recovered memories of childhood sexual abuse: Scientific evidence and public, professional, and personal issues. *Psychology, Public Policy, and Law, 1*, 4, 846–908.

Loftus, E. F. (1993). The reality of repressed memories. *American Psychologist, 48*, 518–537.

Loftus, E., & Ketcham, K. (1994). *The myth of repressed memory: False memories and allegations of sexual abuse*. New York, NY: St. Martin's Press.

Loftus, E. F., Miller, D. G., & Burns, H. J. (1978). Semantic integration of verbal information into visual memory. *Journal of Experimental Psychology: Human Learning and Memory, 4*, 19–31.

Neisser, U. (1978). Memory: What are the important questions? In M. M. Gruneberg, P. E. Morris, & R. N. Sykes (Eds), *Practical aspects of memory* (pp. 3–24). San Diego, CA: Academic Press.

Polusny, M. A., & Follette, V. M. (1996). Remembering childhood sexual abuse: A national survey of psychologists' clinical practices, beliefs, and personal experiences. *Professional Psychology: Research and Practice, 27*, 1, 41–52.

Pezdek, K., & Banks W. P. (1996). *The recovered memory/false memory debate*. (Eds). San Diego, CA: Academic Press.

Poole, D. A., Lindsay, D. S., Memon, A., & Bull, R. (1995). Psychotherapy and the recovery of memories of childhood sexual abuse: U.S. and British practitioners beliefs, practices, and experiences. *Journal of Consulting and Clinical Psychology, 63*, 426–437.

Ross, M. (1989). Relation of implicit theories to the construction of personal histories. *Psychological Review, 96(2)*, 341–357.

Schooler, J. (1994). Seeking the core: Issues and evidence surrounding recovered accounts of sexual trauma. *Consciousness and Cognition, 3*, 452–469.

Schooler, J., Bendiksen, M., & Ambadar, Z. (in press). Taking the middle line: Can we accommodate both fabricated memories and recovered memories of sexual abuse? In M. Conway (Ed). *Recovered Memories and False Memories* (pp. 401–456). Oxford, UK: Oxford University Press.

Schooler, J. W., Fallshore, M. F., & Fiore, S. M. (1995). Epilogue: Putting insight into perspective. In R. J. Sternberg, & J. E. Davidson (Eds.), *The nature of insight* (pp. 559–587). Cambridge, MA: The MIT Press.

Schooler, J. W., Gerhard, D., & Loftus, E. F. (1986). Qualities of the unreal. *Journal of Experimental Psychology: Learning, Memory, and Cognition, 12*, 71–181.

Sternberg, R. J., & Davidson, J. E. (Eds.). (1995). *The nature of insight*. Cambridge, MA: The MIT Press.

Tulving, E., & Pearlstone, Z. (1966). Availability versus accessibility of information in memory for words. *Journal of Verbal Learning and Verbal Behavior, 5*, 381–391.

Tulving, E., & Thompson, D. M. (1973). Encoding specificity and retrieval processes in episodic memory. *Psychological Review, 80*, 352–373.

Yapko, M. (1994). *Suggestions of abuse: Real and imagined memories*. New York: Simon & Schuster.

16

SEXUAL ABUSE MEMORIES

A Medical Perspective from New Zealand

Juliet Broadmore

24 Reading St.
Karori, Wellington 5
New Zealand

1. INTRODUCTION

In New Zealand the social and political climate has affected the application of scientific and clinical research findings on sexual abuse (SA) for medical practitioners as well as psychologists. Contributions from psychiatrists, paediatricians, and general practitioners have been important in the debate, and impacted on their clinical practice.

2. INFLUENCES ON CLINICAL PRACTICE

General practitioner (GP = Family Physician) clinical practice decisions are subject to a range of external influences (see figure 1). This paper addresses those influences with respect to SA. Personal life experiences around SA or memory problems, although important, are not addressed.

2.1. New Zealand Society

2.1.1. General. New Zealand's small size, geographic isolation, sparse population (3 million, 10% Polynesian), government as a parliamentary democracy, and economic performance affect the climate of clinical practice. A limited quantity of good quality scientific research is produced, and there is easy access to research reported internationally.

Stoicism and emotional reserve in the face of traumatic experiences are national characteristics. It is more acceptable to admit to seeing a doctor for physical conditions, rather than a psychiatrist, or a psychologist. Despite increasing political lobbying for women's rights, the prevalence of domestic violence and SA is comparable to other western nations.

Recollections of Trauma, edited by Read and Lindsay
Plenum Press, New York, 1997

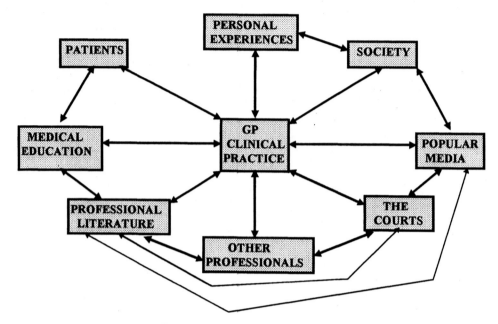

Figure 1. Influences on clinical practice.

2.1.2. Sexual Abuse in New Zealand. The prevalence of SA amongst women in NZ before age 16 years, determined retrospectively, is 19% to 31% depending on whether genital contact, or all types of abuse are included, with full intercourse being reported by 4% (Mullen et al, 1993). Rape or attempted rape of women over age 16 has a prevalence of 12 to 25% (Gavey, 1991; Martin et al, 1992). The Accident Rehabilitation and Compensation Insurance Corporation (ARCIC) has received 12,000 SA claims annually for the last 3 years. Twenty percent of claims are not accepted and males have lodged 20% of the total ARCIC claims (The Manager, ARCIC,* 1996).

2.2. Patients as Educators

In medical practice patient management is influenced by past experiences in treating patients with similar conditions. There have been no NZ surveys of doctors regarding their practice profiles for SA. They may see sexually abused patients:

- in their capacity as gatekeepers for access to services funded by ARCIC
- when they are called on by police to examine rape and SA complainants
- in their routine practice where patients present a variety of disorders, some of which may be correlated to SA (Neumann, 1994; Moeller, Bachmann & Moeller, 1993; Hendricks-Matthews, 1993).

---

* ARCIC was established by statute to provide comprehensive, universal, government funded no fault cover for treatment costs and compensation in all cases of personal injury by accident (PIBA), including cases from criminal injuries. In exchange, victims of PIBA lost the right to sue for damages. The rehabilitation treatment of many SA complainants is thus coordinated through one national organisation other than the police. Research audit projects on this data are being established this year.

Other patients (alleged offenders, or family members affected by an allegation of SA) may also influence GP's clinical practice. The social matrix in which SA occurs, and the community based nature of general practice mean that GPs are more likely to know both "perpetrator" and "victim" and be exposed to conflicts of interest and ambivalence when patients allege SA.

GP's exposure to patient "education" on memories of SA (true and false) is affected by patient recall and communication. An unknown number of patients may falsely believe they have been abused and some will tell their doctor about this "SA". Other patients (38% of SA women in Williams, 1994) may have been abused but not recall the SA. About 20% of the SA women may have long-term psychiatric sequelae that could prompt a GP to enquire about abuse (Mullen et al, 1993). However only 5 - 9% abused women tell their doctor about the abuse (Moeller et al., 1993; Shew & Hurst, 1993).

2.3. Other Professionals

Referrals and case discussions with other professionals affect GP's clinical practice. Information about SA abuse and memories from psychologists and psychiatrists is as varied in New Zealand as overseas (see poster presentation McDougall, this volume).

2.4. Influence of the New Zealand Courts on General Practitioners

In NZ's legal system the accused is deemed innocent until proven guilty. The onus is on the prosecution to produce evidence of guilt beyond reasonable doubt. Standard defence tactics include raising issues of marginal or no relevance to uncover and exploit whatever doubt may exist. If the jury is encouraged to doubt, or left in confusion about matters of fact (e.g., dates, location) or matters of science - fingerprints, DNA testing or memories - it is more likely to acquit. Legal writers on trial advocacy describe this sort of tactic as "increasing the improbabilities" (Ennor, 1989).

When the time between an event and the witnesses evidence in court is substantial, strategies include discrediting the witnesses' perceptions and memory (Ennor, 1989). The absence of memories, or failure to tell others about memories in the intervening years, or poor memory for peripheral information can be used to suggest the witness is unreliable (Henderson, 1996). In the author's opinion this may explain the introduction of "recovered memory" arguments by the defence in some cases when the complainant claims no memory gap, but only delayed disclosure (see 2.4.2.4.).

The courts may influence GPs through their involvement in a particular case, or through cases reported in the media. Acquittal can either be represented as proof that the allegation was false, or leave continuing suspicion of guilt not capable of proof beyond reasonable doubt.

2.4.1. Categories of SA and Memory Cases That Highlight Particular Issues.

2.4.1.1. Child SA Cases. These cases focus attention on the reliability of children's memories (Henderson, 1996). Two NZ preschool childcare centre cases which resulted in convictions continue to receive publicity on this issue (*R v E,* 1993; *R v S,* 1995).

2.4.1.2. Delayed Disclosure Cases. These cases focus on witness credibility because of delayed prosecution.

2.4.1.3. Recovered Memories Cases. There have been few cases where both defence and prosecution have agreed that the complaint arose after the recovery of memory, and no convictions *(R v R,*1994; *R v A* ,1994; *R v G,*1996). They debate "memory repression", and present expert testimony on memory malleability in relation only to complainants.

2.4.1.4. Other "Recovered Memories" Cases. In a few cases since 1994 the defence argued "false recovered memories", while the prosecution claimed the complainants had merely delayed disclosure of events that had never been forgotten *(R v B,* 1994; *R v D,* 1994; *R v D,* 1995). The defence arguments blur the distinctions between ordinary delayed disclosure, and delayed disclosure because of delayed understanding that certain sexual experiences were abusive, and delayed disclosure because of delayed recall (i.e. recovered memories). Media reporting of such cases as "recovered memories" may exaggerate the apparent number of these cases.

2.5. Recovered Memories and False Allegations in the Popular Media

A NZ study on popular media reporting of sexual abuse memories has not yet been done. The media may not accurately reflect the consensus of professional opinion (Galtung & Mari Ruge, 1973; Donaldson & O'Brien, 1995). It is uncomfortable with ambiguity, thus cautious professional non-adversarial answers that do not fit into entertaining "sound bites" may be overlooked. It also promotes the rare and unusual, making this more visible and therefore seem more common in the public eye. Trials of men of influence (charismatic leaders of alternative communities or religious sects, doctors, school teachers etc.) and acts of extreme violence attract attention. The media may represent or distort the real ratio of violent stranger abuse to non-violent coercive SA, or of false memories to corroborated memories of SA.

Doctors may be no less influenced by the public media than patients, particularly where commentary on a topic is provided by a colleague. The first NZ popular book on SA allegations was written by a GP (Goodyear-Smith, 1993). It is controversial (cf. Tyrell, 1994; Freckleton, 1994; Broadmore, 1995; Belton, 1995; Kljakovic, 1995), but the public media has not analysed this professional controversy. Therefore, GPs who are primarily exposed to information on memories of SA in the public media may be unaware of the debate.

2.6. Medical Education and Continuing Medical Education (CME)

Professional education minimises the bias of influences other than evidence-based scientific and clinical research. Medical school undergraduate programs have included information on SA in the last 5–10 years. SA memory dilemmas have been included in the last 2–3 years. Older graduates are professionally informed about these topics through medical journals or attending (CME) seminars.

Doctors for SA Care (DSAC) is a national voluntary organisation of 220 doctors formed in 1988 to improve the standard of medical care available to those affected by SA. DSAC training seminars on the medical management of SA have been attended by 350 regarding forensic examinations of adults, and 260 regarding child SA. A few (2 to 6 per seminar) doctors have attended DSAC sponsored seminars on therapy presented by international experts Lucy Berliner, Toni Cavanagh-Johnson, Jonathan Ross, John Briere, Roland Summit, Jon Conte, Judith Herman, and Mary Koss.

CME seminars on SA, not arranged by DSAC, include locally organised presentations, and national tours such as by Dr. Karen Zelas in 1986, and Dr. Carol Herbert (Canada) in 1994. Dr. Felicity Goodyear Smith, on a Glaxo Postgraduate Medical Fellowship, attended the 1994 False Memory Syndrome Foundation Johns Hopkins conference and gave CME seminars throughout New Zealand on false memories in 1995.

2.7. Medical Literature

Articles in international or local (*New Zealand Medical Journal* (*NZMJ*)) academic journals are read by few GPs. Local pharmaceutical company journals (e.g. *Patient Management*) are more widely read (Barham & Benseman 1984).

Recovered memories and false memories were first mentioned in NZ journals in 1994 when *New Zealand Family Physician* (*NZ Fam Phys*) included brief reviews of articles in *Issues in Child Abuse Accusations* that discussed false recovered memories. This was followed in 1995 by letters in the *NZMJ* (Goodyear-Smith, 1995; Broadmore, 1995; Goodyear-Smith, 1995) and commentaries in *NZ Fam Phys* (Broadmore, 1995; West, 1995). In 1996 *Patient Management* published 3 articles (Goodyear-Smith, 1996 Parts 1 & 2; Gellatly et al, 1996). These articles agreed about the malleability of memory, but offered different perspectives on true/false allegations, and clinical management.

3. THE DEVELOPMENT OF A REPORT AND GUIDELINES FOR DOCTORS

Overall, GPs in New Zealand have been exposed to a varied range of information about SA memories. DSAC is therefore developing a report to address the resultant confusion. Consultation with interested doctors and other professionals is under way. The report will include comprehensive background information on SA and memory. Accompanying clinical management guidelines will cover general principles and provide practical guidelines to follow when a patient discloses previous SA, or when consulted by a family member who is affected by a disclosure of past SA. It is scheduled for completion in 1998, to be taken to the New Zealand Medical Association National Policy Council.

4. CONCLUSION

GPs want sound guidance on how to deal with the uncertainty that follows unsubstantiated disclosure of past sexual abuse. A comprehensive report and practical management guidelines will address some of these problems. It would be useful to have New Zealand research into the relative prevalence of corroborated, uncorroborated, and false allegations, and GPs knowledge and experiences with SA memory cases, as well as an analysis of what is happening in court cases, and in media presentations on these topics.

REFERENCES

Barham, P.M., & Benseman, J. (1984). Participation in continuing medical education of General Practitioners in New Zealand. *Journal of Medical Education, 59,* 649–654

Belton, A. (1995). Book review: First do no harm. *New Zealand Family Physician. 22,*112.

Broadmore, J. (1995).Commentary: False concerns about sexual abuse allegations?: A review of First do no harm. *New Zealand Family Physician,* 107–109.

Broadmore, J.(1995).Letter: DSAC seminars on recovery from the effects of sexual abuse. *New Zealand Medical Journal,* 108,110.

Donaldson, L.J., & O'Brien, S. (1995). Press coverage of the Cleveland child sexual abuse enquiry: A source of public enlightenment? *Journal of Public Health Medicine,* 17, 70–76.

Ennor, S. (1989). Cross-examination. In T. Eichelbaum (Ed.), *Mauet's fundamentals of trial techniques: New Zealand edition* (pp197–247). Auckland: Oxford University Press.

Freckleton, I. (1994). Book review: First do no harm: The sexual abuse industry. *Journal Of Law And Medicine,* 1,261–262

Galtung, J. & Mari Ruge.(1981). Structuring and selecting news. In S. Cohen & J. Young, (Eds.), *The manufacture of news: Social problems, deviance and the mass media.* Great Britain: Constable & Co.

Gavey, N.(1991). Sexual victimization prevalence among Auckland university students. *Journal of Consulting and Clinical Psychology,* 59, 464–466.

Gellatly, R., Broadmore, J., Shand, C., Milford, R., Gray, L., Green, S., Foley, C., & Hurst, C. (1996). Disclosure of past sexual abuse - Management guidelines. *Patient Management,* 25, 53–57.

Goodyear-Smith, F.(1993). *First do no harm: The sexual abuse industry.* Auckland, New Zealand: Benton Guy.

Goodyear-Smith, F.(1995). Letter: Sexual abuse and recovered memories. *New Zealand Medical Journal,* 108, 22.

Goodyear-Smith, F. (1995). Letter: Recovery from the effects of sexual abuse. *New Zealand Medical Journal,* 108,133–134.

Goodyear-Smith, F. (1996). Distinguishing between true and false allegations of sexual abuse - Part I - Adults alleging abuse as children. *Patient Management,* 25, 47–50; Part II - Allegations involving children. *Patient Management,* 26, 61–64

Henderson, E. (1996). Reckless disregard: Cross-examining children in sexual abuse trials. Thesis submitted in completion of Masters in Jurisprudence. University of Auckland.

Hendricks-Matthews, M.(1993). Survivors of abuse. *Primary Care,* 20, 391–406.

Kljakovic, M.(1995). Book review: First do no harm: The sexual abuse industry. *New Zealand Medical Journal,* 108, 515.

Manager, Sensitive Claims Unit, ARCIC, Personal communication and report May 1996.

Martin, J., Anderson, J., Mullen, P., & Romans, S.(1992). Adult sexual assault in a community sample of women. Paper presented at annual meeting of the New Zealand branch of the Australian and New Zealand College of Psychiatrists, Christchurch, New Zealand.

Moeller, T., Bachmann, G., & Moeller, J.R. (1993). The combined effects of physical, sexual and emotional abuse during childhood: long-term health consequences for women. *Child Abuse & Neglect,* 17, 623–640.

Mullen, P., Martin, J., Anderson, J., Romans, S., & Herbison, G.(1993). Childhood sexual abuse and mental health in adult life. *British Journal of Psychiatry,* 163, 721–732.

Neumann, D.(1994). Long-term correlates of childhood sexual abuse in adult survivors. *New Directions For Mental Health Services,* 64, 29–38.

R v A Unreported 25 Nov 1994, High Court, Christchurch T13–94

R v B (1994) 1 HRNZ 1; (1994) 12 CRNZ 417

R v D Unreported 30 September 1994, High Court, Auckland T 149/94.

R v D Unreported 31 August 1995, High Court, Auckland T 79/95

R v Ellis Unreported 1993, Court of Appeal CA 274/93

R v G [1996] 1 NZLR 615

R v R (1994) 11 CRNZ 402

R v Scott [1995] 3 NZLR 674

Shew, R., & Hurst, C.(1993). Should the question "have you been sexually abused?" be asked routinely when taking a sexual health history? *Venereology,* 6, 19–20.

Tyrell, I.(1994). Book review: First do no harm: The sexual abuse industry. *The British False Memory Syndrome Foundation Newsletter,* 10.

West, R.(1995). Commentary: First do no harm: The sexual abuse industry by Felicity Goodyear-Smith. *New Zealand Family Physician,* 22,149–150.

Williams, L.M. (1994). Recall of childhood trauma: A prospective study of women's memories of child sexual abuse. *Journal of Consulting and Clinical Psychology,* 62, 1167–1176.

17

REPORTED AMNESIA FOR CHILDHOOD ABUSE AND OTHER TRAUMATIC EVENTS IN PSYCHIATRIC INPATIENTS

Eve B. Carlson,[1] Judith Armstrong,[2] and Richard Loewenstein[2]

[1]Beloit College
700 College St.
Beloit, Wisconsin 53511
[2]Sheppard Pratt Hospital
Baltimore, Maryland

1. INTRODUCTION

By the close of the NATO Advanced Study Institute on Recollections of Trauma, it appeared that the first hurdle to reaching consensus over the credibility of reports of delayed memory for sexual abuse had been cleared. As the contents of other chapters in this volume show, there seems to be general agreement that both delayed recall of sexual abuse and false reports of sexual abuse do occur. Controversy remains, however, about the prevalence of amnesia for sexual abuse experiences, the prevalence of reports of recovered memories for sexual abuse that did not occur (so-called false memories), the processes involved in forgetting of sexual abuse experiences, and the accuracy of recovered memories of abuse (see Harvey & Herman, 1994; Lindsay & Read, 1993). To clarify our use of the term amnesia throughout this chapter, we mean a lack of recall of life experiences that one would be expected to recall because of their personal salience.

One impediment to progress in understanding memory for traumatic events has been the tendency of researchers and clinicians to focus very narrowly on sexual abuse experiences. By broadening the focus of inquiry to a wider range of traumatic events, we might learn much about the credibility of reports of amnesia for sexual abuse and the processes involved in recall and forgetting of sexual abuse experiences. Specifically, one broader question that might be asked by researchers and clinicians is what patterns of amnesia are reported across different types of abuse experiences and traumatic events? While there is relatively little empirical research on the prevalence of reported amnesia for sexual abuse, some research is available on the prevalence of amnesia for other types of traumatic events. Amnesia for traumatic events has been reported in studies of soldiers, concentration camp victims, rape victims, and refugees (Carlson & Rosser-Hogan, 1991; Loewenstein, 1996; van der Kolk, 1996). In general, these studies have found that a greater

Recollections of Trauma, edited by Read and Lindsay
Plenum Press, New York, 1997

severity of trauma is associated with a greater prevalence of amnesia for the trauma (Loewenstein, 1996).

Given that amnesia for traumatic events has been associated with a variety of traumas, it seems worthwhile to investigate whether patterns of reported amnesia for sexual abuse among various populations are consistent with each other and with patterns of reported amnesia for other types of traumatic experiences. In general, reports of childhood physical abuse experiences and other traumatic experiences have been less subject to controversy than are reports of childhood sexual abuse. Reports of sexual abuse have been questioned because of concern that psychotherapy clients may falsely report sexual abuse as a result of the influence of overzealous therapists and popular books on childhood sexual abuse (Lindsay & Read, 1993).

We do not dispute the point that misleading information on sexual abuse and memory has been widespread in the media (and among some mental health professionals) and that this misinformation has surely influenced some people to make false reports about childhood sexual abuse. These false reports may result either from false beliefs that abuse did occur or because of intentional misreporting. Both types of false reports of sexual abuse might be motivated in some cases by secondary gain. But these factors seem unlikely to be influencing reports of amnesia for other types of childhood abuse or other traumatic experiences. There is almost no popular press or media discussion about amnesia for physical abuse or other traumatic experiences, and we know of no civil litigation involving recovered memories for physical abuse or other traumatic experiences. If amnesia is reported for physical abuse experiences and other traumatic events, this will, in general, lend credibility to reports of amnesia for sexual abuse experiences.

Other questions that might be asked by researchers and clinicians include whether levels of amnesia for experiences are associated with particular aspects of the experiences or with various trauma-related psychiatric symptoms. Findings in studies of diverse populations that support hypothesized relationships between levels of amnesia and aspects of trauma and symptoms would reduce the likelihood that the findings reflect confabulated reports of amnesia. While confabulation of experiences and symptoms is always a possibility in an individual case, it seems unlikely that large numbers of subjects in independent studies at different sites could confabulate their reports in such a way that the hypothesized patterns in relationships between variables would be emerge.

This chapter will report results of a study of psychiatric inpatients that sheds light on the prevalence of amnesia for different types of abuse and other traumatic events. We will also briefly review findings relating to the relationships between level of amnesia for abuse and aspects of abuse experiences and between levels of amnesia for abuse and other trauma-related symptoms.

2. DESCRIPTION OF THE STUDY

The present study was designed to investigate the relationships between aspects of childhood physical and sexual abuse and adult psychological symptoms in psychiatric inpatients. We measured a number of variables that represent aspects of abuse experiences including the severity, duration, and age of onset of abuse experiences. We also measured some variables that are thought to moderate or exacerbate responses to traumatic experiences. These include later traumatic experiences and childhood experiences of neglect, dysfunctional behaviors in caretakers, and social support. Adult psychological symptoms we measured included posttraumatic stress disorder (PTSD) symptoms, dissociation, depression, anxiety, self-destructiveness, somatization, and aggression/hostility. This brief description of the study will include those aspects of the methods and measures used that are relevant to subjects' amnesia reports. A more complete description of the study's methods and findings can be found elsewhere (Carlson, Armstrong, Loewenstein, & Roth, in press).

Subjects for the study were psychiatric inpatients at a large, non-profit, psychiatric hospital serving an urban and suburban population. We attempted to recruit every patient admitted to the hospital during a three and one-half year period who was between the age of 30 and 45 (in order to minimize variation across subjects in the length of the recall period for childhood experiences). Of 2458 patients admitted, were able to obtain therapist permission to interview and to contact a total of 581 patients before they were discharged. Completed interviews were obtained for 217 of these patients. Those not interviewed (364) were unavailable because they declined to participate (180), were discharged before an interview could be completed (126), or for other reasons (58). Of 217 subjects interviewed, 126 (58%) were females and 91 (42%) were males. The average age of subjects was 38 (SD = 4.8). In terms of race, 82% were white, 16% black, and 2% some other race. The sample was socioeconomically diverse and diverse in terms of marital status.

Chart diagnoses was obtained for 178 patients received the following diagnoses: affective disorders (64%), dissociative disorders (30%), substance use disorders (31%), anxiety disorders (25%), other disorders (25%), and schizophrenia (7%). These add to more than 100% because many subjects received more than one diagnosis. The unusually high rate of dissociative disorders is the result of a dissociative disorders treatment unit at the hospital. In order to enhance generalizability of the findings, analyses were also calculated for the subsample of subjects (n=155) who were treated on psychiatric units not specializing in treatment of dissociative disorders. These subjects received diagnoses of affective disorders (75%), other disorders (28%), substance use disorders (26%), dissociative disorders (14%), anxiety disorders (12%), and schizophrenia (8%).

In the context of this study, subjects were administered structured interviews about their sexual experiences and experiences with physical force as children and about their symptoms of PTSD. The interview about sexual experiences inquired about experiences before the age of 18 with an older person or involving force. The interview was a modified version of that used by Jacobson and Richardson (1987). Subjects were asked about specific, behaviorally-defined experiences in a neutral manner. Experiences ranged from less intrusive behaviors such as being kissed or hugged in a sexual way to more intrusive behaviors such as having someone put their penis in the child's vagina or anus. The interview about physical abuse inquired about experiences of physical force before the age of 18 that were not in the context of fighting with other children. Here subjects were asked about physical force experiences using items from the Conflict Tactics Scale (Straus, 1979). These range from experiencing someone throw, smash, hit, or kick something to being threatened with a gun or knife.

Following completion of each abuse interview, subjects were asked "Was there ever a time when you didn't remember these things happening to you or didn't remember part of what happened to you?" Subjects who reported never having a period of not remembering the experiences were classified as reporting having had no amnesia. Those who reported not remembering part of their abuse experiences for some period were categorized as reporting having had partial amnesia. Those who reported not remembering all of their abuse experiences for some period were categorized as reporting having had total amnesia.

Information about amnesia for traumatic events other than childhood abuse was obtained using the Structured Interview for PTSD (SI-PTSD) (Davidson, Smith, & Kudler, 1989). At the beginning of this interview, subjects are asked "Did you ever experience an extremely stressful event, such as serious physical injury, combat, rape, assault, captivity, being kidnapped, being burned, seeing loss of life, your own life being threatened, destruction of property, or threat of harm to you or your family?" As part of the assessment for DSM-III-R Criterion C for PTSD, subjects were asked "Is there an important part of the event that you cannot remember?" Scores for this item were assigned by the interviewer who rated the client's psychogenic amnesia on the following scale: "0" = no problem, "1" = mild; remembers most details, "2" = moderate; some difficulty remembering significant details, "3" = severe; remembers only a few details; "4" = very severe; claims total amnesia for an important aspect of the trauma. For the purposes of this discussion, subjects were categorized as reporting no amnesia if their psychogenic amnesia rating was 0 or 1; they were categorized as reporting partial amnesia if their psychogenic amnesia rating was 2 or 3; they were categorized as reporting total amnesia if their psychogenic amnesia rating was 4.

3. AMNESIA FOR DIFFERENT TYPES OF TRAUMA

Of the 217 men and women interviewed in the study, 136 of them reported childhood forced sexual experiences, 194 reported childhood physical force experiences, and 168 reported one or more traumatic events on the SI-PTSD. Within the group of 168 reporting traumatic experiences on the SI-PTSD, some reported only childhood abuse experiences as traumatic events, some reported both childhood abuse and other traumatic experiences, and some reported only non-abuse traumas. The amnesia reports of the latter group of 75 subjects are of most interest here because they shed light on lack of recall for traumatic events other than abuse. Table 1 shows the rates of no, partial, or total amnesia across sexual abuse, physical abuse, and non-abuse traumas.

These same calculations were conducted for the subset of subjects who were treated on psychiatric units not specializing in the treatment of dissociative disorders. Table 2 shows the results of these analyses.

The results for the subset of subjects is somewhat different from the analysis for all subjects, with fewer subjects reporting total amnesia and more subjects reporting no amnesia. This difference is not surprising given that the units not specializing in treating dissociative disorders would be expected to have patients with less severe trauma histories and less problems with amnesia. Overall, however, the results for both sets of analyses show that, while there are differences in the rates of different reported levels of amnesia across sexual abuse, physical abuse, and other traumas, substantial numbers of subjects report having experienced partial or total amnesia for physical abuse experiences and other traumatic experiences. This finding supports the notion that the phenomenon of amnesia is not unique to sexual abuse experiences. This finding isn't surprising given observations of amnesia in victims of traumas such as disasters, accidents, and combat (for a review of the

Table 1. Levels of reported amnesia across different types of abuse and traumatic experiences

Type of experience	Reported no amnesia	Reported partial amnesia	Reported total amnesia
Sexual abuse (n=136)	38%	21%	41%
Physical abuse (n=194)	57%	23%	20%
Non-abuse traumas (n=75)	61%	19%	20%

Table 2. Levels of reported amnesia across different types of abuse and traumatic experiences for patients from general psychiatric units

Type of experience	Reported no amnesia	Reported partial amnesia	Reported total amnesia
Sexual abuse (n=96)	50%	19%	31%
Physical abuse (n=105)	66%	23%	11%
Non-abuse traumas (n=66)	68%	17%	15%

literature see van der Kolk, 1996 and Loewenstein, 1996) and the fact that severe physical abuse can be quite traumatizing to children.

It is interesting that a larger percentage of those physically abused reported no amnesia for the abuse compared to the percentage reporting no amnesia for sexual abuse. If this finding is confirmed through replication studies with other populations, it might lead us in the direction of asking why people are less likely to have amnesia for physical abuse experiences than for sexual abuse experiences. One possible explanation that awaits further consideration and study points to the secretive nature of sexual abuse experiences. Most often, sexual abuse occurs in private so that there are no witnesses to confirm the experience afterward or to remind the person of the experience. In fact, many people never discuss their sexual abuse experiences with anyone. Physical abuse, on the other hand, is not as likely to be a private act and may be observed by others such as family members who reinforce the memory of the experience in various ways. Furthermore, sexual abuse may leave no physical evidence of its occurrence, while physical abuse often leaves scars or bruises. These physical signs of the experience may serve as cues to remind the person of the experience. They may also serve to inform others of the experiences who, in turn, reinforce the memory of the abuse. Clearly, much more research is needed to confirm our finding of differences in amnesia rates for sexual and physical abuse and to explore possible explanations for them.

Lower levels of amnesia for non-abuse traumatic events than for childhood abuse experiences could be the result of a number of factors. As with physical abuse experiences, traumatic experiences other than abuse are more likely to have been witnessed by others who might provide cues for recall of the events. Furthermore, traumatic experiences other than abuse are less likely to be imbued with the kind of shame and secrecy that often accompanies sexual and physical abuse. Very often, a person's traumatic experience may be publicly acknowledged and openly spoken about, while this is rarely the case for abuse experiences. Support for this hypothesis would be provided if higher levels of amnesia were reported for a "shameful" traumatic event such as rape than for other kinds of traumatic events.

Table 3 shows a comparison of the levels of reported amnesia for sexual abuse in this study to those reported in five other similar studies (Briere & Conte, 1993; Elliott & Briere, 1995; Herman & Schatzow, 1987; Loftus, Polonsky, & Fullilove, 1994; Williams, 1995). In the table, the partial and total amnesia categories are combined because some studies did not distinguish between partial and total amnesia in their questions. This comparison highlights the differences in reported levels of amnesia for sexual abuse across studies. Likely contributing factors to these differences include differences in study methodologies such as how subjects were sampled and the exact question they were asked to determine amnesia level. Though no clear pattern emerges from this comparison in terms of a relationship between reported amnesia and level of mental illness (or population), the rates of partial or total amnesia for sexual abuse in the present study's inpatient population

Table 3. Levels of reported amnesia for sexual abuse across six studies

Study	Population	n	% reporting no amnesia	% reporting partial or total amnesia
Williams (1995)	general	129	53%	47%
Elliott & Briere (1993)	general	116	52%	42%
Loftus et al. (1994)	outpatient	52	75%	25%
Briere & Conte (1993)	outpatient	450	41%	59%
Herman & Schatzow (1987)	outpatient	53	36%	64%
Carlson et al. (1997)	inpatient	136	38%	62%

are roughly comparable to the rates of amnesia reported in two of the three outpatient studies. Again, we clearly need more systematic studies of the prevalence of various levels of amnesia before we can form any conclusions about the relative frequency of the phenomenon.

4. RELATIONSHIPS BETWEEN AMNESIA LEVELS AND OTHER VARIABLES

Results from our study reported elsewhere show that the level of amnesia for abuse is related to characteristics of the abuse experience and to trauma-related psychiatric symptoms (Carlson et al., in press). For example, level of amnesia for sexual abuse was significantly related to the extent of sexual abuse experienced by subjects, and level of amnesia for physical abuse was significantly related to the extent of physical abuse. In both cases, a greater extent of abuse was related to higher levels of amnesia. Furthermore, levels of amnesia for both sexual and physical abuse were significantly related to scores on measures of PTSD and dissociation. Symptoms of PTSD and dissociation have been associated with a wide range of traumatic experiences (see Carlson et al., in press). These findings of hypothesized relationships between level of amnesia and other variables seem to support the genuineness of the amnesia reports and indicate that this approach to the study of amnesia for abuse merits further consideration.

5. CONCLUSION

In conclusion, analyses of reported amnesia for abuse and trauma in our study of psychiatric inpatients indicate that a substantial proportion of inpatient subjects who experienced childhood physical abuse and non-abuse traumas report partial or total amnesia for their experiences. Differences in rates of amnesia for different types of abuse and traumas warrant further research as do relationships between amnesia levels, aspects of abuse, and trauma-related symptoms.

ACKNOWLEDGMENTS

This research was supported by a grant from the Violence and Traumatic Stress Research Branch, NIMH grant number R29 MH49401, Eve B. Carlson, Ph.D., Principal Investigator.

REFERENCES

Briere, J., & Conte, J. (1993). Self-reported amnesia for abuse in adults molested as children. *Journal of Traumatic Stress, 6*, 21–31.

Carlson, E. B., Armstrong, J., Loewenstein, R., & Roth, D. (in press). Relationships between traumatic experiences and symptoms of posttraumatic stress, dissociation, and amnesia. In J. D. Bremner & C. R. Marmar (Eds.), *Trauma, memory, and dissociation* . Washington, DC: American Psychiatric Press.

Carlson, E. B., & Rosser-Hogan, R. (1991). Trauma experiences, posttraumatic stress, dissociation, and depression in Cambodian refugees. *American Journal of Psychiatry, 148*, 1548–1551.

Davidson, J. R. T., Smith, R. D., & Kudler, H. S. (1989). Validity and reliability of the DSM-III criteria for posttraumatic stress disorder: Experience with a structured interview. *Journal of Nervous and Mental Disease, 177*, 336–341.

Elliott, D. M., & Briere, J. (1995). Posttraumatic stress associated with delayed recall of sexual abuse: A general population study. *Journal of Traumatic Stress, 8*, 629–647.

Harvey, J., & Herman, J. L. (1994). Amnesia, partial amnesia, and delayed recall among survivors of childhood trauma. *Consciousness and Cognition*, 295–306.

Herman, J. L., & Schatzow, E. (1987). Recovery and verification of memories of childhood sexual trauma. *Psychoanalytic Psychology, 4*, 1–14.

Jacobson, A. J., & Richardson, B. (1987). Assault experiences of 100 psychiatric inpatients: Evidence of the need for routine inquiry. *American Journal of Psychiatry, 144*, 908–913.

Lindsay, D. S., & Read, J. D. (1993). Psychotherapy and memory of child sexual abuse: A cognitive perspective. *Applied Cognitive Psychology, 8*, 281–338.

Loewenstein, R. J. (1996). Dissociative amnesia and dissociative fugue. In L. K. Michelson & W. J. Ray (Eds.), *Handbook of dissociation: Theoretical, empirical, and clinical perspectives* (pp. 307–336). New York: Plenum Press.

Loftus, E., Polonsky, S., & Fullilove, M. T. (1994). Memories of childhood sexual abuse. *Psychology of Women Quarterly, 18*, 67–84.

Straus, M. A. (1979). Measuring intrafamily conflict and violence: The Conflict Tactics Scales. *Journal of Marriage and the Family, 41*, 75–88.

van der Kolk, B. (1996). Trauma and memory. In B. A. van der Kolk, A. C. McFarlane, & L. Weisaeth (Eds.), *Traumatic stress: The effects of overwhelming experience on mind, body, and society* (pp. 279–302). New York: Guilford Press.

Williams, L. M. (1995). Recovered memories of abuse in women with documented child sexual victimization histories. *Journal of Traumatic Stress, 8*, 649–673.

18

WHY MEMORY IS A RED HERRING IN THE RECOVERED (TRAUMATIC) MEMORY DEBATE

Denis M. Donovan

The Children's Center for Developmental Psychiatry
6675-13 Ave N
Suite 2-A
St. Petersburg, Florida 33710-5483

ABSTRACT

The "rediscovery of trauma" in the late '70s and early '80s, especially the clinical finding of rates of child abuse histories as high as 70% among psychiatrically hospitalized females, presented psychiatry and the as-yet-unnamed field of traumatology with an epiphanous opportunity to spark a profound conceptual paradigm shift in the clinical biobehavioral sciences—and to do so at a time when "the search for traumatic memories" had not yet become a cultural vogue capable of eliciting an organized backlash. The opportunity to develop a revolutionary theory of experience-induced psychobiological change—both pathogenic and therapeutic— was lost as the field adopted the worst of traditional psychiatry's pathocentric categoricism in striving to establish the DSM respectability of categorical trauma-disorders (like MPD) instead of cultivating the richness of the initial clinical observations. The ensuing battle between the diametrically opposed Traumatic Memories camp and the False Memory Syndrome camp has obscured the fact that the literal recovery of traumatic memories ("making the unconscious conscious") was never a necessary feature of good clinical therapeutic problem-solving, while obscuring as well the fact that "Modern Biological Psychiatry" engages in its own version of equally bad thinking producing equally bad results. The actual treatment of trauma-related conditions has suffered greatly as a result.

Science is to see what everyone else has seen and to think what no one else has thought.
Albert Szent-Gyorgyi, 1937 Nobel Prize for Medicine or Physiology

Everything in scientific inquiry should be exposed to remorseless criticism.
Gerald M. Edelman, Nobel Prize for Medicine or Physiology, 1972

Recollections of Trauma, edited by Read and Lindsay
Plenum Press, New York, 1997

1. THE ABSENCE OF THE CHILD FROM PSYCHIATRY AND TRAUMATOLOGY

In 1991, the Canadian Province of Québec asked Jean-Jacques Breton, M.D., director of child psychiatry research at the Rivière-des-Prairies Hospital in Montréal, to conduct a provincial prevalence study of child psychiatric disorders. Breton and his colleagues from the University of Montréal did something practically unheard of in the field: they wondered if children would actually understand the questions on the *Diagnostic Interview Schedule for Children* (DISC-2), one of the most widely used structured interviews developed by David Shaffer, M.D. and his team at Columbia. The results were stunning. *Nine-, 10- and 11-year-old children understood only 38 percent of the questions on the DISC-2.* I was astounded to see Breton's (1993a) presentation in the New Research section of the 1993 annual meeting of American Academy of Child and Adolescent Psychiatry. When I asked Breton what his findings suggested about child psychiatry, he replied with a very sad smile, "That the child is of secondary importance in child psychiatry."

But even when the Academy Journal published a more polished version of Breton's (1995) research, the field missed the point. Mary Schwab-Stone, M.D. of the Yale Child Study Center comments in her *Discussion*: "The endeavor to make the DISC good enough has taken longer than anyone wanted, as work began on it around 1980..." What Breton's findings call into question is not the less-than-polished state of the DISC but, rather, the field's very understanding of children. It is sobering, to say the least, that one of this country's premier academic child psychiatry divisions could be so out-of-touch with a realistic understanding of children that it never even noticed that its instrument was incomprehensible to the very children it was designed to assess.

Far from an isolated example, Breton's findings reflect the overall status of psychiatry and the trauma field. Heir to decades of isolation from academic medicine and the rest of science, psychiatry has become a hermetically sealed, self-contained discipline whose in-house "experts" in everything from child development, cognition and language, memory, and neuroscience to pharmacology obviate the need to be aware of progress in all of those disciplines or study areas (Donovan, 1991b, 1995). Thus, if one examines the *image of the child* as well as the implicit and explicit models of development to be found in psychiatry and traumatology—as represented by the last 25 years of child psychiatry texts, journals such as the *Journal of Traumatic Stress*, *Child Abuse and Neglect* and the *Journal of the American Academy of Child and Adolescent Psychiatry* and works such as *Psychological Trauma* (van der Kolk, 1987) or *Traumatic Stress: The Effects of Overwhelming Experience on Mind, Body and Society* (van der Kolk, McFarlane and Weisaeth, 1996), on the one hand, and those found in the journal *Child Development* and the Monographs of the Society for Research in Child Development, on the other, one finds two non-intersecting conceptual universes: that of psychiatry and traumatology—unrealistic, unchallengeable and essentially unfalsifiable; and that of the greater-child studies field—realistic, challengeable and potentially falsifiable. The invariant serial-sequential abstract-categorical Piagetian stage-model of cognitive development that serves as the foundation for psychiatry and traumatology was long ago abandoned by the greater child-studies field as ecologically unrealistic and invalid (Brainerd, 1974, 1978; Donovan, 1991c, 1996a; Siegel, & Brainerd 1978). Outside psychiatry and traumatology, one finds realistic, contextually relevant, ecologically sensitive *child-oriented* models, such Wellman's (1990) *theory of mind*, or Thelen's application of nonlinear dynamic (self-organizing) system theory to the complex, adaptive, emergent phenomena of development (Thelen, 1992, 1996; Thelen & Smith, 1994). These approaches, represented by thousands of articles in the research literature, are linked vitally to ongoing developments in a wide variety of scientific fields, with much transdisciplinary cooperation and communication. (See Gleick, 1987 and Waldrop, 1992 for two historical accounts of these integrative transdisciplinary developments.) Had psychiatry, traumatology and the allied clinical fields been aware of the striking divergence of their basic theory, methodology and pragmatics from those of much of science, it would have been much harder for them to mistake the road map for the road, as Shaffer and his colleagues did with the *Diagnostic Interview Schedule for Children*.

1.1. Is the Prevailing Model of Traumatogenesis Realistic?

Lacking phenomenal and developmental realism (an understanding of real children), psychiatry and traumatology have developed abstract-categorical *models* of development, so-called "developmental psychopathology" (Cicchetti 1984; Cicchetti & Toth 1995), clinical phenomenology, pathogenesis (traumatogenesis) and treatment that are just as unrealistic, acontextual, depersonalized and immune from challenge, contradiction and falsification as the Freudian-Piagetian foundation upon which the field continues to be grounded (Tanguay 1989, 1991).[*]

This is vitally important because a realistic understanding of the long-term consequences of *childhood* trauma—and the role and fate of "traumatic memories" of *events experienced in childhood*—depends upon a realistic understanding of childhood cognitive-behavioral phenomenology (the meaning of what we see) and how children process experience, including traumatogenic experience (the difference between spontaneous childhood cognitive-behavioral *style* and genuine cognitive-developmental *capacity*), and the results of our interventions (the meaning of what we do).

2. MALIGNANT CAN'TISM

Is this assessment accurate? How can we know? We look. Neurophysiologist Warren McCulloch would tell his students, "When I point, look where I point, not at my finger." The field is obsessed with its finger—categorical models—and fails to see the realities at which it points, in this case, real children. When we do look, what do we find? Instead of real children—and, remember, this is all about the complexities of childhood trauma and its aftermath—we find categorically negative *descriptions* of abused, traumatized and psychiatrically disturbed children. Citing the Piagetian literature, van der Kolk (1987) and his colleagues describe these children:

> [They] were *unable* to conserve and *could not* use the operation of reversibility at an appropriate age; thus they *could not* properly assess other people's intentions. They could manipulate materials but *could not explain* what they had done . . . [they] . . . were *preoperational* and *could not understand* the concept of chance. . . . . They had *poor linguistics skills* and *disturbed symbolic and semiotic functions*. . . . they *seemed to understand* the problem but *could not anticipate or come up with solutions*. . . . To summarize, children in the research studies

---

[*] Lest it be thought that I am taking sides in the "recovered memory debate," let me stress that I include here the epistemologically fragile "broken brain" psychiatry of Andreason (1984) and the depersonalized, decontextualized Kraepelinian categoricism of Spitzer (Bayer and Spitzer 1985; Wilson 1993:p. 400; Young 1995:p. 99) and Goodwin and Guze (Goodwin & Guze 1989; Guze 1992).

reviewed above demonstrated developmental delays in several . . . domains.. (pp. 94–95, emphasis added)

As summed up by van der Kolk, "Thus far, our strongest finding in these abused children has been the inflexibility of organized schemata and structures in all domains. When we studied them, they were at an age when rigid classification boundaries of early preoperational thought should have loosened. Instead, function and structure were frozen so that dynamic change could not take place" (Fish-Murray, Koby & van der Kolk, 1987, p. 101).

The title of the chapter in which these descriptions are found in "Evolving ideas: The effect of abuse on children's thought," so perhaps this categorically negative view has evolved in the intervening 10 years. Not only has it not evolved, the clinical and theoretical descriptions of posttraumatic sequelae remain just as categorical and pessimistically absolutarian—and just as Piagetian. Indeed, this view was mainstream American education and mental health in 1987. (See Hodgins [1987] "You can't help me until you know what I can't do," a paper read at the meeting of the National Association for the Education of Young Children: a list of what children supposedly cannot do, according to Piagetian stages, including distinguishing between fantasy and reality.) And It remains mainstream education and mental health in 1996. The typical "developmental" perspective can be found in Fine (1988, 1990) and Silberg (1996).

Elizabeth Rice-Smith, of van der Kolk's child trauma team at the Human Resources Institute (HRI) in Boston, describes traumatized children in essentially the same words that van der Kolk had used in 1987: "emotionally constricted, developmentally frozen" (Rice-Smith, Pescosolido, Barone & McGettigan, 1995). In fact, the conceptual structure of the HRI child trauma program is not only Piagetian but Skinnerian as well (Rice-Smith et al., 1995): the child is essentially a *locus of pathology* and is described repeatedly in terms of what she supposedly "cannot" do. Complex, dynamic, individual, personal-idiosyncratic, contextually and ecologically relevant *meaning* is absent from this image of the child. "Functions, operations and structures across cognitive domains" are assessed by traditional Piagetian interview methods with questions such as "Where do clouds come from? What makes clouds move? Do you now, or did you ever, think that clouds follow you?" (Rice-Smith et al., 1995). Behaviorally, the focus is on "classical conditioning, counterconditioning and systematic desensitization " (Rice-Smith et al., 1995), while "cognitively," the focus is on adult style verbal-discursive behavior requiring a classical Freudian self-conscious acknowledgment on the part of the child: "'To know together' is what "acknowledgment" means" (Rice-Smith et al., 1995), an adult-style emphasis on conscious awareness and "processing memory" that pervades the field and creates an absolute block to the therapeutic utilization of childhood cognitive-behavioral plasticity. This, then, is the "developmental" context in which we now have to assess the significance and role of "traumatic memory."

Janet (1889) first described how traumatized people become "attached" (Freud would later use the term "fixated") to the trauma: "unable to integrate traumatic memories, they seem to have *lost their capacity* to assimilate new experiences as well. It is .. as if their personality *definitely stopped* at a certain point and *cannot enlarge* any more by the addition or assimilation of new elements." This suggests that traumatized people are prone to revert to earlier modes of cognitive processing of information when faced with new stresses. [. . .] Since the core problem in PTSD consists of a *failure to integrate* an upsetting experience into autobiographical memory the goal of treatment is find a way in which people can acknowledge the reality of what has happened without having to re-experience the trauma all over again. [. . .]

The key element of the psychotherapy of people with PTSD—as perhaps for all psycho-therapy—is the integration of the alien, the unacceptable, the terrifying, the incomprehensible. Life events initially experienced as alien, as if imposed from outside upon passive victims, must come to be "personalized" affectively as integrated aspects of one's history and life experiences [. . .] The treatment of PTSD has three principal components: 1) processing and coming to terms with the horrifying, overwhelming experience, 2) controlling and mastering physiological and biological stress reactions, 3) re-establishing secure social connections and interpersonal efficacy (van der Kolk, van der Hart & Burbridge [no date], emphasis added).

This is Rice-Smith's "*To know together*" *is what* "*acknowledgment*" *means*, above. Traumatic memories are there, in the individual, "engraved" (van der Kolk, 1994; van der Kolk & van der Hart, 1991) in an altered psychobiology, but not "integrated." Trauma therapy thus becomes the pedestrianly conscious verbal-discursive acknowledgment, processing and integration of these memories into the individual's narrative autobiographical memory. (Note van der Kolk's extension of this treatment model to "all psychotherapy." So compelling is this self-contained model that it can be applied to everything.) This same basic view is widely found in the literature on dissociation and the dissociative disorders. Consider:

Pathological dissociation is a complex psychobiological process that results in a *failure* to integrate information into the normal stream of consciousness. It produces a range of symptoms and behaviors including: (a) amnesias; (b) disturbances in sense of self; (c) trance-like states; (d) rapid shifts in mood and behavior; (e) perplexing shifts in access to knowledge, memory, and skills; (f) auditory and visual hallucinations; and (g) vivid imaginary companionship in children and adolescents." [. . .] The disturbances of self characteristic of the dissociative disorders result from a *developmental failure* to integrate differing self-concepts across the traumatically-induced dissociative barriers (Putnam, 1993b, emphasis added).

Note the same absolutarian categorical language: "failure to integrate, "developmental failure."

3. THE SEDUCTIVENESS OF CATEGORICAL MODELS

What can one do with posttraumatic pathological dissociation and other sequelae of childhood trauma? If childhood trauma, and/or the poor parenting that often accompanies it, result in genuine "developmental failures" and the extraordinary range of severe cognitive impairment described by van der Kolk and colleagues, above, would it not make sense to fashion a therapeutic interventionism aimed at remedying each and every categorical consequence of traumatic experience? Indeed, but such is not the case. Instead, we find a categorical explanatory-therapeutic model: "traumatic memory." "This is what psychotherapy is about: You reconstitute the state so that the person begins to retrieve the memories" (Putnam, 1995b).

3.1. Categorical Explanatory Models Assimilate but Do Not Accommodate

When a model becomes paradigmatic, as the traumatic memory model has, other theories, models and data tend to be *assimilated* to it—even when contradictory. Thus, entire developmental theories are adduced to add explanatory power to the model. New findings, such as apparently reduced hippocampal volume in trauma victims, are 1) assigned meaning in terms of the model and then 2) presented as proof of the "reality" and validity of the model itself. Or the predictive validity of instruments, such as the *Dissociative Experiences Scale*, across languages and cultures is adduced to provide the "reality" of the categorical models (Putnam, 1995a). The process is circular, defining the model while the model defines the meanings to be assimilated.

It is easy to get lost in this circular process and be swept along by the logic of the explanations and fail to see alternative meanings and explanations. For example, the unquestioned assumption in Putnam's statement above that recovery of state-dependent memory is *the key* to trauma treatment blinds the field to the significance of the "developmental" issues adduced to support the model. When we switch conceptual lenses and replace the model with a realistic naturalistic understanding of children, we find something troubling in Putnam's description of pathological dissociation, above. First, as any observant parent should know, these are *normative* childhood behaviors: rare is the child who doesn't "forget," display "disturbances" in sense of self, enter into trance-like states, evidence rapid shifts in mood and behavior, perplexing shifts in knowledge, memory and skills, claim to hear voices or have imaginary companions.

What do we find when we focus on children instead of disorders? Let's rethink one of the most cited definitions of dissociation in the literature, one that appears in Putnam's (1989) book on multiple personality disorder: "Dissociative states are characterized by significant alterations in the integrative functions of memory for thoughts, feeling, or actions, and significant alterations in sense of self (Ludwig, 1983; Nemiah, 1981)."

> Any observant adult has seen normative dissociation in children, such as alterations in consciousness (daydreaming, "tuning out") or sense of self: "No, I didn't eat those cookies," replies the adamant five-year-old whose face is still covered with crumbs. ... At the moment he is confronted our five-year-old does not remember the *action* of eating the chocolate chip cookie nor his *thoughts* about getting into the cookie jar that preceded the act nor the *feeling* of enjoyment he experienced as he ate the cookie; his *altered sense of self* is strikingly evident in the absolutely sincere denial that he and the cookie-eater are one in the same person. (Donovan & McIntyre, 1990, p. 59)

Such observations might have pointed back toward real children and how one deals with them. Instead, the model itself becomes a categorical imperative: models point to other models. Thus, we learn that "the modern diagnostic construct of MPD," the paradigmatic dissociative disorder, "is associated with a specific treatment model" (Putnam 1995b), a highly ritualistic and stereotypic structured process of eliciting dissociative symptomatology which includes discovering, meeting, getting to know, and negotiating with alter personalities and then "integrating" them in a long therapeutic process frought with multiple risks and dangers (Putnam, 1989). Note that this is no longer about the would-be cognitive or psychobiological sequelae of trauma in children; it is about categorical treatment models.

Similar models, including the formal use of hypnosis and Spiegel's (1988a, 1988b) "eight Cs," can be found in Fagan and McMahon (1984, 1993), Gould, Graham-Costain, Peterson, & Waterbury, (1993a, 1993b), James (1989), Kluft (1985, 1986) Lewis (1991), Peterson (1996), Shirar (1995), Turkus (no date) and Weiss, Sutton and Utecht (1985). Silberg (1996) offers an adult-MPD model approach to treatment of childhood Dissociative Identity Disorder. Ironically, all of these techniques are intensely *dissociogenic-amnestogenic*, and involve training the patient in complex dissociative and amnestic maneuvers, thereby enhancing and refining the very symptomatic behaviors that were ostensibly the "pathology" to be eliminated (Donovan, 1996b).

4. MISTAKING THE EXPLANATORY MODEL FOR PHENOMENAL DATA

How do dissociative *disorders* develop? "The linkage between the development of a dissociative reaction and the experience of overwhelming psychic trauma is most clear-cut in multiple personality disorder" (Putnam, 1985, p.78). Putnam sees:

> . . . the severe, sustained, and repetitive trauma that occurs during the early to middle childhood of most victims [as playing a decisively pathogenic role by] disrupt[ing] . . . the developmental tasks of consolidation of self across behavioral states and the acquisition of control over the modulation of states, [making it] adaptive for the child to heighten the separation between behavioral states, in order to compartmentalize overwhelming affects and memories generated by the trauma. In particular, children may use their enhanced dissociative ability to escape from the trauma by specifically entering into dissociative states (Putnam, 1989, p. 53).

It is following this formulation that Putnam calls the reader's attention—in passing —to what should have been an epiphanal observation for the entire field.

> In most MPD cases, the abuse is inflicted on the child by a parent or other caretaking figure. One of the most important tasks of a caretaker, particularly in early childhood, is helping the infant or toddler to enter and sustain a behavioral state that is appropriate for the circumstances. One has only to watch good parents feeding a toddler in public to see how they help their child achieve and maintain an appropriate state and how they suppress inappropriate states or help the child recover from disruptions of state. It is easy to speculate that the bad parenting accompanying abuse fails to aid the child in learning to modulate behavioral state (Putnam, 1989, p. 53).

It would appear that Putnam has brought us back to a naturalistic understanding of the developmental substrates of MPD. After all, Putnam notes that "the transitions between alter personality states (switches) closely resemble those seen between infant behavioral states." However, it is the model—not the phenomenal reality—that prevails. While naturalistic observation of the external modulation of biobehavioral state (mothers and infants) points toward a potential realistic problem-solving approach to posttraumatic biobehavioral phenomenology, the model simply points to itself. So, instead of challenging the pathological *appearance* of clinical phenomenology, Putnam returns to the model which specifies that "normal integrative and state-modulating mechanisms have *failed to develop* fully, leaving the MPD victim dependent on more developmentally primitive mechanisms" (1989 p.54, emphasis added). This is an explanation, not a finding. Naturalistic observation and the "developmental" considerations adduced to explain the model actually suggested a testable and potential falsifiable hypothesis—that the biobehavioral style of the individual trauma victim may be *instantaneously* subject to external modulation. The model, however, demands a categorical "developmental failure," dictating that the individual *cannot* modulate biobehavioral state. Which is right?

5. PUTTING THE CHILD BACK INTO "CHILDHOOD ANTECEDENTS"

Let's return to Piaget for a moment. Like the "developmental" model in psychiatry and traumatology, the Piagetian model is negative (it describes what the child *cannot* do until the next stage) and it is rigidly absolutarian. While Piagetians may be willing to admit that Piaget erred in failing to realize that the acquisition of cognitive skills, such as conservation, can occur earlier than he described, they are as adamant as *le patron* ("the boss") that *the serial-sequential order of stages is "invariant."* This is the principle of *décalage horizontal* which maintains that there are invariant sequences of cognitive skill mastery, e.g., that conservation of quantity invariably precedes conservation of weight, which invariably precedes conservation of volume, etc. As Howard Gruber and Jean Jacques Vonèche, editors of *The Essential Piaget* put it: "Piaget's use of the stage concept is an expression of his remorseless anti-empiricism. *During a given stage, the person does thus and so, and he can do no other.* To change as a mere reaction to environmental pressure would be to violate the organized integrity of the individual in his given stage of development" (Gruber &Vonèche, 1977, emphasis added). Thus, one of the enduring features of Piagetian dogma is that children must learn, for example, to conserve quantity ("age 7–8") before volume ("age 11–12"); they *cannot* reverse the order and understand that the volume of liquid in a container does not change when an object placed in the container causes the height of the liquid to rise *before* they learn that physically manipulating the shape of a ball of clay does not alter its quantity.

But Piaget was wrong. Not only can young children, revealed by standard Piagetian interviews to be nonconservers, be taught rapidly to conserve, they can be taught to do so at age 5—years "ahead of time." And follow-up testing demonstrates the durability and robustness of their skill acquisition (Parsonson & Naughton, 1988). These children demonstrated that, once learned at age 5, conservation of quantity generalized to all the other conservations. More important, however, was the finding that children didn't have to wait for biological maturation to proceed sequentially along Piaget's developmental path: they could be taught just as easily to conserve volume—an "11–12-year-old skill"—at age 5, and could do so *prior* to learning to conserve mass. So much for the "invariants of development" that still shape the image of the child as seen by psychiatry and traumatology, while the greater child-studies field has moved on. And what conclusion did Parsonson not include for fear that the article would be rejected outright since its factual conclusions were already seen as "Piaget bashing"? "I would suggest," says Parsonson, "that if development of conservation follows the sequence and timing described by Piaget, then our training study shows that either nature arranges inefficient training experiences or conservation is not an important developmental phenomenon" (personal communication, 1996). Like psychiatry and traumatology, Piaget's abstract-categorical model of epistemogenesis does not reveal children's genuine cognitive-developmental *capacities*; it simply catalogs spontaneous childhood cognitive-behavioral *style*. Good therapy, like good parenting, should maximize childhood potential, not categorize surface appearance.

5.1. Missed Mundane Epiphanies

Now back again to Putnam's apt observation of the effect of good parenting. Putnam's fascinating, accurate and *commonplace* observation of everyday mother-child interaction should have prompted widespread theoretical curiosity and extensive clinical experimentation. After all, any clinician or researcher knows that *mothers routinely modulate infant biobehavioral state.* If naive mothers can do so, and do so routinely and successfully, why couldn't clinicians do so as well? We know that infants cannot spontaneously modulate certain biobehavioral states; they remain dependent upon benevolent external assistance to facilitate such state-modulation. But trauma patients are, with the rarest of exceptions, no longer infants. Therefore, it is up to the clinician to facilitate

1) biobehavioral state-modulation in the present and 2) the acquisition of that autonomous skill as quickly as possible. After all, that is exactly what Barry Parsonson and Kathleen Naughton did with their 5-year-old subjects.

Put more forcefully: If mothers can naively, intuitively and successfully modify their infants' biobehavioral state, and if intelligent and presumably non-naive clinicians and researchers recognize this fact and refer to it in their literature reviews, why was the next logical step—developing an easily described and easily taught approach to the clinical modification of biobehavioral state—not taken? [†]

Had clinicians and researchers conversant with the dissociative disorders and related literature grasped the significance of Putnam's widely cited observation, above (and also found in Putnam, 1989, pp.51–53), the recent history of the trauma field might have been very different. However, instead of exploring and cultivating the potential pragmatic-transformational richness of these mundane naturalistic observations, the field chose to emulate the worst of psychiatric tradition and pressed for official recognition of a static model of the dynamic etiology of trauma-related conditions, as well as for official *DSM* recognition of those conditions themselves. This, in turn, led to, or paralleled, the development of rigid, stereotypic and ritualistic *categorical* approaches to clinical conditions themselves described as rigid, stereotypic and ritualistic. The field quickly lost sight of the fact that the initial rich observations—both clinical and naturalistic—had been of a *dynamic and (initially) adaptive biobehavioral plasticity*. By recognizing the apparently causal role of traumatic experience in the pathogenesis of "traditional" psychiatric disorders (Beck & van der Kolk, 1987; Bryer Nelson, Miller, & Krol, 1987), the trauma field had naively stumbled upon the King Solomon's mine of psychiatry—an appreciation of the role of experience in the genesis of acute and chronic biobehavioral state disorders.

Moreover, whatever role genetic factors may play in the development of traditional psychiatric disorders, clinicians sensitive to the possible role of traumatic experience in psychopathogenesis were beginning to head down a path that could have contributed to a more precocious understanding of the role of experience in the regulation of gene-expression (Kandel, 1992; Kandel & Hawkins, 1989). Unfortunately, in the face of dynamism and plasticity, the trauma field chose the dead-end rigidity of nosological and interventionist categoricism. The rest is history.

6. RETURNING TO SCIENCE

The ideology of repressed or dissociated traumatic memories, and the almost obligatorily *retraumatizing* therapy designed to recover, process, and work through such memories, have blinded the field to the richness and kairotic potential of the initial clinical observations. Trauma victims manifested profound-if-subtle psychobiological change: they were *transformed*. Clearly such experience-induced psychobiological dynamism begged for exploration. Unfortunately, instead of looking where the finger pointed—to the *plasticity* of human psychobiological responsivity and to the unique, idiosyncratic and intensely *personal meaning* of each individual's psychobiological negotiation of "potentially traumatic" experience, the field has, as McCulluch would say, mistaken its own collective finger for the instructive data at which it pointed. Had

---

[†] The step has been taken—but rarely. Our reconceptualization of the concept of inescapable shock and the use of the "therapeutic space" to modify the trauma response is one such application of these mundane and common-sensical observations to experiential interventions (Donovan & McIntyre, 1990, chapters 4 and 6).

psychiatry and traumatology been aware of the conceptual revolutions occurring in realistic child development studies (Thelen, 1992, 1996; Thelen & Smith, 1994; Wellman, 1990) and neuroplasticity research (Barinaga, 1992a, 1992b; Black, Isaacs, Anderson, Alcantia, & Greenough, 1990; Greenough & Black, 1992; Kent, 1991), or had they grasped what Nobel laureate Ilya Prigogine and Isabel Stengers (1984) meant by "the sciences of complexity," it might have become obvious that the complexity in question was not that of the pointing finger but, rather, of the dynamic and transformational biological system at which it pointed. Psychiatry and traumatology failed to recognize in this dynamic plasticity the opportunity for instantaneous transformative interventions and longer-term opportunities to literally change posttraumatic psychobiological style. In the face of the complex dynamic plasticity of the psychobiology of traumatic experience and its sequelae, the field developed static one-size-fits-all models of traumatic memory and trauma treatment.

Remember: Putnam did not tell us, upon observing relatively discrete biobehavioral states and their modulation in human infants, that mothers set out to *prove the reality* of such states and to develop checklists and rating scales to *identify* them, while training parents and caretakers to *document* them (when adults could have been taught to change them on-the-spot). Nor did mothers fashion *one-size-fits-all treatment techniques* for such widely different conditions as trapped esophageal air bubbles (requiring "burping"), exposure to environmental temperature change (requiring clothing change or ambient temperature regulation), hunger (requiring the provision of appropriate nutriments), thirst (requiring appropriate consumable liquids), sleepiness (requiring comforting motion or protection from environmental disturbance), irritability (requiring soothing), etc.

No, mothers just facilitate the modulation of biobehavioral state—without any specialized training. That is where the finger pointed. That was what was there to be seen all along, had the tyranny of categorical explanatory and treatment models not blinded the field to the obvious. So, where was it written that intelligent, observant and sensitive psychiatrists, psychologists, and psychotherapists could not do as well as naive mothers? Virtual revolutions were sweeping across and through scientific fields that *could have* sparked a conceptual-pragmatic revolution within psychiatry and the trauma field. Instead, psychiatry and the trauma field continued in the circular process of mistaking esthetically compelling models for the epiphanous-if-mundane phenomena of real life, resulting in a literalistic ideology of traumatic memory recovery, battles over the "reality" of MPD (Kluft & Spiegel, 1988; Putnam, 1995b) and endless therapies that seem to make things worse, not better. Mothers who successfully modulate their infants' biobehavioral state, including emotional state, do not create stereotypic mystifying one-size-fits-all techniques, nor do they battle with neighbors over the "reality" of their child's condition or create inventories or checklists to identify the eminently changeable. So why should clinicians?

Memory, of course, is inescapably part and parcel of what it is to be human and to have an identity. One cannot do therapy without relying on and using memory. But the myopic pathocentrism and still-Freudian omniscient authority of psychiatry and traumatology have blinded clinicians to the fact that the psychobiological, cognitive-behavioral and affective-affiliative clinical problems brought by trauma victims are potentially solvable, as are those brought by the traditionally depressed, anxious, distracted, obsessed, etc. It is true, as chemist-physicist-philosopher of science Ilya Prigogine has stressed, and as child abuse attorney Andrew Vachss has long insisted, that trauma cannot be "reversed." One simply cannot reverse the arrow of time. But one *can* capitalize on the inherent adaptive-integrative-transformational capacity of "plain old children" and *change* things for the better—and one can often do so quickly (Donovan, 1991a, 1991b, 1991c, 1995, 1996a, 1996b; Donovan & McIntyre, 1990). ‡

REFERENCES

American Academy of Child and Adolescent Psychiatry (1985), Facts for Families from the American Academy of Child and Adolescent Psychiatry: Learning disabilities. November 19, 1996., 11(5). Washington, D.C.

Andreasen, N. C. (1984), *The broken brain: The biological revolution in psychiatry.* New York: Harper & Row.

Barinaga, M. (1992a), Challenging the "No new neurons" dogma. *Science, 255*:1646.

Barinaga, M. (1992b), The brain remaps its own contours. *Science, 258*:216–218.

Beck, J. C. & van der Kolk, B. (1987), Reports of childhood incest and current behavior of chronically hospitalized psychotic women. *American Journal of Psychiatry, 144,(11)*:1474–1476.

Black, J. E., Isaacs, K. R., Anderson, B. J., Alcantara, A. A. & Greenough, W. T. (1990), Learning causes synaptogenesis, whereas motor activity causes angiogenesis, in cerebellar cortex of adult rats. *Proceedings of the National Academy of Sciences, 87*:5568–5572.

Brainerd, C. J. (1974), The concept of structure in cognitive-developmental theory. Paper presented at the annual convention of the American Psychological Association, New Orleans, August-September.

Brainerd, C. J. (1978). The stage question in cognitive-developmental theory. *The Behavioral and Brain Sciences, 2*:173–213.

Breton, J.-J., Bergeron, L., Valla, J.-P. et al. (1993), Do children aged 9 to 11 understand questions from the DISC-2? *Scientific Proceedings of the Annual Meeting of the American Academy of Child and Adolescent Psychiatry, IX,51* (New Research Section, San Antonio, Texas, 29 October 1993). Washington, D.C:AACAP.

Breton, J.-J., Bergeron, L., Valla, J.-P. et al. (1995), Do children aged 9 to 11 understand the DISC Version 2.25 questions? *Journal of the American Academy of Child and Adolescent Psychiatry, 34(7)*:946–954.

Bryer J. B., Nelson B. A., Miller J. B. & Krol P. A. (1987), Childhood sexual and physical abuse as factors in adult psychiatric illness. *American Journal of Psychiatry, 144(11)*:1426–1430.

Cicchetti, D. (1984), The emergence of developmental psychopathology. *Child Development, 55*:1–7.

Cicchetti, D. & Toth, S. L. (1995), A developmental psychopathology perspective on child abuse and neglect. *Journal of the American Academy of Child and Adolescent Psychiatry, 34(5)*:541–565.

Donovan, D. M. (1991a), The real worlds of children. *WELLSPRING, 3(2)*:5–9.

Donovan, D. M. (1991b)The disappearance of the child from child psychiatry. Grand Rounds, Department of Psychiatry, National Children's Medical Center, Washington, D.C., 13 December 1991 *Psychiatry, 30(2)*:333.12

Donovan, D. M. (1991c), Traumatology: A field whose time has come. *Journal of Traumatic Stress, (4)3*:433–436.

Donovan, D. M. (1995), Some thoughts on the conceptual-epistemological foundations of child psychiatry and the future of child psychiatry research and training. St. Petersburg, FL: The Children's Center for Developmental Psychiatry.

Donovan, D. (1996a), "A New Model for 21ˢᵗ Century Traumatology: Why the Field Needs the Greenoughs and Thelens of Science." Plenary paper presented at The New Traumatology Conference, Clearwater Beach, FL, January 12, 1996.

Donovan, D. M. (1996b), A new model of dissociation and dissociogenesis: Putting the child back into "childhood antecedents." Plenary paper presented at The New Traumatology Conference, Clearwater Beach, FL, January 13, 1996.

---

‡ See Hacking (1995) for a brief synopsis of our case of "Sally," a preadolescent case of formally diagnosed MPD on whom more than a million dollars had allegedly been spent in evaluation and treatment. After the first 2-hour evaluation session, Sally found it difficult to dissociate and after the third, could no longer dissociate. That is what one can do with children but not with categorical disorders, dissociative or otherwise. Years later, she is now in normal classes, her "learning disabilities" have disappeared, and her IQ has "risen" to normal and her symptomatic behavior is gone. This is the only case where I have assigned a diagnosis of MPD—and then only strategically, since the parents would accept only "skilled MPD treatment." For reasons known only to himself, Hacking chose to make Deborah McIntyre and myself part of the MPD-DID mainstream, which, of course, we have never been.

Donovan, D. M. & McIntyre, D. (1990), *Healing The Hurt Child: A Developmental-Contextual Approach.* New York • London: W. W. Norton.

Fagan, J. & McMahon, P. P. (1984), Incipient multiple personality in children: Four cases. *Journal of Nervous and Mental Diseases, 172(1)*:26–36.

Fine, C. G. (1988b), Thoughts on the cognitive perceptual substrates of Multiple Personality Disorder. *Dissociation, 1(4)*:5–10.

Fine, C. G. (1990), The cognitive sequelae of incest. In: R. P. Kluft (Ed.), *Incest-Related Syndromes of Adult Psychopathology.* Washington, D.C.: American Psychiatric Press.

Fish-Murray CC, Koby EV & van der Kolk BA (1987), Evolving ideas: The effect of abuse on children's thought. In: BA van der Kolk, (Ed.), *Psychological Trauma.* Washington, D.C.: American Psychiatric Press.

Gleick, J. (1987), *Chaos: Making a New Science.* New York: Penguin.

Goodwin, D. W. & Guze, S. B. (1989), *Psychiatric Diagnosis, 4th Ed.* New York/Oxford: Oxford University Press.

Gould, C., Graham-Costain, V., Peterson, G. & Waterbury, M. (1993a), *Identifying Dissociation in Children* (Videotape). Ukiah, CA: Cavalcade Productions.

Gould, C., Graham-Costain, V., Peterson, G. & Waterbury, M. (1993b), *Treating Dissociation in Children* (Videotape). Ukiah, CA: Cavalcade Productions.

Greenough, W. T. & Black, J. (1992), Induction of Brain Structure by Experience: Substrates for Cognitive Development. In: M. Gunnar & C. Nelson (Eds.), *Developmental Behavioral Neuroscience, Vol. 24, Minnesota Symposium on Child Psychology, 24*:155–200. Hillsdale, NJ: Erlbaum.

Gruber, H. E. & Vonèche, J. J. (Eds.) (1977), *The Essential Piaget.* New York: Basic Books.

Guze, S. B. (1992), *Why Psychiatry Is a Branch of Medicine.* New York: Oxford.

Hacking, I. (1995), *Rewriting the Soul: Multiple Personality and the Sciences of memory.* Princeton, NJ: Princeton University Press.

Hodgins, D. (1987), You can't help me until you know what I can't do. Paper presented at the meeting of the National Association for the Education of Young Children, Chicago.

Jacobson, A., Koehler, J. E., & Jones-Brown, C. (1987), The failure of routine assessment to detect histories of assault experienced by psychiatric patients. *Hospital and Community and Psychiatry, 38,4*:386–389.

James, B. (1989), *Treating Traumatized Children.* Lexington, MA: Lexington Books.

Kandel, E. R. (1989), Genes, nerve cells, and remembrance of things past. *Journal of Neuropsychiatry, 1(2)*:103–125.

Kandel, E. R. & Hawkins, R. D. (1992), The biological basis of learning and individuality. *Scientific American (267)3*:78–86 (September).

Kent, D. (1991), How does learning make physical changes in the brain? *American Psychological Society Observer, 4(4)*:8–9.

Kluft, R. P. (1986), Personality unification in multiple personality disorder: A follow-up study. In: B. G. Braun (Ed.), *Treatment of Multiple Personality Disorder.* Washington, D.C.: American Psychiatric Press, pp. 79–106.

Kluft, R. P. & Siegel, D. (1988): Debate: "Resolved That Multiple Personality Is a True Disease Entity." For: Richard Kluft and David Spiegel. Against: Fred Frankel and Martin Orne. Annual Meeting of the American Psychiatric Association.

Lewis, D. O. (1991), Multiple personality. In: M. Lewis (Ed.), *Child and Adolescent Psychiatry: A Comprehensive Textbook.* Baltimore: William & Wilkins.

Ludwig, A. M. (1983), The psychobiological functions of dissociation. *American Journal of Clinical Hypnosis, 26*:93–99.

Nemiah, J. C. (1981), Dissociative disorders. In Freeman, A. M. & Kaplan, H. I. (Eds.), *Comprehensive Textbook of Psychiatry,* Third Edition. Baltimore: Williams & Wilkins.

Parsonson, B. S. & Naughton, K. A. (1988), Training generalized conservation in 5-year-old children. *Journal of Experimental Child Psychology, 46*:372–390.

Peterson, G. (1996), Treatment of early onset, pp.135–181. In: J. L. Spira (Ed.), *Treating Dissociative Identity Disorder.* San Francisco: Jossey-Bass.

Prigogine, I. & Stengers, I. (1984), *Order Out of Chaos: Man's New Dialogue With Nature.* New York: Bantam.

Putnam, F. W. (1984), The psychophysiologic investigation of multiple personality disorder. *Psychiatric Clinics of North America, 7(1)*:31–39.

Putnam, F. W. (1985), Dissociation as a response to extreme trauma. In: R. P. Kluft (Ed.), *Childhood Antecedents of Multiple Personality* (pp. 66–97). Washington, D.C.: American Psychiatric Press.

Putnam, F. W. (1988), The switch process in multiple personality disorder and other state-change disorders. *Dissociation, 1*:24–32.

Putnam, F. W. (1995a), Dissociative disorders in youth: Assessment and treatment. Workshop presentation, annual meeting of the American Academy of Child and Adolescent Psychiatry, New Orleans, October 22, 1995.

Putnam, F. W. (1995b), Resolved: Multiple personality disorder is an individually and socially created artifact [Negative Position]. *Journal of the American Academy of Child and Adolescent Psychiatry*, 34(7):960–962.

Putnam, F. W., Helmers, K. & Trickett, P. K. (1993), Development, reliability, and validity of a child dissociation scale. *Child Abuse & Neglect, 17*:731–741.

Putnam, F. W. & Peterson, G. (1994), Further validation of the Child Dissociative Checklist. *Dissociation, 7*:204–211.

Rice-Smith, E, Pescosolido, F., Barone, B., McGettigan, M. (1995), Multimodal, phase-oriented application of treatment approaches with traumatized children. Pre-meeting institute, annual meeting of the International Society for Traumatic Stress Studies, Boston, November 3, 1995.

Shirar, L. (1996), *Dissociative Children: Bridging the Inner & Outer Worlds*. New York: W. W. Norton

Siegel, L. S. & Brainerd, C. J. (Eds.) (1978), *Alternatives to Piaget: Critical Essays on the Theory*. New York: Academic Press.

Silberg, J. A. (1996) (Ed.), *The Dissociative Child: Diagnosis, Treatment and Management*. Lutherville, MD: Sidran Press.

Spiegel, D. (1988a), Hypnosis. In: J. A. Talbott, R. E. Hales & S. C. Yudofsky (Eds.), *The American Psychiatric Press Textbook of Psychiatry*. Washington, D.C.: American Psychiatric Press, pp. 907–928).

Spiegel, D. (1988b), Dissociation and hypnosis in posttraumatic stress disorder. *Journal of Traumatic Stress, 1*:17–33.

Tanguay, P. (1985), Piaget: new and improved. *Newsletter of the American Academy of Child Psychiatry*. (Fall, 1985):10–12.

Tanguay, P. (1991), Teaching cognitive development (workshop). Training Symposium: Teaching Child and Adolescent Growth and Development in the 90's (Syllabus). Annual Meeting of the American Academy of Child and Adolescent Psychiatry, San Francisco, 16 October. Washington, D.C.: AACAP.

Thelen, E. (1992), Development as a dynamic system. *Current Directions in Psychological Science, 1(6)*:189–193.

Thelen, E. (1996), A complex adaptive systems approach to the development of cognition and action. Paper presented at the New Traumatology Conference, Clearwater Beach, FL, Jan. 12, 1996.

Thelen, E. & Smith, L. B. (1994), *A Dynamic Systems Approach to the Development of Cognition and Action*. Cambridge, MA: MIT.

Turkus, J. A. (no date), The spectrum of dissociative disorders: An overview of diagnosis and treatment. Found at the Turkus-Cohen-Courtois Psychiatric Institute of Washington World Wide Web home page: http://www.voiceofwomen.com/centerarticle.htm.

van der Kolk, B. A. (1987), *Psychological Trauma*. Washington, D.C.: American Psychiatric Press.

van der Kolk, B. A. (1994), The body keeps score: Memory and the evolving psychobiology of posttraumatic stress. *Harvard Review of Psychiatry*, 1:253–265.

van der Kolk, B. A. & Fisler, R. (1995), Dissociation and the fragmentary nature of traumatic memories: Overview and exploratory study. *Journal of Traumatic Stress, 8(4)*:505–525.

van der Kolk, B. A., McFarlane, A. & Weisaeth (Eds.), *Trauma Stress: The Effects of Overwhelming Experience on Mind, Body and Society*. New York: Guilford Press.

van der Kolk, B.A. & van der Hart, O. (1991), The intrusive past: The flexibility of memory and the engraving of trauma. *American Imago, 48(4)*:425–454.

van der Kolk, B. A., van der Hart, O. & Burbridge, J. (No date,) Approaches to the treatment of PTSD. David Baldwin's Trauma Page on the World Wide Web: http://www.gladstone.uoregon.edu/~dvb/trauma.

Volkow, N. D., Ding, Y., Fowler, J. S., et. al. (1995), Is methylphenidate like cocaine? *Archives of General Psychiatry, 52*:456–463.

Waldrop, M. M. (1992), *Complexity: The Emerging Science at the Edge of Order and Chaos*. New York: Simon & Schuster.

Wellman, H. M. (1990), *The Child's Theory of the Mind*. Cambridge, MA: MIT Press.

Weiss, M., Sutton, P. J. & Utecht, A. J. (1985), Multiple personality in a 10-year-old girl. *Journal of the American Academy, 24(4)*:495–501.

Wolff, P. H. (1987), *The Development of Behavioral States And The Expression Of Emotions In Early Infancy*. Chicago: University of Chicago Press.

Wolraich, M. L., Lindgren, S, Stromquist, Al, Milich, R., Davis, C. & Watson, D. (1990), Stimulant medication use by primary care physicians in the treatment of attention deficit hyperactivity disorder. *Pediatrics, 86*:95–101.

Zito, J. M. (1995), Pharmacoepidemiology meets epidemiology. *Newsletter of the American Academy of Child and Adolescent Psychiatry*, July-August:29, 32, 34.

19

REMEMBERING EARLY EXPERIENCES DURING CHILDHOOD

Are Traumatic Events Special?[*]

Margaret-Ellen Pipe,[1] Gail S. Goodman,[2] Jodi Quas,[2] S. Bidrose,[2] D. Ablin,[2] and S. Craw[1]

[1]University of Otago
Dunedin, New Zealand
[2]University of California at Davis
Davis, California 95616–8686

1. INTRODUCTION

What happens to early memories of childhood trauma? Do children remember stressful and traumatic experiences vividly throughout childhood or are such experiences as likely to be forgotten as more mundane experiences? Because it is sometimes claimed that adults are able to recover long-forgotten memories, the fate of early childhood memories, especially of traumatic experiences, has become a matter of considerable controversy. Until recently, most of what was known about memory for childhood trauma focused on adults' memories of their early experiences, and relatively little was known about the time course of forgetting during childhood. Bridging the temporal gap between childhood memory and later adult recall may, however, be a fruitful approach to understanding the mechanisms by which some memories are forgotten whereas others are retained into adult years (Goodman, Quas, Batterman-Faunce, Riddlesburger, & Kuhn, 1994). Understanding how children remember stressful or traumatic events is also of considerable practical importance, for example, when children are interviewed in clinical and legal contexts and are asked to recount their past experiences.

Several recent studies have explored children's memories of painful and even distressing medical procedures, such as of accidents followed by treatment in hospital emergency rooms (e.g., Howe, Courage, & Peterson, 1994), treatment for cancer (Steward, 1993), and diagnostic procedures such as the fluoroscopic voiding cystourethrogram

* This research is supported in part by a grant from the Health Research Council, New Zealand, to Dr M-E. Pipe, and by grants from SPSSI/Division 9 of the American Psychological Association and the Faculty Research Grant Program of the University of California, Davis, to Dr G. S. Goodman.

(VCUG) (Goodman et al., 1994; Ornstein, 1995). These procedures, although by no means perfect analogues for the kinds of events of interest in the debate concerning memory for traumatic events, include a number of important features that may enhance their ecological validity. A number of aspects of the VCUG procedure, in particular, make it a potentially useful analogue event (Goodman et al., 1994; Ornstein, 1995). The VCUG is used to diagnose such problems as genitourinary anomalies, urinary tract obstruction, or vesicoureteral reflux in children with urinary tract infections. This is an invasive procedure which requires genital exposure and contact for placement of a catheter into the urethra for infusion of liquid contrast into the child's bladder. In some cases children may need to be physically restrained for purposes of catheter placement and performance of the procedure of diagnostic quality. The placement of the catheter may be painful and the procedure stressful for the child. The procedure may also be an embarrassing experience, especially for modest children. Therefore, this kind of event may not be talked about afterwards.

When children are interviewed about the VCUG within a period of a month or 6 weeks of the procedure (Brown, Salmon, Pipe, Rutter, Craw, & Taylor, 1996; Goodman et al., 1994; Ornstein, 1995), they generally remember the procedure very well. Indeed, there is evidence that children remember the VCUG better than a more routine physical examination (e.g., Brown et al., 1996; Ornstein, 1995). These findings are consistent with the possibility that stress experienced during an event enhances memory for that event. Other explanations are also possible, however. For example, medical procedures such as the VCUG may be more organized and the order of actions more constrained by the logical relations between them than is the case in general physical examinations. This organization may contribute to good recall of these kinds of events (Ornstein, 1995; Peterson & Bell, in press). Conversely, more routine procedures such as the pediatric physical examination may be reported in less detail because children are likely to have medical scripts, resulting in less detailed recall of the particular examination of interest (see Hudson, Fivush & Kuebli, 1992).

2. LONG-TERM RECALL OF THE VCUG PROCEDURE: PRELIMINARY FINDINGS

Are stressful and traumatic experiences forgotten more or less quickly than more ordinary or pleasant experiences? Memories for stressful, painful or emotional events and those for other, more mundane experiences may differ not only in terms of their initial memorability, but also the rates of forgetting over time. The mechanisms that lead to a highly salient memory shortly after the event may not be sufficient to ensure that it is remembered over long time periods, and other factors may influence long term retention.

In an on-going study, we are examining children's memories of the VCUG procedure through interviews conducted following very long delays. To date, 29 children, ranging in age at time of VCUG from 29 months to 95 months, have been interviewed about the VCUG. The delays in time between the VCUG and the interview ranged from 9 months to 69 months. The majority (21) of the children had only 1 VCUG, and the remainder (8) had 2 or 3 VCUGs. Age at the time of interview ranged between 41 months and 163 months.

Interviews included free recall, prompts, enactment with anatomically detailed dolls, and direct (specific and misleading) questions. However, only data based on free recall and summarized across the entire interview are described here. Specifically, in our preliminary analyses we asked whether children remembered or accessed the memory for the experience by providing information consistent with the VCUG which was more specific than a general statement (such as "I got fixed") or a repetition of a prompt provided by the interviewer. For example, if the child said "The doctor put the tube in me and it hurt" but provided no further information which would identify the VCUG specifically, the child's memory was classified as ambiguous. If the child said "I got x-rayed and saw a picture on the TV thing," this was taken as evidence that the child remembered the VCUG procedure.

In free recall, children were asked about the test "where they put a tube in you." In response to this very general prompt, 9 children provided some information that identified the VCUG procedure. Across the entire interview and following more extensive cuing and prompting, a total of 17 children reported something about the VCUG procedure and 4 additional children provided information consistent with the VCUG procedure but which did not unambiguously identify it. When they were read a full description of the VCUG procedure and asked whether they had ever had this experience, of the 29 children, 7 still did not recognise the procedure. (Two others also said no, but qualified their answers to indicate they indeed recognised the procedure but disagreed with some details of the description read to them).

Are some children more or less likely to remember the event than others? We examined the effects of the length of the delay between the VCUG and the child's interview, and age of the child at the time of the event. [†] Figure 1 shows the proportion of children interviewed following a delay of less than 30 months who remembered the procedure, and the proportion of those interviewed following longer delays who remembered it. Delay appears to have had little effect on whether or not children recalled the event (Figure 1). Point biserial correlations (controlling for age) confirmed that memory for the event was not significantly related to the delay to the interview, for either free recall ($r = -.06$) or the entire interview ($r = -.18$).

It may seem surprising that delay has so little impact on whether or not children recall the VCUG. However, the shortest delay between the VCUG and the interview in this study was 9 months, and for the majority of children delays were at least 20 months. For all children in the present study, therefore, interviews were conducted following relatively long delays and it may be that including children interviewed within days or weeks since the event will reveal an effect of delay. In the studies by both the Goodman et al (1994) and Brown et al. (1996), for example, all of the children interviewed within days or weeks of the VCUG were able to recall and recount some information about the event after prompting, raising the possibility that at least for some children forgetting takes place within the first year or two.

In contrast to delay, age at the time of the VCUG had a marked impact on recall. Children were aged between approximately 2.5 years and 7 years at the time of undergoing the VCUG and Figure 2 shows the proportion of children younger than age 4 years at the time of the event who later remembered it, and the proportion of children age 4 years and older at the time who later remembered it. Children older at the time of the event were much more likely to remember the event than those younger than 4 years of age at the time of the event. This effect of age was confirmed by point biserial correlations (controlling for delay), with significant correlations between age at the time of the event and memory of the event (VCUG), in both free recall ($r = .41$, $p < .03$) and across the entire interview ($r = .54$, $p<.01$).

[†] We have collected data on a range of variables which may be of predictive value, following Goodman et al. (1994). A more complete description of this study, based on a larger sample of children, will be reported in due course.

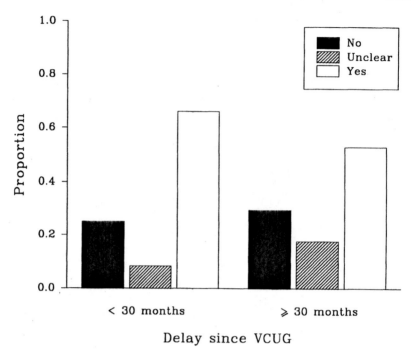

Figure 1. Proportion of children interviewed following a delay of less than 30 months who recalled the VCUG, and proportion of children interviewed following delays of 30 months or longer who recalled the procedure.

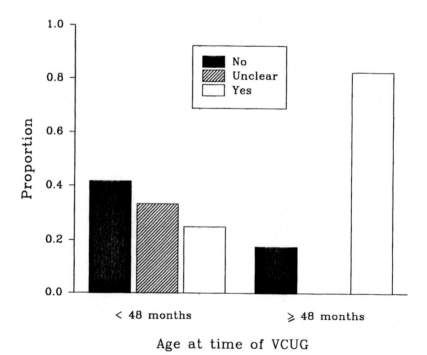

Figure 2. Proportion of children who were less than 48 months at the time of the VCUG who later recalled it and proportion of children who were 48 months or older at the time of the VCUG who later recalled it.

Two other preliminary findings are worthy of note. First, parents were asked to rate the level of distress experienced by their child during the VCUG procedure. There was a tendency for children who suffered more distress to be less likely to recall the procedure although this was not statistically significant at conventional levels of reliability (p< .08). Note that level of distress was not significantly related to the child's age at the time of the event. Second, there was no effect on memory of the total number of VCUG procedures children had, consistent with prior findings of Goodman et al. (1994). Because the sample of children in our study is still relatively small, whether these relationships will emerge as reliable effects in a larger sample will be of interest in the future.

How do these findings compare to those concerning children's long term memory of other experiences? There are no studies directly comparable to our current study, although a number of prior studies have examined children's very long term event memory (e.g., Goodman & Clarke-Stewart, 1991; Salmon & Pipe, in press). Table 1 summarizes 5 of our event memory studies in which we re-interviewed children between 1 and 4 years after they had taken part in the memory event. In four of these studies, the event was fun for the child to participate in and had been contrived especially for the study. In the 5th study, children underwent a routine physical examination. These studies differed from each other and from our current study in a number of ways, for example, in terms of the kind of event experienced, the ages of the children, the numbers of previous interviews, the support provided during interviews, and, importantly, the length of the delay before the interview. These methodological differences must, of course, limit the conclusions that can be drawn from across-study comparisons.

This caution notwithstanding, the data shown in Table 1 indicate that the majority of 5- to 6-year-old children generally recall novel, contrived events, up to 4 years later. The majority of children recall the experiences even in free recall, and following prompting only a very small proportion of the children are unable to report some information about the event. Fivush and colleagues (Hamond & Fivush, 1991; Fivush & Schwarzmueller, 1996) have similarly reported that children can recall distinctive, salient experiences from early childhood when interviewed up to 4 years later. But Table 1 also suggests that in studies based on medical experiences (Salmon & Pipe, 1996, in press), some children had difficulty accessing the event memory, especially in free recall. It is possible that medical procedures are particularly difficult to recall because at least some of their features are familiar and repeated over different examinations. Children may, therefore, have difficulty

Table 1. Percentages of children recalling different events following long delays (numbers in brackets refer to studies listed beneath the table)

Event	Age at time of event	Delay	% of children showing NO memory	
			Free recall	Prompts
(1) visit magician	5-6 years (n=83)	1 year	11	1
(2) visit magician	5-6 years (n=60)	2 years	26	—
(3) visit pirate	5-6 years (n=21)	4 years	9	9
(4) quasi medical	3-4 years (n=32)	1 year	78	19
	5-6 years (n=30)	1 year	67	3
(5) health assessment	5-6 years (n=101)	1 year	46	16
(6) VCUG	2-4 years (n=12)	2.5 - 7 years	92	42
	4 years + (n=17)		47	19

Follow-ups of: (1) Gee & Pipe, 1995; (2) Pipe & Wilson, 1994; (3) Murachver et al., 1996; (4) Salmon, & Pipe, in press; (5) Salmon & Pipe, 1996; (6) current study.

accessing the particular "target" memory. Even though the VCUG was characterized by a number of unique features compared to routine physical examinations, it is possible that over time the VCUG blended with other medical experiences in memory.

There are, however, several other factors that may contribute to the accessibility and recall of experiences such as the VCUG. In particular, Goodman et al. (1994) found that parents' reports of the way in which they had discussed the experience with their children related to errors that children made in response to questions about the VCUG procedure. Further, the way in which events are discussed, either before, during or after an event, may impact on how well the event is represented in memory and later recalled (e.g., Goodman et al., 1994; Tessler & Nelson, 1994). Narrating the event may highlight the specific features that are unique to a particular episode, so that this experience, as distinct from others, is more easily remembered (Tessler & Nelson, 1994). It may also be that meaningful narration provides a framework in which children can interpret the event and increase accuracy by protecting memory from intrusions of other similar experiences (Fivush, Pipe, Murachver, & Reese, 1997). There are some obvious implications of interpretative context for memory of traumatic experiences in particular. Some, if not many, stressful and traumatic experiences are likely to be poorly understood at the time of the event and have little or no accurate interpretive narration. For example, it is highly unlikely that adults provide accurate narrative accounts of abusive experiences; rather they are more likely not to discuss them at all or to provide distorted accounts. This may, in turn, make it difficult for children to form stable, coherent representations of the actual event which would provide the basis for long-term recall.

3. CONCLUSIONS

The clearest effect on whether or not children remembered the VCUG in our study was the age of the child at the time of the event. This finding is consistent with the now well-established finding that adults have particular difficulty recalling experiences from the first years of life, a phenomenon known as infantile amnesia (for review, see Howe & Courage, 1993; Pillemer & White, 1989). Our findings suggest that painful, stressful and even traumatic experiences appear no more likely to traverse the barrier of infantile amnesia than many other early experiences (see also Terr, 1988, for similar findings based on 20 clinical case studies; and Williams, 1994, for similar findings based on an adult sample). Nonetheless, age is not the only factor likely to impact on how well stressful and traumatic experiences are remembered over time. The distinctiveness of the experience and the way in which it is discussed, before, during and even after its occurrence, are among those factors likely to be important. On the basis of his review of adult studies, Christianson (1992) concluded that although there may indeed be differences in the memorability of emotional events on the one hand and more ordinary events on the other, "... the way in which emotion and memory interact is a very complex matter" (Christianson, 1992, p. 303). Similarly, it is unlikely that stressful and traumatic experiences during childhood will simply be either better or less well remembered than other experiences.

REFERENCES

Brown, D., Salmon, K., Pipe, M-E., Rutter, M., Craw, S., & Taylor, B. (1996) *Children's recall of stressful and non-stressful medical procedures: A direct comparison.* Paper submitted for publication.

Christianson, S. A. (1992). Emotional stress and eyewitness memory: A critical review. *Psychological Bulletin, 112*, 284–309.

Fivush, R., & Schwarzmueller, A. (1996). *Children recalling childhood: Eight-year-olds recount their past.* Paper presented at XIVth Biennial Meetings of ISSBD, Quebec City. August.

Fivush, R., Pipe, M.-E., Murachver, T., & Reese, E. (1997). Events spoken and unspoken: Implications of language and memory development for the recovered memory debate. In M. Conway (Ed.), *False and recovered memories* (pp. 34 - 62). London: Oxford University Press.

Gee, S., & Pipe, M-E. (1995). Helping children to remember: The influence of physical object cues on children's accounts of a real event. *Developmental Psychology, 5*, 746–758

Goodman, G.S., & Clarke-Stewart, A. (1991). Suggestibility in children's testimony: Implications for child sexual abuse investigations. In J. Doris (Ed.). *The suggestibility of children's recollections* (pp. 92 - 105). Washington: American Psychological Association.

Goodman, G. S., Quas, J. A., Batterman-Faunce, J. M., Riddlesberger, M. M., & Kuhn, J. (1994). Predictors of accurate and inaccurate memories of traumatic events experienced in childhood. *Consciousness and Cognition, 3*, 269–294.

Hamond, N. R., & Fivush, R. (1991). Memories of Mickey Mouse: Young children recount their trip to Disneyworld. *Cognitive Development, 6*, 433–448.

Howe, M. L., & Courage, M. L. (1993). On resolving the enigma of infantile amnesia. *Psychological Bulletin, 113*, 305–326.

Howe, M. L., Courage, M. L., & Peterson, C. (1994). How can I remember when "I" wasn't there? Long-term retention of traumatic memories and emergence of the cognitive self. *Consciousness and Cognition, 3*, 327–355.

Hudson, J.A., Fivush, R., & Kuebli, J. (1992). Scripts and episodes: The development of event memory. *Applied Cognitive Psychology, 6*, 483–505.

Murachver, T., Pipe, M-E., Gordon, R., Fivush, R., & Owens, L. (1996). Acquiring generalized event memories: The impact of information source. *Child Development, 67*, 3029–3044.

Ornstein, P. (1995). Children's long-term retention of salient personal experiences. *Journal of Traumatic Stress, 8*, 581–605.

Peterson, C., & Bell, M. (in press). Children's memory for traumatic injury. *Child Development.*

Pillemer, D. B., & White, S. H. (1989). Childhood events recalled by children and adults. In H. W. Reese (Ed.), *Advances in child development and behaviour* (Vol. 21, pp. 297–340). Orlando, Florida: Academic Press.

Pipe, M-E., & Wilson, C. (1994). Cues and secrets: Influences on children's event reports. *Developmental Psychology, 30*, 515–525

Salmon, K., & Pipe, M-E. (in press). Props and children's event reports: The impact of a one year delay. *Journal of Experimental Child Psychology.*

Salmon, K., & Pipe, M-E. (1996). *Using props and drawings to facilitate children's event recall following long delays.* Manuscript submitted for publication.

Steward, M. S. (1993). Understanding children's memories of medical procedures: "He didn't touch me and it didn't hurt!". In C. A. Nelson (Ed.), *Memory and affect in development* (pp. 171–225). Hillsdale, New Jersey: Lawrence Erlbaum.

Terr, L. C. (1988). What happens to early memories of trauma? A study of twenty children under age five at the time of documented traumatic events. *Journal of the American Academy of Child and Adolescent Psychiatry, 27*, 96–104.

Tessler, M., & Nelson, K. (1994). Making memories: The influence of joint encoding on later recall by young children. *Consciousness and Cognition, 3*, 307–326.

Williams, L. M. (1994). Recall of childhood trauma: A prospective study of women's memories of child sexual abuse. *Journal of Consulting and Clinical Psychology, 62*, 1167–1176.

20

THE REPEAT AND REVICTIMISATION OF CHILDREN

Possible Influences on Recollections for Trauma

Kevin D. Browne and Catherine E. Hamilton

University of Birmingham and Glenthorne Youth Treatment Centre
Birmingham, United Kingdom

1. INTRODUCTION

Some clinicians assert that memories of adverse childhood experiences, especially those involving severe physical and sexual victimisation, are often repressed, avoided, compartmentalised, or otherwise dissociation from conscious awareness (eg: Briere, 1992). In contrast, it has also been stated that experimental evidence for the existence of repressed memories for trauma is limited and far from convincing (Holmes, 1990; Loftus, 1993), and a recent review by Pope and Hudson (1995) claims that "present clinical evidence is insufficient to permit the conclusions that individuals can repress memories of childhood sexual abuse". However, assuming that repression and dissociation can (and does on occasion) occur, this chapter chooses to focus on how the repeated incidents of abuse (i.e., repeat and revictimisation) may affect the likelihood of such amnesic episodes.

In both clinical and experimental work on memories for abuse, sometimes the assumption is made that a recovered memory for a particular event would be clear, accurate and authentic, such as might be expected when produced as supporting evidence in Court for an allegation against an alleged offender (Wattam, 1991). This assumption is likely to be incorrect for a number of reasons:

1. In most cases abuse is not an event but a process of many events occurring over a certain duration of time.
2. In cases where more than one incident of abuse is experienced, an individual is often subjected to more than one type of abuse.
3. Memories for any one abusive incident would be influenced by other abusive incidents, such that details of any one event would become confused with other events.

An example of the complexity of adverse childhood experiences can be seen from the work of Browne, Falshaw and Hamilton (1995) which found that 74% of young per-

Recollections of Trauma, edited by Read and Lindsay
Plenum Press, New York, 1997

sons in secure accommodation (aged 11 to 18 years) had records showing that they have been victims of abuse and neglect as children. Furthermore, on a larger sample, Falshaw and Browne (1997) found this background in 72% of the young persons. Of those that were sexually abused, 76% had also been physically abused, 46% had also been emotionally abused and 39% had also been neglected. In addition, they had often suffered family breakdown, family criminality, educational failure, health problems and numerous care placements. When working with these young people it is therefore not surprising to find that they have poor recollections of any one event, that memories that are recovered in any detail are often triggered by current events and there is no way of establishing the authenticity of the memory or how much of their recollection has been contaminated by other events of a similar traumatic nature. Therefore, for these kinds of cases the research questions applied to clinical and experimental settings to date appear to have been over simplistic and somewhat unrealistic. Evidence for or against the concept of repressed memory of traumatic events and their recovery may be easier to determine from more sophisticaticated approaches to research.

2. CO-EXISTENCE OF DIFFERENT FORMS OF ABUSE

It may be helpful to the study of recovered memories for trauma to consider a three dimensional model that encompasses the different forms of maltreatment that reflect all possible traumatic experiences. Browne and Herbert (1997) propose that over time violent or coercive interactions may shift along one "dimension of harm" from psychological to physical and another "relationship dimension" from intra to extra familial. At the same time maltreatment, whether it be by a stranger or family member, may occur in an active or passive way within the "dimension of activity" (see Figure I). It has been claimed that less than 5% of the various forms of maltreatment occur in isolation and that emotional and physical neglect often appear to be a precursor to emotional, physical and sexual abuse (Ney, Fung & Wickett, 1994). It is now widely recognised that many children experience more than one form of maltreatment. In fact it can be seen from the Department of Health 1995 figures that 8% of children are placed on the Child Protection Register in the UK for than one type of concurrent abuse and/or neglect by the same perpetrator(s).

3. SUGGESTED CLASSIFICATION FOR VICTIMISATION

Those children who do come to the attention of professionals on more than one occasion or for more than one incident of abuse or neglect can be classified as experiencing repeated abuse. However, a problem with the use of this global term is the lack of reference made to the perpetrator(s) in each incident. Some children experience repeated maltreatment at the hands of the same perpetrator (often an intrafamilial offender), while others are abused by different people at different times in their life. For example, previous literature has suggested that sexual victimisation in childhood increases the risk of further sexual abuse in adulthood (Fromuth, 1986; Russell, 1986; Gidycz, Coble, Lathum & Layman, 1993; Mayall & Gold, 1995). Therefore, it is not enough just to look at repeat victimisation by the same perpetrator, but to investigate whether this vulnerability extends to abuse by different perpetrators *within childhood and adolescence*.

Therefore, a glossary of definitions has been devised to provide a distinction between "repeat victimisation" of abuse by the same perpetrator and "revictimisation" of

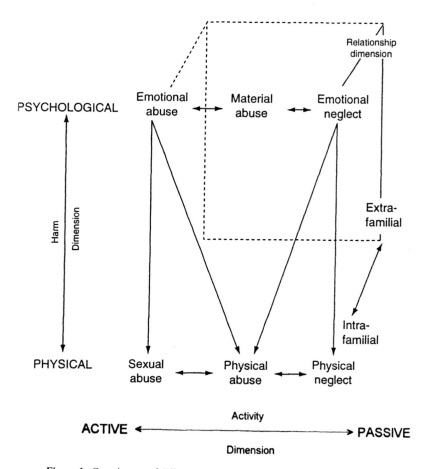

Figure 1. Co-existence of different forms of family violence - three dimensional.

abuse by different perpetrators (see Table 1). The glossary offers a means of standardizing the use of terms within the literature for describing different forms of child maltreatment. At present, these terms appear to be used interchangeably, which limits cross-comparisons and causes confusion.

It is felt that by distinguishing between these different types of repeated maltreatment, it is possible to compare the trauma associated with different occurrences of victimisation. At present it appears that most of the literature considers all these cases as a whole, ignoring the fact that differences occur between number of incidents and the long-term effects each of these may have on the victim.

As each victims's experience of the abuse will differ and their response to it will be determined by their own personal resources and perspective on life, a wide range of different long-term effects can be observed. This makes the prediction of trauma associated with childhood sexual abuse (CSA) very difficult, and much ambiguity exists as to how abuse characteristics influence trauma. Whether the type of abusive act consistently influences trauma is uncertain (Finkelhor, 1979), but evidence for increased trauma and mental health problems resulting from more serious contact, particularly penetration, receives support (Bagley & Ramsey, 1986; Russell, 1986; Beitchman et al., 1992).

Table 1. Glossary of terms

Single victimisation:
  A single incident of maltreatment involving only one perpetrator. This may be intra or extrafamilial.
Multiple victimisation:
  A single incident of maltreatment involving more than one perpetrator. The abusers may be family
  and/or non-family members.
Repeat victimisation:
  Maltreatment on more than one occasion by the same perpetrator(s). This may be either
  intrafamilial or extrafamilial.
Re-victimisation:
  Maltreatment on more than one occasion by different perpetrators. The initial perpetrator may be
  either a family or non-family member, as may subsequent abusers. Incidents of revictimisation may
  also move from intra to extrafamilial abusers, and vice versa.

Most consensus seems to be in relation to the increased traumatising effects of multiple perpetrators and extended duration of CSA (Beitchman et al., 1992). It is suggested that a victim suffering abuse at the hands of several different perpetrators is more likely to blame themselves rather than the offender (Briere, 1992; Peters, 1988).

4. EXTENT OF REPEAT AND REVICTIMISATION

Previous research provides us with estimates of the extent of either repeat victimisation or revictimisation within the general population. Although it is clearly not possible to distinguish the different groupings according to the classifications just presented, it is still of interest to ascertain an idea of an overall incidence level.

Within Britain, official data from the National Society for the Prevention of Cruelty to Children (Creighton, 1992) states that 5% of children placed on the Child Protection Register between 1988 and 1990 had experienced another incident of abuse or neglect by December 1991 (288 out of 6,270). This appears to be rather low but this is a very selective sample, and because these families should be receiving increased support from the various Child Protection Agencies, if the system is working effectively a lower re-referral rate would be expected. Alternatively, a high rate of re-abuse may be occurring, but the detection rate is low.

Studies with longer follow-up periods show higher rates of rereferral. Within the USA, 24,507 children on Colorado's Child Abuse and Neglect Registry between 1986 and 1989 were followed from registration until their first repeat incident or to the end of the study period, i.e., potentially for four years (Fryer & Miyoshi, 1994). In terms of maltreatment type, physical neglect cases had the highest rate of repeats (13%), followed by emotional neglect (12%), lack of supervision (11%), physical abuse (9%) and sexual abuse (8%). However, it was found that girls aged 1 - 6 years were the most vulnerable group, particularly following sexual and emotional abuse.

If the family is considered as a whole for any type of abuse at re-referral (i.e., index child and/or siblings), not surprisingly rates are much higher than when the index child is considered alone. Findings from Hobbs, Hanks and Wynne (1994, from the city of Leeds) show that neglect appears to have the highest rate of re-referral, with sexual abuse the lowest (see Table 2). Possible reasons for the former might be that neglecting parents are either provided with less support by Child Protection Agencies because it is seen as less

Table 2. Child abuse in Leeds (Hobbs, Hanks and Wynne, pers. comm.)

	1st referral of family n	2nd referral of family n	
Neglect	157	81	1/2
Physical	293	92	1/3
Emotional	233	117	1/3
Failure to Thrive	117	42	1/3
Sexual	240	53	1/5

harmful than more active forms of abuse (such as sexual or physical abuse) or because limited resources force them to focus on children experiencing more active forms of abuse. The more likely explanation, however, is that neglect is the form of maltreatment for which interventions seem least effective.

Earlier research found that once a family had been referred to a Child Protection Agency, one in two were re-referred (Magura, 1981), while Cohn and Daro (1987) found a reduced rate of 30% of parents who repeatedly victimised their children while in treatment programmes. Moving to the UK, rates of 20 - 63% have been found for family re-referrals (Baldwin & Oliver, 1975; Lynch & Roberts, 1982) in comparison to 44% in a Canadian study (Greenland, 1987). Overall, therefore, it can be seen that rates of family re-referral are high.

Clearly, the most extreme form of re-referral is that resulting from the death of a child. Indeed, nearly 2/3 of child abuse fatalities in a Canadian study were known to have been previously treated for physical injury as a result of abuse (Greenland, 1986). Furthermore, Creighton (1992) reported that siblings of children registered for physical abuse and/or neglect are also over-represented in fatality cases. So a majority of children killed by a family member were previously known to child protection agencies which highlights the importance of further investigating both repeat and revictimisation.

The fatality figures demonstrate that abuse can quite often become more serious over time (particularly if there is no intervention). Even if the end result is not fatality, it is likely that the greater the number of incidents, the greater the trauma likely to be experienced by the child. In these terms, it would be interesting to look at whether children who suffer revictimisation (i.e., a number of perpetrators at different periods of time within their childhood) experience greater trauma and greater long-term problems.

In terms of revictimisation within amnesic and non-amnesic groups, Cameron (1996) conducted a 9 year longitudinal study with 46 respondents (21 of whom had always remembered the details of their abuse; 25 of whom had amnesic episodes of between 15 and 54 years). In total, 42% of the amnesic women reported being abused by "non-related persons concurrently or sequentially' compared to 29% of the non-amnesic women, although it was not reported whether this was a significantly different rate.

5. FORMS OF REPEAT AND REVICTIMISATION

It does appear that research has yet to fully consider the fact that some children are abused by people both inside and outside the family home, such as the vulnerability in family childhood sexual abuse victims for extrafamilial adulthood rape which was mentioned earlier. Therefore, it is of interest to consider repeat victimisation and revictimisation in terms of the different sequences of perpetrator-child relationships. With respect to the suggested definitions, "repeat victimisation" may involve intrafamilial abuse on the first occasion followed by intrafamilial abuse *or* extrafamilial to extrafamilial, since it will be the same perpetrator offending against the child at different times. However, all permutations of intra- and extrafamilial perpetrators are possible with "revictimisation".

Furthermore, it would be of interest to compare the different characteristics of these groups and, in the long-term, these concepts could prove to be very useful in formulating ideas about memory loss and recovered memory for trauma. This in turn will improve intervention strategies to reduce victim suffering.

6. DEVELOPMENTAL VICTIMOLOGY

One important factor in the response to trauma is the developmental stage of the child at the time the abuse occurred - and as the length of time over which different incidents of abuse increases, the more stages of development which may potentially be affected. Finkelhor (1995) in his paper on "Developmental Victimology" identifies those factors that are likely to influence the possibility of victimisation and its effects on the individual (see Figure 2).

The victim's suitability as a target can be related (amongst other things) to the child's age. For example, young children are more vulnerable than older children to abduction by an estranged parent. However, the consequences of age of victim at the time the abuse occurs is uncertain. Most evidence suggests that younger victims suffer the greater trauma (eg, Baker & Duncan, 1985; Russell, 1986), but some authors claim that trauma may be increased with age of the victim, as a product of social and emotional maturity (Burgess, 1985; Peters, 1988).

The ability for the child to protect themselves will also affect the risk of victimisation; for example, being weaker, smaller or lacking the protection of a guardian or parent. Indeed, trauma resulting from the relationship of the victim and the perpetrator is suggested to be the product of the degree or closeness of the relationship (Conte and Schuerman, 1987; Beitchman et al., 1992), so the closer the relationship the greater the trauma. Finally, the social and physical environment of the child will also influence the chances of becoming a victim, such that Anna Freud (1981) postulates that intrafamilial sexual abuse is more traumatic to the child due to the trust and unquestioning power inherent in the family home. In addition, Baker and Duncan (1985) claim that abuse by strangers results in less long term trauma when the child can tell parents, be believed and not be held responsible for the abuse. It is therefore interesting to note that biological parent as perpetrator and younger age at onset of abuse were both correlated with participants self-reported amnesia about their maltreatment in the study by Cameron (1996).

The above precursors to abuse and victimisation (Figure 2, left stem) in turn will affect the child's vulnerability to further abuse following the initial incident. This vulnerability will be modified to a greater or lesser degree by those factors pertaining to the individual and which influence the child's reaction to the previous abusive incident. These factors represent the developmental stage of the child, whether the abuse occurred at a critical period of development (such as the time of attachment formation to a primary care giver), the child's cognitive appraisal of the abusive incident and what symptoms are present from initial short term effects (Figure 2 - right stem).

Such processes may influence the way a victim behaves which may result in increased vulnerability. For example, many children who have been sexually abused go on to develop

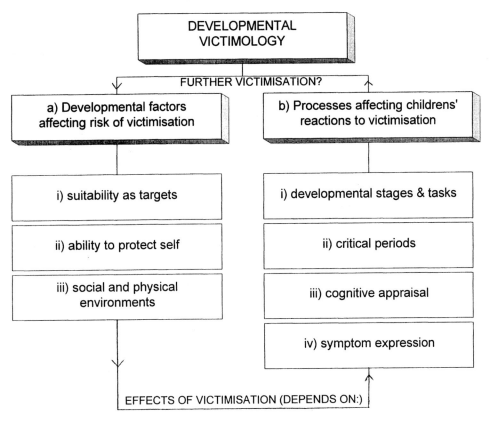

Figure 2. Graphical representation of the developmental perspective of the victimisation of children. Devised from the writings of D. Finkelhor (1995). The victimisation of children: a developmental perspective. *American Journal of Orthopsychiatry,* 65(2), 177 - 193.

age inappropriate sexualized behaviour and acting out which may attract the attention of a potential abuser. The abuser may then use the child's behaviour to justify his or her own actions and make the child feel responsible for their own further victimisation. In addition, it has been established that sex offenders target children and adolescents with certain behavioural characteristics, which identify them as vulnerable (Elliott, Browne and Kilcoyne, 1995). Such behavioural characteristics are often associated with prior victimisation.

7. CONCLUSION

Abusive behaviour towards a child must be considered within context, as a process not an event. In addition, for many children, victimisation occurs on more than one occasion, with the same perpetrator or different perpetrators. It is generally considered that repeat or revictimisation will lead to more severe trauma and that some memory for victimising events may be lost from conscious memory, while those children who experience a single event may be less traumatised and that details of the incident will be remembered (Terr, 1991; Whitfield, 1995). This may be because memories from different abusive incidents become confused, particularly when the same perpetrator is involved and the incidents occur frequently. Furthemore, denial, repression and dissociation may be more associated with repeated victimisation and revictimisation whereas single incidents are more likely to be recollected and talked about freely, particularly if the victim experiences a supportive and understanding environment (Whitfield, 1995). These facts need to be taken into account when designing experiments to investigate the nature of recovered memory.

It is interesting to note that more than a quarter of the non-amnesic women in Cameron's study experienced revictimisation (Cameron, 1996). It is possible that this is occurring because (whether amnesic or not), some victims unconsciously place themselves in situations and environments where the risk of revictimisation is greater (van der Kolk, 1989). So, while it may be useful to employ the concepts of repeat and revictimisation in research into trauma and recovered memory, clearly the relationship is likely to be complex.

In conclusion, it should be remembered that many children who experience repeat or revictimisation do not experience repression or dissociation, but that some factors associated with multiple incidents may increase the likelihood of these amnesic episodes occurring. This is an area where the very occurrence of repression, amnesia and dissociation is under debate and where the full value of considering the concepts of repeat and revictimisation is just beginning to be considered (see Hamilton & Browne, 1997).

REFERENCES

Bagley, C. and Ramsey, R. (1986). Sexual abuse in childhood, psychological outcomes and implications for social work practice. In J. Gripton and M. Valentich (Eds.), *Social work practice in sexual problems* (pp. 33 - 47). New York: Hamworth Press.

Baker, A.W. and Duncan, S.P. (1985). Child sexual abuse: A study of prevalence in Britain. *Child Abuse and Neglect, 8*, 457 - 467.

Baldwin, J.A. and Oliver, J.E. (1975). Epidemiology and family characteristics of severely abused children. *British Journal of Preventative Social Medicine, 29* (4), 205 - 221.

Beitchman, J., Zucker, K., Hood, J., DaCosta, G., Akman, D., and Cassavia, E. (1992). A review of the long-term effects of child sexual abuse. *Child Abuse and Neglect, 16*, 101 - 118.

Briere, J. (1992). *Child Abuse Trauma*. Newbury Park: Sage Publications.

Browne, K.D., Falshaw, L. and Hamilton, C.E. (1995). Characteristics of young persons resident at the Glenthorne Centre during the first half of 1995. *Youth Treatment Service Journal*, 1(2): 52 - 71.

Browne, K.D. and Herbert, (1997). *Preventing Family Violence*. Chichester: Wiley.

Burgess, A.W. (1985). Sexual victimization of adolescents. In A. W. Burgess (Ed.), *Rape and sexual assault: a research handbook*. (pp. 123 - 138). New York: Garland Press.

Cameron, C. (1996). Comparing amnesic and nonamnesic survivors of childhood sexual abuse: a longitudinal study. In: K. Pezdek and W. Banks (Eds.), *The Recovered Memory / False Memory Debate* (pp. 41 - 68). New York: Academic Press.

Cohn, A.H. and Daro, D. (1987). Is treatment too late: what ten years of evaluative research tell us. *Child Abuse and Neglect*, 11, 433 -442.

Conte, J., and Schuerman, J.R. (1987). Factors associated with an increased impact of child sexual abuse. *Child Abuse and Neglect*, 11, 201 - 211.

Creighton, S.J. (1992). *Child abuse trends in England and Wales 1988–1990: and an overview from 1973 - 1990*. London: NSPCC.

Department of Health (1995). *Children and young persons on Child Protection Registers Year Ending 31st March 1995, England*. Department of Health Personal Social Services Local Authority Statistics. London: HMSO.

Elliott, M., Browne, K.D. and Kilcoyne, J. (1995). Child Sexual Abuse Prevention: What offenders tell us. *Child Abuse and Neglect*, 19(5), 579 - 594.

Falshaw, L. and Browne, K.D. (1997). Adverse childhood experiences and violent acts of young people in secure accommodation, *Journal of Mental Health*, (In press).

Finkelhor, D. (1979). *Sexually victimized children*. New York: Free Press.

Finkelhor, D. (1995). The victimisation of children: a developmental perspective. *American Journal of Orthopsychiatry*, 65 (2), 177 - 193.

Freud, A. (1981). A psychoanalyst's view of sexual abuse by parents. In P. Beezley, Mrazek, and C. H. Hempe (Eds.), *Sexually abused children and their families* (pp. 33 - 34). Oxford: Pergamon Press.

Fromuth, M.E. (1986). The relationship of childhood sexual abuse with later psychological and sexual adjustment in a sample of college women. *Child Abuse and Neglect*, 10, 5 - 15.

Fryer, G.E. and Miyoshi, T.J. (1994). A survival analysis of the revictimization of children: the case of Colorado. *Child Abuse and Neglect*, 18(12), 1063 - 1071.

Gidycz, C.A., Coble, C.N., Latham, L. and Layman, M.J. (1993). Sexual assault experience in adulthood and prior victimization experiences: a prospective analysis. *Psychology of Women Quarterly*, 17(2), 151 - 168.

Greenland, C. (1986). Preventing child abuse and neglect deaths: the identification and management of high risk cases. *Health Visitor*, 59(7), 205 - 211.

Greenland, C. (1987). *Preventing CAN Deaths*. London: Tavistock.

Hamilton, C.E. and Browne, K.D. (1997). Repeat victimisation of children: Should the concept be revised? *Aggression and Violent Behaviour*, 2, (in press).

Hobbs, Hanks and Wynne (1994). *Child Abuse in Leeds 1994*. Personal Communication.

Holmes, D. (1990). The evidence for repression: an examination of sixty years of research. In J.L. Singer (Eds.), *Repression and dissociation: Implications for personality, theory, psychopathology and health* (pp. 85 - 102). Chicago: University of Chicago Press.

Loftus, E.F. (1993). The reality of repressed memory. *American Psychologist*, 48(5), 518 - 537.

Lynch, M.A. and Roberts, J. (1982). *Consequences of Child Abuse*. London: Academic Press.

Magura, M. (1981). Are services to protect children effective? *Children and Youth Services Review*, 3, 193.

Mayall, A. and Gold, S.R. (1995). Definitional issues and mediating variables in revictimization of women sexually abused as children. *Journal of Interpersonal Violence*, 10(1), 26 - 42.

Ney, P., Fung, and Wickett, (1994). The worst combinations of Child Abuse and Neglect. *Child Abuse and Neglect*, 18(9), 705 - 714.

Peters, S.D. (1988). Child sexual abuse and later psychological problems. In G. Wyatt and G. Powell (Eds.), *Lasting effects of child sexual abuse* (pp. 101 - 118). Beverley Hills, CA: Sage.

Pope, H.G. and Hudson, J.I. (1995). Can memories of childhood sexual abuse be repressed? *Psychological Medicine*, 25, 121 - 126.

Russell, D. (1986). *The secret trauma: incest in the lives of girls and women*. New York: Basic Books Inc.

Terr, L. C. (1991). Childhood traumas: An outline and overview. *American Journal of Psychiatry*, 148, 10 - 20.

Van der Kolk, B.A. (1989). The compulsion to repeat the trauma: re-enactment, revictimisation, and masochism. *Psychiatric Clinics of North America*, 12(2), 389 - 411.

Wattam, C. (1991). *Truth and belief in the "disclosure" process*. London: NSPCC.

Whitfield, C. L. (1995). *Memory and abuse: remembering and healing the effects of trauma*. Florida: Health Communications, Inc.

21

SEEKERS AFTER TRUTH

Ethical Issues Raised by the Discussion of "False" and "Recovered" Memories

Gwen Adshead

Broadmoor Hospital
Crowthorne Berkshire
United Kingdom

1. INTRODUCTION

The issue of recovered memory has raised strong feelings in professionals, and there has been a tendency for them to align themselves into polarised camps. Some authors have argued that this is not only a clinical, but a political issue (Bloom, 1995). Others have argued that the use of directive, or even coercive techniques, may result in patients recovering "memories" of events which did not occur (what are more accurately called "pseudo-memories" (Laurence & Perry, 1983) and reject the notion of autobiographical memory as essentially accurate (Loftus, 1993; Crews, 1994).

Recent research suggests that a subgroup of therapists exist, who use techniques which are more likely to produce pseudo-memories in their patients (Poole et al., 1995). It is likely that these therapists believe that they are doing their best for the patient (Loftus, 1993 p. 350).

Such therapists might argue that the use of potentially harmful therapeutic techniques (with or without consent) is justified on the grounds that the patient will ultimately benefit. It is this argument that I wish to examine. The argument that patient benefit justifies overriding autonomy and potential harm to the patient implies a fundamental misunderstanding of the duties of mental health care professionals (MHCPs). I will argue that this misunderstanding may be a function of theoretical confusion, an under-estimation of technical difficulty, or a reflection of difficulties or impairment in the therapist. I will also argue that specific psychopathologies caused by childhood trauma may require a type of ethical analysis which places more emphasis on autonomy than benefit.

2. AUTONOMY AND THE DUTY OF THE PSYCHOTHERAPIST

Beuchamp and Childress (1994) suggest the use of ethical principles to determine ethical conduct and identify the following four principles:

Recollections of Trauma, edited by Read and Lindsay
Plenum Press, New York, 1997

Different professional groups have different codes which provide guidance about ethically justifiable practice; most of these codes draw on the four principles in Table 1 which have a wide currency in the bioethics literature (Gillon and Lloyd, 1993).

Although the so-called "four principles" approach has been highly influential it is not without limitations (Toulmin, 1981; Danner Clouser & Gert, 1990). One limitation arises because an emphasis on respect for autonomy may not take sufficient account of the needs of those whose autonomy is reduced by mental distress. However because such patients are especially vulnerable to coercion or pressure, special attention may need to be paid to their claims to respect for autonomy and justice.

A further limitation is the emphasis on beneficence. Clinicians tend to favour the duty of beneficence over the other three principles. This is central to the issue of pseudo-memory generation. If the therapist believes that the good outcome (of recovering memories) outweighs any other consideration, then they will pursue this with vigour. The production of pseudo-memories, however, is not a good outcome; the intended good is in fact harmful to the patient. Both principles 2 and 3 are violated; and principles 1 and 4 appear not to have been considered.

3. CONSENT TO PSYCHOTHERAPY

The question of consent is important. To what do psychotherapy patients consent, regardless of school? At the very least, it might be reasonable to advise patients that they will work hard, and that this work may be uncomfortable at times; for them and their families. Pseudo-memories themselves appear to be a potentially harmful side-effect of some forms of psychotherapy; the risk of which a prudent patient might wish to have been informed.

A further complication is that patients are often much more ignorant about what to expect from psychotherapy than they are from other types of health care service. Psychotherapy has a mystique about it, independent of the relationship with the individual therapist; and patients may assume that a hectoring style, or boundary violations, are part of the treatment.

There are particular problems in the case of adults with suspected histories of childhood abuse. The psychopathology caused by an early breach of trust may have a profound influence on the type of ethical contract arrived at with their therapist. For example, adult survivors find it hard to trust, but very easily become dependent, and compliant in therapy. Therefore, for this group of patients, respect for autonomy may be the most important guiding principle; more even than bringing symptomatic relief or reassurance from anxiety.

Therefore, for adults where childhood trauma is suspected, consent to the therapeutic process is a crucial issue, because it implies a respect for their autonomy which was not given to them before. Respect for autonomy will be the dominating principle, which in turn will entail a special duty on the part of the therapist to let the patient set the agenda,

Table 1. Four principles of health care ethics (Beauchamp & Childress, 1994)

(i)	Respect for the autonomy of the patient
(ii)	The principle of beneficence or welfare, i.e. always doing that which will benefit the patient
(iii)	The principle of non-maleficence
(iv)	Respect for notions of justice.

and NOT to be directive. This might require the therapist to hold back from any directive techniques that take the control of the therapy from the patient.

4. MEMORY WORK: DOING GOOD AND NOT DOING HARM

The complex problems of adults seeking therapy may prompt the question as to why recovery of traumatic memories is thought to be so important. Freud is generally credited with the notion that remembering the painful past is the way to a healthy future, where the past has been left behind; gone, but not forgotten, as it were. However, the conscious recovery of forgotten memories was never accepted as an essential part of the psychoanalytic process (King and Steiner, 1991). It was the treatment of war veterans and traumatised civilians in the 1970s, which lead to a new emphasis on memory. Since Horowitz (1986) described the alternating cycle of intrusive memories and avoidance as a key feature of PTSD, memory work became an essential feature of recovery from traumatic experiences in adulthood.

However, good information is lacking about the most effective treatments for adult survivors of child abuse; it is not clear that memory work is the most effective treatment. It would therefore be just as unethical to use memory work for patients who could not use it or benefit by it, as it would be to prescribe the wrong medication, or employ a useless surgical technique.

5. JUSTICE AND THE VEXED ISSUE OF THIRD PARTIES

Those writers who believe that therapist-induced false-memories are common have argued that therapists have failed in their duty of care; not only to the patient, but also to the patient's family (Applebaum & Zoltek-Tice, 1996). The impact of the therapy on the patient's life is an important issue for therapists to consider, and may well include the impact on the patient's family. To date, psychotherapists, of most schools, have drawn on a medical model which sees only the patient as the object of professional duties.

In the case of psychological disorders and distress, it seems unrealistic to consider the patient outside the context and matrix of the family. One does this when clinically formulating the case; why not then ethically? This is not an argument for the claims of family members to have equal weight with the claims of the index patient. It is an argument that the patient's needs cannot be seen outside that of the family relationship matrix, and that failure to consider these may do the patient harm. This is even more important when the patient experiences negative thoughts and feelings about their family, and is pondering how to relate to them. The relationship with the family, either in vivo or in fantasy, will go on long after the therapy has finished; it is not a question of either the family's or the survivor's interests. Most therapists know that relationships with parents are rarely black and white and this is especially true where there has been sexual abuse between a parent and a child. There is little evidence that adults regularly seek revenge on parents for past wrongs, real or imagined.

Disputes between adults and their parents about the past raise a broader aspect in relation to justice and the therapeutic process. Is it feasible for therapists (or indeed any health care professional) to determine what "really" happened to an individual; especially if that individual themselves does not know? It is hard to see how mental health care professionals could determine the "truth" of what did or did not happen in the past; especially when it is suspected that there has been a crime. Within an adversarial legal framework, there is no crime until conviction, and an allegation is just that; no more and no less. This is equally true for alleged perpetrators; they can no more state categorically that an allegation is false than the alleger can claim it is true.

One of the other difficulties for those who recover memories of abuse is that the adversarial system encourages defendants to deny allegations, but provides no framework for supporting the allegations. One can see how therapists may wish to fill this gap, and indeed the provision of support and space to explore distressing experiences is an essential feature of the therapeutic experience. But advocacy in the legal sense of being partisan is a huge extension of the traditional therapeutic role. In this context, some workers have argued that the current adversarial system is a bad way of resolving disputes within families. Others have argued for the decriminalisation of child abuse altogether. It follows that therapists cannot assume that the therapeutic space is an alternative legal forum, where guilt and innocence can be confirmed. Rather it may be more just (in the sense of fairness) to support the patient in their uncertainty. If patients wish to pursue legal action then this can be explored with them in terms of personal meaning and emotional impact.

6. THE IMPAIRED THERAPIST

One final aspect which deserves discussion is that of the impaired therapist. By definition, impaired therapists are not able to fulfil their professional duties, and must therefore be at risk of acting unethically. There are many ways in which therapists can be impaired; including inexperience, lack of supervision, personality difficulties, and mental illness. Impairment can have an impact on therapy in many ways, most commonly because therapists lose sight of the patient's interests because of their own personal agenda. It is possible that therapist impairment may have played a part in some cases of recovered memory; perhaps because therapists were unskilled in working with possible survivors of child abuse, or because therapists' own feelings about child abuse may have taken over the direction of therapy.

Impaired therapists raise important issues for training and selection for training. Are there people who are not, and never will be, suitable for the psychotherapeutic professions? Perhaps the most acceptable view is that trainees need to have demonstrated that they have survived childhood trauma and loss in such a way that they have the capacity to work professionally and develop professional skills. On this criterion (which is itself complex, and requires an analysis of what it is to be professional), the experience of childhood abuse and trauma would be no bar to training. However, the onus would be on educational institutions.

It is even more complex a task to rid trainee and expert therapists of irrationality and prejudice. The whole area of child abuse appears to polarise people into "it never happens" and "it happens all the time". How many of us can say, in relation to the FMS debate, that we carefully went through the literature on memory, hypnosis, repression and pseudo-memory before we stated our position? In research work, we utilise an intellectual rigour and pay attention to all data which is the basis of scientific technique. That rigorous attitude needs to be part of therapeutic technique as well. This is not an alternative to empathy and attention to feelings; it is an appreciation of the fact that rationality involves analysis, awareness of feelings, and analysis of feelings. One of the biggest difficulties within the FMS debate has been the fact that it polarised so early and so quickly, with more feeling than analysis; more heat than light. A rational approach is vital, both within therapeutic practice, and of course in research. This is a live issue not only for trainees, but also for senior professionals and researchers.

7. CONCLUSION

An ethical analysis, based on a principles approach, is relevant to the false memory debate. I have argued that respect for autonomy is a vital aspect in the treatment of people who are suffering psychological distress; and especially anyone who may have suffered childhood trauma. Such patients are particularly vulnerable to abuse, and I have argued that therapists themselves may become abusers either when they fail to respect patient autonomy in the pursuit of a beneficial outcome, or when their own goals dominate the therapeutic process. In such circumstances abusing therapists may argue that the good consequences justify overriding the patient's autonomy. Interestingly, this is an argument that sexually abusing parents often use to justify their actions.

REFERENCES

Applebaum, P. and Zoltek-Tice, R. (1996). Psychotherapists' duties to third parties, Ramona and beyond. *American Journal of Psychiatry, 153,* 457–465.

Beauchamp, T. and Childress, J. (1994). *Principles of Biomedical Ethics.* (Fourth Edition). Oxford, Oxford University Press.

Bloom, S. (1995). When good people do bad things, meditations on the backlash. *The Journal of Psychohistory, 22,* 273–304.

Danner Clouser, K. and Gert, B. (1990). A Critique of Principilism. *Journal of Medicine and Philosophy, 15,* 219–236.

Crews, F. (1994). *The revenge of the repressed.* (parts I & II). New York Review of Books. (Nov.11 & Dec.1)

Gillon, R. and Lloyd, A. (Eds). (1993). *Principles of Health care ethics.* London, John Wiley & Sons Ltd.

Horowitz, M. (1986). *Stress Response Syndromes.* Jason Aronson Inc. 2nd Edition. p 17. New York.

King, P. and Steiner, R. (Eds). (1991). *The Freud-Klein controversies 1941–1945,* (pp. 926–927). London, Tavistock/Routledge.

Laurence, J. R. and Perry, C. (1983). Hypnotically created memory among highly hypnotisable subjects. *Science, 222,* 523–524.

Loftus, E. (1993). The reality of repressed memories. *American Psychologist, 48,* 518–537.

Poole, D. A., Lindsay, D. S., Memon, A., and Bull, R. (1995). Psychotherapy and the recovery of memories of childhood sexual abuse, U.S. and British practitioners' opinions, practices and experiences. *Journal of Consulting and Clinical Psychology, 63,* 426–437.

Toulmin, S. (1981). The Tyranny of Principles. *Hastings Centre Report, 11,* p 31 - 39.

22

INFORMATION PROCESSING IN COMBAT VETERANS

The Role of Avoidance

Mark Creamer and John Kelly

University of Melbourne
Australia

ABSTRACT

We investigated threat processing in 27 Vietnam veterans. Participants demonstrated a supraliminal attentional bias towards Vietnam words. At a subliminal level, there was a tendency to avoid the processing of Vietnam-related material. Contrary to expectations, the extent of interference was not related to the level of intrusive symptoms. Rather, it was avoidance symptoms that differentiated response styles to Vietnam-related material. Symptomatic avoidance was correlated positively with supraliminal biases, but negatively with subliminal biases. We propose that avoidance strategies may serve to prevent stimuli presented outside conscious awareness from activating traumatic memories.

1. INTRODUCTION

Cognitive models propose that anxiety disorders are associated with a selective processing bias for threat-related material (Williams, Watts, MacLeod, & Mathews, 1988). Empirical support for this hypothesis has been reported for all DSM-IV anxiety disorders using a range of experimental paradigms (Wells & Mathews, 1994). Much of this research has adopted a modified Stroop paradigm in which participants are asked to color-name words of varying emotional valency. It is assumed that increased color-naming latencies reflect an interference effect, indicating that attentional resources have been preferentially allocated to the content of the word.

Post-traumatic stress disorder (PTSD; American Psychiatric Association, 1994) is an anxiety disorder that is etiologically linked to experience of a highly stressful event. Characteristic symptoms include reexperiencing the trauma, avoidance and numbing, and persistently increased arousal. It has been proposed that experience of trauma results in the development of a traumatic memory network and that activation of this network explains

Recollections of Trauma, edited by Read and Lindsay
Plenum Press, New York, 1997

the symptom constellation of PTSD (Creamer, Burgess, & Pattison, 1992; Foa, Steketee, and Rothbaum, 1989). These cognitive models predict that PTSD, like other anxiety disorders, would be characterised by distinct styles of information processing. Indeed, several recent studies have demonstrated an attention bias towards trauma-related stimuli in individuals with PTSD by using a modified Stroop paradigm. Notably, Vietnam combat veterans with PTSD appear to take longer to color-name trauma-related words than neutral, positive, or general negative words (McNally, English, & Lipke, 1993; McNally, Kaspi, Riemann, & Zeitlin, 1990). Cognitive models would propose that delays in color-naming reflect activation of the traumatic memory network.

Several authors have proposed that attentional biases in anxiety may be mediated by automatic, pre-attentive processes which do not involve conscious awareness (Williams et al., 1988). While the available data are not conclusive, it does appear from Stroop tasks using subliminal word exposure conditions that high trait anxious normals, as well as patients with generalized anxiety disorder, may show an attentional bias towards threat stimuli presented outside conscious awareness (MacLeod & Rutherford, 1992; Mogg, Bradley, Williams, & Mathews, 1993). This has intriguing implications for PTSD, since the reexperiencing symptoms that are the hallmark of this condition are often reported to occur in the absence of any obvious reminders or other precipitating stimuli. It is conceivable that activation in such cases results from the processing of trauma-related information of which the patient is not consciously aware. No study to date has reported on the processing of subliminally presented material in PTSD.

The purpose of this study was to investigate processing of Vietnam-related words in combat veterans using both supraliminal and subliminal exposure conditions. The research was not designed to compare participants with and without PTSD. Rather, we assumed that all veterans, regardless of diagnostic status, would possess memory networks formed as a result of their experiences in the Vietnam conflict. We were interested in determining the extent to which those structures in memory direct attentional resources towards the selective processing of one category of stimuli over another within this population. Further, we were interested in the relationship between selective processing of threat information and symptom levels in the three core domains of traumatic stress (intrusion, avoidance, and hyperarousal).

Specifically, we investigated emotional Stroop interference in Vietnam combat veterans using four categories of stimulus word. Both Vietnam threat and social threat categories were included to determine whether processing of threat was selective (and, thus, directly attributable to a "Vietnam memory network") or was more general in nature. Positive words were included to control for emotional valency; that is, to ensure that any attentional bias was threat-related rather than simply a response to any emotional stimuli. Neutral words were categorized (household objects) to control for possible priming effects in the other three lists. We predicted that, for supraliminal exposures, participants would show interference effects on Vietnam threat words only and that the extent of those effects would be positively correlated with symptom severity. Investigation of potential subliminal processing was exploratory in nature.

2. METHOD

2.1. Participants

In order to ensure a range of symptom levels, 27 volunteer Vietnam combat veterans were recruited from both the Department of Psychiatry at a veterans' hospital and a community-based veterans' organization. Levels of intrusion and avoidance were assessed using the Impact of Event Scale (IES; Horowitz, Wilner, & Alvarez, 1979); mean scores for the two subscales were 21.7 for intrusion (SD=11.9, range=0–35) and 21.6 for avoidance (SD=11.4, range=0–38). The Beck Anxiety Inventory (BAI: Beck & Steer, 1990), a scale with strong emphasis on the physical symptoms of anxiety, was used in the current study to assess hyperarousal, the third construct of traumatic stress reactions. The mean score on this scale was 27.6 (SD=14.5, range=0–53).

2.2. Stimulus Materials

Initial word lists were generated from previous research and from clinical experience. Each word was then rated on a Likert-type scale for emotional valence and specificity to combat stress by four independent clinicians experienced with this population. On the basis of these ratings, eight stimulus words in each category were chosen to ensure, as far as possible, that a) the emotional valence of the Vietnam threat, social threat, and positive word lists was approximately equivalent; and b) that the two threat word lists were adequately differentiated in terms of their specificity to combat stress. The words chosen were: a) Vietnam threat (boobytrap, Vietcong, incoming, chopper, ambush, contact, enemy, kill); b) social threat (humiliate, pathetic, hopeless, ashamed, outcast, stupid, loser, fool); c) positive (delighted, splendid, kindness, success, holiday, joyful, pride, good); and d) categorized neutral (bookshelf, doorknob, saucepan, cabinet, curtain, carpet, table, vase). Average word length was identical across the four categories. A pool of stimulus items was created also for use in the awareness check trials (to determine the efficacy of the masking procedure). This stimulus set included all 32 words noted above together with 32 non word letter strings. Each non word was created by randomly rearranging the letters from one of the stimulus words.

2.3. Procedure

The experimental hardware and software was almost identical to that described by MacLeod and Rutherford (1992). Stimuli were presented on an Acorn Archimedes microcomputer. Subjects' responses were detected using a throat microphone and a voice activated relay, with reaction times to each word recorded automatically by the computer. On each trial, a row of white asterisks appeared in the centre of the screen as a fixation point. After 500ms, these were replaced by a stimulus word presented in one of four colours (red, yellow, green, or blue). In the supraliminal condition, the word remained on the screen until the subject made a response. In the subliminal condition the word was replaced after 20ms by a pattern mask, presented in the same colour as the word, which remained on the screen until the subject's response was detected. Following each trial, the screen remained blank for 1000ms before the next trial. The order of stimulus presentation was entirely randomised (word type, colour, masking), with every word appearing in each colour in both masked and unmasked conditions (256 trials). Following the color-naming trials, a series of awareness checks in the form of a lexical decision task was conducted to test the efficacy of the masking procedure. Words and non-words (64 trials) were presented for 20ms followed by a pattern mask. Subjects were asked to press a button labelled "Yes" if they thought they had seen a real word and "No" if they thought the stimulus was a non-word.

Subjects were seated approximately 0.5m from the VDU and were instructed to name the colour in which the word was printed as quickly as possible while ignoring the content. Prior to testing, subjects completed a brief practice session, color-naming a set of neutral words not included in the experimental session.

3. RESULTS

3.1. Awareness Checks and Accuracy

All participants reported that they were unable to see the stimuli presented in the masked condition. On the awareness check trials the proportion of correct responses expected by chance would be 50%, since there was an equal probability on each trial that a word or a non-word would be presented. In fact, the mean proportion of correct responses was 50.5%. It is reasonable to assume, therefore, that the masking procedure effectively prevented awareness of the stimulus content. Although no formal accuracy checks were conducted, observation suggested that errors in color-naming were minimal and no variance across word categories was noted.

3.2. Stroop Interference

For each subject, median color-naming latencies were used to compute a reaction time for each of the four word types; the overall means of these individual scores are summarised in Table 1. These reaction times were submitted to a repeated measures analysis of variance with two within subject factors of word type (Vietnam threat, social threat, positive, neutral) and exposure condition (masked, unmasked). Main effects were obtained for word type ($F[3, 24] = 7.02, p < .01$) and exposure condition ($F[1, 26] = 28.51, p < .001$). Importantly, an interaction effect was apparent for exposure by word type ($F[3, 24] = 8.83, p < .001$).

In order to interpret this interaction effect, three interference indices were computed by subtracting the reaction times to neutral words from the reaction times for each of the remaining word types. Thus, an interference index of zero would suggest that participants responded to the emotional words and the neutral words in the same way. A positive index indicates increased interference, suggesting an intentional bias toward the word type. A negative index suggest an avoidance of that word type. Separate ANOVA's were conducted for masked and unmasked interference indices, with a single within-subject factor of word type (Vietnam threat, social threat, positive). Significant main effects for word type were found in both masked ($F[2, 25] = 3.41, p < .05$) and unmasked ($F[2, 25] = 7.96, p < .01$) conditions. Subsequent univariate t-tests were conducted to determine which indices were significantly different from zero; that is, whether there was actually an attentional bias towards or away from the stimulus type. As shown in Figure 1, a strong bias was found towards Vietnam threat ($t[26] = 5.08, p < .001$) and, to a lesser extent, towards social threat ($t[26] = 2.64, p < .05$) in the supraliminal condition. There was a clear trend towards avoidance of Vietnam threat in the subliminal condition ($t[26] = 2.01, p = .055$). The interference indices for positive words in the supraliminal condition, and for social threat and positive words in the subliminal condition, were not significantly different from zero.

Table 1. Mean color-naming latencies in milliseconds for supraliminal and subliminal word

	Supraliminal		Subliminal	
	Mean	SD	Mean	SD
Vietnam threat	1022	363	817	246
Social threat	945	292	831	250
Positive	906	266	824	238
Neutral	903	274	832	246

3.3. Attentional Bias and Symptom Levels

Following McNally et al. (1990), we were interested in examining the relationship between selective processing of trauma-related stimuli and levels of PTSD symptomatology. Contrary to our expectations, there was no significant correlation between subliminal or supraliminal interference on Vietnam threat words and intrusion or hyperarousal symptoms. Significant correlations, however, were obtained between the Vietnam threat interference indices and the Avoidance subscale of the IES (supraliminal: $r(27) = .40, p < .05$; subliminal: $r(27) = -.43, p < .05$). That is, a high level of PTSD avoidance symptoms was associated with a supraliminal attentional bias towards threat, but with a subliminal avoidance of threat stimuli.

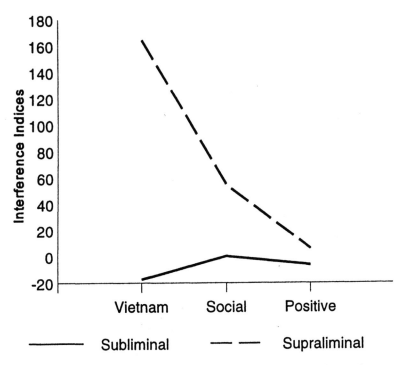

Figure 1. Interference indices for Vietnam threat, social threat, and positive word types.

4. DISCUSSION

In line with previous research, a supraliminal attentional bias towards Vietnam-related threat material was found in our sample of combat veterans, lending support to cognitive models of PTSD. The data are consistent with the existence of a traumatic memory network that not only stores old information, but also plays an active role in the processing of new information. Attentional resources appear to be preferentially allocated to network-congruent stimuli. At a subliminal level, however, an opposite effect was apparent. That is, there was a tendency in this population to avoid the processing of Vietnam-related threat material. This effect was weak and clearly must be interpreted with great caution. Nevertheless, it does suggest the possibility of some kind of pre-attentive semantic processing that allows threatening material to be screened out, preventing further elaboration.

We found no relationship between attention to Vietnam-related threat and either intrusion or hyperarousal symptoms. Rather, it was the avoidance strategies that differentiated response styles to Vietnam-related material. To recap, we found that reported avoidance symptoms were associated with an increased interference effect on Vietnam-related words presented at a supraliminal level (i.e., within conscious awareness). At a subliminal level, the correlation with avoidance symptoms was in the opposite direction. That is, a high level of avoidance symptoms was associated with a tendency to avoid subliminally presented Vietnam-related threat material (a reduced interference effect).

Presumably, individuals who are troubled by high levels of intrusive phenomena are unsuccessful in preventing activation of their traumatic memory networks. It seems likely that a wide range of stimuli in the environment have the capacity to activate the network, even when such stimuli are processed at a pre-attentive or subliminal level. Indeed, many trauma survivors are unable to identify clear precipitants to intrusive episodes (Peterson, Prout, & Schwartz, 1991). Although there is a strong correlation between intrusion and avoidance in traumatic stress reactions, it is widely accepted that the degree of avoidance varies between patients, as well as within the same patient at different times (Horowitz, 1986). This raises an interesting question: how do patients with high levels of avoidance prevent activation of the memory network for such long periods? On the basis of the current data, it seems possible that such patients are able to maintain this avoidant coping style by somehow detecting Vietnam-related material presented outside conscious awareness and screening it out from further processing. This implies that the stimuli are being processed at a semantic level, identified as threatening, and excluded from higher level processing. When patients are confronted with reminders at a conscious, or supraliminal, level, however, the screening mechanism no longer operates. Those strategies that functioned to protect the individual from frequent (and unnecessary) activation of the memories are no longer effective and the network is activated into full consciousness. Indeed, the positive correlation with avoidance suggests that, when such patients are confronted with threat stimuli in a way that makes avoidance impossible, they become even more vulnerable to the preferential processing of Vietnam-related information.

In clinical terms, this conceptualization is most reasonable. High levels of avoidance following trauma are thought to be pathological; while they provide temporary relief from more acute distress, they prevent activation and modification of the traumatic memory network (Creamer et al., 1992). The current findings support this suggestion. While high levels of avoidance symptoms prevent peripheral stimuli from activating the network, they result in greater attention to threat when the individual is confronted with unavoidable reminders of the trauma. Clearly, these hypotheses must remain speculative until the current results are replicated. Nevertheless, these results are consistent with information processing conceptualizations of traumatic stress and suggest an important avenue for future research.

REFERENCES

American Psychiatric Association (1994). *Diagnostic and statistical manual of mental disorders: Fourth edition (DSM-IV).* Washington DC: Author.

Beck, A. T., & Steer, R. A. (1990). *The Beck Anxiety Inventory manual.* San Antonio: Psychological Corporation: Harcourt, Brace, Jovanovich, Inc.

Creamer, M., Burgess, P., & Pattison, P. (1992). Reaction to trauma: A cognitive processing model. *Journal of Abnormal Psychology, 101*, 452–459.

Foa, E. B., Steketee, G., & Rothbaum, B. O. (1989). Behavioral-cognitive conceptualizations of post-traumatic stress disorder. *Behavior Therapy, 20*, 155–176.

Horowitz, M. J. (1986). *Stress response syndromes (2nd Ed.).* New York, Jason Aronson.

Horowitz, M. J., Wilner, N., & Alvarez, W. (1979). The Impact of Events Scale: A measure of subjective stress. *Psychosomatic Medicine, 41*, 209–218.

MacLeod, C., & Rutherford, E. (1992). Anxiety and the selective processing of emotional information. *Behaviour Research And Therapy, 30*, 479–491.

McNally, R., English, G., & Lipke, H. (1993). Assessment of intrusive cognition in PTSD: Use of the modified Stroop paradigm. *Journal of Traumatic Stress, 6*, 33–42.

McNally, R., Kaspi, S. P., Riemann, B. C., & Zeitlin, S. B. (1990). Selective processing of threat cues in posttraumatic stress disorder. *Journal of Abnormal Psychology, 99*, 398–402.

Mogg, K., Bradley, B., Williams, R., & Mathews, A. (1993). Subliminal processing of emotional information in anxiety and depression. *Journal of Abnormal Psychology, 102*, 304–311.

Peterson, K. C., Prout, M. F., & Schwartz, R. A. (1991). *Post-traumatic stress disorder: A clinician's guide.* Plenum Press, New York.

Wells, A., & Mathews, G. (1994). *Attention and emotion.* Hove, UK: Lawrence Erlbaum Associates.

Williams, J. M. G., Watts, F., MacLeod, C., & Mathews, A. (1988). *Cognitive psychology and emotional disorders.* Chichester: Wiley.

23

THE PREDICTION OF ACCURATE RECOLLECTIONS OF TRAUMA

Constance J. Dalenberg

Trauma Research Institute
California School of Professional Psychology
6160 Cornerstone Ct. East
San Diego, California 92121

1. INTRODUCTION

The issue of recovered memories of child abuse has emerged as a lightning rod for rhetoric in the last decade. Clinicians who took these memories seriously in most recent years, sometimes with caution and compassion, at other times with a singleminded bias toward acceptance, were labeled "recovered memory therapists" (Ofshe & Watters, 1994; Wakefield & Underwager, 1994). Arguments were made that these clinicians may deserve condemnation "as a new class of sexual predator, causing psychological trauma equivalent to rape (Ofshe & Watters, p. 7). In response to what they perceive as zealous and negligent acceptance of such memories, some theorists appeared to advocate singleminded rejection of recovered memory of abuse, making categorical statements that "people who experience severe trauma remember it" (Wakefield & Underwager, 1994, p. 182). Exaggerated claims from both "sides" of the controversy culminated in highly biased and non-validated checklists (e.g., Fredrickson, 1992; Gardner, 1995) which purported to be helpful for making legal and clinical decisions despite the absence of supportive scientific research.

Strong existence proof for accurate recovered memory is a very recent phenomenon. Case studies in which partial documentation for accuracy have been offered by several authors reported elsewhere in this volume, individual court cases (in which recovered memory survivors received monetary damages through civil suits) have met repeated legal tests, and news media have brought other documented cases to our recent attention. Williams (1995) found the accuracy of memory of abuse to be equal in groups of women reporting continuous and recovered memory of sexual assault, as documented by their childhood hospital records. It is becoming more clear that recovered memory can be accurate, and may be so in a large percentage of cases.

In many of the cases above, however, the recovery occurred outside of the therapeutic process. Therapy may present risks for the client who believes in his or her own abuse

Recollections of Trauma, edited by Read and Lindsay
Plenum Press, New York, 1997

with no attendant memories of it, or the patient who has partial or vague memories of a known abuse. Some therapeutic interventions, such as hypnosis or guided imagery, may lead the individual to be overconfident in their new memories (McConkey & Kinoshita, 1988), and the well-established need for social approval may produce a motive for patients to offer false stories to gain sympathy or attention from their therapists.

It is not known, however, whether the therapeutic process itself, absent the more risky techniques of guided imagery or hypnosis, would reliably lead to more accurate or less accurate recovered memories. The theory of state-dependent memory, for instance, would predict that the discussion of events that are rarely given cognitive attention and the re-invocation of emotional states that are not commonly experienced, both of which may occur in therapy, might together raise the probability of the phenomenological experience of recovered memory (cf. Dalenberg, Duvenage & Coe, poster abstract, this volume). Freyd's shareability theory (1983) also may be relevant.

2. METHODS

The methodology for the study presented and updated here is described in more detail in Dalenberg (in press). In this study, 17 female subjects, all recruited after their therapies with the author were competed, collaborated in gathering the data. The former patients were contacted in their regular follow-up visits. Patients were asked to give themselves at least one month to consider the potential risks and benefits of undertaking a search for validity or invalidity of their memories.

The following criteria were used to select the subjects:

1. All subjects had some continuous memories of child abuse. Methodologically, it is problematic to test the difference between one group with solely recovered and another group with solely continuous memories of child abuse and subsequently assume that the resulting differences in accuracy are byproducts of the recovery process, rather than due to other aspects differentiating the two groups. If recovered memories are less reliable as a class than are continuous memories, then clinically this is an *intra*-patient issue; that is, my question regarding the patient before me is not whether I should distrust her more than others when she discloses, but instead, if I can trust the *recovered* memories of Patient X less than her *other* memories. This is the first study using such a within-group comparison, testing the difference in the ratio of accurate to inaccurate elements in the recovered and continuous abuse narratives.

2. Only subjects with a substantial recovery percentage (percentage of all abuse memories recalled in therapy) were recruited. Thus, the ratio of recovered to continuous memories in this sample is not normative. The women had recovered two to six distinct episodes of abuse memory; they had discussed four to nine distinct episodes of continuously recalled abuse. Further, subjects were chosen whose recovery substantially changed the rated severity of the abuse that they allegedly experienced. The average severity rating for the abuse *including* the recovered material (8.56 on a 10-point scale) was significantly higher than the rating for the abuse without the new material (M = 6.21, t (16) = 12.67, p < .001). Subjects recovering memories of physical abuse, sexual abuse, or both were included.

3. All subjects had a fully taped therapy which either had been or could be transcribed, and had been assessed pre-therapy on psychological instruments.

4. After contact, patients were eliminated if either they or their parents were involved in abuse "movements" on either side of the controversy. Since both the patients and their fathers were very much involved in this research, it seemed best to eliminate those who may have an existing agenda on the experimental question. Data collection began in 1990; therefore, this criterion did not affect the pool as it might have today. Three subjects were eliminated who would have been otherwise eligible.

5. Two otherwise available subjects were eliminated when fathers denied permission to talk to siblings and alleged witnesses. One of these fathers agreed almost totally with his daughter-subject, but did not wish his other daughter, an attorney, to be reminded of her childhood. The other father remembered the past quite differently than did his daughter, and did not want his son to be contacted. Mothers were not included, due to reports that many had not been fully informed as to the alleged abuse events.

Women who consented and met criteria ($n = 17$), after the thorough informed consent procedure, were given a list of individual pieces of potentially verifiable information on child abuse that they had presented throughout therapy (meaning "facts" as opposed to thoughts or meanings that had not been shared.). Next subjects rated confidence in the truth values of each abuse memory, and attempted to recall the circumstances of their disclosure of each bit of data to me (Was it recovered or continuous? Presented early or late in therapy?) Subjects attempted to track down physical evidence for each element that they would be willing to share with the author.

Fathers were evaluated with a funnel interview, beginning with open-ended questions regarding the general events in question. The final specific questions were revelations of the exact content of the daughter's memories, and a request to state whether the father believed it to be true or false and, if true, whether he had a specific memory of this event. They also participated in locating "evidence." Nine of the father/daughter pairs stated that they had never discussed the abuse in their adult lives and five had been out of contact prior to the study. Informed consent for the fathers was often an extremely long and arduous process, at times taking up to a year and involving discussions with attorneys representing their interests.

After all information had been gathered, the subjects were given access to the tapes and/or transcripts. Various ratings were made (described in Dalenberg, in press) on recalled affect, symptoms, and feelings toward the author.

3. RESULTS AND DISCUSSION

Most subjects and their families located evidence confirming or disconfirming about 65%-75% of their memories. The mean accuracy for recovered memory and continuous memory was identical; on the average approximately 75% of the units were accurate. Four subjects had significantly more accurate recovered memory, four had significantly more accurate continuous memory, and 9 were identical (as tested by z tests for proportions). Seven of the 17 subjects improved in accuracy throughout therapy, a pattern which reaches significance at $p < .001$ using the z for the binomial. Potentially, this finding could indicate that it is possible to teach metamemory skills in psychotherapy, or that the defensive purposes of the distortion shift over time as the subjects improve, or that clients gradually become more honest with their therapists as trust is established.

The definition of accuracy, of course, deserves more concentration and attention than is possible in this brief report. One could certainly argue that a report that is accurate in 90% of the details, but wrong about the identity of the perpetrator (which did occur in at least one case), is in an important sense an entirely false accusation. Thus, the reader might find it relevant that the identity of the perpetrator was confirmed by confession in seven recovered memory cases, supported by other evidence in three cases, largely disconfirmed in two cases, and impossible to establish with any certainty in five cases.

A strong general memory factor appears to run through the data. The accuracy of recovered and continuous memory correlate at .69, $p < .01$. Further, clients were unable to remember with accuracy which of their memories had been recovered in therapy, which recovered elsewhere, and which were continuous. This was particularly true for subjects who were generally inaccurate. The finding, although unsurprising at one level given the literature on source memory (cf., Lindsay, 1994), is disturbing for professionals involved in the already complex area of assessment of the "retractors" engaged in false memory suits, since it would appear that subjects prone to misremembering their childhood might also misremember their therapy experience. In fact, a measure of the accuracy with which patients retained information about therapy topics in general (labelled Session Memory) also correlated significantly with both recovered and continuous memory accuracy (r's > .70). Accuracy in recovered and continuous memory also correlated with reality testing (r's = -.61 and -.53 respectively), as measured by the X-% on the pre-therapy Rorschach.

On a more promising note, subjects did have less confidence in the memories that turned out to be inaccurate, although for a few subjects ($n = 3$) this difference did not reach significance in early months of therapy. Subjects also had less confidence in recovered memories as a whole, whether or not they were accurate. It is unclear whether this client bias against accuracy of recovered memories is due to the memory characteristics of the recovered memories themselves, or to the flood of anecdotes that have been presented as evidence questioning this memory phenomena.

Interesting patterns also are emerging on the therapeutic circumstances in which inaccurate and accurate recovered and continuous memories occur. Briefly, Control Mastery Theory (Weiss & Sampson, 1986) would predict that information would be de-repressed, if that were the mechanism, after a therapist had passed a transference test (healing what the client thought was an overwhelming breach in the relationship). State-dependency or mood-congruency theories would suggest that recoveries would occur during the negative emotion or negative cuing periods, e.g., when the client was angry or experiencing anxiety symptoms. In three sets of sessions — sessions in which the client was experiencing extreme negative affect, a second set in which the an alliance repair occurred, and the remaining group — clients did differ in percentage of accurate and inaccurate memories recovered. Negative affect sessions were defined as the 12% of sessions in which clients reported least positive feelings toward the therapist; alliance repair sessions were either rated in the top 12% or included an event rated by the subject as an alliance repair. Of accurate recovered memories, 27% occurred in negative affect sessions and 38% in alliance repair. For the inaccurate memories, 42% occurred in negative affect sessions and 8% are in alliance repair. Thus, for sessions theoretically linked to de-repression, the base rate for accurate recovered memories was over 3 times the general rate, while the base rate for inaccurate recovered memories did not increase. In the state-dependency sessions, the rates of recovered memories in general increase.

In related work, our research team has been able to achieve stable mood state-dependency in the laboratory (Dalenberg et al., 1996), showing that the degree of state-dependency relates to the severity of physical abuse of the subject. We also find strong predictive power for tests of dissociation, finding subgroups who use dissociation "positively" to hold off the fear and produce remarkable memory, and others who use dissociation "negatively" to become immersed in the fear, producing extreme state-dependency. Both state-dependency and de-repression deserve further study as potential mechanisms for the recovered memory effect. Minimally, the possibility of accuracy in recovered memories apparently related to the therapy process is supported by the present work.

REFERENCES

Dalenberg, C. (in press). Accuracy, timing and circumstances of disclosure in therapy of recovered and continuous memories of abuse. *Psychiatry and the Law*.

Fredrickson, R. (1992). *Repressed memories: a journey to recovery from sexual abuse*. New York: Simon & Schuster.

Freyd, J. (1983). Shareability: The social psychology of epistemology. *Cognitive Science, 7*, 191–210.

Gardner, R. (1995). *Protocols for the sex-abuse evaluation*. Cresskill, N. J.: Creative Therapeutics.

Lindsay, D. (1994). Memory source monitoring and eyewitness testimony. In D. Ross, J. D. Read, and M. P. Toglia (Eds.), *Adult eyewitness testimony: Current trends and developments*. (pp. 27–55). New York: Cambridge University Press.

McConkey, K. & Kinoshita, S. (1988) The influence of hypnosis on memory after one day and one week. *Journal of Abnormal Psychology, 97*, 48–53.

Ofshe, R., & Watters, E. (1994). *Making monsters: False memories, psychotherapy, and sexual hysteria*. New York: Scribners.

Wakefield, H., & Underwager, R. (1994). *Return of the furies: An investigation into recovered memory therapy*. Chicago: Open Court.

Weiss, J., & Sampson, H. (1986). *The psychoanalytic process: Theory, clinical observations, and empirical research*. NY: Guilford Press.

Williams, L. (1995). Recovered memories of abuse in women with documented child sexual victimization histories. *Journal of Traumatic Stress, 8*, 649–674.

24

FORMS OF MEMORY RECOVERY AMONG ADULTS IN THERAPY

Preliminary Results from an In-Depth Survey

Bernice Andrews

Royal Holloway
University of London
United Kingdom

ABSTRACT

Preliminary results are reported from an in-depth survey of 100 qualified therapists with clients who had recently recovered memories in therapy with them. Therapists were questioned about their clients. Around 60% of the recovered memories involved child sexual abuse (CSA), and 40% other traumas. Over half were recovered from total amnesia, with corroborating evidence in 40% of cases. Memories involving CSA took significantly longer to recover than those involving other traumas. Vivid reliving was a common accompaniment, and fear the predominant emotion when memories were recovered.

1. INTRODUCTION

There appears to be at least some consensus between experts from different academic and clinical backgrounds on the issue of whether it is possible to recover previously forgotten memories of childhood trauma. A small but noticeable shift is discernible in the views of protagonists from both sides of the argument, with a certain degree of acknowledgement of the possibility of the other's position. For example, Ceci and Loftus (1994), who take a sceptical position, state that they believe it is possible "to lose contact with memories for long periods of time" (p. 352), and Berliner and Williams (1994) who have argued for the validity of recovered memories, concede that "some individuals, under certain conditions, may come to believe they were abused when they were not.." (p. 381). What is still at issue appears to be the degree to which false versus genuine recovered traumatic memories occur.

So far however there has been little, if any, systematic detailed study of the specific phenomenon. What little information there is on the nature of recovered traumatic memories comes indirectly from surveys of parents accused of child sex abuse (CSA) by their offspring, and directly from scientific investigations of memories of psychotherapy clients and others reporting experiences of child abuse. Surveys of false memory society members in the USA and the UK provide information about the nature of their children's allegations. In the US 39% of the allegations involved sexual abuse beginning before age 3, and 18% involved abuse of a satanic/ritual nature (Freyd, 1993). Rates reported in Gudjonsson's (in press) UK survey were lower (13% and 7% respectively) when recalculated to be comparable with the US data by Andrews (in press). It has been suggested by researchers that these features of recovered memories make them less plausible (e.g. Lindsay & Read, 1994).

Direct investigations of individuals reporting abuse in childhood mainly focus on CSA (e.g., Herman & Schatzow, 1987; Briere & Conte, 1991, and Loftus, Polonsky & Fullilove, 1994). Reported overall rates of total and partial "forgetting" of abuse at some stage in the respondent's life range from 31% (Loftus et al., 1994) to 64% (Herman & Schatzow, 1987). Only one study made explicit the distinction between partial and total forgetting, reporting a rate of 19% total amnesia and 12% partial amnesia (Loftus et al., 1994). The issue of validity has been addressed in two studies, although in one sexual abuse survivors who had forgotten all or part of the abuse were not distinguished from those who had always remembered (Herman & Schatzow, 1987). In the only study that investigated validity in cases of forgotten abuse, 46% of participants who at some stage had partially or completely forgotten the abuse reported corroborating evidence (Feldman-Summers & Pope, 1994). A further study with some bearing on the validity issue investigated documented CSA survivors and reported 38% did not recall the target abuse episode when questioned as adults. Furthermore, 16% of those who did recall the abuse reported some period of prior forgetting (Williams, 1994; 1995).

Even taking into account the varying levels of methodological sophistication, the evidence suggests that the forgetting and later retrieval of traumatic memories is likely to be a real phenomenon. Studies so far, however, have mainly concentrated on rates of forgetting CSA. There has been very little attention to issues of validity and to other types of recovered memories, and none have addressed the issue of plausibility investigated by the false memory pressure groups. In addition there does not appear to be any research into the process of memory recovery in therapy. Systematic information concerning the length of time taken to recover memories, and the accompanying emotions and behaviour, is lacking.

The current study was designed to address these issues. It was prompted by the results of a questionnaire survey of recovered memories in clinical practice, covering the experiences and attitudes of 810 practitioner members of the British Psychological Society (Andrews et al., 1995). As with other similar surveys, (e.g., Poole et al., 1995) memory recovery of past traumatic material was by no means an uncommon feature of clinical practice among these highly trained professionals; overall 36% had at least one client with a recovered traumatic memory in the year before the survey.

2. RESEARCH DESIGN

Around three-quarters of the respondents in the questionnaire survey who reported having recent recovered memory clients identified themselves as willing to take part in further research. To investigate the survey findings in greater detail we planned to carry out between 100 and 120 in-depth telephone interviews. Respondents have been selected

e as representative as possible of all in the original sample who reported having recent
overed memory clients. This preliminary report is based on the first 100 interviews car-
l out between September 1995 and May 1996. A more detailed account of the research
thod and design will be given in a subsequent paper based on all respondents in the
ly.

Prior to interview, details of what was to be covered were sent to the respondents.
ey were initially asked to provide the total number of clients seen since 1993 who had
recovered memories of CSA in therapy with them, b) recovered memories of other
uma in therapy with them, and c) recovered any trauma prior to any therapy, with sub-
uent memory recovery in therapy with them. The 100 respondents generated a total
nber of 671 clients in the above categories. They were then interviewed in detail on up
3 clients in the above memory recovery categories, ideally about one client from each
egory, with instructions to consult their notes in advance about the selected clients.
s procedure generated 217 client cases and in 60% of the cases the information was
ed on the respondent's notes. There were no significant differences in terms of the
iables reported in this chapter between cases where notes were used and cases where
y were not. The tape-recorded interviews covered among other things the features of
overed memories, the process of memory recovery, and the consequences for the cli-
s in terms of the effect on symptoms and current relationships.

RESEARCH QUESTIONS

The questions addressed in this report cover some features and selected elements of
memory recovery process. In terms of features we wanted to know (i) what types of
mories are recovered in therapy, (ii) the degree of amnesia prior to memory recovery,
l (iii) the extent to which such memories are plausible and valid. Regarding process, we
nted to know (i) how long it takes to recover memories in therapy, and (ii) what kind of
otions and behaviour accompany memory recovery.

RESULTS

l. Types of Trauma Recalled

Of the total 671 clients with recovered memories since 1993, respondents reported
t 47% recalled CSA trauma, 39% recalled other non-CSA trauma, and 14% recalled
h CSA and other trauma. To get some idea of what was involved in the memories of
er non-CSA trauma, we looked at the detailed descriptions in the 217 client cases.
ong these memories, cruelty and physical abuse in childhood constituted the largest
egory (36%), followed by traumatic medical procedures (15%). Events surrounding the
s of someone close constituted a further 13%, and another 13% involved witnessing a
th or a trauma happening to someone close. A further 7% involved war events, and 5%
accidents. A final 15% were other events that could not be easily categorised.

The rest of the results in this report are based on the 217 detailed client cases.

4.2. Are Memories Usually Recovered from Total Amnesia?

Respondents were asked whether their client's memory (or first memory in cases where there was more than one) was recovered from total amnesia, or whether the client had some prior vague sense or suspicion, or more definite partial memory, with probes for further details to back up their assertions. The rating of degree of amnesia was made by the interviewer based on the respondent's transcribed comments, on the basis of predetermined criteria for each level of forgetting. The interviewer took into account the respondent's report of what the client said in preference to the respondent's opinion. Inter-rater reliability for the scale was good (weighted kappa = .73), and differences were resolved by discussion. Over half (56%) the clients recovered memories from what was rated as total amnesia, 10% from a vague sense, and 34% already had a partial memory of the experience before recovering further memories. Degree of amnesia was not related to type of trauma.

4.3. To What Extent Are Recovered Memories Plausible and Valid?

To investigate plausibility respondents were asked the age at which the trauma was supposed to have started, whether there were any ritual or cult elements in the memories, or anything else unusual or bizarre. Only a very small proportion of clients (4%) claimed their memories were from the first year of life, with 7% claiming memories from the first 3 years. Memories of ritual cult abuse were recovered by just 11 clients (5%), and 4 of these involved human sacrifice. The only other unusual memory concerned 1 client who claimed a memory of an alien abduction.

Respondents were asked if there was any validating evidence for the memories. Overall corroboration was reported in 40% (86/217) of the client cases, and in 7 (3%) the therapist reported that he or she had actually seen the evidence. In 20% the client reported that someone else had also claimed abuse by the same person, in 17% someone else confirmed that the traumatic event had occurred. Official records confirmed the memory in 8% of cases, and in 6% an abuser confessed. Some reported corroboration from more than one source, which is why the categories sum to more than 40%.

4.4. How Long Does It Take to Recover Memories in Therapy?

The length of time to recover the first memory ranged from less than a week to 11 years, with over 90% recovered inside 2 years. We looked to see if any features of the memories or therapeutic techniques used were related to time taken to recover memories, but the only significant difference concerned the type of trauma. Memories of traumas not involving child sexual abuse took a significantly shorter time to recover than CSA traumas (Kruskall Wallis 1-way ANOVA, $X^2(2) = 11.49$, $p < .004$). The mean number of weeks to recover was 51 for CSA memories, 43 for memories involving CSA and other trauma, and 16 for other traumas.

4.5. What Emotions and Behaviour Accompany Memory Recovery?

The most common emotion observed by the respondents in their clients during recall was fear, expressed by 38%. Other emotions observed were sadness (29%), anger (13%), guilt (13%), and disgust (7%). Vivid reliving of the supposed experience was displayed by 42% of the clients, with 38% showing some reliving, and 20% no reliving. The two emotions distinguishing the reliving groups were fear and distress; nearly two thirds with vivid reliving expressed fear, compared with a third with some and 5% with none, $X^2(2) = 41.2$, $p < .001$. Distress was expressed by 26% with vivid reliving, 48% with some, and 8% with none, $X^2(2) = 21.3, p < .001$.

5. CONCLUSIONS

The results from these in-depth interviews confirm and extend our previous findings that traumatic memories recovered in therapy are not limited to those involving CSA, nor to CSA survivors. In our large scale questionnaire survey similar proportions of therapists reported at least one client recovering memories of CSA (23%) and other traumas (28%) in the previous year (Andrews et al., 1995). The present more detailed study enabled a breakdown of the proportions of actual numbers of clients seen in these categories, which also included those recovering mixed memories of CSA and other traumas.

In only a very small minority of cases were the memories highly implausible. This is at odds with the survey of the U.S. False Memory Foundation (Freyd, 1993). However, the recent British False Memory Society also showed similar small proportions (Gudjonsson, in press; Andrews, in press). One explanation for the different findings may therefore involve cultural variability in the plausibility of the content of recovered memories. Another explanation is that the respondents' clients in the current study are more representative of individuals who claim recovered memories than the accusers in the false memory society surveys. In the relevant cases, over half (55%) had not accused the alleged perpetrators or broken off contact with them.

Corroboration was reported for 40% of the memories, a proportion very similar to that found by Feldman-Summers and Pope (1994) in a direct investigation of abuse survivors. This result should be interpreted with the caution that the reports of corroboration were not collected first hand, but through the therapist. However, it is of interest that in 7 of the cases, the therapist actually saw the evidence.

The study has also illustrated the reality of memory recovery in therapy. For those of us outside therapeutic circles, it is perhaps difficult to imagine what this might entail. It often took an extended period for traumatic memories to emerge, particularly those involving CSA, regardless of whether or not a therapeutic technique was used. This, coupled with the emotion and reliving surrounding traumatic memory recovery can be contrasted with what appears to happen in experimental analogue studies involving deliberately implanted false memories. In these experiments false memories appear to be recalled fairly quickly after being implanted, without accompanying emotion and reliving experiences. This underscores the differences between phenomena generated by analogue studies and the traumatic memories, whether real or imagined, recovered in the clinic.

In conclusion, these in-depth interviews are providing systematic and detailed information about the nature, process and validity of memory recovery that would be difficult to obtain by questionnaire. At this stage of our knowledge exploratory investigations of this sort can reflect the breadth of phenomena that exist, and prevent premature focussing on one particular subset of recovered memories.

ACKNOWLEDGMENTS

The study was supported by a grant from the Economic and Social Research Council ref: ROO0236111, and was carried out in collaboration with Chris Brewin, Debra Bekerian, Graham Davies, Phil Mollon and John Morton. Special thanks are due to Jenny Ochera who carried out the interviewing, and to the therapists involved who gave so much of their precious time.

REFERENCES

Andrews, B. (in press). Can a survey of British False Memory Society members reliably inform the recovered memory debate? *Applied Cognitive Psychology.*

Andrews, B., Morton, J., Bekerian, D. A., Brewin, C. R., Davies, G. M., & Mollon, P. (1995). The recovery of memories in clinical practice: Experiences and beliefs of British Psychological Society Practitioners. *The Psychologist, 8, 5,* 209–214.

Berliner, L., & Williams, L. M. (1994). Memories of child sexual abuse: a response to Lindsay and Read. *Applied Cognitive Psychology, 8,* 379–388.

Briere, J., & Conte, J. (1993). Self-reported amnesia for abuse in adults molested as children. *Journal of Traumatic Stress, 6,* 21–31.

Ceci, S. J., & Loftus, E. F. (1994). 'Memory work': a royal road to false memories? *Applied Cognitive Psychology, 8,* 351–364.

Feldman-Summers, S., & Pope, K. S. (1994). The experience of 'forgetting' childhood abuse: a national survey of psychologists. *Journal of Consulting and Clinical Psychology, 62,* 636–639.

Freyd, P. (1993). False Memory Syndrome Foundation: Family survey results, Summer 1993.

Gudjonsson, G. H. (in press). Accusations by adults of childhood sexual abuse: A survey of the members of the British False Memory Society. *Applied Cognitive Psychology.*

Herman, J. L., & Schatzow, E. (1987). Recovery and verification of memories of childhood sexual trauma. *Psychoanalytic Psychology, 4,* 1–14.

Lindsay, D. S., & Read, J. D. (1994). Psychotherapy and memories of childhood sexual abuse: a cognitive perspective. *Applied Cognitive Psychology, 8,* 281–338.

Loftus, E. F., Polonsky, S., & Fullilove, M. (1994). Memories of childhood sexual abuse: remembering and repressing. *Psychology of Women Quarterly, 18,* 67–84.

Williams, L. M. (1994). Recall of childhood trauma: a prospective study of women's memories of childhood sexual abuse. *Journal of Consulting and Clinical Psychology, 62,* 1167–1176.

Williams, L. M. (1995). Recovered memories of abuse in women with documented child sexual abuse histories. *Journal of Traumatic Stress, 8,* 649–674.

25

TRAUMA MEMORY AND ALCOHOL ABUSE

Drinking to Forget?

Sherry H. Stewart

Dalhousie University
Halifax, Nova Scotia B3H 4J1
Canada

This chapter serves as a theoretical overview of the relationship between trauma memory and alcohol abuse. The chapter commences with a description of the cognitive symptoms of post-traumatic stress disorder (PTSD), followed by a review of the literature on the co-morbidity of PTSD and alcohol abuse/dependence. The bulk of the chapter involves a discussion of mechanisms that may account for the high co-morbidity of PTSD and alcohol disorders, with particular focus on those mechanisms involving memory. Some recommendations for future research and clinical practice are also made.

According to the *Diagnostic and Statistical Manual of Mental Disorders - Fourth Edition* (DSM-IV; American Psychiatric Association (APA), 1994), PTSD is an anxiety disorder which may develop when an individual experiences, witnesses, or confronts an event involving actual or threatened serious injury or death or a threat to the physical integrity of the self or others (e.g., combat, assault, disasters, accidents). There are several sets of symptoms characteristic of the DSM-IV diagnosis of PTSD, which can be broadly classified into four clusters: cognitive, behavioral, emotional, and physiological (Stewart, 1996). The first symptom cluster, cognitive re-experiencing of the traumatic event, is often hailed as the hallmark of the disorder. This persistent reexperiencing can take several forms, including: recurrent and intrusive distressing recollections of the event (intrusive memories); recurrent distressing dreams (nightmares); and/or acting or feeling as if the traumatic event were recurring (flashbacks). Other PTSD symptoms include avoidance of reminders of the traumatic event, emotional numbing, and autonomic hyper-arousal.

Evidence from samples of individuals exposed to a wide range of traumatic events consistently indicates a strong relationship between the diagnoses of PTSD and alcohol abuse/dependence. For example, Green, Lindy, Grace, and Leonard (1992) conducted a long-term follow-up of victims of the 1972 Buffalo Creek flood. A current PTSD diagnosis was statistically related to an alcohol abuse diagnosis, suggesting that participants who were experiencing significant flood-related PTSD symptoms were also likely to be abusing alcohol at the 14-year follow-up. Kilpatrick and Resnick (1993) reviewed data from a large national probability sample of three groups of adult women: those with PTSD who had experienced a violent crime, those without PTSD who had experienced a violent crime, and those who had not experienced a violent crime. All were assessed for the presence of alcohol problems. Those with PTSD were 3.2 times more likely than those without PTSD, and 13.7 times more likely than those not having experienced a crime, to report serious alcohol problems. Thus, those who were exposed to crime and who displayed extreme emotional distress following the crime (i.e., those with PTSD) appeared at highest risk for experiencing major alcohol problems. The majority of research on the relationship between PTSD and alcoholism has been conducted with combat veterans. For example, McFall, Mackay, and Donovan (1992) compared scores on a measure of alcohol abuse problems in a sample of combat-exposed Vietnam veterans and a sample of Vietnam-era veterans who had not been assigned combat duty. No significant differences in severity of alcohol problems were found between the two groups. However, combat veterans with PTSD scored significantly higher overall on the alcohol abuse measure than did combat veterans without PTSD, suggesting greater levels of problem drinking in the PTSD group. Moreover, among the combat-exposed subjects, problem drinking scores were significantly positively correlated with the severity of PTSD symptoms.

In sum, exposure to a wide variety of traumatic events appears to be associated with heightened levels of alcohol abuse. Although some studies provide support for the notion that indices of trauma severity are positively associated with levels of alcohol abuse (Stewart, 1996), even more convincing is the evidence that adverse psychological response to the trauma (i.e., PTSD) may mediate the relationship between trauma exposure and alcohol abuse. PTSD symptom severity appears more highly associated with alcohol abuse than does exposure to trauma or severity of trauma exposure per se (Stewart, 1996).

If the two disorders are causally related, at least two potential pathways may explain the high degree of co-occurrence of PTSD and alcohol abuse/dependence (Stewart, 1996). First, alcohol abuse might heighten the susceptibility to the development of PTSD. Chronic alcohol abuse might increase anxiety and arousal levels through psychological or physiological processes. These effects could serve to induce a hyper-aroused state in which the individual may be more vulnerable to developing PTSD following exposure to a traumatic event. Alternatively, PTSD might be involved in the development of alcohol abuse. Some patients with PTSD might begin abusing alcohol in an attempt to reduce or control (i.e., self-medicate for) their PTSD symptoms. However, it is also possible that there is no direct causal relation between PTSD and alcohol abuse; instead, the two disorders may tend to co-occur simply because both are caused by some third variable, yet to be identified. For example, it could be speculated that poor coping skills might simultaneously increase risk for the development of both PTSD and alcohol abuse, following exposure to a traumatic event.

Several studies have examined the relative order of onset of the co-morbid diagnoses of PTSD and alcoholism, and patients' perceptions of the relationship between their two problems, in attempts to assess the direction of causality. For example, in a large community sample of women who were both sexually assaulted and diagnosed with alcohol abuse/dependence, drinking problems were said to have developed following the assault in every case (Winfield, George, Swartz, & Blazer, 1990). Similarly, in a sample of adolescent alcoholics, Clark and Jacob (1992) found that in the large majority of the PTSD cases (over three-quarters), the PTSD was reported to have developed before the alcohol disorder. These authors also queried the co-morbid PTSD-alcohol abusing adolescents about their perceptions regarding the functional interplay between their PTSD symptoms and drinking problems. In the large majority of cases, the adolescents reported that they perceived that their anxiety disorder was causally linked to the later development of their alcohol abuse problems. Thus, initial results on chronological patterns and perceived relationships provide evidence that PTSD may contribute to the later development of alcohol disorders.

Some researchers have examined the patterns of drinking behaviour in PTSD patients to better understand potential functional relations. For example, Hyer, Leach, Boudewyns, and Davis (1991) examined the typical drinking patterns of Vietnam veterans with alcoholism as a function of the presence or absence of concomitant PTSD. Consistent with the reported clinical impression that PTSD patients tend to drink in an episodic fashion, the PTSD group was found to display higher rates of binge drinking. Although Hyer et al. (1991) speculated that the episodic heavy drinking of PTSD veterans may coincide with periods of intrusive PTSD symptoms, no research has yet examined whether heavy drinking episodes actually overlap in time with PTSD symptoms.

If co-morbid patients do indeed begin drinking in an attempt to reduce or eliminate their PTSD symptoms, there are several potential mechanisms that might account for these effects. It has been variously suggested that alcohol abuse in PTSD patients might represent attempts to control the physiological, behavioral, affective, and/or cognitive symptoms of PTSD. For example, it has been proposed that sexually abused alcoholic women may drink to reduce their avoidance of sexual activity (i.e., a reminder of the trauma; Skorina & Kovach, 1986).

Since intrusive cognitive symptoms are often hailed as PTSD's hallmark, abusive drinking to self-medicate in PTSD patients may involve attempts to control one or more of their cognitive reexperiencing symptoms (e.g., intrusive memories of the trauma, nightmares, flashbacks). Preliminary results do support the notion that alcohol abuse in patients with PTSD may represent an attempt to dampen intrusive cognitive symptoms. For example, in the study by McFall et al. (1992) of veterans exposed to combat, degree of cognitive reexperiencing of the trauma was positively correlated with degree of alcohol related problems. However, these data are correlational and thus do not establish a causal connection between cognitive re-experiencing and alcohol abuse. Some indirect evidence for the efficacy of alcohol in controlling intrusive cognitive symptoms comes from research on the effects of the structurally and functionally similar benzodiazepines (see Stewart, Pihl, & Padjen, 1992) in the treatment of PTSD. For example, Loewenstein, Hornstein, and Farber (1988) report that clonazepam treatment of post-traumatic stress symptoms reduces nightmares and flashbacks.

In a series of case studies of co-morbid PTSD-alcoholic patients, LaCoursiere, Godfrey, and Ruby (1980) noted that these patients drank excessively just prior to bed, reportedly to control sleep disturbances and nightmares. LaCoursiere et al. (1980) postulated that alcohol abuse in patients with PTSD may serve to suppress rapid eye movement (REM) sleep and its associated nightmares, and that the abuse of alcohol in such patients should escalate as tolerance to the REM-suppressant effects of alcohol develops over time. However, traumatic nightmares are not confined to REM sleep (Kramer, Schoen, & Kinney, 1984). Therefore, alcohol's suppression of REM sleep may eliminate some, but not all, nightmares. Failure to succeed in eliminating their nightmares completely may serve to promote heavier drinking in PTSD patients (Stewart, 1996). LaCoursiere et al. (1980) suggested that alcohol use in PTSD might also serve to block intrusive traumatic memories during the waking state.

Researchers have begun to utilize paradigms adapted from experimental cognitive psychology to investigate information processing biases in PTSD patients — biases which may be relevant to explaining the cognitive reexperiencing symptoms characteristic of

PTSD. First, an attentional bias favouring the processing of trauma-related information has been repeatedly demonstrated in patients with PTSD but not controls (e.g., McNally, English, & Lipke, 1993; see also Creamer, this volume). Such findings, using attentional interference tests such as the Stroop colour-naming task, suggest that trauma-related information selectively captures and holds the attention of PTSD patients. It has been proposed that such attentional biases toward trauma-related cues reflect activation of a traumatic memory network (McNally et al., 1993). It is interesting to speculate that alcohol might serve to eliminate this hyper-vigilance toward trauma-related cues in individuals with PTSD, thus providing negative reinforcement for drinking behaviour in this group. Although no research has specifically examined the effects of alcohol consumption on information processing biases in PTSD, a study conducted with analogue anxious students by our research group suggests that alcohol may be an effective agent in reducing anxious subjects' selective attention to threat (Stewart, Achille, Dubois-Nguyen, & Pihl, 1992). The degree to which such findings are applicable to explaining the PTSD-alcohol abuse overlap remains to be established.

In addition, the notion that information about trauma is primed in memory in PTSD has been evaluated more directly using memory paradigms derived from experimental cognitive psychology. Research in this area has used memory tasks such as cued recall to assess relative memory for trauma-relevant versus trauma-irrelevant material in patients with PTSD and controls. Work with such memory tests has demonstrated enhanced memory for trauma-related material in patients with PTSD (see review by McNally, 1994). Although no work to date has yet evaluated this possibility, it might be speculated that alcohol consumption could serve to reduce the memory bias for trauma-relevant material characteristic of PTSD patients. Given much basic science evidence that alcohol impairs human "explicit memory" abilities (e.g., Lister, Gorenstein, Risher-Flowers, Weingartner, & Eckardt, 1991), it might be hypothesized that patients with PTSD may be motivated to drink to reduce their conscious recollection of trauma-relevant material (i.e., a cognitive avoidance strategy). However, this diminished awareness of traumatic memories might be achieved at the cost of a general reduction in their overall memory abilities.

Once abusive drinking is established in PTSD patients, its maintenance could be viewed through the framework of memory network theories of alcohol abuse. One such theory (Baker, Morse, & Sherman, 1987) proposes that alcohol urges or cravings are organized at a cognitive level within a memory network that encodes information on alcohol use eliciting cues, and drug-related responses such as verbal reports of cravings and drug-procurement behaviours. Stimulus information encoded within this type of urge network for alcoholic patients with PTSD might include internal symptoms such as intrusive cognitive symptoms, and/or external stimuli such as events that serve as reminders of the initial traumatic event (Stewart, 1996). This memory network should be activated by exposure to reminders of the trauma, or by the experience of PTSD symptoms such as intrusive memories of the trauma. The responses produced by the activation of this network would include alcohol-seeking behaviour and self-reports of urges or cravings to drink in alcohol abusing patients with PTSD. Researchers have begun to test predictions made by such memory network theories. For example, we recently used a Stroop task in an analogue sample of alcohol misusers to test the prediction that exposure to eliciting cues should lead to enhanced processing of alcohol cues, if alcohol cues are indeed stored in the memory of the alcohol misuser along with eliciting cues (Samoluk & Stewart, 1995). Similar cognitive methods could be used to examine whether alcohol information is stored along with hypothesized triggers (e.g., trauma cues) in the memories of PTSD-alcohol abusing patients.

Alternatively or in addition to the self-medicating role of alcohol abuse in PTSD are notions that alcohol might increase susceptibility to PTSD or worsen PTSD symptoms following exposure to a traumatic event. For example, Greenstein, Kitchner, and Olsen (1986) have suggested that alcohol intoxication-induced disinhibition may contribute to flashbacks and nightmares in patients with PTSD. Similarly, LaCoursiere et al. (1980) have noted that long-term heavy use of alcohol may significantly exacerbate some PTSD symptoms. LaCoursiere et al. (1980) have also commented on the role of the well-known alcohol withdrawal effects that emerge following prolonged drinking. They noted that after chronic use of alcohol, attempts to discontinue this self-medication often lead to an exacerbation of the initial PTSD symptoms. Given the similarities between certain alcohol withdrawal symptoms and PTSD symptoms (e.g., autonomic over-arousal and sleep difficulties) it is possible that PTSD patients misinterpret alcohol withdrawal symptoms as signs of anxiety or that these symptoms serve as reminders of the traumatic event, thereby further increasing arousal levels and motivating continued alcohol consumption.

In conclusion, it appears that a single unidirectional pathway to explain the overlap between PTSD and alcohol abuse is unlikely to be found. Instead it seems possible that both self-medication, and alcohol intoxication- or withdrawal-induced intensification of PTSD symptoms, contribute to the high degree of co-morbidity between alcohol abuse and PTSD diagnoses. Although preliminary evidence suggests that the initial motivation for abusive drinking in patients with PTSD is the relief of intrusive PTSD symptoms, alcohol intoxication and/or withdrawal effects could serve to heighten anxiety in the long run, motivating further heavy drinking to dampen emerging symptoms. Thus, a vicious cycle may be at play in which one disorder sustains the other.

Clearly, additional research on the nature of the relationship between traumatic memory and alcohol abuse is required. First, it remains to be determined whether the experience of intrusive cognitive symptoms actually precedes and motivates drinking binges in PTSD patients. Correlational studies (e.g., McFall et al., 1992) should be supplemented with prospective studies involving patients' monitoring of their intrusive cognitive symptoms in relation to their alcohol use patterns. It also remains to be determined whether alcohol consumption reduces PTSD patients' selective attention, and/or selective memory, for trauma-related cues. These possibilities could be investigated in future by combining selective attention paradigms, such as the Stroop task, and/or selective memory paradigms, such as cued recall of word lists, with the alcohol challenge method in which patients and controls are administered alcohol or placebo (Stewart et al., 1992). These methods could be used to determine whether those PTSD patients administered alcohol show dampening of their sober tendencies to selectively attend to and remember trauma-relevant information. Moreover, the applicability of memory network models to the understanding of the PTSD-alcoholism overlap also remains to be determined. For example, it would be interesting to study whether priming of trauma-related concepts in the memories of PTSD patients leads to selective processing of alcohol related cues, self-reports of alcohol urges/cravings, and/or increased drinking in the lab. Each of these hypotheses could be tested by using McNally, Litz, Prassas, Shin, and Weathers' (1994) method for priming trauma-related concepts in memory, in which patients are exposed to trauma-relevant or trauma-irrelevant videos. This memory priming manipulation could be followed by examination of selective attention for alcohol cues (e.g., using the Stroop task; Creamer, this volume), urges to drink (e.g., using self-report measures of alcohol urges/cravings; Rankin, Hodgson, & Stockwell, 1979), and/or actual drinking behaviour (e.g., using an unobtrusive laboratory-based measure of alcohol consumption; Samoluk & Stewart, 1996).

A number of recommendations for clinical practice also follow from this review. In terms of assessment, when conducting assessments with alcohol abusers, clinicians should always be careful to query about possible exposure to trauma and possible PTSD symptoms. Conversely, when patients present with a history of trauma exposure or PTSD symptoms, clinicians must carefully assess for the potential presence of alcohol abuse (see also Courtois, this volume).

In terms of treatment, both alcohol abuse and PTSD symptoms need to be a focus in therapy. Unfortunately, many anxiety disorder clinicians assume that the motivation for alcohol abuse will subside with successful treatment of the PTSD symptoms. However, independent of etiological factors, once the abusive drinking has begun, the alcohol disorder may take on a life of its own, making drinking discontinuation difficult even after successful PTSD symptom management. Similarly, many substance abuse clinicians focus on treating the alcohol problem while overlooking the PTSD symptoms. However, if the PTSD symptoms are not treated, the patient may experience a reemergence or intensification of PTSD symptoms following sobriety or during detoxificiation, and may again turn to alcohol for temporary symptom relief. Knowledge that these patients tend to drink heavily in an episodic fashion can allow the clinician to assist these patients in identifying high-risk situations that trigger their drinking and to educate them in the use of alternative coping strategies to deal with these situations when they occur (Hyer et al., 1991). Clinicians should also be aware that given the similarity of some alcohol withdrawal symptoms to PTSD symptoms, withdrawal effects such as anxiety, insomnia, and "REM-rebound" (an excess of REM sleep), may present particular difficulties for co-morbid patients attempting to discontinue alcohol abuse (Schnitt & Nocks, 1984). Alcohol intake should be gradually tapered, and patients prepared for withdrawal using psychoeducational and cognitive-behavioral techniques (Stewart, 1996).

REFERENCES

American Psychiatric Association. (1994). *Diagnostic and statistical manual of mental disorders (4th ed.).* Washington, DC: Author.

Baker, T. B., Morse, E., & Sherman, J. E. (1987). The motivation to use drugs: A psychobiological analysis of urges. In P. C. Rivers (Ed.), *The Nebraska Symposium on Motivation: Alcohol use and abuse* (pp. 257–323). Lincoln: University of Nebraska Press.

Clark, D. B., & Jacob, R. G. (1992). Anxiety disorders in 30 adolescents with alcohol abuse and dependence [Summary], *Alcoholism: Clinical and Experimental Research, 16,* 371.

Green, B. L., Lindy, J. D., Grace, M. C., & Leonard, A. C. (1992). Chronic post-traumatic stress disorder and diagnostic co-morbidity in a disaster sample. *Journal of Nervous and Mental Disease, 180,* 760–766.

Greenstein, R. A., Kitchner, I., & Olsen, K. (1986). Post-traumatic stress disorder, partial complex seizures, and alcoholism. *American Journal of Psychiatry, 143,* 1203.

Hyer, L., Leach, P., Boudewyns, P. A., & Davis, H. (1991). Hidden post-traumatic stress disorder in substance abuse inpatients among Vietnam veterans. *Journal of Substance Abuse Treatment, 8,* 213–219.

Kramer, M., Schoen, L. S., & Kinney, L. (1984). The dream experience in dream-disturbed Vietnam veterans. In B. A. van der Kolk (Ed.), *Post-traumatic stress disorder: Psychological and biological sequelae* (pp. 82–95). Washington, DC: American Psychiatric Press.

LaCoursiere, R. B., Godfrey, K. E., & Ruby, L. M. (1980). Traumatic neurosis in the etiology of alcoholism: Vietnam and other trauma. *American Journal of Psychiatry, 137,* 966–968.

Lister, R. G., Gorenstein, C., Risher-Flowers, D., Weingartner, H. J., & Eckardt, M. J. (1991). Dissociation of the acute effects of alcohol on implicit and explicit memory processes. *Neuropsychologia, 29,* 1205–1212.

Loewenstein, R. J., Hornstein, N, & Farber, B. (1988). Open trial of clonazepam in the treatment of post-traumatic stress symptoms in MPD. *Dissociation, 1,* 3–12.

McFall, M. E., Mackay, P. W., & Donovan, D. M. (1992). Combat-related post-traumatic stress disorder and severity of substance abuse in Vietnam veterans. *Journal of Studies on Alcohol, 53,* 357–363.

McNally, R. J. (1994). *Panic disorder: A critical analysis*. New York: Guilford Press.

McNally, R. J., English, G. E., & Lipke, H. J. (1993). Assessment of intrusive cognition in post-traumatic stress disorder: Use of the modified Stroop paradigm. *Journal of Traumatic Stress, 6*, 33–41.

McNally, R. J., Litz, B. T., Prassas, A., Shin, L. M., & Weathers, F. W. (1994). Emotional priming of autobiographical memory in post-traumatic stress disorder. *Cognition and Emotion, 8*, 351–367.

Rankin, H., Hodgson, R., & Stockwell, T. (1979). The concept of craving and its measurement. *Behaviour Research and Therapy, 17*, 389–396.

Samoluk, S. B., & Stewart, S. H. (1995). Attentional bias for alcohol cues as a function of food deprivation and anxiety sensitivity [Summary]. *Convention proceedings for the 29th annual meeting of the Association for Advancement of Behaviour Therapy*, 246.

Samoluk, S. B., & Stewart, S. H. (1996). Anxiety sensitivity and anticipation of self-disclosing speech as determinants of alcohol consumption. *Psychology of Addictive Behaviour, 10*, 45–54.

Schnitt, J. M., & Nocks, J. J. (1984). Alcoholism treatment of Vietnam veterans with post-traumatic stress disorder. *Journal of Substance Abuse Treatment, 1*, 179–189.

Skorina, J. K., & Kovach, J. A. (1986). Treatment techniques for incest-related issues in alcoholic women. *Alcoholism Treatment Quarterly, 3*, 17–30.

Stewart, S. H. (1996). Alcohol abuse in individuals exposed to trauma: A critical review. *Psychological Bulletin, 120*, 83–112.

Stewart, S. H., Achille, M., Dubois-Nguyen, I., & Pihl, R. O. (1992). Alcohol effects on selective attention for threat in anxiety sensitive females [Summary]. *Pharmacology, Biochemistry, and Behaviour, 38*, 309.

Stewart, S. H., Pihl, R. O., & Padjen, A. L. (1992). Chronic use of alcohol and/or benzodiazepines may account for evidence of altered benzodiazepine receptor sensitivity in panic disorder. *Archives of General Psychiatry, 49*, 329–330.

26

IMPLICIT MEMORY, INTERPERSONALITY AMNESIA, AND DISSOCIATIVE IDENTITY DISORDER

Comparing Patients with Simulators

Eric Eich,[1] Dawn Macaulay,[1] Richard J. Loewenstein,[2] and Patrice H. Dihle[3]

[1]University of British Columbia
2136 West Mall
Vancouver, BC V6T 1Y7
Canada
[2]Sheppard Pratt Hospital
[3]Way Station, Frederick, Maryland

Dissociative identity disorder (DID) involves the presence of two or more distinct personality states or identities that recurrently take control of an individual's behavior (see DSM-IV; American Psychiatric Association, 1994). From one DID patient to the next, these identities can vary tremendously in number, complexity, and frequency of emergence, as well as in such fundamental features as age, gender, handedness, and emotional complexion. In general, however, they can be construed as "highly discrete states of consciousness organized around a prevailing affect, sense of self (including body image), with a limited repertoire of behaviors and a set of state dependent memories" (Putnam, 1989, p.103).

Given this definition, one might expect that events experienced in a particular personality state or identity would be more retrievable in the same state than in a different one (see Schacter & Kihlstrom, 1989). In support of this supposition, evidence of interpersonality amnesia was secured in 98 of the 100 DID cases surveyed by Putnam, Guroff, Silberman, Barban, and Post (1986). Less predictably, and hence of greater theoretical interest, is the observation that interpersonality amnesia is more often revealed when memory for past events is assessed using explicit as opposed to implicit measures of retention.

To clarify, consider a seminal study by Nissen, Ross, Willingham, MacKenzie, and Schacter (1988) involving a 45-year-old woman with 22 secondary personality states. One identity claimed to have direct awareness of the core or primary personality and of all the other 21 alternate identities; three reported that they occasionally received "advice" from several of the alternates; and the remaining 18 were densely amnesic for all experiences except their own. Nissen et al. concentrated on eight mutually amnesic identities that could be elicited upon request. The basic strategy was to have one identity study a set of to-be-remembered or target items, and then test either the same or a different identity's retention of these items.

Nissen et al. carried out a series of experiments representing a broad range of target items and retention tests—some explicit in nature, others implicit. The former included tests (specifically free recall and old/new recognition memory) that require deliberate, conscious recollection of past experience, whereas the latter included tests (such as perceptual identification or word-fragment completion) that assess transfer or priming from past experience on tasks that do not demand conscious recollection for their performance (see Roediger, 1990; Schacter, 1987).

Consistent with the patient's clinical presentation, items that had been studied by one identity could not be explicitly recalled or recognized by anyone other than that personality. In contrast, the results of several implicit tests provided evidence of interpersonality priming—the antithesis of interpersonality amnesia. Thus, for example, when the identity called Charles was asked to name words that were briefly flashed on a screen, he was able to correctly identify 75% of the words that had previously been shown to Donna, but only 45% of the words that neither he, she, nor any other identity had seen before. By the same token, having Alice study the word horizon made it easier for Bonnie to solve the fragment h_r_z_n. Thus, the implicit assessment of memory was a necessary condition for demonstrating transfer of information from one identity to another.

Results of a similar sort were obtained in a recent study by Eich, Macaulay, Loewenstein, and Dihle (1997) using an implicit test of picture fragment completion. Culled from norms published by Snodgrass and her associates (Snodgrass & Corwin, 1988; Snodgrass & Vanderwart, 1980), the materials for this test consisted of 20 decks of index cards, each deck comprising 8 cards, and each card carrying a more-or-less complete drawing of a common object (such as a barn). Card 1 in a given deck was the least detailed depiction of the object, offering little more than a few unconnected lines or swiggles. Card 2 provided a bit more visual detail, Card 3 even more, and so on through Card 8 which depicted the object in its most complete—and, hence, readily identifiable—form. The 20 decks were divided into four comparable sets of five pictures each (coded as Picture Sets W, X, Y, and Z).

Participants in the Eich et al. (1997) study were seven DID patients, each of whom was able to alternate, upon the experimenter's nonhypnotic request, between two secondary identities or personality states (designated as P1 and P2), each claiming to have no conscious awareness of the other's experiences.

During the first phase of the study, a clinician (either RJL or PHD) introduced the experimenter (either EE or DM) to the patient's core or primary personality. After reviewing the study's aims and methods, the experimenter obtained the patient's informed consent to participate in accordance with Putnam's (1984) guidelines.

To start the second phase, the patient's primary personality was asked to "step back" so that P1—the first of the patient's two self-selected, mutually amnesic secondary identities—could "come forward" and take control over consciousness and behavior. P1 was then asked to perform a series of tasks, one of which included a test of picture fragment completion involving a total of 10 objects (e.g., a random arrangement of Picture Sets X and Y). The eight cards representing a given object were displayed one at a time in numerical sequence (i.e., from least to most detailed). P1 was asked to look at a card for about 5 sec and, if possible, name the object; guesses were allowed and any incorrect responses were acknowledged as such before the next card in the sequence was shown. The score for a given object equalled the number of cards that had to be seen before the object could be identified; the lower the score, the less detail needed for accurate naming.

In the third phase, P1 stepped back and P2 came forward. Because P2, by definition, claimed not to share conscious experiences with P1, it was necessary to repeat in full the instructions for the picture fragment test. P2 then proceeded to identify 10 objects, following the procedures outlined above. Of these 10 objects, 5 had been previously identified by P1 (e.g., objects in Picture Set W) and 5 were new (e.g., objects in Picture Set Y).

In the fourth and final phase of the study, P2 departed and P1 returned to undertake another series of tasks, including a second round of picture fragment completion. P1 identified a total of 15 objects; of these, 5 had been previously identified by P1 (e.g., Picture Set X), 5 had been identified by P2 (e.g., Picture Set Y), and five were new (e.g., Picture Set Z).

Mean scores for picture fragment completion are depicted in Figure 1 as a function of study/test identity and trial, where "study identity" means which personality state—either P1 or P2—identified a given set of objects initially (on Trial 1) and "test identity" means which personality state identified the same set of objects subsequently (on Trial 2). A 2x3 repeated-measures analysis revealed robust evidence of repetition priming: Having identified a given object on Trial 1, the patients needed to see significantly less pictorial detail in order to do so again on Trial 2 ($F(1/6) = 75.87$, $p < .01$). There was no reliable effect of study/test identity, either alone or in combination with trial ($Fs < 1$), suggesting that priming was as strong between different personality states (P1/P2 or P2/P1) as it was within the same state (P1/P1). Thus, even though P2 claimed to have no conscious or explicit memory of P1's actions, and disavowed ever having done a test of picture fragment completion before, P2's test performance was facilitated by P1's prior test experience. Similarly, objects that had been initially identified by P2 were more readily identified by P1, despite the purported absence of awareness between the two personality states.

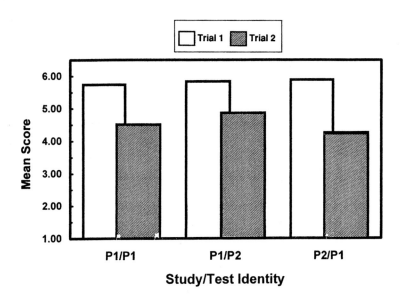

Figure 1. Mean scores in test of picture fragment completion as a function of study/test identity and trial. Source: Eich et al., 1997.

Though our results replicate and extend those reported by Nissen et al. (1988), they leave many intriguing questions unanswered. One is whether the memory performance of DID patients can be reproduced by normal subjects attempting to mimic "multiplicity" (see Schacter, Kihlstrom, Kihlstrom, & Berren, 1989; Silberman, Putnam, Weingartner, Braun, & Post, 1985). More specifically, does repetition priming in picture fragment completion occur between as well as within simulated personality states or identities?

To find out, we recently repeated the test procedures reviewed above with a sample of nine simulator subjects: Mental-health professionals (psychiatrists, psychologists, social workers, dance therapists, etc.) who interact with DID patients on a regular (usually daily) basis. Though every simulator was intimately acquainted with the phenomenology and clinical nuances of DID, none had any formal background in, or detailed knowledge of, contemporary cognitive research and theory on implicit memory. Every simulator was asked (a) draw on his or her own clinical knowledge and professional experience in creating two mutually amnesic DID-like identities (P1 and P2), (b) assume a particular personality state upon the experimenter's request, (c) remain in that state while working on the test of picture fragment completion, and (d) perform the test the way they think "real" DID patients would.

The results are shown in Figure 2. Like the patients, the simulators revealed reliable priming within the same personality state: Objects identified by simulated P1 states on Trial 1 were more readily identified by the same simulated states on Trial 2 ($F(1/8) = 74.34$, $p < .01$). Unlike the patients, however, the simulators showed no significant priming between different personality states: The fact that one simulated state (either P1 or P2) had identified a given object on Trial 1 did not make it easier for the other simulated state to do so again on Trial 2 ($Fs(1/8) < 1.20$, $ps > .10$).

Why did the simulators fail to exhibit evidence of interpersonality priming? Based on extensive postexperimental questioning of the subjects, we think the answer is that when the simulators switched from one personality state to the other (from P1 to P2 or vice versa), they tried to act as if they had not seen a given object before, when in fact they had. Their reasoning was that since P1 and P2 were supposed to be mutually amnesic, the perceptual knowl-

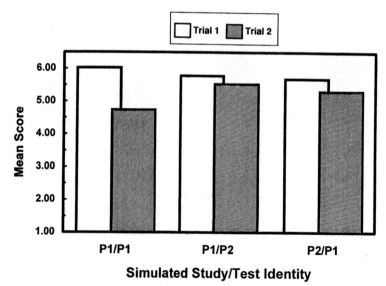

Figure 2. Mean scores in test of picture fragment completion as a function of simulated study/test identity and trial.

edge acquired by one identity neither should nor would carry over to the other identity. Provided that the simulators could keep track of "who" had seen "what," they were successful at showing priming within but not between their sham identities.

Though the present results are suggestive of a qualitative difference in the implicit memory performance of DID patients versus simulators, they should be interpreted with utmost caution. About all that can be said at this point is that, whatever else is going on in DID, interpersonality amnesia does not seem to be simply a matter of deliberate response suppression. Were that the case, no test of retention—including picture fragment completion—would show signs of "leakage" across alternate personality states. Importantly, however, our results do not speak to the reality of DID—one of the most complex, controversial, and emotionally charged issues confronting modern psychiatry (see Lilienfeld, 1995; Schacter, 1996; Spanos, 1994)—nor were they meant to. Moreover, it remains to be seen whether the pattern of implicit memory performance that we observed is specific to DID, or whether emerges in connection with other psychiatric conditions as well. By way of illustration, it is possible that just as the present sample of DID patients (but not the simulators) showed priming in picture fragment completion when they switched between their alternate identities, so too might patients with bipolar affective illness evince priming in the same task when they shift from mania into depression, or vice versa (see Eich, Macaulay, & Lam, 1997). Just how real or remote this possibility is remains to be seen in future studies.

ACKNOWLEDGMENTS

Preparation of this article was aided by a grant (MH48502) from the National Institute of Mental Health to the first author.

REFERENCES

American Psychiatric Association (1994). *Diagnostic and statistical manual of mental disorders, 4th edition* (1994). Washington, DC: American Psychiatric Association.

Eich, E., Macaulay, D., & Lam, R. (1997). Mania, depression, and mood dependent memory. *Cognition and Emotion* (in press).

Eich, E., Macaulay, D., Loewenstein, R.J., & Dihle, P.D. (1997). Memory, amnesia, and multiple personality disorder. (submitted for publication).

Lilienfeld, S.O. (1995). Is multiple personality disorder a distinct syndrome? In S.O. Lilienfeld, *Seeing both sides: Classic controversies in abnormal psychology* (pp.170–172 & 193–195). Pacific Grove, CA: Brooks/Cole.

Nissen, M.J., Ross, J.L., Willingham, D.B., MacKenzie, T.B., & Schacter, D.L. (1988). Memory and awareness in a patient with multiple personality disorder. *Brain and Cognition, 8*, 21–38.

Putnam, F.W. (1984). The study of multiple personality disorder: General strategies and practical considerations. *Psychiatric Annals, 14*, 58–61.

Putnam, F.W. (1989). *Diagnosis and treatment of multiple personality disorder.* New York: Guilford Press.

Putnam, F.W., Guroff, J.J., Silberman, E.K., Barban, L., & Post, R.M. (1986). The clinical phenomenology of multiple personality disorder: Review of 100 recent cases. *Journal of Clinical Psychiatry, 47*, 285–293.

Roediger, H.L. (1990). Implicit memory: Retention without remembering. *American Psychologist, 45*, 1043–1056.

Schacter, D.L. (1987). Implicit memory: History and current status. Journal of Experimental Psychology: *Learning, Memory, and Cognition, 13*, 501–518.

Schacter, D.L. (1996). *Searching for memory: The brain, the mind, and the past.* New York: Basic Books.

Schacter, D.L., & Kihlstrom, J.F. (1989). Functional amnesia. In F. Boller & J. Grafman (Eds.), *Handbook of neuropsychology*, Volume 3 (pp.209–230). New York: Elsevier.

Schacter, D.L., Kihlstrom, J.F., Kihlstrom, L.C., & Berren, M.B. (1989). Autobiographical memory in a case of multiple personality disorder. *Journal of Abnormal Psychology, 98*, 508–514.

Silberman, E.K., Putnam, F.W., Weingartner, H., Braun, B.G., & Post, R.M. (1985). Dissociative states in multiple personality disorder: A quantitative study. *Psychiatry Research, 15,* 253–260.

Snodgrass, J.G., & Corwin, J. (1988). Perceptual identification thresholds for 150 fragmented pictures from the Snodgrass and Vanderwart picture set. *Perceptual and Motor Skills, 67,* 3–36.

Snodgrass, J.G., & Vanderwart, M. (1980). A standardized set of 260 pictures: Norms for naming, agreement, familiarity, and visual complexity. *Journal of Experimental Psychology: Human Learning and Memory, 6,* 174–215.

Spanos, N.P. (1994). Multiple identity enactments and multiple personality disorder: A sociocognitive perspective. *Psychological Bulletin, 116,* 143–165.

27

TRAUMA, MEMORY, AND CATHARSIS

Anthropological Observations on a Folk-Psychological Construct

Michael G. Kenny

Simon Fraser University
Burnaby, BC V5A 1S6
Canada

My interest in catharsis and memory derives from previous research on the cultural history of "multiple personality" in America (Kenny, 1986). In its latest clinical incarnation multiplicity finds a place in the DSM-IV under the heading of Dissociative Identity Disorder. The presence of amnesias "too extensive to be explained by ordinary forgetfulness" is integral to the diagnosis, while "dissociation" figures large in contemporary theorising about the relation between trauma and forgetting. Powerful dysphoric emotion is believed to create disjunctions between consciousness and memory, even to the point of splitting the self into mutually unaware fragments.

But "emotion" is an ambiguous concept. It seemingly refers to passively registered bodily experience, yet emotions cannot be meaningfully discussed without reference to the objects and situations that elicit them. "Emotions" therefore embody meaning and, whatever else they may be, are culturally conditioned *social facts*. "Fear," "anger," and "grief" may be passions, but they are also words, parts of a language. Languages differ from one another, and languages change; therefore we find different languages of emotion, different logics, different performance criteria between cultures and in historically continuous societies at different times.

Our current debates about the relation between trauma and memory are based on propositions about human nature that find one practical expression in psychotherapy. Abreacting or assimilating dissociated emotion is commonly seen as essential in cancelling the pathogenic effects of traumatic memory through a process akin to grieving. This metaphorical extension of a concept derived from bereavement exemplifies the social construction of emotion (Harré, 1986).

Three ethnographic examples illustrate the ideas above. The first, drawn from an 18th century theological dispute in the New England colonies of British North America, pertains to the distinction between "true" and "false" sentiment, an issue of relevance even now. This case (one not involving memory) arose in a religious context strongly influ-

Recollections of Trauma, edited by Read and Lindsay
Plenum Press, New York, 1997

enced by the medical knowledge of the day. My second example is Anna O., Josef Breuer's famous patient so important in the history of psychoanalysis; here the concept of "catharsis" moves to the fore, and I offer observations about how and why a conception derived from the Aristotelian theory of drama took on the connotations it now has, connotations related to my third and final example—present-day theories concerning the relation between dissociated emotion and memory. In this last instance I consider the nature of the therapeutic process via reflections on grief work.

In the early 1740s Connecticut and Massachusetts were seized by a spirit of unusual religious solemnity. Itinerant preachers urged the gathering of reborn congregations and the shunning of unregenerate local pastors. Shoutings, faintings, visions, and convulsions accompanied this wave of spiritual renewal. Historians call it "The Great Awakening," an important phase in the emergence of a distinctly American Protestant religiosity. However, not everyone saw it as an awakening *then*; many interpreted it as a threat to the public order, a Satanic delusion, and the mistaking of medical problems for spiritual insight. It boiled down to an argument about the well-springs of passion.

If a person is overcome by emotion, how is its source to be judged? Calvinist predestinarian theology maintained that, being fallen creatures, redemption or damnation is in God's hands, not our own. Therefore, if we have truly been elected to salvation, the emotional and sometimes visionary experiences accompanying conversion are necessarily of *external* divine origins; if we are merely deluded about the source of our emotional experiences, then it is most probably because of spiritual arrogance or physical weakness, a disturbance of the animal spirits, a mistake. The only way to know for reasonably sure is to see if those reporting or displaying signs of conversion actually lead a changed life.

Opposing views about the spiritual significance of the Awakening were enunciated with great force and clarity by Jonathan Edwards, pastor of the Church of Christ in Northampton, Massachusetts, and Charles Chauncy, pastor of the First Church of Christ in Boston. Edwards's flock had experienced the awakening, and he was a first-hand witness to its effects; he was also philosophically articulate, well able to deploy contemporary British philosophy in his cause. Chauncy was a skeptic who thought that many of the phenomena going on round about him were of not very high order, and that Edwards's philosophical musings were mere casuistry.

These men were well attuned to the mechanical philosophy of their time, of which human physiology was a part. The problem for them both was to untangle what is due to genuine spirituality, what due to disorders of the body, what due to the influence of Satan. As Edwards put it, "all is not from grace, but much from nature. And though the affections have not their seat in the body, yet the constitution of the body may very much contribute to the present emotion of the mind" (Edwards, 1821, pp. 42–43). Persons "of a weak and vapoury habit of body" are particularly susceptible to strong emotional impressions seemingly originating from outside themselves (67). In such persons "the animal spirits are put into such a motion as is wont to be connected with the exhilaration of the mind; and the soul, by the laws of the union of soul and body, hence feels pleasure. The person being surprised, begins to think, surely this is the Holy Ghost coming into him" (212). There is great danger in this, since the Devil cannot affect the soul directly, but only via the medium of the body, and most particularly in those already subject to the disorder of melancholy (234–35).

Chauncy held that extravagant preaching may well produce little more "than a *mechanical Impression on animal Nature*" so strong that the affected cry out in fear, fall down, or swoon. He concluded that "such a Sort of Surprise and Astonishment is affected, not by a rational Conviction of Truth, but a sudden and strong Impression on the *animal*

Oeconomy"—creating an imbalance in the machinery of the body (Chauncy, 1743, p. 80). Many of the most striking physical effects of the Awakening "*have evidently been produced by the mechanical Influence of awful Words and frightful Gestures*" deployed by "over-heated preachers" who favoured the revival and encouraged its enthusiastic manifestations (109). Those vulnerable to such preaching "too commonly mistake the Motions of their *own Minds* for *divine Suggestions*" (216).

Similar in many ways, Edwards and Chauncy differed greatly in their emphasis. Edwards emphasised the affections, holding that religion without spiritual warmth is no religion at all, while Chauncy stressed the necessity of regular preaching and the requirements of public order. The controversy between them is instructive because it seems at once so familiar and yet culturally so distant. If "melancholy" and "animal spirits" were replaced by "depression" and "neuroendocrine imbalance", the dispute would seem far less anachronistic. But an irreducible religious element would still remain.

An atheist might say that Edwards and Chauncy were discussing genuine emotions directed toward *illusory objects*; 18th Century skeptics were concerned about *spurious emotions* directed toward *genuine objects* at the behest of untrained, uncertified, and enthusiastic evangelists (if alive today, Charles Chauncy might well have ended up on the advisory board of the False Memory Syndrome Foundation). What I would say is that these clergymen were sketching a logic of the affections rooted in the theologies and scientific understandings of their time. They were defining what pertains to the self, what to the body, and what to God — guiding their flocks as to what it is appropriate and meaningful to *feel*. No one who reads autobiographical material from that time can doubt the emotional engagement of these New England pietists with the ultimate problems of existence posited by their Christian faith (Kenny, 1994) .

The case of Anna O. (Bertha Pappenheim) witnesses a conceptual shift in the vocabulary of the emotions whereby catharsis and abreaction, as we now understand them, became common currency. The basic features of the case are these: while nursing her dying father a well-educated young woman falls ill with a variety of "hysterical" somatosensory complaints accompanied by episodic amnesia; it is found that these symptoms are symbolically associated with forgotten or repressed traumatic events, and that they are relieved when Anna is able to remember the "chance coincidences" through which the associations arose.

Breuer denied that his own suggestive influence had anything to do with these developments, and adopted an inductivist stance leading to the sweeping conclusion that "hysterics mainly suffer from reminiscences." As he said, "I regard hysteria as a clinical picture which has been empirically discovered and is based on observation, in just the same way as tubercular pulmonary phthsis" (Breuer & Freud, 1955, p. 187). Historians look back on Anna's "hysteria" as a 19th Century culture-bound syndrome that has now more or less evaporated. As for Anna O., recent scholarship has shown that her case—or rather the evolution of Breuer's *account* of her case—is not quite as *Studies on Hysteria* makes it seem (see Ellenberger, 1970; MacMillan, 1991; Borch-Jacobsen, 1996).

Not that Breuer was without reservations, though he managed to convince himself that they were groundless. For example, he noted that the "talking cure" he and his patient had evolved worked with great consistency—one memory recovered, one symptom dissolved—and that Anna's "consistency may have led her (in perfectly good faith) to assign to some of her symptoms a precipitating cause which they did not in fact possess" (Breuer & Freud, 1955, p. 43). Anna, in other words, had a theory of her own, and one wonders why she and Breuer found so congenial the notion that remembering traumatic experiences could alleviate their pathological consequences.

Historians of psychoanalysis point to the influence of the classicist, Jacob Bernays (uncle of Freud's wife, Martha) in popularising a medicalized version of the Greek concept of catharsis (Ellenberger, 1970, p. 484; Sulloway, 1983, p. 57). It is supposed that Anna knew of Bernays's work, and therefore that it could have affected the manner in which she conceptualised what it would take to cure her. Breuer himself was well aware of Bernays, whose *Two Treatises on the Aristotelian Theory of the Drama* had been reissued in 1880, the very year that Anna fell ill (Hirschmuller, 1978, p. 206). This work created quite a stir in German cultural circles, and was widely discussed in the popular press.

What Bernays had done was to re-evaluate some famously obscure passages in Aristotle. Tragedy, said Aristotle, "is an imitation of an action that is serious, complete, and possessing magnitude...effecting through pity and fear what we call the *catharsis* of such emotions" (Aristotle, 1982, p. 50). But he offers no further explanation of why this should be so. Whereas previous interpretations by classical German authors had focused on tragic catharsis as a species of moral education—the education of the sentiments—Bernays saw the concept in medical terms, as the purgation of toxic material (Jackson, 1994, p. 475). Catharsis therefore was a concept closely related to cultural debates of the time. Bernays moved the discussion away from the moral role of catharsis toward a medicalized and deterministic point of view compatible with the positivistic assumptions of late 19th Century neurology.

Ironically, modern classical scholarship has returned to the notion that Aristotelian catharsis is better viewed as "clarification" of the emotions than as their purgation (Belfiore, 1992; Nussbaum, 1986; Rorty, 1992). Aristotle was interested in something far more profound than administering a psychic laxative. As an educator as well as a theorist, he was concerned with the distribution of sentiment in society. Catharsis is an aspect of learning how to love and hate "rightly," such that our souls undergo a change for the better (Aristotle, 1988, p. 191). Aristotelian emotions are therefore motivated cognitions, moral acts, not just irrational responses over which we have no control. Given this fact, one classicist concluded that "an emotion is too complex and world-directed an item for the purgation model to be of significant value" (Lear, 1992, p. 317).

Though catharsis was de-emphasized in Freud's later work, the idea has persisted in other contexts, while recent events have conspired to revive it (Jackson, 1994; Nichols & Zax, 1977; Scheff, 1979). Jeffrey Masson's indictment of Freud for abandoning the seduction hypothesis helped to refocus therapeutic concern on the effects of actual trauma, including trauma long past (Masson, 1985); at the same time renewed interest in multiple personality and the emergence of the concept of Post-traumatic Stress Disorder contributed to a revival of the notion of "dissociation" formulated by Freud's contemporary, Pierre Janet. In combination these developments have led to a theory of the affects highly congenial to the application of cathartic methods.

The effects of sexual trauma are widely seen as lying behind much of the neurotic symptomatology of our own time. Therapies based on this idea focus on recovery and reintegration of dissociated affect-laden material walled off "under conditions of chronic childhood abuse" that "prevents the ordinary integration of knowledge, memory, emotional states, and bodily experience" (Herman, 1992, p. 107). The therapeutic goal is "the integration of affect with recall to achieve resolution of the trauma" (Briere, 1992, p. 41); it is "the recollection, exploration and abreacting of the traumatic material" (Courtois, 1988, p. 184; 1992).

These insights parallel Breuer and Freud, and derive from a critique of what happened to psychoanalysis in later years. Just as Freud maintained in 1896 that "hysterical symptoms are derivatives of memories which are operating unconsciously," so it is now said that "the story of the traumatic event surfaces not as a verbal narrative but as a symptom" (Masson, 1985, p. 280; Herman, 1992, p. 1). Behind the symptom lies a memory deposited as though fossilised, "frozen in time" (Davies & Frawley, 1994, p. 42; van der Kolk, 1994, p. 261; van der Kolk & van der Hart, 1995, p. 177). While Josef Breuer believed that such memories are laid down during special though poorly defined "hypnoid states," current thinking turns to neuropsychology for an account of state-dependent memory (van der Kolk & van der Hart, 1995, p. 174). Specially encoded traumatic memories must be accessed, processed, and incorporated within the conscious life-narrative of the patient. Such memories "are the unassimilated scraps of overwhelming experiences, which need to be integrated with existing mental schemes, and be transformed into narrative language" (176). They need to be fitted into a story; but what kind of story?

Inevitably a story of passion. Traumatic dissociation is the product of extreme events: rape, war, sexual abuse, torture, terrorism, natural disaster. If traumatic memories are laid down under conditions that render them inaccessible to normative consciousness, then—given their state-dependency—perhaps (so the theory predicts) they will reemerge under analogous stressful conditions, say in therapy (van der Kolk, 1994, p. 255). The pain returns with the memory. Accordingly there are moments of high drama—"crises"—as emotion breaks through the dissociative walls that contain it (McCann & Pearlman, 1990, p. 217). "The trauma...will be revived in the therapeutic relationship"; these episodes are "regressive reenactments...which are always intensely passionate," "a recovery and reworking of the early traumatic events" (Davies & Frawley, 1994, p. 5; Putnam, 1989, p. 137; van der Kolk & van der Hart, 1995, p. 179).

Intellectualising one's past is not good enough. Flat affect is itself a symptom of dissociation or post-traumatic stress (Briere, 1992, p. 136). Healing the effects of trauma must take place at gut level. Therefore, "a narrative that does not include the traumatic imagery and bodily sensations is barren and incomplete" (Herman, 1992, p. 177). The emergence of powerful emotion is prima facie evidence that something profound is underway, a "controlled re-experiencing of the trauma" (van der Hart & Brown, 1992, p. 137). The ritual process of therapy takes place in definite stages, among them remembrance and mourning of the trauma and its consequences, followed by reconnection to oneself and the world (Herman, 1992). The healer-client relationship, though creatively interactive, has a theory-driven aim. There must be a visible light at the end of even the darkest tunnel; the process aimed at reaching this light is comprised of an interweaving of "theory, therapy, and transformation" (McCann & Pearlman, 1990).

This process is linked to grief and mourning by something deeper than metaphor. It is not just like mourning, it is a parallel and related process. "The recognition and expression of long-suppressed memories and emotions...result in grief and require mourning" (Courtois, 1988, p. 181). As with grief, there are a number of stages—denial, anger, acceptance, transcendence—to be gone through in coping with the hidden effects of dissociated trauma: "Grieving, a necessary therapy component, brings to the surface feelings of sadness, depression, and anger which must be encouraged and supported by the therapist"; "mourning and reconstruction" are essential "in the resolution of traumatic life events." Painful energy "must be expressed, grieved and processed" (Courtois, 1988, p. 226; Herman, 1992, p. 69; Whitfield, 1995, p. 124). And it is difficult: "the descent into mourning is at once the most necessary and the most dreaded task" of the stage of recovery involving the return of traumatic memories (Herman, 1992, p. 188). "The way to move beyond the grief and pain is to experience them fully" (Bass & Davis, 1994, p. 131). Like the workings of the Holy Ghost preparatory to religious conversion, the pain washes over one unbidden as though of external origins.

I am uncertain as to how these became commonplace notions. Perhaps they are ultimately derived from Freud's observations on "Mourning and Melancholia" where he drew an explicit parallel between the active process of normal grief, and the impacted or aborted grief manifest in depression (Freud, 1957). John Bowlby's research on attachment and loss in children and the rise of the concept of PTSD are significant factors as well (Briere, 1992; Davies & Frawley, 1994; Herman, 1992, p. 69). However it came about, a widely-shared expectation has arisen that demonstrative grief-like emotion will and should occur as a normal part of therapy. Among other things this model establishes an expectation that—like grieving—trauma therapy actually has a terminable course, thus providing a sense of order and progress.

Writers on traumatic stress and dissociation are concerned with the nature of extreme experiences. So were Jonathan Edwards, Charles Chauncy, and Josef Breuer. But the beliefs and practices mentioned above are markedly peculiar to their own times and places, a fact that is somewhat harder to see in our own situation because these are our own times (see Kenny, 1986; Hacking, 1995; Young, 1995). The healing potential of therapy is undeniable, but I think we would be wrong to assume that the trauma-dissociation theory underlying much current practice is "scientifically" proven. Ours being a scientific age, the theory is couched in terms that allow it to be presented and legitimated as a new departure in the explanation of old human ills, a new bio-psychological paradigm that is simultaneously good science and social critique (Kenny, 1995).

In my view, retroactive trauma therapy evinces the same creative and interactive processes seen in the Great Awakening and the case of Anna O, and for that matter in the trauma-oriented therapeutic practices of other cultural traditions (Kenny, 1996). We enter an "as-if" world of metaphor. We grieve "as if" we really are abused children once more; we experience the past as if really there. Emotion *is* transformative, but this does not mean that affect-laden traumatic memories are somehow being hauled up out of a dissociated mnemonic abscess. Instead—if things go well—affect is *created, facilitated, and manipulated* in a dramatically plausible manner consistent with the actual experiences, present situation and world-view of the client, *and* the structural requirements of the therapeutic process. Our authorities wish to help the sufferer toward a coherent and satisfying life story that points forward, not back. We are not dealing with the cathartic expression and purging of emotions, but rather with their *domestication* and *cultivation*. Dramatic emotive performances mark one phase in a complex rite of passage. The relation of these socialised emotions to the "actual" past is a deep question.

Trauma theory may be more scientifically adequate than its predecessors, but I for one doubt it and will let history be the judge. What I *would* say is that, notwithstanding the trappings of positivistic science, trauma therapists who focus on memory are engaged in an education of the sentiments, guiding their clients in how to feel *rightly* so as to establish an experiential consistency between thought, feeling, and action. This is not the mechanistic psychology of Breuer and Freud. It is far closer to Aristotle, and should be regarded as such—as another example of the intimate relation between culture, morality, and self-experience.

REFERENCES

Aristotle (1982). *Aristotle's poetics* (James Hutton, Trans.). New York: W.W. Norton.
Aristotle (1988). *The politics*. Cambridge: Cambridge University Press.
Bass, E., & Davis, L. (1994). *The courage to heal* (3 ed.). New York: Harper Perennial.

Belfiore, E. S. (1992). *Tragic pleasures: Aristotle on plot and emotion*. Princeton: Princeton University Press.

Borch-Jacobsen, M. (1996). Remembering Anna O.: A century of mystification (Kirby Olson, Trans.). New York: Routledge.

Breuer, J., & Freud, S. (1955). *Studies on hysteria*. London: Hogarth Press.

Briere, J. (1992). *Child abuse trauma: theory and treatment of the lasting effects*. Newbury Park: Sage Publications.

Chauncy, C. (1743). *Seasonable thoughts on the state of religion in New England*. Boston: Rogers & Fowle.

Courtois, C. A. (1988). *Healing the incest wound: adult survivors in therapy*. New York: W.W. Norton.

Courtois, C. A. (1992). The memory retrieval process in incest survivor therapy. *Journal of Child Sexual Abuse, 1(1)*, 15–31.

Davies, J. M., & Frawleyp M. G. (1994). *Treating the adult survivor of childhood sexual abuse: a psychoanalytic Perspective*. New York: Basic Books.

Edwards, J. (1821). *A treatise concerning religious affections*. Philadelphia: James Crissy.

Ellenberger, H. F. (1970). *The discovery of the unconscious*. New York: Basic Books.

Freud, S. (1957). Mourning and melancholia. In J. Strachey (Ed.), Standard Edition, v. 14 (pp. 243–258). London: Hogarth Press.

Hacking, I. (1995). *Rewriting the soul: multiple personality and the sciences of memory*. Princeton: Princeton University Press.

Harré, R. (Ed.). (1986). *The social construction of emotions*. Oxford: Basil Blackwell.

Herman, J. L. (1992). *Trauma and recovery*. New York: Basic Books.

Hirschmuller, A. (1978). *Physiologie und psychoanalalyse in leben und werk Josef Breuers*. Tubingen: Verlag Hans Huber.

Jackson, S. W. (1994). Catharsis and abreaction in the history of psychological healing. *Psychiatric Clinics of North America, 17(3)*, 471–491.

Kenny, M. G. (1986). *The passion of Ansel Bourne: multiple personality in American culture*. Washington D.C.: Smithsonian Institution Press.

Kenny, M. G. (1994). *The perfect law of liberty: Elias Smith and the providential history of America*. Washington D.C.: Smithsonian Institution Press.

Kenny, M. G. (1995). The recovered memory controversy: an anthropologist's view. *Journal of Psychiatry and Law, 23(3)*, 437–460.

Kenny, M.G. (1996). Trauma, time, illness, and culture: an anthropological approach to traumatic memory. In P. Antze & M. Lambek (Eds.), *Tense past: cultural essays in trauma and memory* (pp. 151–171). New York: Routledge.

Lear, J. (1992). Katharsis. In A. O. Rorty (Ed.), *Essays on Aristotle's Poetics* (pp. 315–340). Princeton: Princeton University Press.

MacMillan, M. (1991). *Freud evaluated: the completed arc*. Amsterdam: Elsevier.

Masson, J. M. (1985). *The assault on truth: Freud's suppression of the seduction theory*. New York: Penguin Books.

McCann, I. L., & Pearlman, L. A. (1990). *Psychological trauma and the adult survivor: theory, therapy, and transformation*. New York: Brunner/Mazel.

Nichols, M. P., & Zax, M. (1977). *Catharsis in psychotherapy*. New York: Gardner Press.

Nussbaum, M. C. (1986). *The fragility of goodness: luck and ethics in Greek tragedy and philosophy*. Cambridge: Cambridge University Press.

Putnam, F. (1989). *Diagnosis and treatment of multiple personality disorder*. New York: Guilford Press.

Rorty, A. O. (Ed.). (1992). *Essays on Aristotle's Poetics*. Princeton: Princeton University Press.

Scheff, T. J. (1979). *Catharsis in healing, ritual, and drama*. Berkeley & Los Angeles: University of California Press.

Sulloway, F. J. (1983). *Freud, biologist of the mind*. New York: Basic Books.

van der Hart, O., & Brown, P. (1992). Abreaction re-evaluated. *Dissociation, 5(3)*, 127–140.

van der Kolk, B. (1994). The body keeps the score: memory and the evolving psychobiology of posttraumatic stress. *Harvard Review of Psychiatry, 1(5)*, 253–265.

van der Kolk, B., & van der Hart, O. (1995). The intrusive past: The flexibility of memory and the engraving of trauma. In C. Caruth (Ed.), *Trauma: explorations in memory* (pp. 158–182). Baltimore: Johns Hopkins University Press.

Whitfield, C. L. (1995). *Memory and abuse: remembering and healing the effects of trauma*. Deerfield Beach: Health Communications, Inc.

Young, A. (1995). *The harmony of illusions: inventing post-traumatic stress disorder*. Princeton: Princeton University Press.

28

THE SOCIAL CONSTRUCTION OF MULTIPLE PERSONALITY DISORDER

Steven Jay Lynn[1] and Judith Pintar[2]

[1]State University of New York at Binghamton
Binghamton, New York 13902
[2]University of Illinois, Champaign–Urbana
Champaign–Urbana, Illinois 61820

In the first part of this paper, the senior author (SJL) provides a first-person account of his observations as a supervising psychologist at a state mental hospital that specialized in the treatment of multiple personality disorder (MPD). These observations encompass a fertile and influential period in the history of the evolving conceptualization and treatment of serious dissociative disorders. In the second part of the paper, Judith Pintar and the senior author maintain that MPD can be understood in terms of the way narratives of multiplicity are embedded in social interactions and emerge within the discourse of a psychotherapeutic relationship. The paper retains the conversational tone adopted in presenting an earlier version of the manuscript as a spoken commentary on Sherrill Mulhern's talk on the topic of sociocultural factors in the treatment of multiple pesonality disorders.

1. A PERSONAL ACCOUNT

In the late 1970's I had the opportunity to sit on the sidelines as I observed what I now know to be history in the making. The stage was the Athens Mental Health Center, where I served as a supervising psychologist from 1978 until 1992, and where a patient of some notoriety was residing and being treated by Dr. David Caul, a compassionate general practitioner physician with little formal training in psychiatry. The patient, William ("Billy") Milligan was the first individual in the United States to be found not guilty of a crime (in this case, sexual assault) because he was diagnosed as a multiple personality. Milligan's life was the topic of a best-selling book and the subject of a movie made some years ago. Largely as a result of his treatment of Milligan, Caul became one of the pioneers of the MPD movement, and along with other individuals such as Cornelia Wilbur and Ralph Allison, organized the first American Psychiatric Association courses on MPD in 1978.

Recollections of Trauma, edited by Read and Lindsay
Plenum Press, New York, 1997

Within a few years of Milligan's arrival at the hospital, the facility became known as a treatment center for multiple personality disorder. My perception was that increasingly, borderline and histrionic patients at the hospital were being diagnosed as multiples, while patients were referred from other facilities who were suspected multiples. Milligan became quite a controversial patient, who was viewed by some as a calculating antisocial personality, and by others as person with a terrible history of abuse who was rightly an object of sympathy. Caul steadfastly defended Milligan against his critics and began to have critics of his own.

Indeed, many of the staff were skeptical not only of Milligan but also of the techniques Caul was using. The psychology staff had an opportunity to view a number of Caul's tapes of his work with diagnosed multiples. We were, with no vocal exceptions, convinced that the procedures used were leading and highly suggestive. Sodium amatyl and hypnosis, for example, were used to diagnose multiplicity, and suspected multiples attended group therapy sessions in which they observed other multiples tell stories of horrific abuse, and parade their different personalities before the group following the hypnotic command, "the door is open." Each personality was viewed as a separate entity, with a distinct history; with certain patients, signs of resistance to the diagnosis were interpreted as the product of a secretive or fearful alter and as direct confirmation of the diagnosis. According to Caul's treatment model, confronting such signs of resistance was of paramount importance because he believed that the first step in the treatment of MPD was to convince patients that they suffered from the condition.

What evidence of multiplicity was used to convince patients? Some patients kept journals, and changes in handwriting were interpreted as a manifestation of an emergent alter personality, as were episodes of acting out. Subtle changes in behavior or nonverbal expressions were taken as evidence of "switching" personalities or the struggle of one personality to dominate the host personality. Not only did Caul use group therapy with multiples, but he pioneered a technique called "inner group therapy" in which the personalities introduce themselves, are helped to interact with one another, and eventually negotiate how feelings and actions will be handled and personalities will be integrated. In these sessions, patients had ample opportunity to observe other patients and to model the expression of symptoms consistent with MPD. Many of the procedures that Caul and others in that first generation of workers in the field pioneered are now part of mainstream treatment of dissociative identity disorder. Unfortunately, my impression is that many of these procedures can reinforce, if not create from whole cloth, the symptoms of MPD (see also Merskey, 1992; Spanos, 1996).

One aspect of the treatment that particularly concerned me were the symptoms that were supposed to raise the index of suspicion regarding the diagnosis of MPD. In 1980, Cornelia Wilbur, who was one of the original consultants on the Milligan case, visited the hospital and gave a talk to staff members. During this visit, she advanced a simplistic model of dissociation, arguing that "missing time" was the sine qua non of dissociation, and contending that the combination of missing time and puzzling, unpredictable, or irrational behaviors were danger signals that very likely indicated the presence of MPD. The problem was that many of the patients, including borderline and psychotic patients, as well as patients with organic disorders, fit this symptom picture: missing time is a nonspecific symptom reported by many patients across diverse diagnostic categories. Unfortunately, the presence of these and a checklist of other symptoms of dissociation justified the use of invasive and leading hypnotic procedures and amytal interviews, on occasion, to exhume a history of abuse that could account for the dissociative symptoms. Not surprisingly, an abuse history was often uncovered under these conditions.

Wilbur's talk stoked the flames of the therapists and staff who approached the treatment of multiples with missionary zeal. Around this time, I remember a conversation with a master's level clinician who asked me, "What diagnosis do you think most schizophrenics who hear voices really have." I said, "beats, me, probably schizophrenia." He said, "No, 80% of these people are multiples." This turned out to be a rather short conversation.

Staff members like the one who accosted me came to view themselves as trauma specialists, a status they did not otherwise have in the hospital hierarchy. They seemed to thrive on the skepticism of their colleagues, which only seemed to fuel their fervor. New staff were recruited to work with multiples, and were indoctinated into a subculture of avid, unquestioning belief in the diagnosis and prescribed treatments. I was privy to one staff meeting in which a staff member raised some questions about the appropriateness of the diagnosis of MPD, and was told that he was becoming a "nonbeliever." Pride and a sense of accomplishment were apparent when certain staff played a role in uncovering personalities, and patients were carefully observed for subtle signs of "switching" indicative of personalities lurking in the background.

Not surprisingly, the staff became deeply polarized in terms of the "believers" versus the "skeptics" on the topic of multiple personality. Unfortunately, the patients appeared to get caught up in the staff conflict. There was a perception that the diagnosed multiples received more attention and were treated better than patients not so diagnosed. I learned from staff members that certain patients were jealous of diagnosed multiples, and some even confided they were tempted to try to receive a multiple diagnosis; a few even tried to mimic symptoms of MPD, one with apparent success.

I had an opportunity to get to know a number of female patients who were diagnosed as multiples, two women in particular. Both impresssed me as very fragile, insecure, and desperate for love. One of the patients seemed to revel in the diagnosis. She said it was the first time in her life she felt special. She reported that she would sit in the laps of various staff members and play childlike games with them in sessions during which she was encouraged to regress to a childlike state and "be herself" as she really was when she was a child with understanding adults in the present. Unfortunately, her behavior was also regressed on the ward and she attempted to mutilate herself and commit suicide on a number of occasions. Her treatment course was bumpy, at best, and in the end she was transferred to another facility.

The other patient told me she was diagnosed a multiple after she reported she was sitting in a class and wrote a note to herself when she was doodling. She then underwent a hypnosis interview and several personalities were elicited. When I spoke with her, she said that she never fully believed she was a multiple, but that the hypnosis and therapy sessions allowed her to talk about a lot of feelings that were ordinarily difficult to express. She stated that she "played along" in many of the therapy sessions because she did not want to disappoint her physician, whom she felt great affection for. After a number of "integration rituals" she reported she felt better than she had in years and had resolved many of her angry feelings toward her parents and forgiven them.

Were these patients better off than they were before the treatment? Perhaps one patient was, better off, yet I fear she was in the great minority of individuals who received the diagnosis. The treatment of most persons who received the diagnosis was protracted and tumultuous. The other patient was definitiely worse for the therapy. Yet perhaps the important point for our discussion is that the two patients constructed very different narratives about the self, the treatment, and the healers who worked with them.

2. A SOCIAL NARRATIVE MODEL OF DISSOCIATION

The psychological distress of the patients at Athens Mental Health Center, and the course of their symptoms, actions and treatment cannot be accurately interpreted apart from the historic events occurring within the Athens Mental Health Center, the ongoing debates within the larger medical community at that time, and in the volatile imagination and normative power of popular media. We believe that the patients' diagnosed disorder was not theirs alone, a straightforward reflection of their subjective psychological processes, but was also an explicitly cultural construction (see also Spanos, 1996 for an excellent discussion of cultural issues).

The underlying phenomena of MPD rest on cultural assumptions about the nature of the self. We, in Western society, share a social narrative of the identity as a complex, but essentially unitary phenomenon, beside which an apparent "multiple" agency must appear pathological. Jumping off from this basic insight, we can shift the unit of analysis from society and culture, back down to the individual to consider just why and how individuals in recent years have come to interpret their subjective experience in terms of multiplicity. Specifically, we will focus on the performative aspect of MPD, recognizing the therapeutic relationship to be the principle mechanism of socialization which facilitates an individual's identification with the diagnosis.

A body of psychological literature (e.g., Meichenbaum & Fong, 1993; Sarbin, 1986; Spence, 1984) that can be loosely identified as narrative social psychology considers personal identity not just as an attribute of an individual but as a dynamic process constructed within social relationships through the mechanism of shared narratives. These narratives give personal identity continuity in the past and the future. When a woman becomes a mother, for instance, the factors that determine the extent of her identification with motherhood include her memories of her own mother, as well as cultural images and discourse about motherhood. Most importantly, others will treat her as a mother, and will expect her to act in a "motherlike" way, defined by shared narratives. In this way, identity is constructed and maintained through relationships. Motherhood is performed.

An interesting aspect of our social identities is that we can have many such roles, which can exist together without discontinuity. A woman can be a mother, a daughter, a doctor and a wife, a complex set of roles which may wear her out, but will probably not confuse her sense of herself. A child who is sexually abused, on the other hand, finds herself in the position of having experiences which not only exist outside of shared social narratives, but which blatantly contradict them. Elsewhere (Lynn, Pintar, & Rhue, in press; Rhue, Lynn, & Pintar, 1996) we have suggested that the phenomenon of dissociated identity may be a straightforward reflection of traumatic and contradictory social conditions; in other words, if personal identity is constructed through social relations, and if those social relations are ruptured in traumatic fashion, then the construction of identity is accordingly disrupted. In this view, the dissociation itself is not a pathology, but the particular manifestation of a normal cognitive capacity under abnormal circumstances.

A narrative view of dissociation—in contrast to mechanistic conceptualizations which locate the phenomenon within an individual as a symptom of a disorder, or as a defense mechanism outliving its usefulness—locates the phenomenon in the social relations of the victim, both at the moment of the trauma and as a continuing or recurring process. We might ask the question, if identity is constructed within social relations, what type of social relations would lead to the subjective experience of multiple or partial selves? In attempting to answer this question, it is necessary to distinguish in greater detail between dissociated multiple identities, and the multiple identities we all experience that are merely complex.

A child who lives in separate households may develop a complex sense of self that encompasses two distinct narratives: "I am a responsible big sister," in one household and "I am just a little kid" in the other. This is a multiple personal narrative, but it is occurring within a larger social narrative which may be stressful but is not traumatic. The child has toys and clothes at Mom's and different toys and clothes at Dad's, and she can bring the toys from Dad's house to Mom's house if she wants to. But what if she is being abused at Dad's house? There are still two personal narratives, but something is different: what Dad is doing is no longer reflected in a shared social narrative. What does the child do now? Who is she when she's with her Dad? Not the same person she is when she is with her Mom where personal and social narratives match. She can't bring Dad's toys with her to Mom's house. She may say that she "split" at that point, but the crucial thing to note is that the world split first.

The social narrative upon and through which she constructed her identity ruptured. It lost coherence and consistency. We would suggest that rather than being a way to separate from reality, dissociation may well be, under some circumstances, a way to bring identity in line with those circumstances. Trapped between a broad social narrative that says, "fathers care for their daughters and don't hurt them" and a personal narrative based on the experience of being repeatedly raped by her father, the child's construction of a multiple identity is a realistic reflection of her actual social condition, and her subjective experience of having many selves which appears to be a distortion of reality may be an accurate reflection of lived experience.

Multiplicity is perhaps the only way that both narratives can be true at the same time. She can be both a nine-year-old school girl and her father's lover. It may be true, as many have postulated, that pathology arises because she cannot "integrate" the two identities within one coherent self. But the reason the identities cannot co-exist is that the social world does not acknowledge that they might both be true. It may be accurate to suggest that the world and she are mutually dissociated from one another.

The important point to note is that what the experience of trauma disrupts is not identity itself but the social process through which identity is constructed. Correspondingly, in this view, the phenomenon of multiplicity is not so much a disorder of identity, but a disorder of identity construction. The suggestion that multiplicity is in part, or whole, iatrogenic becomes less surprising (though no less problematic) in this light. Multiple identity, like unitary identity, is performed, that is to say, it is dynamically constructed through social relationships.

Therapists treating multiples share with their clients a narrative about identity that includes a belief in the existence of MPD/DID (dissociative identity disorder, the current nomenclature for what was once multiple personality disorder). They engage in discussions with alters, developing relationships with them within which the alters come alive. The therapist-client relationship may not be the only one in which the alters perform, but it is often the most important one.

The meaning of whether therapists convince their clients that they are multiples varies as a function of what the client believes in advance. If the client believes "Oh I'm not a multiple; that's just a mood that I'm in sometimes," that's one thing. It's another if the client's belief is "Oh I'm not a multiple, Jane is a physically distinct other person, rather than another personality." In the first case, the therapist's effort can legitimately be construed as iatrogenic creation of MPD. In the second, it can be construed as countering a delusion and not at all iatrogenic, but a reflection of the subjective conviction of multiplicity.

The process in which multiple identities are constructed or maintained within the discourse of a therapeutic relationship will be even more powerful in a relationship between therapists and their highly suggestible and fantasy-prone clients. Research in our laboratory (Lynn, Rhue, & Green, 1988) has shown that there are many parallels between persons with a profound history of fantasy involvements that date to early childhood and individuals diagnosed with multiple personality (now termed dissociative identity disorder). Indeed, when we look at what measures of dissociation index, one prominent component is fantasy and imaginative proclivities. Fantasy prone persons report that they play with imaginary companions during childhood, often pretend to be other people during times of stress, report out of body experiences to deal with traumatic and nontraumatic experiences, and create absorbing imaginative narratives during which time stands in abeyance. In short, we might say they dissociate.

These individuals are also more suggestible, even in nonhypnotic situations, than their less fantasy prone counterparts. To say that a client is suggestible is also to say that he or she is particularly sensitive to the immediate social relationship, so that the influence of a hypnotherapist can override other preexisting social beliefs; for instance, if the therapist suggests that a woman's arm is getting lighter and will rise on its own, that narrative suggestion replaces, at least for the moment, the shared social belief that arms don't ordinarily do that.

In ordinary conversations, many of us talk about ourselves as having different parts or as feeling as if one part of ourselves is in conflict with another part. So suggestions for one part to "come out" in the context of psychotherapy or hypnosis may, in fact, conform more closely to one's ordinary experience of oneself than the feeling of nonvolition and involuntariness that often accompanies responses to hypnotic suggestions for one's arm to rise, for example.

The majority of hypnotizable participants can easily get in touch with so-called hidden parts of the mind, or "hidden observers" that can comment on imaginative and hypnotic dreams and age regression suggestions and afterward report complete or partial amnesia for what the "hidden part" revealed during hypnosis, awake imagining, and relaxed nonhypnotic conditions (Mare, Lynn, Kvaal, Segal, & Sivec, 1994). It is not likely, however, that suggestibility or imaginative tendencies alone can explain why an individual would take on and participate in the ongoing construction of multiple identities. It may be necessary for the therapist and the relationship to provide incentives (e.g., feeling of being special, meeting important needs of the client and therapist, and so forth) for construing the self in terms of having multiple, discrete identities, a conceptualization reinforced and legitimized by therapeutic procedures (e.g., repeated suggestions for alters to emerge during hypnosis) that give fiber and body to nascent aspects of the self.

However another, yet by no means mutually exclusive possibility, is that the narrative of multiple identity that underlies DID may be comfortable to many survivors of traumatic abuse because it fits their subjective experience of their disrupted identities more closely than than the dominant cultural narrative of ordinary unitary identity which assumes non-traumatic social conditions and relations. A woman who accepts the diagnosis of DID and engages in complex interactions through a group of altered personalities cannot be said simply to be "faking it," unless we are willing to consider our more mundane construction of unitary identity to be fake as well. The bottom line is that identity is a malleable narrative construct, exquisitely sensitive to social conditions.

In attempting to outline the ways in which social and cultural forces acted together to "create" multiple personality disorder as a category of psychological distress, Mulhern (1992, 1994) persuasively argues that the medicalization of child abuse shifted the locus of control over the meaning of traumatic experience from the survivors of the trauma to a "corps of experts;" with the resulting shift in interest from remembered stories of abuse to repressed memories, accessed only with the help of these experts. Memories of abuse became, in short, a "mediated discourse." An intrinsic part of that discourse is the process of diagnosis. There is a self-recursive irony in the diagnosis of DID as an "identity disorder," since the dynamic process of diagnosis itself confers identity.

In diagnosing physical illnesses Western medicine traditionally has maintained a distinction between sickness and wounding. There is a big difference between having arthritis in the knuckles, and having a sore thumb because you hit yourself with a hammer. The pain may be comparable, but the sickness confers identity (you have become an arthritis-sufferer) in a way that the wounding does not. A patient who learns that she has cancer, for instance, becomes at that moment a "cancer patient," a label that comes with a lot of baggage. Relationships will be negotiated, and she will have to decide to what extent she wishes to take on or reject this label as an aspect of personal identity, to identify with other cancer patients as a group. Identity after remission involves a similar process of negotiation, both internal and external as she decides whether she wants to think about herself as a "recovered cancer patient" or just as an ordinary person again, the person she was before the cancer.

The distinction between sickness and wounding exists in the treatment of mental health problems, but it is a slippery one. In coming to speak about the consequences of psychological trauma in medical terms, the symptoms of psychological wounding become a sickness, so that a woman diagnosed as DID is not only suffering from having been abused, but from the fact that she is now "a multiple." A psychiatric diagnosis actually confers identity in a much more powerful way than a medical diagnosis. A psychiatric patient, especially one who is diagnosed as having an identity disorder, is under an exceptionally strong compulsion to identify with the category of diagnosis since multiplicity is not something you have, like cancer; it is something you are. The existence of an authoritative diagnosis for DID creates a contested category of identity increasingly contingent on the criteria of spontenaity and non-volition, so that we now must distinguish between real multiples, those who are faking it, and those whose personalities are iatrogenic concoctions.

A patient's identification with the diagnosis is made more likely when it is a contested status. MPD and now DID (dissociative identity disorder) are trendy diagnoses which may, in some instances, bring more or better attention from mental health workers and insurance companies. A diagnosis of DID also provides a boost of self-esteem since multiples are supposed to be creative individuals with high IQs. Examined through the lens of multiplicity, behaviors such as self-mutilation, promiscuity, and infantile regression, which in other contexts may have been viewed as repugnant or deviant, can come to be seen as understandable and even heroic. Another factor that may have encouraged identification with the disorder was the political climate of "identity politics" during the 1980s, when it became fashionable and politically expedient to identify with membership of a group with a grievance. As survivors of sexual abuse organized, so did the subgroups who identified themselves as multiples or as survivors of satanic abuse. When one is born into a racial minority, membership is uncontested; however, membership in the psychological communities of "multiples" or "satanic abuse survivors" requires evidence of shared suffering and identification with the community involves conscious choice.

As we implied earlier, identification with a diagnosis also results from the therapeutic relationship, a culturally constructed relationship that has both medical and what we might call ritual components. The ritual aspect of therapy is particularly explicit when hypnosis is involved. And the rhetoric of "belief" in debates about multiplicity lends the whole discussion a mythical tone "Do we believe in false memories?" "Do we believe in multiplicity?" "Do we believe in the existence of satanic cults?" Diagnosis acts on these beliefs and confers a status change in identity. To be pronounced a multiple by a medical authority invokes the ritual power of the spoken word, in much the same way that a priest can pronounce a couple to be married. With that kind of authoritative power a psychiatrist can "create" a multiple at the moment of diagnosis in the same way that the leader of a possession cult can decide whether a possession is authentic by identifying and authenticating the appearance of a particular spirit. The "diagnosis" confers upon the possessed individual a change in status within the cult. The combination of medical and religious structure and authority makes the therapeutic relationship into a powerful mechanism of socialization.

Mulhern's (1994) analysis of the historical, cultural and sociological mechanisms that facilitated the construction of the MPD model, is a clarion call for self-reflection. For researchers, this means greater awareness of the historical biases and cultural influences that may affect the way that theoretical models are developed; for clinicians it means coming to terms with the fact that in spite of our best intentions our methods can hurt as well as heal. And so we return to the two women whose experience was described at the beginning of this paper, one who seems to have been helped by the diagnosis of MPD and one who may have been hurt by it. We think it is fair to say that the diagnosis of multiplicity — with its narrative of separation and integration, can be a useful therapeutic tool for a few patients, but that for most patients it opens a veritable Pandora's box, and can lead to an exacerbation of symptoms, a breakdown of relationships and social networks and a tangled conflation of fantasy images with actual memories.

To believe unconditionally in clients' recovered memories can be as damaging to them as it is to write off their authentic memories as oedipal-based fantasies. It is simply bad therapy to fail to recognize the highly suggestible nature of the subsample of abuse survivors who can be identified as fantasy-prone. It is also a mistake to suggest to dissociative clients that multiplicity is a category of identity that one can be, rather than a narrative of identity that one can use. There is a world of difference between saying to a client, "the experience of trauma made you feel as if you were three people, let's imagine what they would say to one another," and saying "the experience of trauma made you into three people, let me talk to them."

Multiplicity is a narrative of identity that is compelling for certain trauma survivors because it comes closer to reflecting their subjective experience of self than other shared social narratives. It becomes problematic when it ceases to be just a useful metaphor, and becomes (through the process of evaluation/suggestion/iatrogenic procedures leading to a medical diagnosis) a category of identification. This is especially dangerous for those whose presenting symptoms have to do with disruptions in identity to begin with. It appears, in this light, that the "epidemic" of DID during the last twenty years is not the deliberate product of a conspiratorial movement of therapists to construct a chronic disorder in a highly-suggestible and fantasy-prone subpopulation, but the byproduct of a compelling metaphor run wild.

REFERENCES

Lynn, S.J., Pintar, J., & Rhue, J.W. (in press). Fantasy proneness, dissociation, and narrative construction. In S. Powers & S. Krippner (Eds.), *Broken Selves: Dissociative Narratives and Phenomena*. New York: Bruner/Mazel.

Lynn, S.J., Rhue, J., & Green, J. (1988). Multiple personality and fantasy proneness: Is there an association or dissociation? *British Journal of Experimental and Clinical Hypnosis*, *5*, 138–142.

Mare, C., Lynn, S.J., Kvaal, S., Segal, D., & Sivec, H. (1994). Hypnosis and the dream hidden observer: Primary process and demand characteristics. *Journal of Abnormal Psychology*, *103*, 316–327.

Meichenbaum, D., & Fong, G.T. (1993). How individuals control their own minds: A constructive narrative perspective. In D. M. Wegner & J. W. Pennebaker (Eds.), *Handbook of mental control* (pp. 473–490). Englewood Cliffs, New Jersey: Prentice Hall.

Merskey H. (1992). The manufacture of multiple personalities: The production of multiple personality disorder. *British Journal of Psychiatry*, *160*, 327–340.

Mulhern, S. (1992). Ritual abuse: Defining a syndrome versus defending a belief. *Journal of Psychology and Theology*, *20*, 230–232.

Mulhern, S. (1994). Satanism, ritual abuse, and multiple personality disorder: A sociohistorical perspective. *International Journal of Clinical and Experimental Hypnosis*, 42, 265–288.

Rhue, J., Lynn, S., & Pintar, J. (in press). Narrative and imaginative storytelling: Treatment of a sexually abused child. In S.J. Lynn, I. Kirsch, & J.W. Rhue (Eds.), *Casebook of clinical hypnosis*. (pp. 251–270) Washington, DC: American Psychological Association.

Sarbin, T. (1986). *Narrative psychology: The storied nature of human conduct*. New York: Praeger.

Spanos, N.P. (1996). *Multiple identities and false memories*. Washington, DC: American Psychological Association.

Spence, D. (1994). *Narrative truth and historical truth: Meaning and interpretation in psychoanalysis*. New York: W.W. Norton & Co., Inc.

29

THE ROLE OF LEGAL RULES IN RECOLLECTIONS OF TRAUMA

An Overview and Introduction to the Legal Panel

Daniel W. Shuman

Southern Methodist University
P.O. Box 750116
Dallas, Texas 75275-0116

It is tempting in a discussion about recollections of trauma dominated by psychologists to assume that the role of the legal system in addressing recollections of trauma is at best irrelevant and at worst anti-therapeutic. Not only does this thinking ignore explicit pro-therapeutic legal efforts, as for example in the recognition of a psychotherapist-patient privilege limiting compelled disclosure of relational communications (*Jaffee v. Redmond*, 1966), but it also inaccurately assumes the existence of a monolithic world legal system. The wide differences in world legal systems, and the wide differences in the experiences of different countries to the issues surrounding recollections of trauma addressed in this conference, fuel speculation about the role that these legal systems may play in explaining, for example, the varying frequencies with which allegations of "recovered repressed memories" of childhood sexual abuse arise in different countries. For example, does the availability of tort damages provide an incentive for patients to remember forgotten traumatic tortious events; does the availability of tort damages provide an incentive for therapists to encourage patients to remember traumatic tortious events to fund therapy; and, does the availability of tort damages provide an incentive for researchers to conduct studies that may enhance their prestige as expert witnesses? By their response to issues surrounding recollections of trauma, legal systems may shape not only the behavior of those who identify themselves as abuse survivors, but also the behavior of therapists who treat them and the researchers whose work addresses this treatment and related phenomena.

While legal systems occasionally explicitly communicate to classes of claimants that they are or are not welcome, more typically a constellation of pragmatic considerations combine to produce these incentives or disincentives. The pragmatic considerations that combine to encourage or discourage criminal prosecutions and civil damage claims on behalf of adults who identify themselves as having recently discovered recollections of childhood trauma, as well as to shape the behavior of therapists and researchers include: the legal model (adversarial, inquisitorial, etc.), along with its rules for assigning the re-

Recollections of Trauma, edited by Read and Lindsay
Plenum Press, New York, 1997

sponsibility to investigate allegations of wrongdoing and presentation of evidence at trial (judge or the parties), and the mode of presentations at trial (live witnesses or documentary presentations of witnesses testimony); the fact finder (judge or jury); whether the system's substantive law recognizes a right to recover damages for mental and emotional harm; whether the system uses court appointed experts or retained experts, or both, and the standard or process the system uses to scrutinize the testimony of these experts; and, the length of and exceptions to statutes of limitations that govern the time within which claims must be brought or abandoned. In addition, other factors such as the existence of national health insurance to pay for lengthy mental health care and social security to provide income support for those unable to work because of psychological disabilities may explain differences in the behavior of patients, therapists, and researchers.

To examine these differences, especially as they relate to the presentation of expert testimony about recollections of trauma, and assist exploration of their impact on how recollections of trauma have played out differently in different countries, we present discussions of the inquisitorial legal system from the perspective of the Netherlands by Hans Crombag, the Nordic legal system from the perspective of Denmark by Eva Smith, and the adversarial legal system from the perspective of the United States by Daniel Shuman. One approach to determining whether rules are just asks people to decide whether they would be willing to live by them if they did not know what role fate had in store for them, in this case whether they would be someone claiming to be a victim of abuse or someone claiming to have been wrongly accused of abuse. Likely most individuals considering the possibility that they may find themselves in the role of victim would see the benefits of the inquisitorial system that places the responsibility for the trial in the hands of a neutral judge and limits both the necessity for live trial testimony and cross-examination at the hands of the lawyer for a hostile adversary. Likely most individuals considering the possibility that they may find themselves in the role of wrongly accused abuser would see the benefits of the adversary system that permits the accused to play an active role in the discovery and presentation of evidence and grants the accused the opportunity to confront his or her accuser at trial and to cross-examine adverse witnesses at trial. While our personal histories and professional or national cultures may not permit us to suspend disbelief about the role we might find ourselves playing if the cosmic dice were re-thrown, the way in which these legal systems differ fundamentally on these basic issues makes clear not only that these differences matter but also that they are not incidental features of these legal systems. This exploration of the inquisitorial, adversarial, and Nordic legal systems offers us the opportunity to see their benefits and costs as they relate to recollections of trauma.

While their roles and affiliations may vary, in all world legal systems it is necessary for someone to question child witnesses and for someone to offer available expert guidance in sorting out information about the cases that would not otherwise be properly understood by a lay judge or jury. While their experience is in the United States, Nancy Walker's discussion of research on questioning of children and Spencer Eth's discussion of the role of an expert witness address issues that transcend specific legal systems. These presentations offer a direct link from the work of the conference to the work of the legal system. Not only do these presentations span psychological/psychiatric research and practice, but they address an area in which courts are often most receptive to psychiatric and psychological assistance.

REFERENCE

Jaffee v Redmond, 116 S. Ct. 1923 (1966).

30

FRAMING THE QUESTION OF THE ADMISSIBILITY OF EXPERT TESTIMONY ABOUT RECOLLECTIONS OF TRAUMA IN THE UNITED STATES

Daniel W. Shuman

Southern Methodist University
P.O. Box 750116
Dallas, Texas 75275-0116

To understand the rules of any legal system it is necessary to understand the constructs that underlie that system. Similarly worded rules may have vastly different consequences in different legal systems based on unspoken values and assumptions that underlie the operation of the legal system. This is nowhere more apparent than in seeking to understand the American legal system. The American legal system is built on a common law system inherited from England, informed by a revolutionary, rugged individualistic heritage of distrusting authority. This heritage is reflected in the U.S. Constitution which does not give citizens the right to receive anything from the government but rather grants them the right to protection from the government. This same heritage of distrust of authority is reflected in contemporary American political debates, for example those involving governmental assurances of health care for all citizens, in which the rejection of universal health care (unique among western democracies), is tied, in part, to the assumption that the government cannot be trusted to get it right.

The adversary legal system American style is a product of this distrust of authority, designed with multiple checks on authority, including using different fact finders (jurors) for each case, and placing responsibility for presenting and challenging evidence in the hands of the parties whose fate is at stake rather than accepting the investigation of a single governmental entity. It follows from this distrust of authority and attempt to spread the responsibility for investigating and presenting evidence, that the U.S. legal system permits the parties to select their own expert witnesses and rarely uses court-appointed experts. By permitting parties to select their own expert witnesses and challenge their opponents' experts, the American adversary system seeks to avoid the presentation of a single narrow, unchallenged perspective. However, because the American legal system's support for the jury's competence is not unbridled, it is thought necessary for the judge to address the competence/qualification of the expert as a question of law before the jury addresses the

Recollections of Trauma, edited by Read and Lindsay
Plenum Press, New York, 1997

weight/believability of the expert as a question of fact. The American adversary system's distrust of and checks on authority necessitates that it articulate standards and procedures to guide the judge in deciding the admissibility of expert testimony and to assist in reviewing the judge's performance.

The debate about the legal implications of recollections of trauma frequently focuses on the standard of admissibility for expert testimony, which is understandable because it is often dispositive of claims and defenses in civil and criminal suits alleging recovered memories of abuse, and civil suits claiming negligent therapy giving rise to false memories of abuse. Exclusion of a party's expert may result in dismissal of a claim based on an inability to prove that an exception to the statute of limitations should apply to a claim brought long after the statute has run or based on the failure to prove a prima facie case sufficient to get to the jury. While it is tempting to criticize particular court decisions on the subject of the admissibility of expert testimony about recollections of trauma for missing the underlying scientific question or analyzing it incorrectly, that is not the focus of my discussions here; rather I maintain that the debate has framed the question too narrowly and simplistically. My concern is with the issues that have been left out of the debate.

The debate about the standard for admissibility and its application to expert testimony addressing recovered memories of child abuse is usually framed by the clinical/research dichotomy (Sales, Shuman, O'Connor, 1994). While supporters of the admissibility of therapist's clinically based expert opinions seeking to validate claims of recovered memories of abuse do cite research for the validity of recovery of repressed memories, they also argue that a rigorous scientific threshold for clinical/behavioral science expert testimony is neither possible nor desirable, nor done elsewhere in the law. For example, rigid independent judicial scrutiny of the validity of the methods and procedures underlying the expert's testimony is not applied to clinician's testimony in child custody cases about "the best interests of the child" or insanity defense cases about a clinician's ability to reach an accurate and meaningful diagnosis of an individual on some past occasion when the expert had not seen the defendant (Shuman, 1994a). And, they maintain that a competent clinician's use of therapeutic techniques accepted by at least a respectable minority of the profession and their resulting opinions that patients suffer from real harm that they have experience assessing is sufficiently helpful to satisfy standards of admissibility that are applied across the legal system (Lorenzen, 1988). A number of courts have responded favorably to this approach (*Herald v. Hood*, 1993; *Isely v. Capuchin*, 1995; *Shahzade v. Gregory*, 1996).

Proponents of rigorous scientific screening of all expert testimony that invokes the mantle of science, whether natural or social science, argue that it is necessary and appropriate due to risks that decisionmaking errors (heuristics) cause us to give undue regard to anecdotal, clinical information that is likely to be wrong because researchers find no scientific proof of repression and recovery of repressed memories as claimed and, as well, because of evidence that some therapies used to recover these claimant's memories taint memories. This approach to rigorous independent scrutiny of the science underlying the expert testimony has been reinforced by the United States Supreme Court's decision in *Daubert v. Merrel Dow Pharmaceuticals, Inc* (1993) which requires federal judges to make a "preliminary assessment of whether the reasoning or methodology underlying the testimony is scientifically valid and of whether that reasoning properly can be applied to the facts in issue." Proponents of rigorous scrutiny argue that there is no scientifically valid basis to conclude that therapists' testimony about these memories are reliable/helpful and therefore they should be excluded (Loftus, 1993). A number of courts have responded favorably to this approach. (*Gier v. Educational Service Unit No. 16*, 1994; *State v. Hungerford*, 1994; *State v. Morahan*, 1993).

What frames this debate is an assumption that reaching truth is the only acceptable goal of the judicial system and the only acceptable question in that debate is how high it is necessary to raise the threshold of scrutiny to reach the truth. Of course, if the truth was the only acceptable goal of the judicial system we would never recognize a privilege that results in the exclusion of relevant communications between a therapist and patient, for example. Truth is only one of many goals of the judicial system. The determination of the threshold for the admissibility of expert testimony and the approach that is taken to setting it does more than decide the results of a particular case; its symbolism shapes our confidence in the judicial system and the competence of psychologists, psychiatrists, and other mental health professionals that extend beyond cases involving recollections of child abuse.

One of the sobering lessons of the 20th century is that democratic societies lack the resources to identify and prosecute more than a small percentage of proscribed acts. Thus, for most people the decision to obey the law turns on whether the law legitimizes their values and justifies their confidence (Tyler, 1990). Several of the many factors that shape this confidence are the judicial system's accuracy, impartiality, and availability.

Trust in the judicial system is related to a belief that the legal result accurately answers disputed factual questions. This concern is central in the debate over the degree of scrutiny that should be applied to expert testimony about recently recovered memories of childhood sexual abuse and the assumption that there is a direct correlation between the height of the admissibility bar and the accuracy of the result. But higher threshold standards of admissibility do not correlate with accuracy in the simplistic manner often assumed. Where there is sound research that helps to resolve the disputed question of fact and we admit only expert testimony that is properly grounded in that research, we are more likely to get it right. However, at least in this area of social science, because the facts of each case are unique so that the expert must extrapolate from the research to the case and because of the ethical/methodological limitations on research that might address the most directly relevant of these questions, it is unlikely that there will be sound research to resolve all of the disputed questions. Abusing children to determine the course of their memories of abuse or attempting to suggest to children who were not abused that they were, are experiments that no ethical researcher would ever contemplate or sane society would ever tolerate. Where there is not sound research addressing the disputed question of fact or where the research says that we cannot be certain, both admitting and excluding expert testimony leaves us uncertain whether we got it right. Thus, where there is not relevant sound research that resolves the issue, both the decision to admit or exclude expert testimony proceeds from a bias about where the risk of error should fall.

This bias about the risk of error is important because people's willingness to comply with the law turns, in part, on their trust in the impartiality of the judicial system. However, in civil/tort damage claims, where the system claims neutrality, higher evidentiary admissibility standards, which are facially neutral, have a disparate impact on plaintiffs and lower evidentiary standards have disparate impact on defendants. Indeed, civil defendants typically argue that juries cannot be trusted to get it right and that therefore we need higher standards of admissibility and civil plaintiffs typically argue that juries can be trusted to get it right and that therefore we need lower standards of admissibility to give juries all of the relevant evidence to assist their decision.

Plaintiffs must bring or lose claims within a specified time (the statute of limitations for personal injury actions in the U.S. is typically 1–3 years from the date that the wrongful conduct occurs) in which researchers may not yet have extensively researched the question. Indeed, there is an inherent tension between the development of scientifically validated knowledge and timely legal demands for the use of that knowledge. Thus demands for greater rigor and higher threshold scrutiny prejudice plaintiffs and benefit defendants, particularly in claims based upon new phenomena like "recovered repressed memories of child sexual abuse." We justify this because it is the plaintiff who seeks to change the status quo, but this is an ultimately semantic game that begs the question who first changed the status quo and places a premium on extra-judicial activities.

The legal system's history and legitimacy is rooted in its evolution as an alternative to blood feud and other forms of self-help. This history provides powerful evidence of a primal need of injured persons to seek vindication for their injuries (Shuman, 1993). If the legal system is to serve as a viable substitute to temper this primal need, it must be available for participation by citizens with disputes. Yet, without regard to its impact on accuracy, a higher evidentiary threshold standard for expert testimony that results in summary dismissal of claims bars certain classes of plaintiffs from the trial process and risks a perception that the judicial system is not available to give voice to persons who claim to suffer harm. These legally voiceless persons are then left to fashion their own remedy (Shuman, 1994). The impact of this more demanding scrutiny in the case of recollections of trauma is not neutral and falls disproportionately upon women and children (Enns, McNeilly, Corkery & Gilbert, 1995), which bolsters the feminist critique that the legal system consists of rules made by privileged white males that operate to disadvantage women and children (Bender, 1990).

Thus, more rigorous evidentiary standards have a complex relationship to confidence in the judicial system — they may result in increased accuracy, but only where they result in the presentation of testimony grounded in an existing body of relevant sound research that helps to answer the disputed question in the case. However, even in this case, they risk signaling the judicial system's partiality and limited accessability.

The standard for scrutiny of the information experts may offer in these cases also has important consequences for psychologists, psychiatrists, and other mental health professionals. Because judicial proceedings often dramatically publicize questions that are otherwise addressed in confidential settings or arcane intra-professional debate, the professions have a keen interest in how they are viewed through the lens of the judicial system and often argue for more demanding scrutiny in an effort to bolster the profession's image (Sales & Shuman, 1993). Yet rigorous/demanding scrutiny is a double edged sword, which even when wielded wisely, simultaneously excludes and publicizes the extent of unreliable practices in the diagnosis and treatment of mental disorders.

Those whose research or experiences cause them to doubt the ability of the lay public serving as jurors to get it right in resolving disputed scientific questions have no greater reason to expect the lay public to do any better in their role as patients. Thus, by identifying and publicizing such practices as unreliable, judicial rejection of clinically based testimony risks sowing more seeds of generic doubt about the therapeutic competence of mental health professionals and increases the risk of deterring people with real problems from seeking out competent therapists who use empirically grounded methods and procedures.

The standard for admissibility also has an important potential to affect the expert's privacy. Increasingly, attorneys have demanded that experts in abuse and custody cases disclose their personal mental health/abuse histories, based on the belief that this history may bias or prejudice the expert's decisions (*Cheatham v Rogers*, 1992). Although there is no empirical validation for the claim that an expert's abuse history, for example, may affect the expert's interpretation of ambiguous information in abuse cases, it corresponds to other common sense legal paradigms. For example, it is a legal article of faith that it is important to discover a prospective criminal juror's personal and familial experiences with the criminal justice system both as a victim and a suspect to exercise challenges to that juror because it is assumed that these experiences may affect the juror's decision in the case (Gobert & Jordan, 1990).

Intuitively, the strength of the argument in favor of compelling disclosure of the expert's mental health/abuse history seems most persuasive in the case of clinically rather than research based opinions. If expertise rests on validated methods and procedures, then the source of knowledge that forms the foundation for claims of expertise is, at least in theory, external to the expert and possessed equally by all informed and qualified experts. Thus, questions about whether the expert witness was abused as a child, is currently in counseling, or has had a difficult relationship are seemingly irrelevant to claims of scientifically based professional knowledge.

Expert testimony based on experience which is not uniform and not likely equally possessed by all informed qualified practitioners demands acknowledgment that experiences that may affect the development of the expert's theories and their application may well be relevant to the foundation for and impeachment of the expert. Thus, questions about whether the expert was abused or is currently in counseling are intuitively relevant to clinically/experientially based expertise. Of course, philosophers of science remind us that no science is value neutral, and thus any attempt to restrict this inquiry to experts who ground their expertise in experience is ultimately artificial. Moreover, there are significant risks that compelling disclosure of personal abuse/mental health histories will chill participation by experts with child sexual abuse histories and that because this is more likely to occur among women they will appear less frequently as experts thus providing courts with a skewed perspective. Thus, without regard to confidence in the judicial system, claims that clinical/experientially based expertise should be sufficient transforms expertise into a personalized claim and risks placing a fuller range of the experiences of the expert at issue which threatens the expert witness' own privacy interests and the availability of the full range of expert opinions to the courts.

In contrast with societal scrutiny of psychotherapy which is based on a competent adult/free market approach, in the crucible of the adversary system, courts now increasingly scrutinize the admissibility of expert opinion testimony based on the quality of the science that underlies the testimony and psychologists and psychiatrists should expect courts to demand evidence of the research that supports their opinions (*Daubert v. Merrell Dow Pharmaceuticals, Inc.*, 1993). Individual theories and practices of psychotherapy simply do not ordinarily undergo this level of judicial or societal scrutiny. More rigorous standards for admissibility may spillover to therapeutic practice and cause them to be grounded in more defensible or better research/avoid inappropriate, i.e., avoiding suggestive hypnotic techniques for refreshing memory (*Borawick v Shay*, 1995). And, more rigorous scrutiny may reinforce the importance of avoiding therapeutic/forensic role conflicts (Greenberg & Shuman, 1996)[*].

---

* The therapeutic and forensic roles demand different and inconsistent orientations and procedures. The therapist is a care provider—usually supportive, accepting, and empathic; the forensic evaluator is an assessor—usually neutral, objective, and detached as to the forensic issues. A forensic evaluator's task is to gain empathic understanding of the person but to remain dispassionate as to the psycholegal issues being evaluated. For therapists, empathy and sympathy—generating a desire to help—usually go hand-in-hand.

Thus, while a higher, more rigorous evidentiary standard may spill over to therapy increasing the scientific/ethical scrutiny of therapeutic practices and protecting therapist's privacy, it risks raising generic public doubts about therapeutic competence of mental health professionals.

The work of this NATO ASI teaches that successful efforts to address recollections of trauma must be inclusive and collaborative. For example, they must involve a collaborative effort that appropriately integrates clinical experience in experimental research and experimental research in clinical practice. This same lesson of inclusion holds true for the approach courts take to addressing the admissibility of expert testimony about recollections of trauma. Admissibility criteria have a more complex impact on the judicial system and psychology and psychiatry than is often understood and involve a range of consequences that demand our consideration. Only by recognizing and addressing this full range of complexities can we successfully address these questions.

REFERENCES

Bender, L. (1990). Feminist (Re)torts: Thoughts on the liability crisis, mass torts, power, and responsibilities. *Duke Law Journal*, 1990: 848–912.

Cheatham v. Rogers, 824 S.W.2d 231 (Tex. Civ. App. - Tyler 1992)

Enns, C. Z., McNeilly, C. L., Corkery, J. M., & Gilbert, M. S. (1995) The debate about delayed memories of child sexual abuse: A feminist perspective. *The Counseling Psychologist 23*: 181–279.

Daubert v. Merrell Dow Pharmaceuticals, Inc., 113 S. Ct. 2786 (1993).

Gobert, J. J. & Jordan, W. E. (2nd ed 1990) *Jury Selection: The Law, Art, and Science of Selecting A Jury.* Colorado Springs, CO: Shepard's/McGraw-Hill.

Greenberg, S. A. & Shuman, D.W. (1996). Irreconcilable conflicts between therapeutic and forensic roles. *Professional Psychology: Research and Practice* (forthcoming)

Herald v. Hood, 1993 Ohio App. LEXIS 3688

Isely v. Capuchin, 877 F. Supp. 1055 (S.D. Mich. 1995).

Loftus. E. (1993). The reality of repressed memories. *American Psychologist*, 48: 518–537.

Lorenzen, D. (1988). The admissibility of expert psychological testimony in cases involving the sexual misuse of a child. *University of Miami Law Review*, 42: 1033–1072.

Sales, B.D., Shuman, D.W., & O'Connor, M. (1994). In a dim light: Admissibility of child sexual abuse memories. *Applied Cognitive Psychology*, 8: 399–406.

Sales, B. & Shuman, D. (1993). Reclaiming the integrity of science in expert witnessing. *Ethics & Behavior*, 8: 223–229.

Shahzade v. Gregory, 1996 US Dist LEXIS 6463 (D Mass 1996)

Shuman, D. (1993). The psychology of deterrence in tort law. *University of Kansas Law Review*, 42: 115–168.

Shuman, D. (1994). The psychology of compensation in tort law. *University of Kansas Law Review*, 43: 39–77.

Shuman, D. (1994a). *Psychiatric and Psychological Evidence* 2nd ed. Colorado Springs: Shepards-McGraw Hill.

State v. Hungerford, No. 94-S-045 (N.H. Super. Ct., Hillsborough County 1994)

State v. Morahan, No. 93-S-1734 (N.H. Super. Ct., Hillsborough County 1993)

Tyler, T. (1990). *Why people obey the law.* New Haven, CT: Yale University Press.

31

EVIDENTIARY STANDARDS IN SEXUAL ABUSE CASES IN CONTINENTAL EUROPEAN LEGAL SYSTEMS

Hans F. M. Crombag

University of Limburg
P.O. Box 616, 6200 MD
Maastricht
The Netherlands

Before coming to the real subject of my contribution, which is the way in which continental European legal systems in general and the Dutch Legal system in particular handle evidentiary problems in sexual abuse cases, it is important to consider some general features of continental European legal systems, as they differ in significant ways from the Anglo-American way. All continental European legal systems have civil law systems as opposed to the Anglo-American common law system. Both are actually families of systems, with different pedigrees, different family traits and based on radically different philosophies concerning what the law is about.[*]

The most relevant difference between civil law and common law legal systems is procedural, in particular with respect to criminal procedure. Common law systems follow an adversarial procedure, civil law systems an inquisitorial procedure. In an adversarial procedure a case, even a criminal case, is considered to be a contest between two parties, who present their case in a partisan way to an independent and mostly passive third party, which in principle consists of a jury of the defendant's peers.[†] Under an inquisitorial procedural regime a criminal case is an inquest by an independent state authority of an alleged infringement of its rules. This independent state authority in a simple case is a single professional judge, and in complicated cases a panel of three professional judges. These different views of how a criminal case must be handled, has implications for the position of expert witnesses, whose role is particularly important in sexual abuse cases.

In an adversarial procedural system it is the duty of the parties, the prosecution and the defense, to see to it that all evidence necessary for the trier of fact to decide the case is gathered and presented in court. In preparation for trial both the prosecution and the de-

---

[*] For more details and their meaning see: M. Damaska, *The Faces of Justice and State Authority: A Comparative Approach*

[†] I am aware that nowadays most criminal cases in the UK are dealt without a jury.

Recollections of Trauma, edited by Read and Lindsay
Plenum Press, New York, 1997

fense investigate the case. There are, however, strict rules for this — the rules of evidence — and it is the judge's task during the trial to exclude all information that was gathered in an illegal or improper manner. All evidence admitted during the trial and therefore considered proper evidence, is subject to challenge through cross-examination of testimonial evidence and the introduction of contradicting evidence by the opposing party. On the basis of this the trier of fact is assumed to be able to value the evidence and to decide the case on the basis of it. I say "assumed", because juries do not have to give reasons for or otherwise to explain their verdicts. We have no reliable way of knowing whether a jury took only proper evidence into account or whether it weighed the various pieces in a sensible manner.

Under an inquisitorial regime only the prosecution actively investigates a case. It is expected to do so in an even handed manner, not only gathering incriminating, but also exculpatory information. Although the prosecution is required to refrain from illegal investigative practices — i.e. manners that violate the constitutional rights of the defendant — there are few rules restricting the prosecution and the police in their investigatory activity.

In an inquisitorial criminal procedure it is considered highly improper for the defense to investigate a case actively. The defense is expected to wait for whatever the prosecution comes up with. Before a case goes to trial the defense is entitled to see all the evidence gathered by the prosecution, which is available for its inspection in documentary form in the dossier.

During the trial the defense may try to rebut this evidence by asking the court to call certain witnesses, whose statements are already available in the dossier, to appear in court in person and suggest the presiding judge to put certain critical question to those witnesses. The court, however, does not have to comply with such a request; at any point it may decide that it is already sufficiently informed and refuse to consider any more evidence.

In the Netherlands as well as in Germany courts are required to give reasons for their verdicts, but this is not true in all inquisitorial systems; in Belgium and France the courts can decide without giving reasons. In practice it does not make much of a difference, because the reasons that Dutch courts usually give for their verdicts are so scant, that they might as well have given no reasons at all.

During trial the defense may want to rebut evidence presented by the prosecution by proposing that witnesses of its own choice be called and heard. Again, the court is under no obligation to comply with such a request. However, if it does, even a witness heard on the initiative of the defense is in principle considered to be the court's witness.

All this is also true for expert witnesses. Whenever deemed necessary, an expert witness is appointed by the court. In practice this is most of the time done by the investigating judge in the preparatory phase. An expert witness thus appointed is considered the court's own expert, working under its authority. It is the appointing judge who instructs the expert what is to be the subject of his or her investigation. The expert reports, usually in written form, to the court. Whether such a court appointed expert is also heard in person during trial, is also the court's decision.

The defense, reading the expert's report before the trial, may want a second expert opinion. To this purpose it may propose to the court to appoint "a counter-expert", but this name sits uneasily with the idea that every witness is the court's witness.

When the defense proposes the appointment of a second expert witness, the court may refuse to do so. But the court may also decide to adopt such a "counter-expert" proposed by the defense. When the court refuses to adopt the "counter-expert", it may yet allow such a witness to submit his report and even to testify in person. But again this is by no means certain, although in recent years the courts in my country, under the influence of the due process clause (Article 6) of the European Convention on Human Rights, have become more lenient in this respect.[‡]

Let us now consider the role that behavioral expert witnesses may and actually do play in sexual abuse cases in my own and neighboring countries. When young children are involved in sexual abuse cases, the police often calls on a child psychologist or person of similar training to question the alleged victim. Such an expert is assumed to have two advantages over a common police officer: she is assumed to be better able to make the child talk and also to interpret better what the child is saying.[°] Her conversation with the child is usually recorded on audio - or even videotape. Next she writes a report, relaying what the child has divulged and whether she considers this reliable information. The report becomes part of the case dossier.

The good thing about this procedure is that the court itself as well as anyone else, e.g., a "counter-expert" proposed by the defense, can examine the videotaped recording and make up their own minds as to its content. However, hardly ever do courts take the time to watch such recordings themselves. Instead they rely on the written reports of experts and, if any, "counter-experts".

This procedure, often followed in the Netherlands, raises a number of problems. First, what about the right of the defendant "to examine or have examined witnesses against him," as guaranteed by Article 6 of the European Convention on Human Rights? It is almost universally assumed, even in the United States, that alleged child victims of sexual abuse must not be examined, let alone cross-examined, in court.[+] But what is the alternative if one is to take the defendant's right to cross-examination seriously? To my mind at least that interviews of alleged child victims of abuse are **always recorded** on videotape, that these recordings are always made available to a "counter-expert" proposed by the defense, and that the report of the "counter-expert" is always admitted into evidence and treated by the courts on an equal footing with the report of the expert who interviewed the child for the prosecution.[□] Obvious as this "rule" may seem, it is by no means always accepted and adhered to in inquisitorial criminal proceedings.

Even if this "rule" would be generally accepted in continental European countries, there is the problem of hearsay evidence. It may yet come as a surprise to those accustomed to the Anglo-American way that in practice hearsay evidence is by no means excluded from most inquisitorial criminal proceedings. In the Netherlands the statute of criminal procedure of 1926 in Article 341 explicitly forbids hearsay evidence in criminal cases, but by 1927 the Dutch Supreme Court had shelved this rule. The same thing happened in Belgium. As a result most inquisitorial criminal proceedings have gradually degraded into paper proceedings; criminal cases are decided on the basis of the written documents, mostly consisting of statements of witnesses' testimony taken by the police or

---

‡ For more details see: H.F.M. Crombag, On the Europeanisation of criminal procedure; In: B. de Witte & C. Forder, *The Common Law of Europe and the Future of Legal Education*; Deventer: Kluwer, 1992, 397–414.

° In my country nowadays we have some police officers specially trained for questioning child witnesses. The interrogations are usually videotaped.

+ G.S. Goodman, M. Levine, G.B. Melton & D.W. Ogden, Child Witnesses and the Confrontation Clause: The American Psychological Association brief in *Maryland v. Craig, Law and Human Behavior*, 1991, *15*, 13–29.

□ I have said so before; see: H.F.M. Crombag, Contra-expertise in de strafrechtelijke afwikkeling van gevallen van vermoed sekueel misbruik van kinderen (Counter-expertise in criminal cases concerning suspected sexual abuse of children); In: L.P. Raijmakers, F. Wafelbakker, O.H. van der Baan-Slootweg, R.A.R. Bullens & D. Wouters (eds.), *Handelen bij Vermoeden van Seksueel Misbruik van Kinderen en Jeugdigen II*; Assen: Van Grokum/Dekker & Van de Vegt, 1995, 55–57.

the investigating judge prior to the trial and reports by expert witnesses. During the trial the court usually works its way through these documents, occasionally asking the defendant whether "all this is true". A defendant who contradicts (parts of) the documentary evidence, is simply reminded by the presiding judge that the dossier contains evidence to the contrary.

One last point should be mentioned. In cases of sexual abuse of children the experts called on by the prosecution are usually members of a rather small group of experts known to the courts. In France expert witnesses are even taken from an official list of experts drawn up yearly by the criminal authorities. Being a member of the pool of "official" expert-witnesses, however, does not guarantee real expertness, so some colleagues and I have learned from bitter experience in our own country.[¥] Even so, since the courts know these experts well, their credentials are hardly ever questioned. Moreover, the "official" expert witnesses are not available to the defendant, who must therefore rely on "counter-experts" of lower notoriety to the courts. This may well lead to inequality of arms during the ensuing "battle of experts", even if this battle is mostly fought on paper.

Under inquisitorial criminal proceedings the defendants in cases of alleged sexual abuse in general and of children in particular are quite vulnerable. The defendant or his counsel are never allowed to confront the alleged victim directly. It is, moreover, by no means certain that he will be allowed to examine a recorded version of the child's testimony or to criticize the expert who interviewed the child victim. This is especially worrying since charges of sexual abuse of children have been brought in increasing numbers in continental Europe. In so far as these are real cases, of course, these must be prosecuted diligently. But one may well ask whether inquisitorial criminal proceedings, as they are practiced nowadays in most continental legal countries, are really up to this task.

¥ W.A. Wagenaar, P.J. van Koppen & H.F.M. Crombag, *Anchored Narratives: The Psychology of Criminal Evidence*; Hemel Hempstead: Harvester Weatsheaf, 1993.

32

EVIDENTIARY STANDARDS IN SEXUAL ABUSE CASES IN NORDIC LEGAL SYSTEMS

Eva Smith

University of Copenhagen
6, Studiestraede, DK-1455
Copenhagen K
Denmark

Like the other papers addressing the legal system's response to recollections of trauma, I will begin with some general remarks about the difference between the Anglo-American system and the Nordic system. A very significant difference in the Nordic system is that our judges are legally obliged to seek the truth. I believe that is current for central Europe as well.

In the Anglo-American legal tradition this approach would probably be regarded as rather naive. The truth is regarded as God's department. All a mortal judge can do is establish whether the requisite quantum of proof has been presented. If it is, the person should be convicted, if it is not, the person should be acquitted. But in Europe we worry about finding the truth. We believe innocent men and women should be acquitted and we also think that guilty men and women should be convicted. We get upset when we see someone who is apparently guilty is acquitted, while an Anglo-American might just shrug his or her shoulders: well, the defendant might have done the act charged, but if evidence sufficient to satisfy the standard of proof has not been presented the defendant should be acquitted.

I am not arguing which system is the better, but it is important to be aware of this difference because it has important implications. For instance, Nordic law is not as harsh on formalities as Anglo-American law. If the police, for instance, have overstepped their boundaries, Nordic law does not automatically ignore the evidence. The judge will carefully consider whether it will be unfair to the defendant to use the evidence under those particular circumstances. Nevertheless, the Nordic legal system abides by international rules about rights of the defendant. In criminal cases, guilt should be proven beyond reasonable doubt and, like Anglo-American law, the Nordic legal system expresses a preference in favour of acquitting 10 guilty people rather than convicting 1 innocent person.

The Nordic system is a mix of the adversary system found in the Anglo-American systems and the inquisitorial system found in central Europe. On a number of points the Nordic legal system resembles the Anglo-American system: First, it always uses lay judges in criminal cases. In Denmark we use a jury if the prosecution is asking for more than 4 years imprisonment. If the prosecution asks for less than four years the court consists of one judge and two lay judges.

In the Nordic countries we firmly believe that the question of inflicting punishment should not be left entirely to the legal profession. That kind of pain and bereavement should not be inflicted unless other members of the public agree both that the defendant is guilty and with the punishment inflicted. Furthermore because of the use of lay judges, Nordic criminal cases are always oral. Finally the questioning of the defendant and the witnesses is done by prosecution and defence - not by the judge. In some other ways the Nordic legal system resembles the inquisitorial system: the investigation is done by the police and the appointment of experts rests with the court.

Table 1 provides a useful overview of the different systems. Starting with the investigation, in the Nordic countries as in central Europe, the investigation is done by the police. However, in Denmark a number of defence rights exist designed to create some degree of equality between the prosecution and the defence even before the trial. The defence has a right to know of all investigative steps being taken by the police. The defence can also request the police to take certain investigative steps such as trying to locate a witness. If the police refuse, the defence counsel may take the matter to court for the judge to decide.

When very important steps are taken which are likely to become evidence in the trial to follow, like a line-up or a video-questioning of a child witness, the defence counsel has a right to be present. I have already discussed the judge and the proceedings.

Medical doctors are often appointed as experts in these proceedings. And, as you all are very well aware, medical doctors often differ significantly in their views. In accordance with our principle of trying to uncover the truth we believe that we are not helping matters by confusing the jury with a lot of different ideas such that they do not know which to believe.

Therefore, a board of 12 experts has been set up involving medical doctors from various fields. The board is set up by the government, but the members are supposed to be independent experts. They can call upon a number of other experts if a question is too specialized. The board has been criticised for being old-fashioned and not very experimental in its views. Demands for a second opinion are more often heard nowadays. Unless the claim for a second opinion can be substantiated with some evidence of high medical standard and will add important knowledge to the court's deliberations, however, it will often not be allowed.

Table 1. Comparison of relevant features across three legal systems

	Anglo-American	Central Europe	Nordic
Investigation	Police + defense	Police/investigating judge	Police (rights for defense)
Judge	Jury	Judge	Jury/lay judges + judge
Proceedings	Oral	Partly written	Oral
Appointment of experts	Prosecutor + defense	Court	Court
Questions to experts, witnesses and defendant	Prosecution + defense	Court	Prosecution + defense
Children's testimony	(Court) questioning by prosecution + defense	Written report from child psychologist	Video in court from police interview

The questioning of the board or any other experts is normally done in writing. The prosecution and the defence prepare a line of questions to be put before the board and these are given to the court for examination. They will generally be approved by the court unless they are unclear or not relevant. The questions are then put before the board and the answers are read out during the court proceedings.

Occasionally a member of the board will appear in person in front of the court. I personally do not find this procedure completely satisfactory. To my mind the opportunity for the defence to bring in a second opinion should be less restricted especially in areas where the question is not purely medical and the answer depends to a greater or lesser degree on an assessment on the part of the expert.

As far as Denmark and Norway are concerned, the system concerning psychologists as witnesses is the same as I described with the board of doctors. The attorneys may pose a line of general questions and a psychologist may answer them.

The questions to the board have to be general if they touch the credibility of a witness. This is because it is up to the court to decide whether evidence with the purpose of assessing a witness' credibility may be brought before the court. Normally the court will not allow this. Only the court assesses the testimony. In Danish and Norwegian law there is even a statement assuring this procedure.

Let me give you an example to illustrate the meaning of "general" questions. In one case the following question was put to the board of doctors (by the counsel for the defendant).

"Are there any signs in a young child like displaying sexual behaviour, excessive washing of the body, being afraid of men or any other sign that unmistakably states that a child has been abused?"

And the board answered of course that no signs to that effect exist. But it would not have been allowed for the defence counsel to ask the board, "Is it likely that this child, with the specific symptoms she has, was sexual abused?"

Recently in another case counsel for the defence asked the court for permission to put a line of questions before a psychologist. One of these questions was:

"Is it psychologically likely that a person who has just committed a murder would sit in his car near the place of the murder and when approached by the victim's husband would volunteer to help him find his missing wife?"

This kind of behaviour was of course just what the counsel for the prosecution alleged that the defendant had done. His request to put these questions before an expert was denied. It is strictly up to the court to assess whether this was a likely behaviour or not seen in the light of the other evidence.

In the cases we are dealing with at this meeting you may for instance ask whether it is possible that memories can be barred and forgotten by the conscious mind - to pop up at a much later time in one's life. Or, how is a trauma defined? What are its manifestations?

The situation is the same in Norway but you should know that Sweden has a different tradition. In Sweden psychologists (called witness psychologists) are used in a very special way. Their job involves doing what one could call "good policemen's work". They study all the police interrogations and they will typically re-do all the interviewing all over. They question witnesses, the defendant, the policeman who did the first interview—anybody who can help the psychologist put together what actually happened. Then the psychologists offer a statement for the court. The statement may say the evidence collected points to the defendant being guilty. It may also say the child is not to be trusted, because very likely there has been a misunderstanding or the child has reasons for not telling the truth. But, as mentioned, this is a very special Swedish way of assessing children's testimony which, as far as I know and is not found anywhere else in the world.

The last point from my table concerns the obtaining of children's testimony. I was in Great Britain 6 months ago and witnessed an abuse case. The victim - a nine-year old girl - was being interviewed on closed circuit television. This means that the child is in another room of the court building, answering questions from the two counsels. The two counsels were in the courtroom and the child was shown on a screen when answering the questions. The case involved a number of different incidents of indecent behaviour. The child knew the defendant and had on numerous occasions accompanied him to different places.

One line of questioning ran like this:

Counsel for the defence: On this particular afternoon the two of you went in a different car. What colour was the car?

Child: I am not sure. I think it was black.

Counsel: Well, I am asking you a direct question. What colour was the car?

Child: I think it was black.

Counsel: Was it black or was it not black?

Child: It was black.

Counsel (pulls out police file): Well according to what you said to the police 6 months ago it was dark-blue?

Child: Well, I am not sure about the colour of the car. It has been so long...

Counsel: So you are not sure about the colour of the car? Are you sure about any of all this you have been telling us?

You lied to us about the car. Are you one of these children that quite often lie about things?

And so on...

I was appalled. To me it is very disrespectful not only to the child but also to the court. It makes a mockery out of something much too serious - to the defendant and to the child - to be treated that way. Such a line of questioning would never be allowed in the Nordic countries. Certainly not with a child witness but not with any witness for that matter. This again has to do with our principle about trying to find the truth. Intimidating a witness this way is assumed to be counterproductive to that search.

When it comes to children's testimony, older children are questioned in court. Children under the age of 12 or even older if the facts are very distressing, are questioned by a policeman in a taped interview. The counsel for the defence will sit in a nearby room following the interview on a monitor. When the interview is finished the policeman will leave the child and ask the defence counsel if he or she has any questions for the child. The policeman will then ask these questions as well. The whole interview will be taped and shown in court, where the counsels may challenge its content.

They do not have exactly the same procedure in the other Nordic countries. In Norway the child is normally questioned by the judge in the judge's chamber with the counsels present. I must admit that I much prefer the Danish way both to the Anglo-American system and to the central European. I have seen a number of court videos and it makes a powerful impression when you see small children cuddling their favourite toy animal and struggling to convey these painful memories. Most of them seem very honest and convincing, but once in a while you listen to one and you wonder.

Still I think our system can be improved. For instance, I think the counsel for the defence should be allowed to put the questions to the child himself rather than letting a policeman do it. As we all know, it makes a difference to the answers how the question is put and what the interviewer's opinion is. Of course it may confuse a very young child to be confronted with a new person, but around the age of 6 I think most children can handle it. I am not worried for the child. Danish defence counsels are very gentle with children. Primarily because of our tradition not to bully witnesses. But they also know that if the jury thinks they are trying to intimidate a child, the jury will almost certainly turn against them (and their clients).

Finally I think it was a very good idea to have a legal panel on this conference. It is very difficult to find the delicate balance between the interest of the vulnerable child witness and the interest of the defendant. It is important to learn from the ways other countries have approached the problem.

33

THE PSYCHIATRIC EXPERT WITNESS

Spencer Eth

UCLA School of Medicine
11301 Wilshire Boulevard
Los Angeles, California 90073

Forensic mental health professionals serving as expert witnesses are regularly asked to opine whether an alleged traumatic incident caused psychological harm, and if so what type of treatment may be indicated. When the plaintiff in a personal injury lawsuit is a child and the incident involves sexual abuse, these clinical determinations can become quite difficult. A further complicating factor is the nature of the United States judicial system. In the majority of civil tort cases involving putative psychiatric injuries, different expert witnesses are separately retained by the attorneys for the defendant and plaintiff. Given the prevailing adversarial system of law, there are considerable incentives for the expert to offer opinions favorable to the hiring side. In some instances experts are selected because of their reputation for advocating a particular point of view (e.g., "false memory" authorities). In other cases more "neutral" appearing experts are chosen, but even the most independent minded of expert witnesses will experience subtle pressure to conform their opinions to fit the attorney's theory of the case.

The challenge for the expert is to infuse scientific objectivity into the practical task of providing judgments regarding etiology, psychopathology, and therapeutics. Fortunately, clinical experience is an important teacher that will guide this complex work. Consider the following case vignettes and the lessons they offer, cognizant of the fact that in each of these three cases I served as an adviser to the defendant insurance company with regard to the validity and value of the plaintiff's injuries. Although I believe that I examined each case on its merits, I cannot exclude the possibility that I may have been subject to a defense-oriented bias, despite the fact that my writings in general reflect a pronounced sympathy for the traumatized child (Eth, 1988). The case histories have been constructed from accounts of the events in question obtained from court records, including police investigations and transcripts, and from interviews with the children.

CASE 1: JEREMY AT SUMMER CAMP

Jeremy is a nine-year-old boy who was sexually accosted on several occasions at night by his summer camp director. The incidents became more intrusive and upsetting,

Recollections of Trauma, edited by Read and Lindsay
Plenum Press, New York, 1997

and eventually culminated with an act of forced oral copulation accompanied by threats of death if he told anyone. A few days later, a group of boys escaped from the camp and notified the police. Jeremy was reunited with his mother and stepfather, but he was too scared to mention the abuse until he was questioned by the police several days later. Only then did he disclose the initial incidents, but not the act of fellatio. Several months later the camp director was successfully prosecuted for sexual molestation.

Jeremy began to have nightmares of the director chasing him with a knife, while he was still at the camp. The nightmares increased in frequency and intensity over the ensuing months. In addition, Jeremy became fearful of being alone in his bedroom and would seek refuge at night in his sister's bed. His fears generalized to the point where he was "afraid of everything," and he demanded to stay at home for protection. About a year after his molestation Jeremy developed thoughts of killing himself with a knife. Jeremy was hospitalized and revealed to his therapist all of the details of his sexual abuse.

Jeremy's early childhood was unremarkable until age five years, when his father committed suicide by carbon monoxide poisoning in his car in the family garage. When Jeremy became suicidal five years later, he wondered if he would end up like his father. A month after his father's suicide a man broke into the home and attempted to rape Jeremy's mother at knife point. Jeremy witnessed this attack, and the perpetrator was later apprehended and convicted.

The case of Jeremy reminds us that disclosure of child sexual abuse is best conceived of as a process rather than as a single event. Jeremy at first told no one, then described some of the incidents to the police, and finally revealed the most embarrassing aspects to his therapist. Given the fact that Jeremy's full account of his molestation was shared first with his therapist over the course of several sessions, there is an inherent danger that the therapist's own views towards this emotionally charged subject influenced the nature of Jeremy's disclosures and perhaps even his own memories of the events. The powerful effect of demand characteristics on human memory has been well documented by experimental cognitive psychologists, and this research has direct relevance to psychotherapy and to the legal arena (i.e., Ceci & Bruck, 1995). It is, therefore, incumbent upon child therapists, and especially child forensic experts, who work with possibly sexually abused children to be well versed in the various interviewing techniques that enhance accurate recollections and minimize memory distortions (i.e., Jones & McQuiston, 1988).

Jeremy appears to be a legal "eggshell," insofar as significant predisposing factors can be identified (Rosenberg & Eth, 1994). It is likely that his father's suicide placed Jeremy at risk for suicidal ideation. However, the proximate cause of his psychiatric decompensation appears to be the sexual abuse, since there is no reason to believe he would have become so ill at that time had the molestation not occurred. The early emergence of incident-specific post-traumatic symptomatology, that progressed to include a depressive syndrome, certainly supports that conclusion. One is left to wonder what would have happened if Jeremy had been the only child molested at camp — would he have had the courage to disclose when he returned home; would he then have been believed by his parents and the police; and would his solo testimony have been sufficient to convict the generally well liked camp director?

CASE 2: ANNABELLE'S NURSERY SCHOOL

The next case involves the children who attended Annabelle's Nursery School and the owner's husband, Joseph. Joseph took a series of children from the nursery to his nearby home, undressed the child, positioned the child, and photographed the child naked, usually with a genital closeup and sometimes in a sexually provocative pose. The child was then dressed, bribed with a cookie to remain silent, and returned to the nursery school.

Eventually, one child confided to his parents, who subsequently notified the police. The police searched the house and found a file cabinet containing approximately 2,000 pictures of nude children, taken over a two year period and affecting about 15 different children, two of whom were the subject of 85% of the pictures. Joseph was arrested and convicted of felony child molestation at trial, during which the parents but not the children testified.

It is important to note that the discovery of the photographs precipitated a crisis in the families of current and former students. The parents commonly exhibited anxiety, anger, shame, guilt, blame and sadness. This stress seemed to exacerbate parental psychopathology, including depression, alcohol abuse, and marital discord. It also affected parental attitudes and behaviors regarding their children, with some mothers becoming overprotective and some fathers believing that their children had become "damaged goods." The publicity over the trial was particularly painful for parents.

At least 23 former students filed lawsuits, of whom 14 had been the subject of recovered photographs and 9 had not. Those children who were not in the pictures used the theory that there was, in fact, no evidence that these children had not been abused, and that they were suffering from a behavior syndrome associated with sexual abuse. In general the children who had the worse psychological outcomes were the ones who had retained memories of being photographed, or who had other unpleasant memories of the nursery school, or who had problems during their attendance at the preschool. Several children with happy memories of school and no memories of being photographed were not symptomatic at follow up, despite the existence of nude pictures of them.

The case of Annabelle's Nursery School underscores the salience of the child's perspective of the event. A young child might experience being taken on a special trip to Joseph's house, being photographed like a naked movie star, and being rewarded with a cookie as enjoyable. Such a child would not be expected to react to the incident with symptoms of post-traumatic stress, and indeed the entire event might readily fade from memory. Of course, another child might respond to the same sequence with humiliation, fear, and severe distress. It is likely that the latter child would have a very different psychological response and could well retain robust recollections of the incident.

Not only is the child's subjective appraisal critical, but so too are the post-event factors to which the child is exposed. The emotional reactions of the families to the discovery of the photographs, the closing of the preschool, and Joseph's trial were often profound. Many children developed psychiatric symptoms for the first time in the aftermath of the revelation of child pornography, which in turn validated their parents' fear and expectation that they had been seriously harmed, and further served to stress the family system and worsen everyone's distress. These families might have benefited from a prompt intervention designed to interrupt this vicious circle of self-fulfilling prophesy of mental damage.

The daunting challenge for the forensic psychiatrist is to distinguish the early sequelae of sexual abuse from the alter reciprocal and nonspecific symptoms that arose after the discovery of the pictures and in the context of family upheaval. A nagging clinical and ethical question remains unanswered — should the children who have no memories of being photographed be told about the pictures, when, by whom, and in what way?

CASE 3: MR. MARTIN'S FIRST GRADE CLASS

The final case study concerns an accusation by five children that their first grade teacher, Mr. Martin, showed pornographic movies in their classroom. When the children were in the third grade a girl, who was by then living out of state, told her mother that she had been shown a dirty movie while in Mr. Martin's class two years before. Her mother called a former classmate's mother to seek confirmation of her daughter's story. That woman asked her son if a teacher ever showed dirty movies, and was "told everything." Three other mothers were contacted and asked to question their children. Those children, two boys and one girl, also admitted that they had viewed pornographic movies in Mr. Martin's first grade class. The police were notified and conducted a search of Mr. Martin's apartment. No pornographic materials were found, and Mr. Martin adamantly denied the accusation. Consequently, no criminal charges were brought against Mr. Martin, though civil lawsuits were filed against the school district on behalf of the four local children who claimed to have been shown pornography in class.

When interviewed by the psychiatric expert, all four children recalled disliking Mr. Martin, who was described as mean. The first boy recalled that on the day of the lunar eclipse Mr. Martin shut the door to the classroom, pulled down the shades, and showed a video to the entire class of a naked man lying on top of a naked woman. The child thought he saw this same video on other occasions, but "it's hard to remember." He also recalled seeing an army movie of people and animals getting killed. The second boy also reported reviewing a movie with his class of a grown man, a woman, and several girls all undressed. The third boy described being brought to a shed to see movies of "a lot of killing." He also recollected being shown sex videos, including one in which a man stuck his penis into a woman's behind and his fingers into her vagina. The girl remembered seeing a film of a naked man and woman lying on top of each other. Three of these children recall Mr. Martin threatening to hurt their families if they told anyone about the movies. The threats were particularly frightening because all of these children lived in a fatherless home. At the time of their psychiatric examination each of the children presented with school performance and behavioral difficulties. However, none suffered from post-traumatic stress disorder or depression.

The case of Mr. Martin's first grade class contrasts sharply from the previous two cases in that there exists considerable dispute about the validity of the unsubstantiated allegation of sexual exploitation, especially since no other child from the first grade class of over twenty children confirmed the account of exposure to pornographic movies. However, it also possible that the other children forgot or repressed seeing the movies, and that no implication should be drawn that the movies had not been shown in class (see Williams, 1994 and Pope & Hudson, 1995 for conflicting data on the reliability of later recollections of childhood sexual trauma). In the final analysis, it may not be possible for the forensic mental health expert to conclude with reasonable medical certainty that the incident actually occurred. Clearly, if the abusive event did not happen, then it could not have caused any direct psychological harm. Although these four children display psychiatric symptoms, they do not conform to the classic, post-traumatic syndromes. Rather, the absence of a father in the home may have rendered these particular children more sensitive to negative interactions with Mr. Martin, and may be a salient etiological factor in their subsequent maladjustment.

These three cases illustrate that the "truth" is often elusive; the psychiatric expert must strive to collect relevant data, consider possible bias, and be able to accept uncertainty (Eth & Leong, 1993). Ultimately, it is the court and not the expert who is the final arbiter of justice in an imperfect and ambiguous world.

REFERENCES

Ceci, S. J. & Bruck, M. (1995). *Jeopardy in the courtroom: A scientific analysis of children's testimony*. Washington, DC: American Psychological Association.

Eth, S. (1988). The child victim as witness in sexual abuse proceedings. *Psychiatry 51*:221–232.

Eth, S. & Leong, G. B. (1993). Ethics and psychiatry. *Current Opinion in Psychiatry 6*:795–798.

Jones, D.P.H. & McQuiston, M. G. (1988). *Interviewing the sexually abused child*. London: Gaskell.

Pope, H. G. & Hudson, J. I. (1995). Can memories of childhood sexual abuse be repressed? *Psychological Medicine, 25*:121–126.

Rosenberg, J. & Eth, S. (1994). Post-traumatic stress disorder in children. In R. Rosner (Ed.), *Principles and practice of forensic psychiatry*. New York: Chapman and Hall.

Williams, L. M. (1994). Recall of childhood trauma: A prospective study of women's memories of child sexual abuse. *Journal of Consulting and Clinical Psychology, 62*:1167–1176.

34

SHOULD WE QUESTION HOW WE QUESTION CHILDREN?

Nancy E. Walker[*]

Creighton University
Omaha, Nebraska 68178

1. THE PROBLEM

Children appear in court following trauma in both adversarial and inquisitorial legal systems. Although some countries (e.g., Israel) spare children the necessity of appearing at trial by questioning specially trained youth investigators in their stead, most systems require that, absent special circumstances, when a case proceeds to trial children provide testimony following victimization. In addition, children who allege that they have been victimized must be questioned at some point during legal proceedings, whether during criminal investigations, depositions, and/or at trial. It is important, therefore, to investigate children's comprehension of the various types of question forms they are likely to encounter during legal proceedings. The purpose of this section is to integrate legal policy, clinical practice and empirical findings regarding the questioning of child witnesses following trauma.

2. THE RATIONALE

There are three major reasons why we should be concerned with how we question children during legal proceedings. The first reason is ethical or moral: Both the welfare and safety of children and the reputations and liberty interests of alleged perpetrators depend upon the accuracy of the questioning process. The second reason is scientific: The results of recent empirical studies demonstrate that the nature of the interview process itself contributes substantially to the relative accuracy and completeness (or inaccuracy and incompleteness) of accounts provided by children (Walker & Hunt, in press; Warren, Woodall, Hunt, & Perry, 1996). The third reason is pragmatic: Poor questioning proce-

[*] Nancy E. Walker, Ph.D., is Professor of Psychology at Creighton University, Omaha, Nebraska 68178, USA. She may be contacted by telephone at (402) 280–3181, by fax at (402) 280–4748, or by e-mail at nwalker@creighton.edu. Formerly she published under the name of Nancy W. Perry.

dures can lead to an interviewer being "on trial" in a child victimization case (cf., *People v. Buckey* [1984]; *State v. Michaels* [1994]).

3. THREE CENTRAL QUESTIONS

This section addresses three central questions: First, what are the statutory guidelines for interviewing children? Second, what do we know about how specific question forms affect the quality and quantity of children's responses? Finally, how are interviews of children actually conducted in the "real world"?

3.1. What Are the Statutory Guidelines for Interviewing Children?

Walker and Nguyen (1996) reviewed statutes from each of the 50 U.S. states that pertained to questioning children. They found that 30 states (60%) had enacted legislation that was in some way pertinent to questioning child witnesses; however, the content of those statutes varied widely. For example, some statutes addressed the issue of protecting children from harassment during questioning, whereas others designated that interviewers must have specialized training. Still other statutes delineated where children may testify, whether they may testify via closed circuit television or videotaped deposition, whether support persons may be present, and so forth.

Walker and Nguyen's (1996) article included a features analysis of statutes that pertained specifically to the interview process with children which revealed that U.S. statutes provided very little useful guidance regarding how to question children. Only seven states (14%) required that proceedings be explained to children in age-appropriate language, and just four states (8%) specified that interviewers receive special training in child development. Only two states (4%) recommended limiting the amount of time the child spends on the witness stand. And only the state of California required that questions posed to children be in language the child can understand!

3.2. How Are Interviews of Children Actually Conducted?

Both Walker and Hunt (in press) and Warren et al. (1996) analyzed the linguistic features of 42 transcripts of Child Protective Services (CPS) interviews of children (30 females and 12 males) aged two to 13 years who alleged to have been sexually abused. The researchers conducted both quantitative and qualitative analyses of interview structure and of question form and content, examining the effects of several question forms on children's responses. They found that the CPS interviewers engaged in a number of questioning practices that might be considered suspect. For example, 40% of the interviewers never attempted to establish rapport with the children. Those who did try to build rapport primarily used specific questions (e.g., "What school do you attend?") rather than open-ended questions (e.g., "What do you like to do after school?"). As a result, interviewers talked three times more than children during the so-called rapport-building phase. These results are particularly troubling given the fact that Lamb and colleagues (in press) in Israel found that when interviewers spent adequate time on rapport-building activities, the first substantive open-ended questions regarding abuse produced four times as much information as when inadequate time was spent on rapport-building.

Empirical studies have demonstrated clearly and repeatedly the importance of obtaining an uninterrupted free narrative account of the alleged events, because children's spontaneous free recall reports, although typically less detailed than those elicited by specific questioning, tend to be more accurate than reports obtained through direct questioning. In the CPS sample, however, only 2% of the interviewers began the incident-relevant portion of the conversation with open-ended questions. Strikingly similar results (2.2%) were obtained by Lamb et al. (in press) when they analyzed interviews conducted by Israeli youth investigators who had been specially trained. In contrast, 100% of the interviews in the CPS sample involved the use of direct questions regarding the forensically-relevant incidents, despite the fact that direct questions often are fraught with suggestive potential.

Finally, 59% of the CPS interviews ended abruptly, with no formal closing. In fact, one interviewer simply stated, "The end." Interviewers were significantly more likely to formally close interviews with children aged eight to 13 than with children aged two to seven years.

These results suggest that at least some (and perhaps a large proportion) of interviewers engage in poor questioning procedures when interviewing child victim-witnesses.

3.3. How Do Specific Question Forms Affect the Quality and Quantity of Children's Responses?

In a laboratory study, Perry, McAuliff, Tam, Claycomb, Dostal, and Flanagan (1995) investigated five "lawyerese" question forms, that is, questions involving negatives, double negatives, complex syntax, multi-part questions, or difficult vocabulary. They found that children and adults alike had difficulty responding to all "lawyerese" forms, although they could respond correctly to simply phrased questions asking for the same substantive details. Multi-part questions were the most difficult form for all interviewees to answer, adults as well as children. Use of the multi-part question form reduced correct responses by nearly 100%.

Walker and Hunt (in press) investigated a variety of specific questioning techniques used in a sample of 42 Child Protective Service (CPS) interviews, including multi-part questions, forced- choice questions, and modifications. The researchers defined a modification as an instance in which an interviewer reworded a child's statement in a way that changed its meaning, or claimed that the child made a statement that he or she had not made. The following is an example of a modification:

Interviewer: What did Daddy do when you went to bed at night?
Child: He tucked me.
Interviewer: Oh, he sucked you.

Walker and Hunt found that modifications occurred in 74% of the CPS interviews and, on average, an interview contained 2.6 modifications. The researchers also assessed children's responses to modifications. They found that children agreed with modifications 46% of the time, disagreed 26% of the time, and ignored the interviewers' modifications 28% of the time. Interviewers were more likely to continue repeating modifications with which children had agreed and rarely continued to refer to modified statements when children overtly disagreed with them. Overt disagreement, however, occurred in only one-fourth of the cases. Moreover, interviewers seemed to regard a child's failure to comment on a modification as tacit agreement with the modification, and therefore continued to repeat the modified-but-ignored statements.

Walker and Hunt defined a multi-part question as one in which two or more inquiries with potentially different responses were contained within the same question. The following is an example of a multi-part question: "Did you like doing that or did it happen later?" Multi-part questions occurred in 86% of the interviews, with an average of 4.5 multi-part questions per interview. In 61% of the cases, children's responses to multi-part questions did not appear to answer any of the questions asked by the interviewer.

Walker and Hunt defined a forced-choice question as one presenting a limited number of response options. For example, the question, "Was her coat red or blue?" fit this category. Forced-choice questions are considered leading because they suggest that there is a limited number of correct responses to a question. Forced-choice questions ocurred in 88% of the CPS interviews, with an average of 5.2 forced-choice questions per interview. Although forced-choice questions amounted to only 1% of the total inquires, they often were used to obtain critical information, such as details about the alleged abuse or perpetrator. Children chose one of the answers suggested by the interviewer 65% of the time. Only 21% of the time did children provide a meaningful alternative answer.

In a laboratory study of forced-choice questions, Walker, Lunning and Eilts (1996) found that children were likely to choose one of the options presented by the interviewer, even when none was correct. In fact, kindergarten, second- and fifth-grade children alike were significantly more likely to choose the most recently heard alternative regardless of correctness.

4. IMPLICATIONS FOR LEGISLATORS, INTERVIEWERS, AND RESEARCHERS

4.1. Implications for Legislators

The research reviewed in this section provides evidence that interviewers' questioning techniques can have a profound impact upon the quality and quantity of children's responses. How, then, should such empirical findings inform legal policy? To enact statutes endorsing particular questioning techniques probably would be both cumbersome and inappropriate. However, it seems prudent to enact statutes requiring that interviewers receive adequate specialized training in the areas of child development and child interviewing, and that questioning of children be developmentally appropriate.

Some U.S. statutes currently serve as models in this regard. For example, the Minnesota statute notes, "A child describing any act or event may use language appropriate for a child of that age" (§592.02(m)). The Wisconsin statute states, "Counties are encouraged to provide . . . advice to the judge, when appropriate and as a friend of the court, regarding the child's ability to understand proceedings and questions" (§950.055(2)(b); see also Pennsylvania §42–5983(a) and Washington §7.69A.030(1)). And the California statute reads, "With a witness under the age of 14, the court shall take special care to protect him or her from undue harassment or embarassment, and to restrict the unnecessary repetition of questions. The court shall also take special care to insure that questions are stated in a form which is appropriate to the age of the witness. The court may in the interests of justice, on objection by a party, forbid asking of a question which is in a form that is not reasonably likely to be understood by a person of the age of the witness" (§765(b)).

4.2. Implications for Interviewers

Interviewers must keep abreast of empirical findings regarding how questioning procedures and specific question forms affect the quality and quantity of children's responses following trauma. It should be encumbent upon interviewers to read the relevant literature, to attend special training sessions, and to have their interviews of children evaluated on a regular basis by knowledgeable professionals. In addition, interviewers need to communicate with researchers about the special challenges associated with questioning children in the "real world" context.

4.3. Implications for Researchers

Research on the topic of interviewing children needs to be continued. In particular, further investigation of the effects of specific question forms is warranted. Furthermore, researchers need to establish and maintain good lines of communication with practitioners so that empirical investigations can be conducted in pragmatically useful and ecologically valid ways.

In addition, knowledgeable researchers in this area need to create, publish, and disseminate agreed-upon empirically-based guidelines for questioning children (see, for example, American Professional Society on the Abuse of Children, 1990). Researchers also need to develop viable means for disseminating research findings regarding interviewing children to a variety of relevant professionals including clinicians, law enforcement personnel, child protection workers, attorneys, and judges. Publishing articles in esoteric research journals likely is not the best method to reach such audiences. Instead, it might be more useful to employ the following methods: (a) publish findings in trade publications widely read by practitioners, (b) distill research articles into "executive summaries" distributed to large numbers of professionals, and (c) conduct workshops designed to train interviewers in empirically-based questioning procedures and to maintain open communication lines between interviewers and researchers.

REFERENCES

American Professional Society on the Abuse of Children (APSAC). (1990). *Guidelines for psychosocial evaluation of suspected sexual abuse in young children.* Chicago: Author.

California Codes, §765(b).

Lamb, M. E., Herschkowitz, I., Sternberg, K. J., Esplin, P. W., Hovav, M., Manor, T., & Yudilevitch, L. (in press). Effects of investigative utterance types on Israeli children's reponses. *International Journal of Behavioral Development.*

Minnesota Statutes, §592.02(m).

Pennsylvania Statutes, §42–5983(a).

People v. Buckey, No. A750900 (filed Mar. 22, 1984).

Perry, N. S., McAuliff, B. D., Tam, P., Claycomb, L., Dostal, C., & Flanagan, C. (1995). When lawyers question children: Is justice served? *Law and Human Behavior, 19,* 609–629.

State v. Michaels, 625 A.2d 489 (N.J. App. 1993), aff'd, 1994 WL 278424 (N.J. Sup. 1994).

Walker, N. E., & Hunt, J. S. (in press). Interviewing child victim-witnesses: What you ask is what you get. In C. P. Thompson, D. Herrmann, J. D. Read, D. Bruce, D. Payne, & M. Toglia (Eds.), *Eyewitness Memory: Theoretical and Applied Perspectives.* Mahwah, NJ: Erlbaum.

Walker N. E., & Nguyen, M. (1996). Interviewing the child witness: The do's and the don't's, the how's and the why's. *Creighton Law Review, 29,* 1587–1617.

Warren, A. R., Woodall, C. E., Hunt, J. S., & Perry, N. W. (1996). "It sounds good in theory, but . . . ": Do investigative interviewers follow guidelines based on memory research? *Child Maltreatment, 1,* 231–245.

Washington Revised Code Annotated, §7.69A.030(1).

35

AGENDA FOR RESEARCH

Clinical Approaches to Recollections of Trauma

Lucy Berliner[1] and Judith McDougall[2]

[1]University of Washington
325 9 Ave.
Seattle, Washington 98104
[2]Victoria University
P. O. Box 600 Wellington
New Zealand

1. INTRODUCTION

The Working Groups approached the development of a clinical research agenda on recollections of trauma from two perspectives: general considerations and specific research topics. Recommendations are directed both at the way that research on memory and trauma is conducted and at areas for study that will enhance knowledge and clinical practice.

2. GENERAL CONSIDERATIONS

Scientific investigations of the accuracy of memory and of beliefs about the accuracy of memory cannot be entirely separated from the societal context. To date, much of the research on recollections of trauma has focused on the fallibility of memory. This emphasis may have the effect of undermining the hard-won progress in creating a climate that encourages children and adults who have suffered trauma to come forward, to receive support, to seek therapy and to secure justice. The potential implications of such research confer a special responsibility for precision in language, attention to generalizability, and care in discussion sections that contain recommendations for policy and practice.

Research on memory for traumatic events is especially likely to have real world consequences. In part, this is because the extant research has often made specific reference to sexual abuse reports. There is no question that recent research on the susceptibility of young children to suggestive influences and the questions raised about the validity of recovered memories have increased skepticism about sexual abuse reports from young chil-

Recollections of Trauma, edited by Read and Lindsay
Plenum Press, New York, 1997

dren or adults who claim a period of forgetting of childhood abuse experiences. This research has raised important issues and has identified circumstances under which the probability of memory distortion is increased. However, clinicians and trauma researchers are concerned about spill-over effects to all abuse reports, as well as the impact on legitimate sexual abuse reports from young children or adults with delayed recall.

The fact that sexual abuse claims and reports of other traumatic events may result in legal actions has a significant bearing on the implications of research as well. Results that unduly heighten skepticism may influence policy makers, practitioners, jurors and judges in ways that are harmful to crime victims. Excessive caution in investigations, evaluations or clinical practice may leave children and the community unprotected. Expert testimony about the fallibility of memory can create an impression that memory is invariably suspect, in spite of the ample evidence that memory, especially memory for personally significant and unusual events is generally strong.

The study of trauma and memory is further complicated by the nature of the phenomenon. True trauma and its accompanying emotions cannot be induced in a laboratory, but the factual accuracy of memories for traumatic events can rarely be established. On the other hand, investigations of factors that influence memory require that the elements of the event in question be known. This means that research will need to be directed at a broad range of relevant dimensions, from basic science on the biologic and cognitive processes of memory to the phenomenology of remembering and forgetting in real life circumstances. Investigations must employ a variety of methodologies and designs. They should be conducted in the laboratory and in the field; involve observation, physiologic measurement and self report; and use general population and clinical samples. Creativity in research designs and careful integration of findings from different kinds of studies will be necessary to produce a complete and valid understanding of trauma and memory.

Dialogue and collaboration among memory researchers, trauma researchers, clinicians, forensic experts, and lawyers would produce substantial benefits. Greater mutual appreciation of the principles, assumptions and methods that obtain in clinical practice and in scientific inquiry is likely to reduce the contentiousness that has so marked the pursuit of knowledge in this area. Research that is informed by the experience and expertise of practitioners will be more meaningful. Practice that incorporates scientific findings will pose fewer risks and be more effective. Terms that have caused confusion and led to misunderstandings can be clarified and common definitions developed. Researchers who explicitly seek to influence practice and policy are most successful when research findings provide useful answers to relevant questions.

3. RESEARCH RECOMMENDATIONS

3.1. Memory for Trauma

Memory research should not be restricted to sexual abuse, but include other types of events that are potentially traumatic and investigate both remembering and forgetting.

Prospective studies that inquire about various aspects of memory for a range of traumatic events experienced by children and adults would provide important information about the impact, over time, of such experiences. There is evidence that trauma does affect the nature and accuracy of memory in general and for the traumatic events (e.g., Bremner, et al, 1993; Koss, Figueredo, Bell, Tharan, & Tromp, 1996; Pynoos & Nader, 1988; Williams, 1995). While the ground truth could not be established in many of these studies, it would be possible to identify individual, trauma, and contextual variables that are correlated with how events are remembered and possibly with types of distortions. It is especially important to know more about memory-related coping strategies, including active efforts such as intentional forgetting and thought suppression (e.g. Koustaal & Schacter, in press) and less voluntary processes such as dissociation. Measures of memory might be incorporated into prospective investigations of the impact of traumatic events and examined in relation to psychological and other outcomes.

3.2. Non-Reporting of Trauma and Negative Events

Studies of situations where traumatic or negative events are not reported would help establish the incidence of the phenomenon and clarify the role of psychological and emotional factors, as well as effects on memory.

The available evidence confirms that sexual abuse is not always reported when it undoubtedly has occurred (e.g., Elliott & Briere, 1994; Lawson & Chaffin, 1992). Non-reporting in response to open-ended questioning also occurs in laboratory studies of embarrassing (e.g., Saywitz, Goodman, Nicholas, & Moan, 1991) or aversive events (e.g., Bruck, Hembrooke, & Ceci, this volume) and events that involve adult wrongdoing (e.g., Bussey, Lee, & Grimbeek, 1993; Pipe & Goodman, 1991). In addition to parental support which has been implicated in non-reporting, other variables may be important. Although social and emotional factors that inhibit reporting may not be directly implicated in questions about memory or lack of memory for truama, they are relevant because traumatic events may not be disclosed spontaneously. Questioning may be necessary to learn about trauma, and questioning increases the possibility of memory error.

3.3. Questioning about Traumatic Events

Studies are needed to investigate how children and adults can be asked about experiences without unduly increasing memory errors or false reports.

It is commonly accepted practice to take a trauma history in clinical situations (e.g. APSAC, 1996) and investigations of child abuse or crimes require questioning about the possible events. A large literature exists that describes interviewing practices and the types of questioning that can distort memory or produce confabulation in children (e.g., Ceci & Bruck, 1993; Goodman & Saywitz, 1994; Lamb, Sternberg, & Esplin, 1995; Myers, Goodman, & Saywtiz, 1996; Saywitz, 1995; Warren & McGough, 1996). At the same time, there are barriers to reporting and possibly to remembering sexual abuse and other traumatic events. Some commentators and researchers have addressed the complexities of eliciting accurate information under such circumstances (e.g., Lyons, 1995; Marxsen, Yuille, & Nisbet, 1995) and strategies to inoculate children from potential sources of influence have preliminary support (e.g., Mulder & Vrij, 1996; Poole & Lindsay, 1995). Further development and testing of methods that permit sufficient exploration of the possibility of abuse or traumatic events in children and adults is urgently needed.

3.4. Psychological Sequelae of Disconfirmed Reality

The specific impact on memory and psychological status of trauma victims who are not believed or are told their experiences are illusory has not been fully investigated.

There is substantial evidence that belief and support following a report of sexual abuse is associated with better outcome (e.g., Conte & Schuerman, 1987). There are no studies of the impact of denial of the experience on the quality and nature of memory. It would also be useful to explore what happens to memories under conditions where children are repeatedly abused, fail to tell, and both the abuser and the victim carry on everyday life as if the abuse is not occurring. Investigations might examine relationships between characteristics of the disconfirmation (e.g., active versus passive, relative importance of source), the extent to which various conscious (e.g., intentional forgetting) or less conscious (e.g., dissociation) processes are used, and the impact on recollection and on psychological status.

3.5. Memory and Meaning of Uncertain or Unproven Cases

Prospective studies of children in cases where evaluations determine there was no abuse, the abuse could not be proven or disproven, or there was no official action would help clarify the impact on children of adult suspicions or persistent inquiry regarding possible abuse.

There is currently no information available about the impact of investigations or inquiries that are inconclusive on children's memories or psychological status. It is unknown whether children recall these events, or the extent to which beliefs about these experiences are sustained or diminish over time.

3.6. The Phenomenology of Recovered Memory

There is insufficient information about the process of remembering and the nature of memories in situations where there was a period of not remembering.

It appears that in some cases remembering is gradual and begins with dreams or fragmented memories (Williams, 1995), while in other cases remembering occurs as a sudden, dramatic experience (Schooler, this volume). The memories may be hazy and the rememberer may lack confidence in their validity (Williams, 1995). Much more needs to be known about the precipitants and the evolution from initial vague recollections or symbolic representations to detailed memories. The sources of influence on recall and possible confabulation could be explicated by prospective field studies of remembering subjects.

3.7. The Role of Therapy in Recovered Memory

Experimental studies of clinical responses to recovered memories could shed light on the remembering process and the importance of remembering for symptom reduction or restoration to healthy functioning.

Controlled studies might be designed in which responses to remembering clients were systematically manipulated. Approaches that focus on remembering could be compared with those that acknowledge past experiences, but emphasize treatments for current distress. While there is evidence that remembering traumatic experiences in detail in therapy is a central ingredient of effective therapies for PTSD (Foa, Rothbaum, Riggs, & Murdock, 1991; Resick & Schnicke, 1992), it is not clear what the function of remembering is for clients who have previously not recalled traumatic experiences, or who do not suffer from PTSD.

3.8. Reported False Memory

The prevalence of false memory for autobiographical events, especially potentially traumatic events, needs to be ascertained. Experiments with children and adults have demonstrated that it is possible to induce memories for events that have not occurred (e.g., Ceci, Loftus, Leitchmen, & Bruck, 1994; Hyman, Husband, & Billings, 1995, Loftus & Pickrell, 1995). But it appears that the type of event matters; subjects do not succumb to suggestions about very unusual, physically invasive events (Pezdek, 1995). In addition, there are individual differences in susceptibility to false beliefs. Ecologically valid and creative studies are required before generalizations about the creation of false memories of trauma can be made from studies of memory for word lists, and common or relatively benign events. It is especially important to investigate variables associated with efforts to implant memories for implausible events with significant negative consequences.

3.9. The Validity of Memories of Alleged Perpetrators

Questions have been raised about the possibility that offenders may not recall their crimes. While there are strong reasons to believe that in most cases reported lack of memory is simply denial or lying, there may be instances where the nature or circumstances of the event produce loss of memory or memory distortions. Investigations of memory with convicted offenders may shed light on this phenomenon.

3.10. Impact of False Allegations

Systematic studies of the effects of accusations that are subsequently determined to be false, or asserted to be false, on the accused and/or their families would provide empirical data to supplement the currently available anecdotes.

One study has attempted to investigate this question (e.g., DeRivera,). Although the ground truth could not be fully established, prospective studies of representative samples would provide information about the psychological consequences, the impact on family relationships and community reputation of being accused. The actual course of response to accusations, including rates of legal involvement, retraction and family resolution have yet to be established.

3.11. Individual and Family Characteristics in Cases Where a False Accusation Is Alleged

Studies of the psychological make-up of individuals who make false accusations and the dynamics of their family environments would provide valuable information regarding the social and emotional climate in which false allegations occur.

Hypotheses have been offered to explain the occurrence of these accusations (e.g. Haaken & Schlaps, 1991; Lindsay & Read, 1994) but systematic investigations have not yet been conducted. Retractors and their families could serve as a population for study.

3.12. Beliefs about Memory

There is insufficient information regarding beliefs and attitudes about memory in general, memory for traumatic events, or delayed recall.

A few studies have specifically compared the effect of delayed recall versus always remembered memories of sexual abuse on belief (e.g., Garry, Loftus, & Brown, 1994). Subjects believe in repression and subjects ratings of belief are affected by whether memory has been repressed or was always present. It is particularly important to extend investigations to traumatic events other than sexual abuse and to determine whether the type of event is associated with systematic differences in beliefs about memory. These studies should also inquire about the meaning ascribed to terms such as repression or amnesia. They should be undertaken in general population samples, as well as key groups that become involved with reported cases including clinicians, investigators, lawyers and judges.

3.13. The Societal Impact and Response to Memory and Trauma Controversies

Sociological/anthropological investigations examining how recovered memory cases emerge as a salient public issue would provide important insights.

It seems clear that the emergence of sexual abuse as an issue and various aspects of sexual abuse reports are influenced by cultural and historical factors (e.g., Mulhern, 1994; Olafson, Corwin, & Summit, 1993). Identifying the social and political forces that may be a sub-text or serve as the vehicle for making the issue resonate so strongly in some countries, or parts of countries, and not others, could be helpful in disentangling the influence of these factors from other variables. Comparative studies of countries with different cultural values about sexual misconduct and historical responses to sexual abuse, different forms of media and popular press outlets, or different legal systems might be revealing. It might be particularly instructive to undertake such research in a country that has not yet experienced the full force of the controversy, but where the early presumed relevant factors are present (e.g., a high level of awareness of abuse, the availability and acceptance of treatment for adult survivors of child sexual abuse).

REFERENCES

APSAC. (1996). *Statement of Therapist Roles and Responsibilities*. Chicago, IL: American Professional Society on the Abuse of Children.

Bremner, J. D., Randall, P., Scott, T. M., Capelli, S., Delaney, R., McCarthy, G., & Charney, D. S. (1995). Deficits in short-term memory in adult survivors of childhood abuse. *Psychiatry Research, 59*, 97–107.

Bussey, K., Lee, K., & Grimbeek, E. J. (1993). Lies and secrets: Implications for children's reporting of sexual abuse. In G. S. Goodman & B. L. Bottoms (eds.) *Child Victims, Child Witnesses: Understanding and Improving Testimony.* (pp. 147–168). New York: Guilford Press.

Ceci, S. J., & Bruck, M. (1993). Suggestibility of the child witness: A historical review and synthesis. *Psychological Bulletin, 113*, 403–439.

Ceci, S. J., Loftus, E. F., Leichtman, M. D., & Bruck, M. (1994). The possible role of source misattributions in the creation of false beliefs among preschoolers. *International Journal of Clinical and Experimental Hypnosis, 42*, 304–320.

Conte, J. R., & Schuerman, J. R. (1987). Factors associated with an increased impact of child sexual abuse. *Child Abuse & Neglect, 11*, 201–212.

de Rivera, J. (1994, December). Survey of retractors' families. Paper presented at the Memory and Reality: Reconcilliation Conference sponcered by the False Memory Syndrome Foundation and Johns Hopkins Medical Institution, Baltimore, MD.

Elliott, D. M., & Briere, J. (1994). Forensic sexual abuse evaluations of older children: Disclosures and symptomatology. *Behavioral Sciences and the Law, 12*, 261–277.

Foa, E. B., Rothbaum, B. O., Riggs, D. S., & Murdock, T. B. (1991). Treatment of Posttraumatic Stress Disorder in rape victims: A comparison between cognitive-behavioral procedures and counseling. *Journal of Consulting and Clinical Psychology, 59*, 715–723.

Garry, M., Loftus, E. F., & Brown, S. W. (1994). Memory: A river runs through it. Special Issue: The recovered memory/false memory debate. *Consciousness & Cognition: An International Journal, 3*, 438–451.

Goodman, G. S., & Saywitz, K. J. (1994). Memories of abuse: Interviewing children when sexual victimization is suspected. *Child & Adolescent Psychiatric Clinics of North America, 3*, 645–660.

Hyman Jr, I. E., Husband, T. H., & Billings, F. J. (1995). False memories of childhood experiences. *Applied Cognitive Psychology, 9*, 181–197.

Haaken, J., & Schlaps, A. (1991). Incest resolution therapy and the objectification of sexual abuse. *Psychotherapy, 28*, 39–47.

Koustaal, W., & Schacter, D.L. (in press). Intentional forgetting and voluntary thought suppression: Two potential methods for coping with childhood trauma. *Review of Psychiatry.*

Koss, M. P., Figueredo, A. J., Bell, I., Tharan, M., & Tromp, S. (1996). Traumatic memory characteristics: A cross-validated mediational model of response to rape among employed women. *Journal of Abnormal Psychology, 105*, 421–432.

Lamb, M. E., Sternberg, K. J., & Esplin, P. W. (1995). Making children into competent witnesses: Reactions to the Amicus Brief In re Michaels. *Psychology, Public Policy, and Law, 1*, 438–449.

Lawson, L., & Chaffin, M. (1992). False negatives in sexual abuse disclosure interviews: Incidence and influence of caretaker's belief in abuse in cases of accidental abuse discovery by diagnosis of STD. *Journal of Interpersonal Violence, 7*, 532–542.

Lindsay, D.S., & Read, J.D. (1994). Psychotherapy and memories of childhood sexual abuse: A cognitive perspective. *Applied cognitive Psychology, 8*, 281–338.

Loftus, E. F., & Pickrell, J. E. (1995). The formation of false memories. *Psychiatric Annals, 25*, 720–725.

Lyon, T.D. (1995). False allegations and false denials in child sexual abuse. *Psychology, Public Policy and the Law, 1*, 429–437.

Marxsen, D., Yuille, J. C., & Nisbet, M. (1995). The complexities of eliciting and assessing children's statements. *Psychology, Public Policy, and Law, 1*, 450–460.

Mulder, M. R., & Vrij, A. (1996). Explaining conversation rules to children: An intervention study to facilitate children's accurate responses. *Child Abuse and Neglect, 20*, 623–631.

Mulhern, S. (1994). Satanism, ritual abuse, and multiple personality disorder: A psychohistorical perspective, *International Journal of Clinical and Experimental Hypnosis, 42*, 265–288.

Myers, J. E. B., Goodman, G. S., & Saywitz, K. J. (1996). Psychological research on children as witnesses: Practical implications for forensic interviews and courtroom testimony. *Pacific Law Journal, 27*, 1–82.

Olafson, E., Corwin, D.L., & Summit, R. C. (1993). Modern history of child sexual abuse awareness: Cycles of discovery and suppression. *Child Abuse and Neglect, 17*, 7–24.

Pezdek, K. (1995, November). *Planting false childhood memories: When does it occur and when does it not?.* Paper presented at the 36th Annual Meeting of the Psychonomic Society, Los Angeles.

Pipe, M. E., & Goodman, G. S. (1991). Elements of secrecy: Implications for children's testimony. *Behavioral Sciences & the Law, 9*, 33–41.

Poole, D. A., & Lindsay, D. S. (1995). Interviewing Preschoolers: Effects of nonsuggestive techniques, parental coaching, and leading questions on reports of nonexperienced events. *Journal of Experimental Child Psychology, 60*, 129–154.

Pynoos, R., & Nader, K. (1988). Children's memory and proximity to violence. *Journal of the American Academy of Child and Adolescent Psychiatry, 27*, 567–572.

Resick, P. A., & Schnicke, M. K. (1992). Cognitive processing therapy for sexual assault victims. *Journal of Consulting and Clinical Psychology, 60*, 748–756.

Saywitz, K. (1995). Improving children's testimony: The question, the answer, and the environment. In M. S. Zaragoza, J. R. Graham, G. N. C. Hall, R. Hirschman, & Y. S. Ben-Porath (eds.), *Memory and Testimony in the Child Witness* (pp. 113–140). Thousand Oaks, CA: Sage.

Saywitz, K. J., Goodman, G. S., Nicholas, E., & Moan, S. F. (1991). Children's memories of a physical examination involving genital touch: Implications for reports of child sexual abuse. *Journal of Consulting & Clinical Psychology, 59*, 682–691.

Warren, A. R., & McGough, L. S. (1996). Research on children's suggestibility: Implications for the investigative interview. *Criminal Justice and Behavior, 23*, 269–303.

Williams, L. M. (1995). Recovered memories of abuse in women with documented child sexual victimization histories. *Journal of Traumatic Stress, 8*, 649–674.

36

INVESTIGATING ALTERNATIVE ACCOUNTS OF VERIDICAL AND NON-VERIDICAL MEMORIES OF TRAUMA

Jonathan W. Schooler[1] and Ira E. Hyman, Jr.[2]

[1]University of Pittsburgh
635 LRDC
Pittsburgh, Pennsylvania 15260
[2]Western Washington University
Bellingham, Washington 98225

1. INTRODUCTION

We summarize the discussions of the two Cognitive Working Groups of the NATO ASI meeting on memory and trauma. The groups found that an understanding of the processes that contribute to veridical and nonveridical memories of trauma will require clarification of the relationship between clinical and cognitive constructs, and a variety of research approaches. The groups concluded that advancement will require greater communication and collaboration among researchers interested in memory of trauma

This report represents the summation of discussions of two working groups that met at the NATO workshop on memory and trauma to consider cognitive and neurocognitive research issues. As it happened, the two groups adopted different, but complimentary, approaches. One group (hereon called Group A) took a conceptual approach, identifying central clinical constructs and considering how they might relate to existing cognitive and neurocognitive ideas. The second group (hereon called Group B) took a more research oriented approach, breaking the issues down into general research domains and identifying specific research questions and methodologies within each domain. A fortuitous consequence of the distinct approaches taken by the two groups is that they lend themselves to sequential consideration, with Group A's analysis identifying a number of key conceptual issues that are then fleshed out by specific research suggestions by Group B. In this chapter, we summarize the discussions of the two groups and then close with several general observations about the strategies and goals that we believe productive research on this topic might profitably adopt.

Recollections of Trauma, edited by Read and Lindsay
Plenum Press, New York, 1997

2. COMPARING CLINICAL AND COGNITIVE CONSTRUCTS

Group A took as its starting point the premise that successful research endeavors require the clear definition and operationalization of the constructs in question. Unfortunately, such clarity of constructs has been sorely lacking in discussions of recovered and fabricated memories of trauma. Clinical and cognitive psychologists often use different terms and, worse yet, use the same terms but with different meanings. This state of affairs suggests that an important step is the development of a common terminology and the assessment of the relationship between pertinent clinical and cognitive constructs. Towards this end, Group A explored the relationship between cognitive psychological theory and four constructs that have been central in clinical discussions of memory for trauma: the sensory/narrative memory distinction, repression, dissociation, and PTSD.

2.1. The Sensory/Narrative Memory Distinction

A common clinical claim dating back as far as Janet (1889) is that some traumatic memories are often recollected in a purely sensory form "without any semantic representation... experienced primarily as fragments of the sensory component of the event" (van der Kolk & Fisler, 1995, p. 513.) In contrast, other traumatic memories are incorporated into a narrative framework that involves symbolic verbal interpretations of experience. Sensory/affective and narrative memories of trauma have been speculated to differ with respect to their formation, susceptibility to change, and retrieval conditions. Sensory memories have been hypothesized to form under conditions of severe trauma, be relatively invulnerable to change, and be invoked automatically in response to certain environmental cues. In contrast, narrative memories have been hypothesized to form under less severe trauma conditions, be more vulnerable to change, and be retrieved volitionally (for a review see van der Kolk & van der Hart, 1991.)

Claims associated with the sensory/narrative memory distinction share both similarities and differences with a variety of cognitive constructs. For example, many cognitive models posit distinctions between sensory/perceptual processes and verbal/conceptual processes (e.g. Atkinson, Herrmann, & Westcourt, 1974; Paivio, 1986; Jacoby & Dallas, 1981, Mandler, 1980.) Indeed, this distinction seems fundamental to many information processing models and continues to be popular, (though there is certainly plenty of variation in how sharply the distinction is drawn and in the precise manner in which the two types of knowledge are presumed interact.) Although such models share the assumption that it is useful to distinguish between perceptual and verbal memory representations, these models differ from the sensory narrative distinction in a number of important respects. For example, in contrast to the assumptions of sensory traumatic memories, standard cognitive models assume that sensory/perceptual memories are not exclusively generated under extremely arousing conditions. Many (e.g., Paivio, 1986) standard cognitive models also differ in that they assume that perceptual memories can be volitionally retrieved. However, this premise is not shared by all theories, as some cognitive theories (e.g., Jacoby & Dallas, 1981) suggest that perceptual memories may be under less volitional control then conceptual memories. Finally, unlike the sensory/narrative distinction many cognitive theories assume that perceptual memories are formulated in addition to rather than instead of more verbal explicit knowledge (e.g. Paivio, 1986.) However, once again this assumption varies across theories with other theories suggesting that implicit perceptual memories can be formed in the absence of explicit verbal memories (see discussion of implicit memory below.)

Another partial mapping between cognitive theory and the sensory/narrative distinction is the notion that sensory memories are exclusively elicited by encoding cues that, in some manner, resemble the trauma experience. This premise resembles in some respects the cognitive principle of encoding specificity (Tulving & Thompson, 1973), which states that memory performance is maximized when retrieval conditions approximate encoding conditions. Like claims of sensory memory retrieval, encoding specificity predicts that cues similar to the trauma experience could prompt recollection of trauma. This claim is mirrored by the related construct of state dependent memory (e.g., Eich, 1980) which holds that memories are most apt to be retrieved when individuals are in similar states (e.g., sad) during encoding and recollection. However, in contrast to the sensory/narrative traumatic memory distinction, which assumes that environmental cues are uniquely relevant to the retrieval of particularly traumatic sensory memories, the encoding specificity principle is not exclusively limited to traumatic nor sensory materials, and indeed most demonstrations of encoding specificity have involved semantic associations with rather mundane materials.

A third cognitive construct that bears a resemblance to the sensory/narrative memory distinction is the frequently used cognitive distinction between implicit and explicit memories. Implicit memories correspond to memories that influence performance without awareness, whereas explicit memories involve conscious recollective experiences (for reviews see, Roediger, 1990; Schacter, 1987; Schacter, Chiu, & Ochsner, 1993.) Over the last 20 years cognitive psychologists have amassed substantial evidence that implicit memory can influence behaviors without conscious recollection. Moreover, like sensory memories, implicit memories are hypothesized to involve perceptual knowledge, be exclusively prompted by environmental cues, and to be relatively less vulnerable to disruption. Indeed, implicit memories have been shown to be extremely sensitive to the fine grained perceptual characteristics of stimuli. Explicit memories also bear some resemblance to the sensory/narrative distinction. Like narrative memories explicit memories are hypothesized to emphasize semantic/conceptual knowledge, to be more vulnerable to disruption, and to be volitionally recalled. These parallels have led some clinicians to use the two constructs interchangeably (e.g., van der Kolk & Fisler, 1995.) However, Group A observed a number of important differences between the implicit/explicit and sensory/narrative memory distinction that suggests caution in drawing parallels between them. For example, in contrast to the alleged vivid experiential quality of sensory traumatic memories, the phenomenological quality of implicit memories is quite subtle (e.g. slightly increased perceptual fluency or familiarity), if it is perceived at all (cf. Jacoby, Kelley, & Dywan, 1987.) Implicit memories also differ from sensory narrative memories in that they can be conceptual as well as perceptual (cf. Roediger, Weldon, & Challis, 1989.) Moreover, in contrast to the characterization of sensory trauma memories, implicit memories can be generated in response to even the most mundane of experiences. In addition, unlike sensory memory which are hypothesized (at least sometimes) to become integrated into narrative memories (i.e., recovered), implicit memories are generally not believed to transform themselves into explicit memories. (Although it possible that one could have access to implicit memories but not explicit memories under one set of conditions, yet be able to retrieve the corresponding explicit information if properly cued.)

A final, albeit controversial, construct in the cognitive literature that bears a resemblance to the sensory narrative distinction, is the hypothesized distinction between standard autobiographical memories and flashbulb memories of very emotionally salient experiences (Brown & Kulik, 1977). Like sensory traumatic memories, flashbulb memories are hypothesized to be very vivid, sensorially rich, and relatively invulnerable to change and forgetting. Indeed, a further similarity between flashbulb memories and sensory traumatic memories is that flashbulb memories' status as uniquely inviolate memories has also been questioned (e.g., Neisser & Harsch, 1992, showed a high proportion of large errors in supposedly flashbulb memories). However, even if we grant the possibility that flashbulb memories do exist, they still have a number of fundamental differences from sensory traumatic memories. Unlike sensory memories, flashbulb memories are volitionally recalled and easily recounted in the context of a narrative memory. Indeed, one explanation for why flashbulb memories seem so vivid is that they are so frequently rehearsed in the context of narrative discourse (Neisser, 1982).

In sum, after significant consideration of the sensory/narrative distinction, it was concluded that although the distinction shares some similarities with a number of cognitive constructs, there is no construct within cognitive psychology that adequately captures all of the characteristics hypothesized to be associated with sensory traumatic memories. This disparity caused some in Working Group A to express skepticism towards the construct of unique sensory memories, and in particular towards the claim that sensory memories are especially invulnerable to change and distortion. Others however, viewed these disparities as further evidence of the uniqueness of sensory memories.

Although there was a lack of consensus in Group A regarding the likelihood that sensory traumatic memories qualitatively differ from more standard types of memories, there was general agreement that the status of sensory traumatic memories is a pressing research issue. More generally, the analysis of the sensory traumatic memories in the context of standard cognitive distinctions provided a powerful example of the lack of alignment between clinical and cognitive constructs. This disparity illustrated the need for clinical and cognitive psychologists to work collectively to develop systematic, research based, approaches for operationalizing and comparing their respective constructs.

2.2. The Construct of Repression

A second clinical construct that Group A considered from a cognitive psychological perspective was repression. Group A noted a variety of opinions regarding what repression means and what types of memory behavior constitute evidence of repression. Sometimes repression is used as a label for the forgetting of traumatic experiences. Other times it is used to define a particular mental mechanism involving an often complex constellation of forgetting, storage and remembering processes. Moreover, even within each of these usages there is considerable lack of agreement. When used as a label for a type of forgetting, repression can refer to the forgetting of any unwanted memories, or limited to the forgetting of severely traumatic memories, or limited to the forgetting of repeated incidents of severe trauma. Similarly, when used as a specific mechanism of forgetting, repression can involve a variety of different processes. Repression mechanisms are sometimes characterized as being intentional and other times as being automatic. Repression has been postulated to cause the immediate forgetting of trauma, but it has also been suggested to operate over an extended period of time. In addition to these seemingly contradictory characterizations of the mechanisms underlying repression, there is also a significant subset of assumptions that sometimes are, and sometimes are not, viewed as defining properties of the repression mechanism. Examples of such claims include: 1) repressed memories are entirely unavailable; 2) repressed memories are maintained in a pristine uncontaminated form; 3) although forgotten, repressed memories nevertheless cause a specific set of mental disturbances; 4) these mental disturbances are so distinctive that their presence can reliably be used to diagnose the existence of repressed memories;

5) repressed memories are only retrieved when the ego is capable of coping with the disturbing recollection; 6) repressed memories are uniquely responsive to memory retrieval therapies, and; 7) these various attributes of repressed memories are the consequence of special ego defense mechanisms that are distinct from standard memory processes.

With respect to the notion that repression involves special ego defense mechanisms, it was noted that the operationalization of such processes remains difficult and that despite substantial effort, little direct cognitive evidence for such mechanisms has been produced. Nevertheless, clinical suggestions of such mechanisms continue to be generated (see Brewin, this volume, and Briere, this volume) and thus further efforts to cognitively pin down unique repression mechanisms seems warranted. At the same time however, group A noted a variety of more standard cognitive operations that individually or in combination might account for the forgetting and remembering of trauma without the postulation of special repression mechanisms. These include: lack of verbal rehearsal (e.g., Atkinson & Shiffrin, 1969, Nelson, 1993), delay (e.g., Ebbinghaus, 1913), directed forgetting (e.g., Bjork, 1989), re-interpretation (e.g., Anderson & Pichert, 1978), encoding specificity (e.g., Tulving & Thompson, 1973), state-dependent memory (e.g., Eich, 1980), thought suppression (Wegner, 1994), and hypermnesia (e.g., Erdelyi & Kleinbard, 1978.) In addition, it was noted that both post-event suggestion (see Loftus, this volume) and other types of source confusions (e.g., Johnson, Hashtroudi, & Lindsay, 1993) are likely to contribute to the generation of non-veridical memories of abuse.

Group A concluded that a scientific assessment of repression will require a much clearer operationalization of the construct, with a precise specification of its hypothesized conditions and processes carefully considered in the context of basic cognitive constructs. Only then will it be possible to determine whether, and to what degree, repression represents a unique memory mechanism that is distinct from more standard cognitive operations.

2.3. Dissociation

Another clinical construct that Group A considered particularly apt to benefit from cognitive analysis is the notion of dissociation. As with repression, the construct of dissociation has been associated with a number of different meanings. However, unlike repression, there seems to be some consensus regarding the alternative appropriate usages of the term. Specifically, three common usages were identified: 1) the intentional dissociation of oneself from unpleasant experiences (e.g., I imagined I was somewhere else while it was happening); 2) experiential distortions during encoding, (e.g., the experience seemed a like a dream) and; 3) memory for experiences becoming partitioned from one another (i.e., the alleged amnesia associated with multiple personality disorder and fugue states.) Group A noted the dearth of cognitive research into the construct of dissociation in the context of memory for trauma and identified several areas for further research. One important step will be determining the cognitive constructs that might relate to dissociation. Potentially related cognitive constructs include divided attention (e.g. Jacoby & Dallas, 1981, Spelke, Hirst, & Neisser, 1976), daydreaming (Singer, 1993), thought suppression (Wegner, 1994), and the tendency of some autobiographical memories to be recalled from the third person perspective (Nigro & Neisser, 1983.) A second important consideration is assessing the impact of dissociation on both actual forgetting (see Eich, this volume) and memory fabrication (Hyman et al. 1996.) In addition, an understanding of the cognitive underpinnings of dissociation would also benefit from further specification of the relationship between the various forms of dissociative experiences mentioned above and other related clinical constructs such as hypnosis (e.g., Hilgard, 1992) and absorption (Tillegen & Atkinson, 1974).

2.4. Post-Traumatic Stress Disorder

A final clinical construct that Group A sought to clarify from a cognitive perspective was Post Traumatic Stress Disorder. PTSD diagnosis requires the encountering of trauma and the subsequent symptoms of re-experiencing symptoms (e.g., intrusive memories), protective reactions (e.g., emotional numbing, amnesia), and arousal symptoms (e.g., hypervigilance.) One issue upon which there was marked differences of opinion was whether PTSD symptoms can be viewed as a useful indicator that recovered memories correspond to actual abuse experiences. Some suggested that the existence of PTSD symptoms in conjunction with recovered memories of abuse indicates exposure to some type of traumatic experience. Others, however, strongly objected to the use of clinical symptomatology in the assessment of the likely authenticity of recovered memories.

This discussion led to the formulation of a number of future research questions such as: Can PTSD symptoms accompany false memories (e.g., alien abductions)? If so, might such false recollections involve source confusions (e.g. Johnson et al., 1993) in which fragments of authentic and fabricated events become muddled together? Alternatively, might the formation of a false memory of a traumatic event itself be sufficient to elicit PTSD symptoms? Although little consensus on these issue was reached, there was general agreement that an understanding of the relationship between PTSD and memory will be an additional key component of a deeper understanding of the relationship between memory and trauma.

3. AN OVERVIEW OF RESEARCH DOMAINS

Group B focused on outlining some areas that would benefit from research by clinical, cognitive, and neurocognitive psychologists. The view of this group was that in order to understand the existing memory controversy, several areas of research need further examination. At the least, additional research is needed concerning how trauma affects memory, how the phenomenon of recovered memory occurs, how false memories are created, and how both adults and children can be asked about the past in nonleading fashions. These domains are not only important for disambiguating the current controversy, but also for applied concerns and for untangling theoretical issues. Several different methodologies will be useful in each of the different topic domains.

3.1. Memory for Trauma

Research on how trauma is remembered should help discriminate among several theories — repression theory arguing for memory loss, flashbulb theory arguing for better memory for trauma, and other theories suggesting more complex relationships between arousal and memory. Repression theory argues that when people experience trauma they are likely to place that memory in the unconscious until the anxiety is sufficiently relieved (Freud, 1915/1957). There are also several modern versions of special memory mechanisms, such as dissociative tendencies, that are thought to cause some traumatic events to be forgotten (or perhaps only be available as sensory rather than narrative memories.) How these mechanisms differ from repression and what predictions they make for traumatic memories needs to be more clearly defined.

In contrast to theories arguing for some form of memory loss, flashbulb memory theory (Brown & Kulik, 1977) claims that extremely emotional experiences are better remembered than other experiences. In essence, during very arousing and important events, a special brain mechanism is activated and records a lasting record of current brain activity. Although several studies have shown surprisingly large errors in memories for such experiences (e.g., Neisser & Harsch, 1992), the idea that traumatic experiences tend to be very well recalled remains popular (e.g., Terr, Bloch, Michel, Shi, Reinhardt, & Metayer, 1996; Tromp, Koss, Figueredo, & Tharan, 1995).

Other theories have predicted more complex relationships between arousal and memory. For example, the Easterbrook Hypothesis makes a different prediction regarding the relationship between trauma and memory — namely that as arousal increases, attention narrows (Easterbrook, 1959). Thus as events become traumatic, less information will be attended to and subsequently available for recall. The loss of information will be noted particularly in peripheral features of the event. As still another idea about trauma and memory, Post-Traumatic Stress Disorder researchers have noted that memories of traumatic experiences may frequently be experienced as intrusive memories (e.g., Horowitz & Reidboard, 1992). Thus, there are several suggestions for how traumatic events will be recalled (or forgotten), but the existing research does little to discriminate among them.

Group B believed this was cause for an increased effort to study memories for traumatic experiences. Future research should emphasize memory for a variety of traumatic experiences, partly because there is no reason to assume that all trauma will affect memory in the same fashion. For example, some forms of traumatic experiences are shared and thus may be rehearsed while others are private. In addition, different forms of emotions (fear, shame, guilt, etc.) may accompany traumatic experiences and these emotions may have differing effects on memory. Future research should also consider individual differences related to memory for trauma: differences in what the individual brings to the experience (such as a history of trauma), in how the individual responds to the trauma (this might include immediate emotional, cognitive, and behavioral responses), and in the outcome of the traumatic experience (no long-term negative consequences compared with a variety of negative outcomes such as PTSD, depression, anxiety, or fear development.) In addition to studying how traumatic experiences are recalled, researchers should also continue to investigate how people who develop PTSD differ from others (e.g., Yehuda, this volume.) In order to better understand the effects of trauma on memory, baseline studies of other memories need to be conducted. For example, how well and how long are non-emotional, mildly emotional, strongly positive, and other comparison experiences remembered?

Research on trauma and memory will necessarily involve a variety of methodologies. Everything from animal studies to controlled laboratory studies with humans experiencing mild forms of emotion to naturalistic studies of memory for very emotional experiences will be needed. This domain of inquiry provides an opportunity for experimental researchers to collaborate with clinical practitioners to study how people remember extreme trauma.

3.2. Recovered Memories

Group B and the conference as a whole came to an agreement that people can forget and later remember a variety of experiences, including traumatic experiences. Unfortunately, there was less agreement concerning how that phenomenon occurs. Do recovered memories occur because people repress or dissociate memories for traumatic experiences? Are there other inhibitory mechanisms in memory, such as directed forgetting or partial-list cueing (e.g., Anderson, Bjork, & Bjork, 1994), that account for forgotten and recovered memories? Does encoding specificity, the fact that events are retrieved in the presence of only particular cues, explain the recovery of some traumatic experiences? Or is it the case that people mistakenly believe that a memory has been unavailable for a period of time in which they actually discussed the experience (see Schooler's, this volume, "forgot-it-all-along effect")?

In this domain, there was agreement that more descriptions of recovered memories are needed. When dealing with recovered traumatic memories, researchers should attempt to document that the event occurred, that there was a period of non-memory, and how the memory was recovered. Although descriptions of recovered traumatic memories will aid in explaining the phenomenon, a description of the base rate of memory recovery experiences for other types of events (e.g., Read, this volume) and for a variety of traumatic experiences (e.g., Elliott, this volume) would help. Although much of this research will rely on surveys, there is the opportunity to study some of the basic mechanisms (such as directed forgetting, part-list cueing, encoding specificity, and the forgot-it-all-along effect) in controlled laboratory studies. In addition, as Brewin (this volume) has noted, there may be individual differences in inhibitory processes. These differences can be studied in both laboratory and naturalistic settings.

3.3. False Memories

As with the existence of recovered memories, there was little disagreement over the existence of false memories. The focus of discussion here was also on the mechanisms involved in the creation of false memories and how the findings can be applied to a variety of clinical settings. In essence, the existing research (Bruck, this volume; Hyman, Husband, & Billings, 1995, Hyman and Pentland,1996; Lindsay, this volume; Loftus, this volume; Loftus & Pickrell, 1995) has indicated that in repeated interviews, with misleading information and some social pressures, some people can create memories of events that did not happen. What needs to be defined is the exact roles that the different pressures play in the creation of false memories. In addition, although researchers have found that a variety of false memories can be created, there likely are some limits in the nature of false events that people can be led to believe occurred. Is it possible that people can create memories of traumatic experiences? Must events be related to personal experiences in order for false events to be created? Group B felt that several other factors related to memory construction should also be explored, including: beliefs concerning memories, social pressures, group processes, emotion, and individual differences.

Group B also felt that future research should explore how people can be asked about the past in non-leading fashions. This issue is particularly important in interviewing children. Future research should investigate further the cognitive interview (and other techniques) and its application to interviewing child witnesses and adults remembering their childhood. How leading is too leading is a question that repeatedly surfaced in a variety of conversations at the NATO conference. In addition, future research should continue efforts to discriminate true from false memories.

Research on memory errors should take a variety of approaches. It can involve careful lab studies of small memory errors in which it is possible to manipulate variables and note their effects. It can also involve naturalistic studies that investigate the application of existing knowledge to the creation of full memories in a variety of contexts. In addition, case studies of recantors, people who claim that memories they previously claimed as recovered are actually false, would be valuable.

4. CONCLUSION

There are several important conclusions to be drawn from the conversations that occurred in the work groups. Group A's discussions illustrated the need for systematic cognitive analyses of the specific assumptions and mechanisms underlying various clinical constructs. Group B's discussion revealed the plethora of research directions that will be necessary for understanding veridical and non-veridical memories of trauma. Finally, both discussions highlighted the value of conversation and collaboration among the various types of researchers interested in memory for trauma. The independent approaches so often taken by researchers studying these issues has reached the point where we no longer speak the same language or even agree on the basic questions. To counter this alarming trend, we must open avenues of intellectual exchange between cognitive, clinical and neurocognitive psychologists (among others) so that we can overcome, without overlooking, differences as we systematically disentangle the complex issues in which the field is currently ensnared. We hope that one outcome of the NATO ASI generally, and the work groups in particular, is the beginning of such cooperative exchanges.

REFERENCES

Anderson, R.C., & Pitcher, J.W. (1978). Recall of previously unrecallable information following a shift in perspective. *Journal of Verbal Learning and Verbal Behavior*, 17, 1–12.

Anderson, M.C., Bjork, R.A., & Bjork, E.l. (1994). Remembering can cause forgetting: Retrieval dynamics in long-term memory. *Journal of Experimental Psychology: Learning, Memory and Cognition*. 20(5), 1063–1087.

Atkinson, R.C., Herrmann, D.J. & Westcourt, K.T. (1974) Search processes in recognition memory. In R.L. Solso (Ed.) *Theories in cognitive psychology: The Loyola Symposium* (pp. 101–146). Hillsdale, NJ: Lawrence Earlbaum Associates.

Atkinson, R. C., & Shiffrin, R. M. (1969). Human memory: A proposed system and its control processes. In K. Spence & J. Spence (Eds.), *The psychology of learning and motivation* ((Vol. 2). New York: Academic Press.

Brown, R., & Kulik, J. (1977). Flashbulb memories. *Cognition*, 5, 73–99.

Bjork, R.A. (1989). Retrieval inhibition as an adaptive mechanism in human memory. In H.L. Roediger., & F.I.M. Craik. (Eds). *Varieties of memory and consciousness: Essays in honor of Endel Tulving.* (pp. 309–330). Hillsdale, N.J.: Erlbaum.

Easterbrook, J. A. (1959). The effect of emotion on cue utilization and the organization of behavior. *Psychological Review*, 66, 183–201.

Ebbinghaus, H. (1913 (1885)). *Memory: A contribution to experimental psychology.* New York: Columbia Teacher's College.

Eich, J.E. (1980) The cue dependent nature of state dependent retrieval *Memory and Cognition*, 8, 157–158.

Erdelyi, M.H. & Kleinbard, J. (1978). Has Ebbinghaus decayed with time ? The growth of recall (hypermnesia) over days. *Journal of Experimental Psychology: Human Learning and Memory*, 4, 275–289.

Freud, S. (1901/1974). Childhood memories and screen memories. In J. Strachey (Ed.), *The standard edition of the complete psychological works of Sigmund Freud* (Vol. 6, pp. 43–52) London: Hogarth Press.

Freud, S. (1915/1957). Repression. In J. Strachey (Ed.), *The standard edition of the complete psychological works of Sigmund Freud* (Vol. 14, pp. 141–158). London, Hogarth Press.

Hilgard, E.R. (1992) Dissociation and theories of hypnosis. In Fromm, E. & Nash, M.R. *Contemporary Hypnosis Research* N.Y., N.Y.: Guilford Press Horowitz, M. J., & Reidboard, S. P. (1992). Memory, emotion, and response to trauma. In S. Christianson (Ed.), *The Handbook of Emotion and Memory: Research and Theory* (pp. 343–357). Hillsdale, NJ: Erlbaum.

Hyman, I. E., Jr., Husband, T. H., & Billings, J. F. (1995). False memories of childhood experiences. *Applied Cognitive Psychology, 9,* 181–197.

Hyman, I. E., Jr., & Pentland, J. (1996). Guided imagery and the creation of false childhood memories. *Journal of Memory and Language, 35,* 101–117.

Janet, P. (1889). L'automatisme continue. *Revue génerale des sciences*, 4, 167–179

Jacoby, L.L., & Dallas, M. (1981) On the relationship between autobiographical memory and perceptual learning. *Journal of Experimental Psychology: General*, 3, 306–340

Jacoby, L.L., Kelley, C.M. & Dywan, J. Memory Attributions. in H.L. Roediger and F.I.M. Craik (Eds) *Varieties of memory and consciousness: Essays in honor of Endel Tulving.* (pp. 391–422)Hillsdale, N.J.: Erlbaum.

Johnson, M. K., Hashtroudi, S., & Lindsay, D. S. (1993). Source monitoring. *Psychological Bulletin*, 114, 3–28.

Loftus, E. F., & Pickrell, J. E. (1995). The formation of false memories. *Psychiatric Annals, 25*, 720–725.

Mandler, G. (1980). Recognizing: The judgment of a previous occurrence. *Psychological Review*, 87, 252–271.

Neisser, U. (1982). *Memory observed: Remembering in natural context.* San Francisco: Freeman.

Neisser, U. & Harsch, N. (1992). Phantom flashbulbs: False recollections of hearing the news about *Challenger.* In E. Winograd & U. Neisser (Eds.), *Affect and accuracy in recall: Studies of "flashbulb memories"* (pp. 9–31). Cambridge: Cambridge University Press.

Nelson, K. (1993). The psychological and social origins of autobiographical memory. *Psychological Science*, 4, 1–8.

Paivio, A. (1986). *Mental representations: A dual coding approach.* New York: Oxford University Press.

Roediger, H.L. (1990). Remembering reconsidered: Ecological and traditional approaches to the study of memory. *American Journal of Psychology.* 103(3), pp. 403–407.

Roediger, H.L., Weldon, M.S., & Challis, B.H. (1989) Explaining dissociations between implicit and explicit measures of retention: A processing account. In Roediger, H.L., & Craik, F.I.M. (Eds) *Varieties of memory and consciousness: Essays in honor of Endel Tulving.* (pp. 1–41). Hillsdale, N.J.: Erlbaum.

Schacter, D. (1987). Implicit Memory: History and current status. *Journal of Experimental Psychology: Learning, Memory, and Cognition.* 13(3), 510–518.

Schacter, D., Chiu, C.Y.P., & Ohcsner, K.N. (1993). Implicit memory: A selective review. *Annual Review of Neuroscience*, 16, 159–182.

Singer, J.L (1993) Experimental studies of ongoing conscious experience. In Bock, G.R & Marsh, J (Eds) *Experimental and Theoretical Studies of Consciousness*, N.Y., N.Y.: John Wiley and Sons.

Terr, L. C., Bloch, D. A., Michel, B. A., Shi, H., Reinhardt, J. A., & Metayer, S. (1996). Children's memories in the wake of *Challenger. American Journal of Psychiatry, 153*, 618–625.

Tromp, S., Koss, M.P., Figueredo, A.J. & Tharan, M. (1995). Are rape memories different? A comparison of rape, other unpleasant, and pleasant memories among employed women. *Journal of Traumatic Stress*, 8, 607–628.

Tulving, E., & Thompson, D. M. (1973). Encoding specificity and retrieval processes in episodic memory. *Psychological Review, 80*, 352–373.

van der Kolk, B.A., & Fisler, R. (1995). Dissociation and the fragmentary nature of traumatic memories: Overview and exploratory study. *Journal of Traumatic Stress*, 8, 505–525.

van der Kolk, B.A., & van der Hart, O. (1991). The intrusive past: The flexibility of memory and the engraving of trauma. *American Imago*, 48, 425–454.

Wegner, D. (1994) Ironic processes of mental control. *Psychological Review,* 101, 34–52.

Winograd, E. & Neisser, U. (1992), *Affect and accuracy in recall: Studies of "flashbulb memories."* Cambridge: Cambridge University Press.

37

PROFESSIONAL GUIDELINES ON CLINICAL PRACTICE FOR RECOVERED MEMORY: A COMPARATIVE ANALYSIS

Fran Grunberg[1] and Tara Ney[2]

[1]British Columbia Ministry for Children and Families
Vancouver, BC V6J 1C4
[2]Island Psychological Services
Health Care Consultants
Ste. 214–2187 Oak Bay Ave.
Victoria, BC V8R 1G1
Canada

1. INTRODUCTION

At the NATO- ASI a work group was organised to identify and discuss key components of guidelines for clinicians working with adults who allege a trauma history or who have recovered memories of past trauma. We have sifted through the minutes of these discussions, as well as the existing guidelines developed by professional organisations (see Table 1), and present here a comparative analysis of the issues and conclusions contained within them.

Over the past few years, a number of guidelines have been developed by various professional organisations, with considerable expert involvement, to give guidance to practitioners regarding clients' memories of traumatic experiences (see Table 1). In this paper, guidelines developed by experts from the following organisations have been examined: The Canadian Psychological Association (CPA), 1996; The Canadian Psychiatric Association (CPsychiatricA), 1996; The American Psychological Association (APA), 1996; The American Psychological Association, Division 17, Committee on Women, Draft (APA-DIV 17), 1995; The American Society for Clinical Hypnosis (ASCH), 1995 ; The British Psychological Society (BPS), 1995; The International Society for the Study of Dissociation (ISSD), 1994; The American Medical Association, (AMA), 1994; The Australian Psychological Society (APS), 1994; and, The American Psychiatric Association (APsychiatricA), 1993.

Development of these guidelines was sparked by controversies in the late 80's and early 90's surrounding cases in which psychotherapy clients experienced recovery of previously unavailable memories of past trauma, especially childhood sexual abuse: specifi-

Table 1. Description of the categories in the guidelines

	CPA (1)	C. Psychiatric A. (2)	APA (3)	ASCH (4)	BPS (5)	APA Div 17 (6)	ISSD (7)	AMA (8)	APS (9)	A. Psychiatric .A. (10)
Specialized knowledge & competence	✓	✓	✓	✓	✓	✓	✓	✓	✓	✓
Consideration of alternative Diagnoses		✓	✓	✓	✓	✓		✓	✓	
Memory enhancing techniques	✓	✓	✓	✓	✓	✓	✓	✓		✓
Emotional competence						✓	✓	✓		✓
Objectivity/Neutrality in forensic context	✓		✓			✓				
Record-keeping	✓			✓		✓			✓	
Informed consent	✓		✓	✓		✓			✓	
Confrontation/Legal action	✓	✓		✓		✓		✓	✓	✓
Awareness of personal beliefs	✓			✓	✓	✓	✓			✓

Note — The presence of a check-mark indicates that this issue is referred to in the guidelines

*Association Guidelines:

Canadian Psychological Association (1996)
Canadian Psychiatric Association (1996)
American Psychological Association (1996)
American Society of Clinical Hypnosis (1995)
British Psychological Society (1995)
American Psychological Association Div. 17, Committee on Women - Draft (1995)
International Society for the Study of Dissociation (1994)
American Medical Association (1994)
Australian Psychological Society LTD. (1994)
American Psychiatric Association (1993)

cally, determining whether recovered memories are always, often, or rarely reasonable approximations to historical truth, or whether such memories are always, often, or rarely pseudomemories manufactured during therapy, has been a topic of considerable contention (see Enns, McNeilly, Corkery, & Gilbert, 1995, for a review from a feminist perspective). During this time, "trauma treatment" was relatively new, and a standard of practice, or even professional training as a specialty, had not yet developed when the "memory controversy" emerged (Courtois, 1996). In response to both the "memory controversy" and the newness of "trauma treatment," knowledge, and ethics, guidelines were developed to assist clinicians with the complexities of treatment in this area of practice. Generally, as the guidelines indicate, there is a developing concern (albeit with increasing consensus) among clinicians about how memory works and how clinicians should conduct themselves in their work with trauma survivors and with clients who may or may not be trauma survivors.

Debate about the reliability of recovered memories, and about the potential risks of therapeutic approaches used to foster memory recovery, has created a litigious climate for clinicians who work with trauma survivors. Unfortunately, there are reasons to fear that many talented clinicians are now choosing not to work with family violence cases due to increased scrutiny of their work and fear of being caught up in a whirlwind of legal cross-fire (see Caudil, 1996 for a description of the various kinds of litigations in this area). This is an unfortunate trend for an already under-served and vulnerable client population. In order to practice risk management in a climate that is unfriendly to therapists working with abuse survivors, clinicians need to be well informed about the knowledge, ethics, and practice of this specialty.

2. EVALUATING KNOWLEDGE, PRACTICE, AND ETHICS ISSUES IN GUIDELINES ON RECOVERED MEMORIES

General codes of professional conduct and ethics provide insufficient detail and direction for clinicians working with the issues of memory for trauma. Based on our discussions with the NATO Work group, our analysis of existing guidelines, as well as readings of other discussions on this topic (see for example, Adshead, this volume; Courtois, this volume, 1996; Lindsay and Read, 1994; Pope & Brown, 1996; Yapko, 1994), we argue here that there are several issues related to professional training and competence in the practice of psychotherapy that require unique attention when working in this area. These include: knowledge about the scientific research on memory, suggestibility, and trauma; awareness of the necessity of considering alternative diagnoses; caution in the use of memory enhancing techniques; emotional competence; objectivity and impartiality when presenting forensic evidence; maintenance of descriptive and accurate records of therapy; use of informed consent procedures; appropriate advice to clients regarding confrontations and legal action; and awareness of one's own personal beliefs and their potential impact on therapy (see Table 1). The aim of this brief paper is to compile and compare ten sets of guidelines developed by experts of major professional organisations since 1993. The strengths and limitations of each set of guidelines is evaluated on each category described above using the following criteria: present or not present; the degree of caution that is advised; degree of comprehensiveness and explicitness; and, up-to-dateness.

2.1. Specialized Knowledge and Competence about Memory, Suggestibility, and Trauma

Enns et al. (1995) identified a number of content areas in which practitioners must be educated to work competently with trauma survivors. These include knowledge of memory research, including: suggestibility research (Ceci & Bruck, 1993; Lindsay & Read, 1994); autobiographical memory (Brewin, Andrews, and Gotlib, 1993); childhood memory and infantile amnesia (Howe & Courage, 1993); hypnosis and memory (Lynn, this volume; Nash, 1987); and, delayed memory for trauma (Dalenberg, Coe, Reto, Aransky, & Duvenage, 1995; Freyd, 1996; Loftus, Polonsky, & Fullilove, 1994; Van der Kolk & Saporta, 1991; Williams, 1994; Yates & Nasby, 1993). Of course, knowledge about trauma, Post-Traumatic Stress Disorder (PTSD), and dissociation is also necessary (Briere & Runtz, 1993; Davies & Frawley, 1994; Herman, 1992; Rowan, Foy, Rodriguez, & Ryan, 1994; Terr, 1994). It is beyond the scope of this paper to provide this information, but excellent reviews of each of these areas can be found in the references cited. An integrated, working knowledge of each of these content areas is essential for practitioners working in this field.

Since issues related to trauma, interpersonal victimisation, and delayed recovered memory are not likely covered in most practitioners' formal clinical training, the need for specialised knowledge is appropriately recommended in all of the guidelines, with an emphasis on the personal responsibility that a practitioner must take for developing competence through consultation, reading, supervision, research, and networking with other knowledgeable professionals. This is a dynamic, high-risk, and ever-changing field of practice which demands continuing education.

2.2. Consideration of Alternative Diagnoses

Throughout assessment, psychotherapists must remain cognizant that a multiplicity of experiences or traumas other than incest can contribute to a profile that is suggestive of abuse (Briere, in press; Cole & Putnam, 1992). Cole and Putnam noted that "virtually every psychological symptom and many medical symptoms have been associated with incest, including some reported cases of no symptomatology" (p. 175). Lindsay & Poole (1995) cautioned psychotherapists to avoid the cognitive errors of "confirmatory bias" and the "representativeness heuristic," which may encourage therapists to over predict the relationship of some disorders to childhood sexual abuse. Therapists must not make premature conclusions about the meaning of symptoms and must maintain an open mind about the wide range of factors that could contribute to a client's distress.

The APA (1996) document suggests that therapists consider an array of alternative hypotheses.[*] The APA, as well as the CPsychiatricA and BPS caution there is no one symptom, or set of symptoms specific to a kind of abuse and that therapists must not conclude that child sexual abuse has occurred based solely on symptom presentation. The APA-DIV 17 guidelines are consistent with APA, CPsychiatricA, and BPS on this issue, but also provide constructive guidance adding that the therapist "assist the client in ex-

---

[*] These alternatives are: a) that the retrieved material is a reasonably accurate memory of events; b) that it is a distorted memory due to developmental factors or source contaminations; c) that it is a confabulation emerging from underlying psychopathology or difficulties with reality testing; d) that it is a pseudo memory emerging from exposure to suggestions; or e) that it is a form of self-suggestions emerging from the client's internal suggestive mechanism.

ploring various circumstances and experiences that may be related to his or her symptoms." The APS is brief, but to the point stating that alternative causes of any problem should be explored. The ASCH guidelines consider the scenario of a client who believes abuse may have occurred: the therapist is encouraged to evaluate how the patient came to hold these beliefs, thus recognising more how clients may be influenced (as opposed to the therapist). Together these guidelines urge practitioners to be open to alternative interpretations, and certainly, no one symptom is pathognomic of a history of abuse. Therapists must neither suggest nor suppress reports of abuse and trauma in their assessment and in their treatment.

2.3. Use of Memory Enhancing Techniques

Hypnosis and hypnosis-like procedures such as guided imagery often make memory more confident but less reliable (Lynn, this volume; Nash, 1987). While it is not known which clinical techniques are most likely to lead to the creation of pseudomemories, it is known that pseudomemories have been created in trance states, and that such memories can be held with considerable confidence. It is also known that memory is not perfect and that a number of other factors influence the memory process. For example, the passage of time influences the strength and organisation of stored information. A person's prior knowledge also affects memory in that it affects the individual's ability to understand an experience and encode it accurately and can also influence reconstruction of memories during attempts to recollect the past.

For reasons described above, there is a general consensus, in both the clinical and academic communities, that using hypnosis to retrieve memories of child sexual abuse involves unnecessary risk (see Briere, this volume). Many jurisdictions have ruled that if evidence is acquired from a witness under hypnosis, or if hypnosis was used in therapy or elsewhere prior to a court proceeding, that evidence will not be admitted in court (Lindsay and Read, 1995). Clinicians must be aware that use of hypnosis could jeopardise ongoing or anticipated legal actions.

Guidelines that address memory enhancement strategies are typically focused on the use of hypnosis. The AMA recommends that hypnosis be used only for investigative purposes (and concludes that amytal "has no legitimate use in recovered-memory cases," p.11). The CPA is less committal but recommends awareness about the benefits and risks particularly where legal action is being considered by the client. The CPsychiatricA is specific but brief, and recommends avoidance of the use of hypnosis and other memory enhancing techniques which are directed at lost material. The APA recommends that hypnosis not be used for clients who are attempting to retrieve or confirm recollections of abusive histories and provides a number of reasons for this including: risk of creating pseudomemories; risk of increased confidence with inaccurate memories; potential to jeopardise future legal actions; and individual variability in proneness to suggestibility and proneness to fantasy. The BPS does not explicitly address the hypnosis issue in the "guidelines for therapists," although one of the guidelines states that the therapist must be "alert to the dangers of suggestion." There is also discussion in the text of the BPS document on how hypnosis makes memory more confident and less reliable. The APsychiatricA states that "...special knowledge and experience are necessary to properly evaluate and/or treat patients who report the emergence of memories during the use of specialised interview techniques (e.g. the use of hypnosis or amytal), or during the course of litigation." No specific guidance is given in this respect, and unfortunately there is no guidance on how or when to use hypnosis (or amytal).

The most extensively developed guidelines for using hypnosis are the ASCH guidelines: they provide guidance on when to, how to, and who should use hypnosis (but see Lynn, this volume, for criticism of the ASCH guidelines). The supposition here is that problems with hypnosis lie more in the manner in which hypnosis has been used rather than the procedure per se. However, the guidelines are unclear regarding the critical issue of hypnosis. Although exploratory hypnotic techniques (e.g. encouraging insight into interpersonal dynamics, adaptive functions, or feelings of earlier life experiences) are discouraged in more severely disturbed patients (i.e. serious borderline conditions, psychosis), permission is granted to experienced hypnotherapists, if used with caution. Unfortunately, no rationale is provided for this caution, and it is not clear to the reader whether memory recovery is supported. Further, exploratory hypnosis is indicated in "patients who present with long-standing and complex symptoms that have generalised to a larger number of life areas, where the initial assessment suggests adaptive functions and conflicts [that] may be associated with patient problems, and where the patient's present life stressors and relationships do not seem to adequately account for symptomatic complaints..." and where "patients possess adequate impulse control and ability to tolerate affect involved in exploration, who are psychologically-minded, verbal, intelligent and who have capacity for insight, and in patients who enter treatment with the expectation that insight will be curative and who wish to pursue a therapeutic goal of self-awareness." (p.26).

The exploratory hypnotic approach is also said to be indicated for "resistant" patients. In contrast to the ASCH guidelines, the APA-DIV 17 guidelines state that hypnosis should be used only "to support and strengthen the self-care activities, but should not be used for memory recovery." The reasoning given, as stated by other organisations, is that hypnosis can result in increased confidence, but decreased reliability of recollected events. The APA-DIV 17 guidelines also provide guidance on how to treat emerging memories without using hypnosis. Finally, the ISSD guidelines describe a number of functions of hypnosis including: crisis management, ego strengthening, aiding safe expression of feeling, cognitive rehearsal, skill building, and relief of somatic memory pain. The guidelines go on to describe the divergence of opinions concerning the role of hypnosis in psychotherapy: "[s]ome believe that hypnotic techniques are useful in memory retrieval; others believe that hypnotically facilitated memory processing increases the patient's chances of mislabelling fantasy as real memory..." (p.8). Ultimately, the clinician is advised to be aware that trance states can confuse a patient about reality.

In sum, all sets of guidelines have addressed the hypnosis/suggestibility issue. Clearly, the recent research suggests that practitioners must understand the degree to which some clients can create pseudomemories and the legal implications of using hypnosis. The guidelines vary in the degree of cautiousness that the practitioner should exercise and the reasons why such techniques should not be used. The bottom line is do no harm.

2.4. Emotional Competence

It is increasingly understood that counselling and psychotherapy can be hazardous to the physical and mental health of practitioners (Arvay, this volume; Arvay and Uhelmann, 1996). This is particularly true when working with trauma survivors: *the demands of the clinician who works with traumatised individuals or those who retrieve memories of trauma is above and beyond the demands of more general psychotherapy.* Specifically, when clients' traumatic experiences are shared with a therapist, and when the therapist is empathically engaged with the client, similar symptoms of intense vulnerability, overwhelming affect, and disrupted beliefs may be experienced by the therapist (Saakvitne & Pearlman, 1996). In other words, the therapist too can become traumatised. This phenomenon has been labelled as compassion fatigue (Figley, 1995), secondary traumatization (Herman, 1992), or vicarious traumatization (McCann & Pearlman, 1990).

Vicarious traumatization is now seen as an occupational hazard (Saakvitne & Pearlman, 1996). Previous lack of attention to this phenomenon has not only been misleading, but dangerous to both client and therapist (Pearlman & Saakvitne, 1995). Both counter transference and vicarious traumatization are powerful phenomena when working with trauma survivors and, as noted by Pearlman and Saakvitne (1995), "if unacknowledged or unexamined, they can damage both client and therapist" (p.xv).

In spite of the importance and uniqueness of this category, as described above, only three sets of guidelines address the issue of emotional competence as it relates to therapist self-care and boundaries. In two sets of guidelines this issue is inadequately detailed (i.e. APsychiatricA and ISSD). The APsychiatricA states that the clinician should "...vigilantly assess the impact of their conduct on the boundaries of the doctor/patient relationship." While this concern is recognised at the end of the document, there is no discussion or rationale in the text of the document. Subsequently, the importance of this concern is downplayed. The ISSD guidelines refer to the therapeutic boundary issues (e.g. length of therapy sessions, therapist availability in between sessions, the use (or non-use) of physical contact with the therapist) that may arise with a client who has experienced trauma, but this is not related to the broader issue of vicarious traumatization. On the other hand, the APA-DIV17 provides more thorough and explicit guidance for practitioners on how to minimise potential vicarious traumatization. In summary, these recommendations include: avoid isolation; avoid too many trauma history caseloads; maintain an awareness of personal life status; pay attention to self-care; seek personal therapy during personal crises; seek consultation or support when necessary; and, for therapists with a similar history, be aware of over- or under identification with the client's abuse history.

Emotional competence in this work is also a training and training ethics issue (Courtois, this volume). Supervisors must work to assist supervisees to develop emotional competence and maturity and to be aware of blind spots and personal issues that interact with patient issues and dynamics. In our opinion this content area is highly under-addressed in all but the APA-DIV 17 guidelines.

2.5. Objectivity and Impartiality when Presenting Forensic Evidence

Clinical forensic psychologists and memory researchers in forensic settings must be cautious in making generalisations about memory for traumatic child abuse based on the available research (e.g., Enns et al., 1996; Loftus, 1996; Pope & Brown, 1996): None of the research studies conducted to date can in themselves conclusively discount or confirm a particular recovered memory, and it is likely that limitations of the scientific evidence will always preclude definitive statements regarding individual cases. Memory research has often demonstrated the fallibility of memory (Lindsay & Read, 1994), but such memory research usually takes place either in a laboratory or some everyday setting. Thus, there is still considerable controversy among memory researchers as to whether memories of traumatic events are encoded and stored differently from memories of non-traumatic events (e.g. Bremer, Randall, Scott, Bronen, et al., 1995; Ornstein, Ceci, & Loftus, 1996; Yehuda, Kahana, Binder-Byrnes, Southwick, et al., 1995). Some recent studies have demonstrated pseudomemories of mildly distressing childhood events (e.g. Hyman, Husband, & Billings, 1995; Loftus, 1993; see also Lindsay, this volume; Loftus, this volume). However, there are also studies that indicate that traumatic experiences can be forgotten and later accurately remembered (Feldman-Summers & Pope, 1994; Loftus, Polonsky, & Fullilove, 1994; Schooler, Ambadar, & Bendiksen, this volume; Williams, 1994), although in these studies there are limitations due to lack of experimental control and validation (Briere, 1995). At present, there is a converging opinion that "some recovered memories for childhood abuse are true and some are suggestively planted" (Pezdek & Banks, 1996, p. 1).

The bottom line is that memory researchers, forensic psychologists, and other mental health professionals must avoid speaking to the truth of a particular case, because this is neither their role nor expertise. The forensic psychologist is rather an educator of the judge and jury. Forensic psychologists should also rely on a variety of converging data to make their formulations. This is particularly true when testifying in cases in which trauma memories are at issue, because biased reporting of research evidence by forensic psychologists can add unnecessary fuel to an already heated fire. In sum, forensic psychologists should always exercise caution, and be aware of both the limitations and the strengths of their methodologies and of the existing scientific evidence.

The CPA emphasise the need for psychologists to maintain professional objectivity and impartiality in presenting legal evidence, recognising that this is not always easy to do when emotionally charged scenarios are being presented. The only other document to discuss this matter is the APA encouraging forensic psychologists and expert witnesses to consider multiple sources of information and contamination, and to be aware of the limitations of the research that may be used. Only the CPA and APA refer to this issue. The APA provides a great deal more detail on conduct, whereas the CPA is more general.

2.6. Record Keeping

Most clinicians have record-keeping guidelines that require them to keep records of client contact and treatment. Because each file is a medical-legal chart, the documentation should be systematic, regular, and comprehensive. Every chart should of course have a detailed history, which includes the presenting concern(s), assessment information, and psychosocial history, as well as the diagnosis, treatment goals and objectives, and progress towards goals. This is critical so that any diagnostic formulations are evidence-based and not just subjective whims.

At minimum, good progress notes should include the date on which treatment was provided, what happened, and any significant interventions undertaken. The notes should be behaviourally descriptive—here is what was done in this session. Thus, a brief, behaviourally-focused record should contain pertinent information regarding the patient's mood, progress, and action taken by the therapist for each session (Courtois, 1996). Pope & Brown (1996) have an excellent demonstration of the kinds of notes that will protect both the therapist and client should they need to be used for legal purposes.

Clinicians working with trauma survivors, as with all patients, are best to operate under the assumption that any record could be subpoenaed.[†] It has become increasingly

---

[†] In Canada, for example, the Supreme Court has recently set out guidelines concerning the circumstances in which confidential documents must be disclosed to an accused in criminal proceedings. Essentially, the Supreme Court has broadened the disclosure test from that set out by the Court of Appeal, and it is now likely that confidential records will be ordered more often. Specifically, and most relevant here, the conclusion is that one reason that documents may be used is if "they reveal the use of a therapy which influenced the complainant's memory of the alleged events" (Boyd & Tetrault, 1996). Thus, notes should clearly document exactly what went on during therapy when a disclosure was made.

advised that process notes (i.e. those notes which refer to the clinicians' transitory formulations) should not become a part of the record, because there have been numerous instances in which process notes about the client have undermined a legal proceeding against the client (Caudill, 1996) (although Courtois, this volume, recommends process notes when the patient is struggling with unclear memory or reporting recovered/delayed memory). In this climate of litigation it is critical that therapists keep their notes brief and behaviourally descriptive, in order to protect clients, third parties and themselves.

Both the CPA and APS make general statements on maintaining systematic, regular, and comprehensive records. The AMA guidelines insist on careful record keeping during hypnosis. The ASCH guidelines say that the more serious or unusual the memories and allegations of the patient, the more thorough the treatment notes should be. The APA-DIV 17 suggests audio-or video-taping sessions, as well as noting client misinformation or erroneous expectancies and the therapists' efforts to convey accurate information. Generally, the guidelines lack adequate detail and rationale to be helpful to clinicians. We believe that in this area the focus should be on brief, behaviourally descriptive notes, and that practitioners should be cautioned about the dangers of process notes in the legal system. This would serve to protect therapists, clients, and third parties.

2.7. Informed Consent

It is increasingly advised that informed consent be in writing. This is particularly true with any therapeutic approach that may be viewed as controversial. Informed consent should also continue throughout the therapy process, to ensure the client is always making an informed decision to participate in therapy and to receive the interventions offered (Courtois, this volume; Pope & Brown, 1996). The risks associated with any procedure should be described in full, and the client must know how the procedures work. This is especially so with any controversial intervention such as hypnosis or age regression, or new procedures such as Eye Movement Desensitisation Reprocessing (Shapiro, 1996) that may undermine or lead to litigation. The therapist must always know that the client knows that participation in the therapy process is voluntary and is aware of his/her rights and privileges. Thus, informed consent should be discussed throughout the therapy process.

The CPA, APA, and APS all make general, brief comments about informed consent. The APS states that informed consent be obtained at the beginning of therapy as it relates to the therapeutic procedures and process; the notion of informed consent is only implicit in the the CPA guidelines which refer to the importance of discussing particular therapeutic techniques with clients; the APA similarly states that all clients be provided with informed consent for treatment. The ASCH guidelines refer to informed consent as a routine procedure except of course in emergency situations where it may not be feasible. The APA-DIV 17 discusses informed consent as an ongoing process, and not a one-time contract that is negotiated at the outset of treatment or a particular treatment intervention.

Given the kinds of concerns that have arisen in legal cases, it is important that the therapist approach the entire treatment process with an attitude that the client needs to know that she is participating in the treatment voluntarily. Most of the guidelines have indicated that informed consent be obtained either at the beginning of therapy or for particular techniques. One set of guidelines argues that informed consent go on throughout therapy.

2.8. Confrontation

Disclosing the secret of familial abuse can facilitate healing when family members (and the abuser) validate the survivor and provide social support. However, while confrontations can be empowering and exhilarating for survivors, they can also be disappointing and another source of pain (Cameron, 1994). Family members have been known to attack the survivor for revealing abuse, reject the survivor, or engage in other actions that may revictimize the client (Daniluk & Haverkamp, 1993). Because of the potential for so much harm, many practitioners believe that therapists should carefully explore with their client whether to confront in pursuit of healing, and if so, when and how to do so.

Written accounts of confrontations suggest that a number of issues must be considered, including: the responsibility of the therapist toward a client who is considering confrontation; the physical and psychic risks that a survivor may encounter in doing so; the possibility of uncovering multiple victims within a family; and the crucial nature of realistic goals, preparation and readiness (MacFarlane & Korbin, 1983). Others have suggested that at the very least therapists should assess client motivation and prepare the client for best and worst possible outcomes of seeking justice through the legal system (Enns et al., 1995). In some instances, confrontation has been completely discouraged, and some clinicians suggest that therapists offer their clients meaningful alternatives such as letter-writing (unsent), the "empty chair" to enact an imaginary confrontation, psychodrama, or becoming involved in prevention programs and volunteer organisations that deal with abuse (Cameron, 1994).

Arguably, confrontations with clear/available memory are risky enough for reasons described above; they are all the more so when there is no corroborative evidence available, which is sometimes the case with a recovered memory. Although primary concern for the welfare of the client is always paramount, a secondary consideration of harm must also be given to third parties (especially those who may be important in the life of a client). In the interest of all parties, confrontations should probably not be undertaken if the evidence/corroboration is unavailable. In response to increasing numbers of legal suits against therapists by their clients, Caudill (1996) suggests that all confrontations be done by a third party. Or, if done by the client's therapist, it should be done after signing a Waiver of Conflict which informs the third party of the potentially distressing situation. While primary duty is to the client, therapists must also consider the degree of distress that is being inflicted upon third parties when confronting. A combination of sensitivity and realism is necessary with confrontation: confrontation is a choice, not a necessity.

The AMA recognises that restoring control to the victim is an important part of therapy, and supports lawsuits which "help an abuse victim retake or reassert control of his or her life." The only caution made by the AMA is that standards of proof might need to be considered. Other guidelines are considerably more cautious. For example, both the CPA and CPsychiatricA bring attention to the secondary importance of no harm to others who may be important to the client, The CPsychiatricA, contrary to the AMA, argues there is no evidence that confrontations which are solely designed to express anger, are therapeutic, and both of these guidelines caution that therapists must protect the interests of patients and their supportive relationships. The APsychiatricA states that if patients desire to take legal action or confront "attachment figures," the role of the clinician is to support patients to assess all ramifications of such actions and adapt to any uncertainty of emotional issues. The ASCH guidelines urge clinicians to caution patients who decide to confront an alleged abuser based upon information retrieved solely under hypnosis, emphasising that veridicality is not essential. Clinicians are advised to keep clear, written records on the advice given and discussions which ensued around confrontation. APS insists on caution in responding to questions from clients about pursuing legal action, although no comment is made about confrontation per se. The APA-DIV 17 provides the most comprehensive discussion on the issue of confrontation and discusses if, when, and how a confrontation could take place and the role of the therapist.

In sum, guidelines are most cautious when memories are recovered using hypnosis, and if there is no corroborating evidence of abuse. There is apparent divergence of emphasis on the value of confrontation to the patient, ranging from recognition of the value of empowerment resulting from a confrontation, to avoiding confrontation which serves to express anger towards alleged abusers.

2.9. Awareness of One's Personal Beliefs

Because clinical work is to a large extent a subjective experience, it is necessary for clinicians involved in assessment and treatment to be constantly aware of their own beliefs and biases (Ney, 1995). Our beliefs incorporate our knowledge about the world around us and our own attitudes. Therapists who are mindful of the potential authority/parental role they may play will be aware that clients are particularly vulnerable to suggestive influence. Therapists must balance being supportive, empathic, and concerned, on the one hand, with avoiding being leading, on the other. This delicate balance is a challenge to all therapists. Seigel (1995) concluded that the "principles of clinical interest, compassion, and open-mindedness can help optimise therapeutic progress and minimise iatrogenic distortions" (p. 112).

The CPA guidelines include an ethical principle which describes the importance of being aware of personal beliefs and values to avoid advancing personal agendas. The APsychiatricA and ISSD similarly caution clinicians not to impose beliefs and values on patients, and the APS advises clinicians to critically evaluate their own assumptions or biases. The BPS guidelines are more narrow in this respect and state the therapist should avoid imposing conclusions about what took place in childhood, and the ASCH guidelines specifically advise therapists who themselves are abuse victims to have their own issues resolved. The APA-DIV 17 does not deal explicitly with this issue, but throughout the document insists on increased awareness of personal agendas and issues. Since much of a clinician's practice is driven by personal beliefs, awareness of what these are contributes to a reduced likelihood of imposing personal agendas on clients. The majority of guidelines have highlighted this issue, although most often in a cursory manner.

3. CONCLUSION

This paper has provided a compilation of guidelines developed by numerous organisations since 1993 and which deal with trauma-memory issues in therapy. The development of these guidelines has been undertaken in response to personal, political, and legal controversies about the nature and validity of recovered memories of childhood sexual abuse. The importance of nine specific issues has been discussed, and the degree to which each set of guidelines has addressed each issue has been evaluated. None of the guidelines provide recommendations on all nine issues, perhaps reflecting the need for organisations to consider the particular relevance of each issue for their members when developing guidelines. We believe that associations that represent mental health workers, crisis intervention workers, child protection workers, medical practitioners, legal and police workers all need to consider guidelines to suit their special working circumstances.

Perhaps not surprisingly, there is a high degree of consensus among the guidelines on the importance of addressing Specialised Knowledge and Competence (10), Considering Alternative Diagnoses (6), Memory Enhancing Techniques (9), Confrontation (7), and Awareness of Personal Beliefs (7). This consensus only indicates that the issue is of importance, not that there is agreement on how the issue is to be dealt with in therapy. For example, the consensus on Memory Enhancing Techniques indicates that all but one set of guidelines has recognised the importance of this issue. However, while all guidelines advise caution in the use of hypnosis (and other memory enhancing techniques), this differs between guidelines. The AMA states that it should only be used for investigative purposes, others advise that it not be used for memory retrieval (e.g. APA-DIV 17), and yet others focus on the need of the clinician to be aware of the implications of using memory enhancing techniques ques. A lack of consensus also exists on the use of amytal (see AMA vs APsychiatricA). Thus, while there is consensus that this is an important issue, there is not consensus on how hypnosis and other memory enhancing techniques should be used in therapy.

Regarding confrontation, all but three of the guidelines address this contentious issue, suggesting a high degree of consensus on the importance of this issue. Generally, caution is urged when memories are recovered using hypnosis, or if there is no corroborating evidence of abuse. There is apparent divergence of emphasis on the value of confrontation to the patient, where the AMA recognises therapeutic empowerment from a confrontation, while the CPsychiatricA argues there is no evidence of therapeutic value of expressing anger to alleged abusers. Perhaps this is an area where more systematic research is required to determine the conditions under which confrontation has been therapeutic or not.

Lack of clear record keeping and informed consent procedures has created a great deal of conflict for therapists with their clients and and third parties. Informed consent is discussed in a general and almost trivial way in most guidelines, except the APA-DIV 17, where descriptions of the importance and rational of obtaining informed consent are woven throughout the document. The rationale for and the most effective way to keep records is usually not detailed in the guidelines (except APA-DIV 17), and so the value to the clinician is not necessarily convincing.

We have deliberately separated Emotional Competence from Awareness of Personal Beliefs. Most (all but three) of the guidelines have commented on the importance of being aware of personal beliefs and values, recognising how preexisting personal agendas can interfere with respect and rights of the client. However, only one set of guidelines fully addresses Emotional Competence. Combining these two categories would have disguised this observation. The lack of adequate commentary in the guidelines on Emotional Competence is a concern given our current knowledge of vicarious traumatization to therapists who work with this population.

There are many different reasons for greater/lesser consensus in each of the categories. The absence of consensus may be explained by a number of factors: there may be a stronger research foundation on some factors; methodological differences have produced non-comparable findings; and, theoretical divergence may contribute to different interpretations of findings. For example, is there theoretical congruence in the areas where there is consensus, or does this mean there is theoretical congruence where there is consensus? Future developments in this field will likely depend on theoretical coherence. This is an area where disciplinary boundaries may interfere with the development of coherent theory. Movement forward requires an integration of theory pertaining to human development, learning, trauma, elaboration of mental constructs, and their relationship to memory as interpretation. In many cases there is no "right" or "wrong" way to act; aspects of the situation must be weighed and a combination of sensitivity and realism must be considered in all clinical practices. We anticipate that guidelines will evolve in conjunction with developments in clinical practice and research in this area. There is still much that is not yet understood, and guidelines which are overly prescriptive will not likely survive the test of time; however, without sufficient detail and rationale in the guidelines, the clinician is left without adequate reason for acting in particular ways. Clinicians are best to operate from a position of "there are no absolutes."

It has been suggested that it is no longer productive to debate whether recovered childhood memories are true or false. It now seems clear that some recovered memories for childhood abuse are true and some are suggestively planted (Pezdek & Banks, 1996). Current research is investigating the conditions under which traumatic events are or are not likely to be repressed and the conditions under which recovered memories are or are not likely to be true.

The general consensus is that the problem of child sexual abuse cannot be underestimated; the problem is grave and prevention and treatment is critical. Yet, while it is necessary to be open to the emergence of (previously unremembered) memories, the accuracy of recovered memories cannot be ascertained. Thus, most professional organisations have urged caution on this matter. The way and degree to which caution is recommended between organisations, professions, and countries varies, as can be observed in our analyses of the guidelines. Organisations wishing to develop their own guidelines may find this compilation and analysis useful. Numerous complementary writings have recently emerged that provide important recommendations and comprehensive rationales for competent practice in working with trauma survivors (e.g., Courtois, 1996, this volume; Enns et al., 1995; Lindsay & Read, 1995; Yapko, 1994). These are not included in the current analysis but have been used to create the categories to evaluate existing guidelines.

REFERENCES

American Medical Association (1994, June 16). *Report of the Council on Scientific Affairs: Memories of childhood abuse.* CSA Report 5-A-94.

American Psychiatric Association (1993, December 22). *APA issues statements on memories of sexual abuse, gun control, television violence.* News Release No. 93–58.

American Psychological Association, Division 17 Committee on Women, Division 42 Trauma and Gender Issues Committee (1995, July 25). *Psychotherapy guidelines for working with clients who may have an abuse or trauma history.*

American Psychological Association (1996, February 14). *Working group on investigation of memories of childhood abuse: Final report.*

Arvay, M., & Uhlemann, M. (1996). Counsellor stress in the field of trauma: A preliminary study. *Canadian Journal of Counselling, 30(3)*, 193–210.

Australian Psychology Society (1994, October 1)

Bremer, J.D., Randall, P., Scott, T.M., Bronen, R.A., Seibyl, J.P., Southwick, S.M., Delaney, R.C., McCarthy, G., Charney, D.S., & Innis, R.B. (1995). MRI-based measurement of hippocampal volume in patients with combat-related post traumatic stress disorder. *American Journal of Psychiatry, 152*, 973–981.

Brewin, C. R., Andrews, B., & Gotlib, I. H. (1993). Psychopathology and early experience: A reappraisal of retrospective reports. *Psychological Bulletin, 113*, 82–98.

Briere, J.N. (1995). Child abuse, memory, and recall: A commentary. *Consciousness and Cognition, 4*, 83–87.

Briere, J.N. (in press). *Psychological assessment of adult post traumatic states.* Washington DC: American Psychological Association.

Briere, J.N., & Runtz, M. (1993). Childhood sexual abuse: Long-term sequelae and implications for psychological assessment. *Journal of Interpersonal Violence, 8,* 312–330.

Brown, L. S. (1996, November). *Expert testimony and forensic evaluations.* Paper presented at Trauma and Controversy, International Society for Traumatic Stress Studies, 12th Annual Meeting. San Francisco, CA.

British Psychological Society (1995, January). *Recovered memories: The report of the Working Party of The British Psychological Society.*

Cameron, C. (1994). Women confronting their abusers: Issues, decisions, and outcomes. *Journal of Child Sexual Abuse, 3,* 7–35.

Canadian Psychiatric Association (1996, March 25). Position statement: Adult recovered memories of childhood sexual abuse. *Canadian Journal of Psychiatry, 41(5),* 305–306.

Canadian Psychological Association (1996, October) *Ethical guidelines for psychologists addressing recovered memories of abuse.*

Caudil, O. B. (1996, November). *New legislation and case law effecting trauma therapy.* Paper presented at Trauma and Controversy, International Society for Traumatic Stress Studies, 12th Annual Meeting. San Francisco, CA.

Ceci, S. J., & Bruck, M. (1993). Suggestibility of the child witness: A historical review and synthesis. *Psychological Bulletin, 113,* 403–439.

Cole, P., & Putnam, F. (1992). Effect of incest on self and social functioning: A developmental psychopathology perspective. *Journal of Consulting and Clinical Psychology, 60,* 174–184.

Courtois, C.A. (1988). *Healing the incest wound: Adult survivors in therapy.* New York: Norton.

Courtois, C. A. (1996). Informed clinical practice and the delayed memory controversy. In: K. Pezdek and W. Banks (Eds.),*The recovered memory/false memory debate.* New York: Academic Press.

Dalenberg, C., Coe, M., Reto, M., Aransky, K., & Duvenage, C. (1995, January). *The prediction of amnesic barrier strength as an individual difference variable in state-dependent learning paradigms.* Paper presented at the conference, Responding to Child Maltreatment, San Diego, CA.

Daniluk, J. C., & Haverkamp, B. E. (1993). Ethical issues in counselling adult survivors of incest. *Journal of Counselling and Development, 72,* 12–22.

Davies, J. M., & Frawley, M. G. (1994). *Treating the adult survivor of childhood sexual abuse: A psychoanalytic perspective.* New York: Basic Books.

Enns, C., McNeilly, C., Madison Corkey, J., & Gilbert, M. S. (1995). The debate about delayed memories of child sexual abuse: A feminist perspective. *The Counselling Psychologist, 23,* 181–279.

Feldman-Summers, S., & Pope, K. S. (1994). The experience of "forgetting" childhood abuse: A national survey of psychologists. *Journal of Consulting and Clinical Psychology, 62,* 636–639.

Figley, C. R. (Ed.). (1995). *Compassion fatigue: Coping with secondary traumatic stress disorder in those who treat the traumatised.* New York: Brunner/Mazel.

Freyd, J.J. (1996). *Betrayal trauma theory: The logic of forgetting abuse.* Harvard: Harvard University Press.

Herman, J. (1992). *Trauma and recovery.* New York: Basic Books.

Howe, M. L. & Courage, M. L. (1993). On resolving the enigma of infantile amnesia. *Psychological Bulletin, 113,* 305–326.

Hyman, I. E., Jr., Husband, T. H., & Billings, F. J. (1995). False memories of childhood experiences. *Applied Cognitive Psychology, 9,* 181–197.

Lindsay, D. S., & Poole, D. A. (1995). Remembering childhood sexual abuse in therapy: Psychotherapists' self-reported beliefs, practices, and experiences. *The Journal of Psychiatry and Law,* Fall, 461–476.

Lindsay, D. S., & Read, J. D. (1994). Psychotherapy and memories of childhood sexual abuse: A cognitive perspective. *Applied Cognitive Psychology, 8,* 281–338.

Lindsay, D.S., & Read, J.D. (1995). "Memory work" and recovered memories of childhood sexual abuse: Scientific evidence and public, professional, and personal issues. *Psychology, Public Policy and Law, 1,* 846–908.

Loftus, E. F., Polonsky, S., & Fullilove, M. T. (1994). Memories of childhood sexual abuse: Remembering and repressing. *Psychology of Women Quarterly, 18,* 67–84.

McCann, I. L., & Pearlman, L. A. (1990). Vicarious traumatization: A framework for understanding the psychological effects of working with victims. *Journal of Traumatic Stress, 3,* 131–149.

MacFarlane, K., & Korbin, J. (1983). Confronting the incest secret long after the fact: A family study of multiple victimisation with strategies for intervention. *Child Abuse & Neglect, 7,* 225–237.

Nash, M. (1987). What, if anything, is regressed about hypnotic age regression? A review of the empirical literature. *Psychological Bulletin, 102,* 42–52.

Ney, T. (1995). Assessing allegations in child sexual abuse: An overview. In Ney, T. (Ed.), *True and false allegations in child sexual abuse: Assessment and case management* (pp. 3–20). New York: Brunner/Mazel.

Ornstein, P.A., Ceci, S.J., & Loftus, E.F. (1996, Febuary). Reply to the Alpert, Brown, and Courtois document: The science of memory and the practice of psychotherapy. In: *American Psychological Association (1996, February 14). Working group on investigation of memories of childhood abuse: Final report.*

Pearlman, L., & Saakvitne, K.W. (1995). *Trauma and the therapist: Counter transference and vicarious traumatization in psychotherapy with incest survivors.* New York: Norton.

Pezdek, K., & Banks, W. P. (1996). Childhood trauma and memory. In Pezdek, K., & Banks, W. P. (Eds.), *The recovered memory/false memory debate* (pp. 1–2). New York: Academic Press.

Pope, K.S., & Brown, L.S. (1996). *Recovered memories of abuse: Assessment, therapy, forensics.* Washington, DC: American Psychological Association.

Rowan, A. B., Foy, D. W., Rodriguez, N., & Ryan, S. (1994). Post traumatic stress disorder in a clinical sample of adults sexually abused as children. *Child Abuse and Neglect: The International Journal, 18,* 51–61.

Saakvitne, K., & Pearlman, L. (1996) *Transforming the pain: A workbook on vicarious traumatization.* New York: Norton .

Seigel, D. (1995). Memory, trauma, and psychotherapy. *Journal of Psychotherapy Practice and Research, 4,* 93–122.

Shapiro, F. (1996). Eye Movement Desensitisation and Processing (EMDR): Evaluation of controlled PTSD research. *Journal of Behavioural Therapy and Experimental Psychiatry, 27*(3), 1–10.

Terr, L. (1994). *Unchained memories: True stories of traumatic memory loss.* New York: Basic Books.

Van der Kolk, B.A., & Saporta, J. (1991). The biological response to psychic trauma: Mechanisms and treatment of intrusions and numbing. *Anxiety Research, 4,* 199–212.

Williams, L. M. (1992). Adult memories of childhood abuse: Preliminary findings from a longitudinal study. *The Advisor, 5,* 19–20.

Williams, L. M. (1994). Recall of childhood trauma: A prospective study of women's memories of child sexual abuse. *Journal of Consulting and Clinical Psychology, 62,* 1167–1176.

Yapko, M. (1994). *Suggestions of abuse: True and false memories of childhood sexual trauma.* New York: Simon & Schuster.

Yates, J.L., & Nasby, W. (1993). Dissociation, affect and network models of memory: An integrative proposal. *Journal of Traumatic Stress, 6,* 305–326.

Yehuda, R., Kahana, B., Binder-Byrnes, K., Southwick, S., Mason, J.W., & Giller, E.L. (1995). Low urinary cortisol excretion in Holocaust survivors with post traumatic stress disorder. *American Journal of Psychiatry, 152,* 982–986.

38

PERSONAL PERSPECTIVES ON THE DEVELOPMENT OF THE CONCEPT OF SEXUAL TRAUMA IN FRANCE

Comparisons to the North American Experience

Marie-Christine Simon de Bergen

La Residence Sociale
Levallois-Perret
17 rue du Hameau
75015 Paris
France

1. INTRODUCTION

Discussions of "sexual trauma" have raised different issues concerning reported or unreported trauma, the recollection of mistreatment and abuse, the psychological impact of such memories, and the difficulties in distinguishing between false and true allegations. Although the following discussion will not include a point-by-point comparison of the French and American approaches to the issue of trauma, we nonetheless want to describe the French perspective for taking sexual trauma into account in the social, clinical, foren-sic, and judicial fields, and the methodological and ethical problems posed by sexual trauma. One could say that the notion of "sexual trauma" has only just emerged in France, while the US seems, on the contrary, to have overdetermined this notion. Let us explore the differences.

2. FRANCE: THE SOCIAL EMERGENCE OF THE NOTION OF SEXUAL TRAUMA

2.1. France: Late Media Awareness of Sexual Abuse

The emergence of the theme of sexual abuse, notably incest, in the media dates from the late 1980's and explains the relative lateness of the awareness of these questions by some professionals and, on a larger scale, by the public at large. It is clear that equating "sexual assault on a child" with "trauma" was not an object of debate but rather taken for granted during the NATO-ASI Conference. It is, however, difficult for French professionals who care for abused children or adults to have others accept the idea of criminal sexual activity when there are no physical signs. For example, during the 1994 Conference, "Taking charge of child victims of sexual violence in France," organised by the French Government,[1] one child psychiatrist described a child abused by his mother in this way: (p.72): "this child could not even say that he was mistreated, because he was well-treated..." Another said of a girl being abused by her stepfather, "We are the ones who think that it is not good" (p. 76). Later, "it depends if there is violence or not." Indeed, sexual mistreatment is so rarely considered as a trauma that one also heard: (p.75) "That is to say, that one of the questions we can ask is how the child participates.. to what happens in the body/body relationship and the dimension of enjoyment, which is shared or not."

In fact, when the notion of physical violence, measured by its physiological consequences, is taken into account by French professionals, sexual violence is often considered non-existent, if there are no physical signs. Only physical evidence is considered as proof of child abuse.

2.2. Proving the Crime, Not the Trauma

According to French criminal law, the accused is innocent until proven otherwise. It is therefore the responsibility of professionals to bring forward the proof of guilt, which is central to the French criminal system. In practice, doubt seems systematically to protect the adult, to the detriment of the child. Statistics attest to the importance of physical proof. In the Hauts de Seine area, located near Paris, it was reported[2] in 1994 that, of sixty criminal complaints recorded following a phone call to the local hotline, 93.5% of the complaints of physical abuse resulted in a criminal trial and a conviction carrying a prison sentence, whereas only 53% of the complaints of sexual aggression did.

Other figures (according to unofficial sources) state that in France, only 25% of incest cases are prosecuted. When neither physical proof nor confession is present, the French court system relies on the files of the administrative evaluating committee which is composed of social workers and educators. These professionals, by each considering the separate historical information they have about a child, can reconstruct a dossier of clues that supports a guilty finding by the judge.

Unfortunately, many children, who have been designated as having been abused, do not benefit from regular meetings of committees that act on their behalf. We even see children, in emergency placement (generally through a judge), for whom there have been no evaluation committes meetings at all[3]. This failure can sometimes be observed in over 50% of the cases. The quality of the files that come before judges depends then on the quality of the investigation (police, forensic, psychiatrist, medico-legal experts, etc.), which itself, unfortunately, is frequently traumatic for the child, because of the way it is carried out most of the time.

2.3. The Word of the Child Is Not Proof

The word of the child, as it is actually taken into account, does not really allow for the truth to come forward either. Social workers are supposed to state facts, nothing more, and they are generally never allowed to question the children, unless the child herself first speaks. In that case, words are allowed to flow and are quoted as part of the charges. For their part, psychiatrists and psychologists rely mainly on listening and, therefore, do not ask questions.[4]

The confrontation between the victim and the accused in the police station provides dubious proof, even for adult victims. The training of police has just begun to include interviewing techniques in the interrogation of children[5]. Until recently, the questioning was often suggestive and frequently included leading questions. When adult and child confront one another in front of a judge, the child commonly retracts the accusation, although we cannot know whether it is the adult's threatening look or the falseness of the child's former allegations that has produced such a retraction.

Until recently, the French justice system had very few protocols to protect children. For example, 20% of French departments have signed agreements to limit the number of hearings, since it is known how unbearable they are for the child. Children and adolescents often go through hearings and trials alone, without the mandated presence of a social worker. There is no video recording of the child's testimony and no protective screen between the child and the adult. Nothing is done to protect the child, because many professionals have only recently been sensitised to the possibility of sexual trauma.

2.4. Fear of Reporting Cases

France has only very recently (early 1990's) been sensitised to the drama of sexual abuse and similarly, the notion of "sexual psychic trauma" has only recently begun to emerge. Even if the law is explicit and describes clearly that rape, and rape by a older relative, is a serious felony (art. 62, 226–14 of the Penal Code and art. 375 of the Civil Code), a number of psychiatrists and social workers still hesitate to bring it to the attention of the authorities, for fear of its consequences for families and the social fabric. Among the leading arguments they adduce, professional confidentiality or priviledged communications (art. 226–13 of the Penal Code and art. 375 of the Civil Code) is most common. Nevertheless, recent trials show that this is not always an acceptable argument (e.g., Trial in Le Mans, 1994), when the child is in danger. Another argument adduced by professionals is the necessity of caring for the pedophiles, who consider themselves former victims. Stated in more general terms, professionals agree that the rights of the family surpass the rights of the individual in the family, although the situation has evolved considerably in the last years.

2.5. Media Dramatisation

We must recognise that, today, it is most often the media that promote public awareness of abuse-related trauma, notably in the dramatisation created around news. In France, events such as the Affair Dutroux (Belgium) and the rumour of pedophile networks in the South of France increase public awareness. The prime-time television program "Bas les Masques" (Put Down the Masks) and information campaigns have had a direct impact on the number of cases reported through hotlines.

2.6. Trauma as Proof

The media have successfully brought about public recognition of the traumatic impact of sexual aggression. One could say that sexual trauma also has to be publicised trauma to be recognised, and that, in order for this to happen, shocking pictures are usually needed. Violence and physical traces are part of these icons. In their absence, other displays feed the media, for example, the direct testimony of a victim, visibly upset by the experience. The "visible" trauma thus becomes one of the criteria of recognising sexual mistreatment. To play a role in clinical and psychological evaluation, the trauma must be seen by the society, the public must agree upon its importance, and only then will clinicians pay attention to it. The 1996 book by Darves-Bornoz entitled "Syndromes traumatiques du viol et de l'inceste" ("Traumatic Syndromes of rape and incest") clinically establishes the syndrome and gives French clinicians helpful information on diagnosis.

3. THE RISK OF OVERDETERMINATION

While collective awareness of the trauma caused by incest or sexual mistreatment of a child is important, we nonetheless need to ask ourselves about the risk of overstating the trauma, a risk that we were able to recognise throughout discussions held during the ASI Conference.

3.1. Trauma: A Cause and an Effect

Is it sound to use the term "trauma" to represent both the behaviour and its consequences such as "sexual abuse," "psychological marks left by this event on a victim," or "identity problems/behaviour disorders"? Confusing the three makes sense in the cases where an event, such as war, proven rape, or accident has been demonstrated. But when the reality of the event is not certain, should we use such a term?

Similarly , the PTSD (Post-Traumatic Stress Disorder) diagnosis itself leads to confusion; because it does not differentiate between the cause (a traumatic event) and its effects on behaviour, such as, identity problems/ behavioural disorders.[6] This failure to differentiate means that the symptoms may either be a cause or an effect. Here a shortcut that should not be taken has been taken: inferring causes from symptoms. However, symptoms do not belong to their causes. By definition, symptom description allows the establishment of a diagnosis, but only a diagnosis, not the cause.

Thanks to this shortcut, the reasoning follows: every person who has lived through traumatic events has the symptoms of PTSD. But certain other persons have symptoms identical to those of traumatised persons. Therefore, these others also have been traumatised. This kind of reasoning by analogy is obviously questionable. After all, are there any behaviour disorders that could not plausibly be linked to a specific event?

3.2. The Recollection of Trauma

Does not the recollection itself, rather than the event, become the point of reference? Is it not because of this confusion that certain practitioners have looked for any means of uncovering a memory of the actual event, an event that has the value of a reference point in supporting the existence of the trauma, so that they can then explain the PTSD diagnosis? Through the aid of recollective processes professionals have attempted to discover this forgotten, hidden trauma. The alleged victim's subsequent remembering therefore becomes proof of existence of the original traumatic event. If a criminal charge is laid, strong pressure is automatically put on behavioural professionals to find proof, so much so that they may be under unconscious pressure to discover an event and thereby validate the trauma.

3.3. Recollection: The Metaphor of the Trauma

If the therapist uses hypnosis to assist the client act out the recollection, by suggestion (through abreactions or medically induced trances), the therapist may transform the nature of the recollection. As described above, the recollection may be in itself "the event", the metaphor of the traumatic event. In effect, if the process of recollection is accompanied by visible symptoms (tears, strong emotion, etc.), a suggested, "forced", and dramatised recollection can present itself as traumatic expression: panic attacks, D.I.D. (Dissociative Identity Disorder) symptoms, and abreaction. It is through these experiences that the recollection may become a traumatic event. If so, one could speak of the "trauma of recollection", instead of the "recollection of trauma". The event that constituted the memory is then considered by professionals as a repeat of the original trauma and has a quasi-ritual value: to (re)live the trauma confirms her or his status as victim.

3.4. True or False Allegations

If there is a suggestion and resulting false allegations, they alone could very well represent the only traumatic event. But who knows? For this reason it is very important to differentiate between "reinstated memories and recollected memories" (see Shimamura, this volume). Otherwise, the patient and therapist risk belief in false memories, merely by wanting to provoke remembered events but these may be unfounded.

The event of recollection that is dramatised/and such dramatisation favours the emergence of visible symptoms. But how does one know in this case if the recollection is real or made up? Physiological signs of psychological trauma may allow us to make such a determination (see this volume, commentary by J. Briere). But for now, psychological trauma is still the result of public and professional belief and the vocal complaints of the patient. Trauma is put on stage and it receives attention by the media: it is the result of a social process. Through no fault of patients or therapists, the history of trauma is not only a psychiatric history; it is also history of the media and political influence.

4. CONCLUSION

4.1. Trauma, an Indicator of Crime

The NATO-ASI Conference emphasised the central idea of trauma, a phenomenon that has received more media coverage in the United States than in France. We understand the relevance of trauma and PTSD to criminal justice and as a basis for explaining emotional suffering. To some extent, usage of these concepts establishes through psychological symptoms the reality of non-visible acts. How otherwise can one prove violence against a child, when there are no visible signs and when one is trying to save the child from her/his aggressors? It is difficult to prove a crime without bringing in the trauma of the victim, the psychological indication that she is a victim. Because of the acceptance of the nature of trauma, children's rights have finally been recognised.

4.2. The Risk of the Trauma of Recollection

It is difficult to show crime without also showing the emotional trauma it produces. Nonetheless, paying this price is not without a risk, notably the risk known as the trauma of recollection. If the indicators of real trauma are lost, or if the trauma never existed, it is the act of recollection that will be the traumatic event in the file, allowing charges to be brought or a program to take charge. For example, in New Zealand, among other countries, the act of remembering is recognised as sufficient reason for access to free therapeutic care.

It is important that we be understood. We have no doubts that there are subjective recollective phenomena that may be interpreted as the events themselves. However, if we dramatise these scenes of memory, we take a risk. If there is suffering, then there are certainly visible symptoms. However, the use of other techniques to arrive at proof (hypnosis, abreaction) may amplify this suffering and create distress where there was little and cause the patient to lose contact with the reality of his memory. For the victim, losing his/her reference points and no longer being aware of the difference between reality and imagination or fantasy is the worst thing that can happen in therapy. In effect, the therapeutic strategy is radically different, according to whether it is a matter of softening the pain of a person who suffers real pain or treating the root cause of mental disease trauma and its symptoms. The therapeutic contract is different; the very outcome of therapy depends on this difference. Apart from the potentially negative consequences of recollection upon the client, it is important to remember that a false accusation has serious consequences for the person and his/her family. For those assumed guilty of abuse and accused of wrongdoing, the consequences are also important; let us remember that judicial error may have serious person and family consequences.

The foregoing discussion shows that the notion of "trauma" could be meaningless when there is no evidence of the causative event. If, however, the event is proven, the notion is no longer meaningless, because one can legitimately work on the relationship between the cause and the effect. Would it not be useful to return to a description of symptoms that allows for a disassociation of the sexual assault from the intense psychological response of the victim? If we did, we might finally know what we refer to when we speak of trauma.

REFERENCES

1. *Actes du Colloque "la prise en charges des enfants victimes d'abus sexuels - l'intervention du pedopsychiatre"* - 24 octobre 1995 - Ministere de la Sante publique et de l'Assurance Maladie - Direction de l'Action sociale - D.S.F.2 Direction Generale de la Sante - ED. I.D.E.E. sous la direction de P. Kassis - Paris 1996
2. *Rapport d'Activite 1994 - SOS Enfance 92* - Direction de la Vie Sociale (Aide Sociale a l'Enfance) - Publication du Conseil General des Hauts de Seine - Nanterre - 1995
3. *Rapport d'etude - Mineurs en difficultes - Document thematique* Direction de la Vie Sociale - Schema departemental - Conseil General des Hauts de Seine - Nanterre - Fevrier 1991
4. *Guide de signalement, "Signalement judiciaire d'enfant en danger - Elements d'analyse et modalites pratiques* Direction de la Vie Sociale Conseil General des Hauts de Seine - Nanterre - Mars 1994
5. *L'audition de l'enfant : la Police Francaise a la recherche de nouvelles methodes et techniques* - Carole Mariage-Cornali - Actes des Journees d'etudes et de reflexion de l'Unite de Formation et de Recherche de la Fondation pour l'Enfance - Paris - Unesco - 2 fevrier 1996
6. *PTSD. Diagnostic and Statistical Manual of Mental Disorders.* Fourth Edition. Washington DC. American - Psychiatric Association.

39

ASI PARTICIPANTS QUESTIONNAIRE

D. Stephen Lindsay and Jonathan W. Schooler

[1]University of Wales-Bangor and University of Victoria
[2]University of Pittsburgh

Shortly before the ASI, Steve Lindsay and Jonathan Schooler threw together a questionnaire, with the aim of collecting descriptive data on participants' opinions on issues related to adults' recollections of childhood abuse. The questionnaires were distributed at the beginning of the ASI, and respondents were asked to complete and return them within the first few days of the meeting. The phrase "threw together" is used advisedly here—the questionnaire was written very quickly and consequently suffered from numerous ambiguities and belied the cognitive-psychology backgrounds of its authors. One consequence of this was that many participants chose not to return the questionnaire (total returns = 49 out of 95, for a 52% return rate) and varying numbers of respondents left particular questions unanswered. The shortcomings of the questionnaire also sparked considerable discussion both during and after the ASI, which was of value in its own right.

Despite the limitations of the questionnaire, three aspects of the results are worth reporting. The most striking aspect of the findings is the tremendous variability in responses to virtually every question. For example, respondents were asked to estimate "What percentage of clients seeking psychotherapy for common psychological problems (e.g., depression, anxiety, relationship difficulties, eating disorders, sleep disorders, etc.) suffer from after-effects of CSA (remembered or not)?" Responses ranged from 2% to 55%, with a mean of 20% and a standard deviation of 14%. Similarly, responses to a question regarding the percentage of clients seeking psychotherapy for common psychological problems who experienced childhood sexual abuse that they do not remember ranged from 0% to 90%. These disparities in opinions were not limited to a few extremists; rather, on a number of issues substantial proportions of the participants clustered on each end of the issue. For example, on a question regarding the essential accuracy of recovered memories of childhood abuse that arise outside of therapy, nearly 20% of respondents estimated that less then 10% of such memories are accurate, whereas an equal percentage estimated that more then 90% are accurate. Similarly, on a 7-point scale rating whether the processes that lead to forgetting and remembering of traumatic memories are definitely the same as (1) or definitely different from (7) those involved in non-traumatic memories, approximately 25% of the participants responded that traumatic memories were definitely the same (circling 1 or 2) whereas 35% indicated equally strong views that such memories were definitely different (circling 6 or 7).

Recollections of Trauma, edited by Read and Lindsay
Plenum Press, New York, 1997

Although there were striking disparities in the opinions of many participants on a number of the central issues regarding memory for trauma, these differences did not divide neatly between practitioners and researchers. Indeed, comparisons of respondents who self-identified primarily as researchers versus those who self-identified primarily as practitioners revealed few if any statistically reliable differences. Separate independent-groups t-tests conducted on a total of 23 items yielded only two reliable differences. Relative to practitioners, researchers indicated a larger role of "ordinary forgetting" in recovered-memory cases, $t(43) = 2.65$, $p < .02$. Similarly, compared to practitioners, researchers indicated that "self-help suggestions" play a larger role in recovered-memories cases, $t(41) = 2.43$, $p < .02$. In view of the large number of t-tests, it is possible that these two findings are Type I errors rather than real differences (the Bonferroni-adjusted alpha to obtain a p value of .05 across 23 tests is approximately .002). In any case, the point we want to emphasise is that these two subgroups did not come anywhere near to differing reliably on the vast majority of questions. For example, responses from the two subgroups were very similar on ratings of how often childhood trauma is a major cause of psychological problems in adulthood, how often it is useful to help clients work through memories of childhood trauma in general practice, how often it is appropriate for psychologists in general practice to ask clients if they experienced CSA, estimates of the percentage of people who experienced an isolated instance of extreme trauma in childhood who forget that they had that experience, or estimates of the percentage of clients seeking psychotherapy for common psychological problems who experienced CSA that they do not remember (all $ps > .23$). Responses on these and many other items covered the full range. It may be that the ambiguity of some of the questions contributed to the wide variability in responses, but we suspect that to a large extent it accurately represents the state of affairs among the ASI participants: opinions varied widely both between and within subgroups of participants.

It must be emphasised that these data should not be generalised; applicants to the ASI were not selected with an eye to obtaining representative samples of researchers and practitioners. The data may not even be representative of the ASI participants, given the disappointing return rate and the likelihood that those ASI participants who were most put off by the questionnaire were least likely to return it. It is also important to note that, although we dichotomised "researchers" and "practitioners" in the foregoing analyses, these categories may be misleading. For example, of the 29 respondents who self-identified primarily as researchers, 4 also indicated a secondary identification as practitioners; of the 19 respondents who self-identified primarily as practitioners, 9 also indicated a secondary identification as researchers. A related point is that both sub-groups of respondents were relatively diverse in other ways (e.g., practitioners included psychiatrists and psychologists with a variety of backgrounds and orientations, and researchers included anthropologists, legal scholars, etc., as well as psychological researchers).

In summary, the central message of this survey is that participants at the ASI who returned the questionnaire varied widely in their opinions on issues related to the controversy regarding recovered memories of childhood abuse. Researchers and practitioners showed at least some tendency to divide on some issues, but on very few, and no differences were statistically reliable by the Bonferroni adjustment. Despite the limitations of the questionnaire, we think that there are important grains of truth in these data: Opinions vary widely, and do not divide neatly between researchers and practitioners. Acknowledging this sets the stage for a less polarised and more constructive consideration of the issues than has been typical of the controversy surrounding recovered memories.

POSTER SESSION ABSTRACTS

SECONDARY TRAUMATISATION: A PRELIMINARY STUDY OF THERAPISTS WORKING IN THE FIELD OF TRAUMA

Marla Arvay

University of Victoria, Canada

A random sample of therapists (N=161) working in the field of trauma were surveyed to study levels of stress. Therapists were assessed on measures of general life stress, burnout, and traumatic stress. Twenty-four percent were experiencing high levels of general life stress, 16% reported high levels of emotional exhaustion, 26% felt ineffective in terms of personal accomplishment at work and 14% were experiencing high levels of traumatic stress similar to clients with post traumatic stress disorder. Relationships between measures and demographic variables were reported, a profile of traumatised therapists was identified, and implications of these findings of therapists were presented.

SATANIC RITUAL ABUSE (SRA) STORIES AS RECOVERED MEMORIES

Benjamin Beit-Hallahmi

University of Haifa, Israel

Some recovered memories include reports of abuse which are alleged to have occurred as an integral part of a secret religion that worships Satan. Transmitted across generations for hundreds of years, it demands the most gruesome deeds humans can imagine (e.g., child sacrifice), as components of its rituals. If such a secret religion exists, we will be forced to revise everything we know about human history and human behaviour. Fortunately, there is no need for such a revision. Such allegations cannot reflect reality, and the vast underground network of Satanists is just a delusion. When mental health professionals promote such allegations they demonstrate poor judgment, incompetence, or delusional thinking.

CIRCUMSTANCES AND THE PHENOMENOLOGY OF A RECOVERED MEMORY: A CORROBORATED CASE STUDY

Miriam Bendiksen

Clinical Practice, Bendiksen and Bendiksen, Norway

A case study of recovered memory of sexual abuse is presented. The recovery occurred prior to and outside the context of therapy. The original incident and the circumstances surrounding the recovery experience are corroborated. The case is presented as a time line. It includes the original incident, the interim period when the memory was not available and the recovery experience. Directed forgetting and encoding specificity are memory mechanisms that can explain the phenomenon. The distinctive and startling quality of this recovered memory is highlighted. It can be understood as emotional flooding and as an insight experience.

DIGGING UP THE PAST: HARMFUL OR HELPFUL?

Ellen Berah and Penny Brabin

Monash University, Australia

Our study focused on the common concern of ethics committees of whether reviving memories of past traumas adversely affects research subjects. At the conclusion of intensive interviews with 416 parents who had a stillborn baby some years earlier, parents reported the extent to which they found the interview (a) distressing and (b) helpful/unhelpful. Of the small proportion who found the interview distressing, nearly all reported that it was also helpful. This suggests that, in evaluating research which may evoke painful memories, ethics committees should focus on whether the experience will be positive rather than on whether it will cause distress.

DOES PANIC DISORDER RESULT FROM MEMORY DYSFUNCTION?

Oguz Berksun

University of Ankara, Turkey

Following fear-induction, 74 patients with ($n=30$) or without ($n=44$) panic disorder attempted to recall a fearful episode from their life. Whereas all but one of controls were successful in recalling such an episode, none of the panic disorder patients did so. The results suggest that one central notion of the cognitive theory of panic, the misinterpretation process (Beck et al., 1985), may be a secondary defence mechanism to the emotional-autonomic recollection. That is, an attempt is made to control recalled emotional-autonomic activity (like fear) by the misinterpretation process, but the process fails to control the autonomic-emotional activity. In short, panic attacks may result from the recollection of dissociated emotional-autonomic activity.

EXAMINING DIFFERENCES BETWEEN INVOLUNTARY AND VOLUNTARY RECOLLECTIONS

Dorthe Berntsen

University of Aarhus, Denmark

Involuntary recollections recorded in a diary study are compared to voluntary recollections, retrieved in a cue word study. The cue words matched the cues that triggered the involuntary memories. Non-specific events were less frequent among the involuntary memories. Contrary to psychoanalytic theory, the involuntary memories were rated as less rehearsed (i.e., less repetitive) and as more emotionally positive than the voluntary memories. For both types, rehearsal ratings correlated with emotional intensity, not with valence. The findings indicate that stressful, repetitive memories, as observed in PTSD, form an unusual class of everyday involuntary memories.

MEMORY OF EMOTIONAL TEXTS ABOUT AIDS: EFFECTS OF TRUTH AND OPINION VALUE

Denis Brouillet

University of Montpellier III, France

Participants who had or did not have a close relationship with someone with AIDS learned emotional sentences about AIDS. The content of these sentences had a truth value or an opinion value. Before learning they had to recall and to recognise them. Results showed that people concerned with AIDS easily recalled opinion value sentences but were less successful in the recall of truth value sentences. However, the two types of sentences were equivalent in recognition for these participants. Participants who were not concerned with AIDS recalled and recognised opinion and truth value sentences with the same success.

CHILD SEXUAL ABUSE: THE TRAUMATIC EXPERIENCE OF AMNESIC AND NON-AMNESIC SURVIVORS

Catherine Cameron

University of La Verne, USA

Three consecutive posters report a ten-year longitudinal study of 46 women who reported childhood sexual abuse (CSA) as adults. It was hypothesised that amnesics (who until recently had lived in ignorance of their trauma) would report more serious sexual abuse than non amnesics (who had always remembered it but without full recognition). Significant findings: Amnesics were more likely than non amnesics to report abuse by parents, penetration, and sexual violence. Their CSA began at a younger age and they were less likely to claim even one adult on whom they could count.

THE CRISIS OF RECALL: RECOLLECTIONS OF TRAUMA

Catherine Cameron

University of La Verne, USA

In the study described on the previous page, it was also hypothesised that amnesics would experience a more serious "crisis of recall" than non amnesics upon recognising trauma's impact on their lives. Significant findings: Amnesics were more likely to report disillusionment, horror, sexual upset, and suicidal ideation. They were also more likely to need all available support and more likely to cycle into denial of CSA. Memories (more fragmentary and sensory than for non amnesics) gradually yielded adequate recall of trauma, and harassed them less. Usually the women reported some external validation of their abuse.

RESOLVING THE TRAUMA

Catherine Cameron

University of La Verne, USA

The study described above presented questions (about respondents' self-concept, coping, health and PTSD symptoms) at two points in time: prior to confronting their past CSA and six or more years later. Each woman was compared with herself over time, and it was hypothesised that more amnesics would show less improvement. Significant findings: Both groups showed high endorsement of negative items in 1986 (a nonsignificant difference) and low endorsement in 1992 (also nonsignificant). Both showed significant recovery.

MEMORY DISTURBANCES IN THE ACUTE AFTERMATH OF DISASTERS

Etzel Cardeña, Thomas Grieger, Jeffrey Staab, Carroll Fullerton, and Robert Ursano

Uniformed Services University of the Health Sciences, USA

A reanalysis of data on the aftermath of an earthquake, an oil rig collapse, and a sky walk collapse (cf. Cardeña, Holen, McFarlane, Solomon, Wilkinson, & Spiegel, in press) showed that intrusive memories were very common (range = 39–88%), followed by difficulties with everyday memories (range = 26–44%), and amnesia for the event (range = 6–24%). Another study focused on 43 rescue workers for US Air Flight 427, which crashed near Pittsburgh. As compared with unit members not involved in the operation, rescue workers reported significantly more intrusive memories, difficulties with everyday memory, and partial amnesia ($p<.005$ for all analyses). These symptoms were, however, very infrequent.

TRAUMA, HYPERVENTILATION, AND MEMORY

Ashley V. Conway

Bowden House Clinic, England, U.K.

Hyperventilation (breathing in excess of metabolic requirements) is a normal part of the 'fight or flight' response, and is therefore likely to occur during trauma. Physiological consequences include a reduction in cortical blood flow and oxygen availability, interference with normal neuronal function, and gross disruption of electroencephalogram. Little is known about the effects of hyperventilation on memory, but it could cause disruption by interfering with encoding and/or recall, and possibly produce a state-dependent effect. Level of activity during trauma would influence carbon-dioxide levels and therefore, possibly the encoding of memories. Manipulation of breathing could influence recall of trauma.

REPRESSION AS A CONSENSUAL PHENOMENON

Hans F. M. Crombag

University of Limburg, The Netherlands

It is argued that the decisive question is not whether repression of traumatic memories is a psychological reality, but whether most people believe that it is a real phenomenon and act accordingly. If so, then repression is a social, or consensual phenomenon and as such to be reckoned with irrespective of its validity. Data are presented that belief in repression is widespread among lay people as well as mental health professionals. However, this belief is not entirely free of ambiguity, as many who readily believe that repression occurs in others, do not believe it may have happened to themselves. As the discussion about the validity of the concept, whose empirical validity is by no means established as yet, goes on, repressed memories and expert testimony on repressed memories should not be admitted as evidence in criminal cases.

CLIENTS' AND THERAPISTS' PERCEPTIONS OF THE PSYCHOTHERAPEUTIC PROCESS: A STUDY OF ADULTS ABUSED AS CHILDREN

Peter Dale

National Society for the Prevention of Cruelty to Children, East Sussex, U.K.

Fifty three interviews were undertaken with a sample which included i) adults who were abused as children, ii) therapists, and iii) therapists who were abused as children. Findings indicate that it is simplistic for adults who were abused as children to be categorised as a unitary group. Nevertheless, certain issues merit particular attention to minimise the possibility of therapy being ineffective, unhelpful, or retraumatising. Whilst the "False Memory' Societies may be seen as providing a necessary corrective to specific forms of bad therapy practice, from the evidence available such pressure groups overgeneralise their indictment against therapy as a whole.

FANTASTIC DETAILS IN THE CHILD SEXUAL ABUSE DISCLOSURE

Constance J. Dalenberg

Trauma Research Institute, California School of Professional Psychology, San Diego, USA

At present, fantastic details within the child sexual abuse disclosure leave the interviewer in a quandary regarding the appropriate future course of the interview. Using stratified samples, child abuse interviews were coded as severe/non severe abuse, and as containing/not containing fantastic detail. Contrary to the assumptions of many authors, fantastic allegations were positively related to strength of physical evidence. Further, within the "gold standard" group (confessions + medical evidence), fantastic details were associated with severity of known abuse, but not with presence of leading questions in young children.

PHYSICAL ABUSE HISTORY AND DISSOCIATION AS PREDICTORS OF INDIVIDUAL DIFFERENCES IN THE STATE-DEPENDENCY OF MEMORY

Constance J. Dalenberg, J. Cathy Duvenage, and Michael T. Coe

Trauma Research Institute, California School of Professional Psychology, San Diego, USA

The classic mood state dependency paradigm was used to study the phenomenon of dependency as an individual difference variable. Subjects experience one fear induction, 1–3 neutral mood inductions, and 1–3 sad mood inductions totalling 4 inductions for each subject. Physical abuse history was associated with fear state-dependency. Three types of dissociation -- isolation, absorption, and amnesia -- related to state dependency in divergent ways. Results were discussed in terms of the mechanism of dissociation as the mediator for production of increased or decreased state-dependency, and thus increased amnesia or hypermnesia, for abuse victims.

CONTROVERSIAL ORIGINS OF SEXUAL ABUSE ALLEGATIONS: WHAT DO PROFESSIONALS BELIEVE?

Matthew Dammeyer, Narina N. Nightingale, and Monica McKoy

University of Wyoming, USA

Professionals in the United States answered survey questions regarding repressed memory and techniques used to uncover childhood sexual abuse. The results demonstrated that, overall, professionals who are conducting research or who have obtained degrees that reflect clear empirical training are more skeptical about repressed memory or in the helpfulness of anatomical dolls in interviewing children. Conversely, these same professionals are more likely to believe that false allegations can arise from leading questions or from the therapeutic techniques used to recover memories than those whose degrees reflect less empirical training or who are not currently active in research.

A RECOVERED MEMORY OF A TRAUMATIC EVENT—A SINGLE CASE STUDY

Graham Davies and Noelle Robertson

University of Leicester and Leicester General Hospital, U.K.

Mr. B, a schoolmaster, experienced lapses of consciousness triggered by stimuli such as a sudden noise or the sight of a handgun on television. This in turn was linked to nightmares during which he referred to a shooting and a demand for money. Over the ensuing months he recovered a memory of having been held up and shot in the school office. Partial corroboration existed in the form of a contemporaneous note in his own hand and damaged clothing consistent with being hit with an air rifle pellet. The implications of this case for theories of memory and trauma are discussed.

MEMORIES OF CHILD ABUSE, ATTRIBUTIONAL STYLE, EMOTIONS, AND CHILD ABUSE POTENTIAL

Joaquín De Paúl, N. Alday, Y. Mocoroa, P. Paz, and A. Pérez de Albeniz

University of Basque Country, Spain

Despite documented pathological consequences of child abuse in adults, many abused children are asymptomatic as adults and most do not abuse their own children. The research explored adults with recollections of physical or sexual abuse the relationships between attributional style (internal vs. external), intensity of emotions, and the potential to physically or sexually abuse children. Only adults who recalled physical abuse obtained higher scores for child abuse potential than non-abused adults. Recollections of sexual abuse showed no such relationship. Compared to those with sexual abuse recollections, adults who recalled physical abuse less frequently provided external attributions, had more intense memories of anger and sadness, but less shame.

IN BITS AND PIECES: A BIOGRAPHICAL STUDY ON CHILD SEXUAL ABUSE EXPERIENCES OF FIFTEEN MALES

Sietske Dijkstra

University of Utrecht, The Netherlands

In this retrospective PhD study of fifteen males (average age 31.4) in depth-interviews well transcribed on the nature and consequences of sexual abuse, inside and outside the family. The abuse started before the age of sixteen, involved bodily contact and needed to be perceived as involuntary from the concurrent perspective. Twenty-eight perpetrators (five female) are mentioned, half of them family members. Two-thirds mention temporary states of no recall of (part of) the abuse. Memories were activated principally by triggers of similar situations. Most reported consequences: low self esteem, sexual problems, trauma-specific fears, distrust, depression, and confusion of sexual orientation.

CHILDREN REMEMBER CHILDHOOD: AUTOBIOGRAPHICAL MEMORY FROM AGE 3 THROUGH 8

Robyn Fivush and April Schwarzmueller

Emory University, USA

Adults clearly have difficulty recalling events that occurred before the age of 3 or 4, yet children this young have detailed memories of their past. To date, however, no one has investigated the developmental fate of these early memories. We assessed 8-year old children's memories of events that they had recalled in previous interviews at 40, 46, 58, and 70 months of age. Children recalled almost all of the events queried, and in as much detail as in the original interviews. Although retention interval was related to amount recalled at age 8, rehearsal was not. These results call into question current conceptualisations of "childhood amnesia" and demonstrate that memory for distinctive personally experienced events may endure from early childhood.

DISSOCIATION IN ADOLESCENT GAMBLERS

G. Ron Frisch and Richard Govoni

University of Windsor, Canada

Jacobs' (1982) "General Theory of Addictions" proposes that a common dissociative-like state is found among compulsive gamblers, alcoholics and compulsive overeaters when they are involved in their respective addictive behaviours. One of the conditions that the theory proposes in the development of the addictive pattern is a childhood and adolescence marked by "deep feelings of inadequacy, inferiority, shame, guilt, and low self-esteem, plus a pervasive sense of rejection by parents and significant others (Jacobs, 1993, p. 288)". The theory proposes that the addictive behaviour is purposefully designed as a means for the individual to enter into a dissociative-like state. The dissociated state has aspects of functional amnesia or memory blackouts although they are incomplete and even under some level of volitional control.

HOW RELIABILITY OF THE MISINFORMING PERSON AND OF REPEATED QUESTIONING VS. REPEATED SUGGESTIONS AFFECT CHILDREN'S MEMORY OF EVENTS

Camilla Gobbo, Carla Fregoni, and Luigina Pau

University of Padova, Italy

The research project investigated the effects of some variables on children's memory trace and suggestibility, concerning specific events they observed. We looked at: (a) reliability of the source of knowledge available to the misinforming person and completeness of her report; (b) centrality of the suggested information; (c) repeated questioning over time vs. repeated suggestion; (d) modality of testing, verbal vs. visual tasks. The results showed that suggestibility varies according to some of the variables considered. Repeated questioning after a one week delay improved children's recall, showing that the original trace had not been deleted. Repeated suggestion, after further delay decreased performance.

PARENTS AND OTHER RELATIVES ACCUSED OF SEXUAL ABUSE ON THE BASIS OF RECOVERED MEMORIES: A NEW ZEALAND FAMILY SURVEY

Felicity Goodyear-Smith, Tannis M. Laidlaw, and Robert G. Large

University of Auckland, New Zealand

Demographic and other characteristics were collected where an accusation of sexual abuse based on recovered memories had been made in 73 New Zealand families. Truth or falsity of individual accusations could not be established, but many allegations involved very low probability events, including memories under age 2, full penetrative rape or sodomy of a young child, objects inserted in the child's vagina or anus, sexual abuse by a mother, or satanic ritual abuse. Memories recovered during therapy should be treated with respect as part of the patient's narrative truth, but not assumed to be factually accurate without corroborative evidence.

STRATEGIES TO DEAL WITH SUGGESTIVE PRE-INTERROGATIONS IN ASSESSING THE CREDIBILITY OF CHILDREN'S TESTIMONIES

Luise Gruel

University of Bremen, Germany

Complaints of child abuse first evoked by therapists or other professionals (e.g., kindergarten teachers, social workers), which have not been spontaneously made by the children themselves, are a great problem in the practical work of expert witnesses assessing statement credibility. The main question is: Is the statement under consideration based upon a real trauma experience or based upon suggestion? First, certain conditions must be present in order to apply the method of Criteria-Based Statement Analysis. As a result, scientific credibility assessment often is not practical in specific cases. Second, the question is raised: What shall be done when the quality of a statement indicates a true memory, whereas the origin of the statement suggests a possible distortion of memory? Specific criteria are discussed that may differentiate between true and false trauma memories in such problematic cases.

FACTORS INFLUENCING BELIEF IN FALSE MEMORY AND IN ABUSE ACCUSATIONS: A STRUCTURAL EQUATION MODEL

Evan Harrington and Brian Altman

Temple University, USA

Structural equation modelling was used to assess a model explaining belief in false memory and in abuse accusations. Psychology students ($N = 62$) were tested with scales relating to authoritarianism, belief in a just world, feminism, erotophobia-erotophilia, attitudes toward sexual abuse, belief in false memory, and belief in abuse accusations. Kristiansen, Felton and Hovdestad (in press) suggest that belief in false memory is driven by authoritarianism. The model failed to provide support for this hypothesis: no factor significantly predicted belief in false memory. Belief in abuse situations was predicted by high-authoritarianism, feminism, erotophilia, and a lack of belief in a just world. High and low authoritarians estimated the prevalence of sexual abuse at identical levels. The vast majority of subjects believed that experts can discern true from false accusations.

PROFESSIONALS' ATTITUDES TOWARD CHILD ABUSE: A COMPARISON OF TWO GROUPS

Evan Harrington and Bruce Rind

Temple University, USA

Mental health professionals answered a questionnaire regarding children's typical reactions to abuse. Subjects were recruited from two conferences: a false memory conference and a conference on the treatment of abused children. The survey assessed respondents' attitudes about the resilience abused children have, confidence that abuse is causal for a client's presenting symptoms and the degree to which clinical samples may be generalised to the population. The samples did not differ on the resilience of abused children, nor on the generalizability of clinical samples. The false memory group was more skeptical that abuse can be assumed to be causative of adult client's presenting symptoms. The false memory group was older, was more male, and had taken fewer statistics classes.

THE EFFECT OF EXPERT WITNESS TESTIMONY, PLAINTIFF GENDER, AND AUTHORITARIANISM IN A MOCK CHILD SEXUAL ABUSE CASE

Evan Harrington and Bruce Rind

Temple University, USA

In an mock jury experiment consisting of a 2 (child gender) X 4 (type of expert testimony) factorial design subjects read of an ambiguous child sexual abuse allegation where the alleged victim initially refused to disclose, after repeated interviews the child lodged accusations, and later retracted them. Testimony was supplied relating to either suggestibility, the child sexual abuse accommodation syndrome (CSAAS), or both. Each testimony type biased verdicts and when presented together cancelled each other out. Suggestibility testimony did not bias jurors beliefs about the credibility of the accusation nor the credibility of the retraction, but CSAAS testimony biased both of these beliefs. Additionally, belief in the defendants guilt and right-wing authoritarianism were highly correlated.

THE PROCESS OF RECOVERING MEMORIES OF ABUSE

Daphne Hewson

Macquarie University, Australia

Grounded theory analysis of interviews with 20 women, accessed through survivor support networks, who had recovered childhood abuse memories after a period of amnesia. Most started to recover memories before starting therapy. Most did not believe memories at first, many reacting with shock or terror; six remain ambivalent in belief. Nine have used active memory recovery methods (eg. hypnosis), but only three recovered any memories this way (one of those corroborated by perpetrator confession). Seven reported periods of re-forgetting and re-remembering after earlier memory recovery (eg. as shown in past diaries). Body memories and physical signs (eg. bruising) were reported by 16.

SOURCE MONITORING AND THE MISINFORMATION EFFECT: REMEMBERING THE SOURCE OF SUGGESTED INFORMATION DOES NOT ELIMINATE FALSE MEMORIES

Philip A. Higham

University of Northern B.C., Canada

Participants viewed a videotape of a simulated armed robbery, were asked misleading questions about it, and later were tested for their memory of its contents. A "know" response category was included on the memory test, to remove guesses regarding the source of objects, and to ensure that misattributions to incorrect sources were caused by false recollection. The results indicated that, at short questions-test delay, even though participants recollected suggested items from the questions, they falsely believed they also occurred in the video. However, at long delay, participants more often falsely believed that suggested items occurred only in the video.

PERCEPTUAL FLUENCY CAN PRODUCE FALSE RECOLLECTIONS

Philip A. Higham and Robert M. Cochrane

University of Northern B.C., Canada

Participants memorised a list of words, subsequently attempted to identify brief displays of old and new words (which were displayed individually for variable durations), and then made a memory judgment on each clearly presented item after trying to identify it. In Experiment 1, the memory judgment was an "old/new" decision followed by a "remember/know" judgment if the item was rated "old". In Experiment 2, the memory judgment involved separate "recollection" and "familiarity" ratings on Likert scales with no overt "old/new" judgment. In both experiments, participants were more likely to indicate that test items displayed for longer durations were recollected.

MEMORY LOSS FOR CHILDHOOD SEXUAL ABUSE: DISTINGUISHING BETWEEN ENCODING AND RETRIEVAL FACTORS

Elaine Hunter

Royal Holloway, University of London, U.K.

Memory loss for childhood sexual abuse is frequently attributed solely to deficits in retrieval processes. This poster describes the findings from interviews with 16 female patients who were asked about three factors which could affect memory encoding at the time of the abuse: emotional arousal, level of understanding and dissociative reactions. A majority of women reported deficits in all three factors. Lack of understanding was found to be significantly correlated to later periods of forgetting, suggesting an inability to locate the abuse within existing cognitive schemata. These findings illustrate the need to investigate encoding, as well as, retrieval deficits in traumatic memory loss.

MEMORY FOR THE ONSET OF FEAR AND PHOBIA

Ira E. Hyman, Jr., Ron Kleinknecht, E. Kheriaty, and P. Solomon

Western Washington University, USA

College students recalled the onset of their fears and phobias using either a leading questionnaire (Phobia Origins Questionnaire--POQ) or less leading interview (Phobia Origins Structured Interview--POSI). Significantly more individuals provided original experiences in response to the POQ than the POSI. The parents, however, verified significantly fewer of the experiences obtained using the POQ than the POSI, indicating that although the POQ resulted in more information being obtained, that information is less reliable. We concluded that several experiences may contribute to fear development but people may only remember a few as part of their narrative. In the second study, we surveyed students about positive and negative experiences associated with possible fear objects. Trauma with the stimulus did not by itself predict fear. Instead, it appears that trauma and other negative experiences without any positive experiences predicts the development of fear.

MANIPULATING JUDGMENTS OF WHETHER AN EVENT IS REMEMBERED: THE ROLE OF REALITY MONITORING IN FALSE MEMORY ACCEPTANCE

Ira E. Hyman Jr., L.L. Gilstrap, K. Decker, C. Wilkinson, and M. Brennan.

Western Washington University and Cornell University, USA

The creation of a false autobiographical memory involves at least three processes: the acceptance that an event could have occurred, the construction of a memory, and the reality monitoring error of coming to believe that the event is personally remembered. College participants described one of three types of childhood experiences: remembered, known but not remembered, and unsure whether remembered or known. In Experiments 1 through 3 some participants formed a mental image of the event while control participants did not. Those individuals who formed mental images of events they originally claimed to only have known and not personally remembered rated their knowledge of the events as being closer to something remembered than did those who did not form images. In Experiments 4 and 5, we found evidence that reality monitoring plays a critical role in remember versus know judgments for autobiographical memories. The information to which individuals attend can influence their claims about whether or not they personally remember an event.

CHILDREN'S SUGGESTIBILITY: THE EFFECT OF MISINFORMATION VS. INCONSISTENT INFORMATION

Kerry Lee

Macquarie University, Australia

To examine the extent to which the misinformation effect is caused by misinformation acceptance, twenty-eight 7 year-olds were exposed to either misinformation (i.e., misleading instructions and inconsistent information) or inconsistent information once or thrice. Children exposed to misinformation once remembered significantly more about the target event; no differences were found between those who were exposed to either type of information thrice. These findings are believed to be caused by two processes. When children were initially exposed to misinformation, they were affected by a facilitative process that improved their performance. Subsequent exposure to misinformation resulted in a detrimental process that attenuated this facilitative effect.

SYMPTOM PATTERNS OF PATIENTS WITH RECOVERED AND CONTINUOUS MEMORIES OF CHILD SEXUAL ABUSE

Colleen Masters and Constance J. Dalenberg

Trauma Research Institute, California School of Professional Psychology, San Diego, USA

Therapists referred one sexually abused and one non abused patient to participate in this research. A profile was developed which maximally distinguished the two groups using measures of depression, anxiety, dissociation, and post-traumatic symptoms. Next, patients with recovered and continuous memories of abuse were compared. In general, recovered memory patients were more symptomatic, particularly on those measures which related most highly to the overall dissociation factor. The largest differences were noted on those measures of dissociation which were least obviously associated (had low face validity, although strong predictive validity) with abuse history.

THE QUALITY OF FALSE MEMORIES

Giuliana Mazzoni

University of Florence, Italy

A high rate of false memories for personal dream words (Dream-self) was obtained with a modified misinformation procedure (Mazzoni & Loftus, 1995). Dream-self words were mistaken for words seen in a previously presented list. In addition, Dream-self words had a special "Remember" quality (Gardiner, 1988; Tulving, 1985). An additional experiment on dream sentences has confirmed that false memories of Dream-self items have a special quality. Dream-self false memories cannot be distinguished from original memories in that they have the same "recollective" quality of true memories. These findings have important implications for the evaluation of recovered memories of traumatic events.

APPLES AND ORANGES: MEMORY OF TRAUMA. ISSUES AND QUESTIONS FOR CLINICAL PSYCHOLOGY AND RESEARCH

Judith McDougall

Victoria University of Wellington, New Zealand

The difficulties of the scientist/practitioner model of clinical practice are identified. The credibility of clinical practice - who decides? The efficacy, validity and reliability of methods of intervention - are research laboratory methods appropriate? The paucity of relevant clinical research - should clinicians take more responsibility for initiating research? Do researchers have a social responsibility to address questions of public interest as well as following their own interests? Standards of truth - are different levels of evidence necessary/acceptable? The assumptions of science and the assumptions of clinical practice - are they compatible? Are we trying to understand apples by studying oranges?

JUROR PERCEPTIONS OF RECOVERED MEMORIES: DOES PRIOR KNOWLEDGE INFLUENCE DECISION MAKING?

Amina Memon, Gill Wedge, and Rachel Beese

University of Texas at Dallas, USA and University of Southampton, U.K.

The effects of providing an *amicus* brief (pretrial information) on mock jurors' reactions to a case summary involving a hypnotically elicited recovered memory for childhood sexual abuse was examined. The pretrial information summarised scientific evidence surrounding the likely validity of hypnotically recovered memories. The latter resulted in significantly fewer guilty verdicts. Males showed greater leniency towards the accused than females with fewer guilty verdicts and lower believability ratings. Participants tended to deliver fewer guilty verdicts with increased age and mock jurors who came from "professional" backgrounds showed greater skepticism in evaluating the victim's testimony.

MISLEADING METAPHORS: ASSUMPTIONS OF STUDENTS AND PSYCHOTHERAPISTS ABOUT MEMORY

Harald Merckelbach and Ineke Wessel

Limburg University, The Netherlands

One position taken in the debate about the phenomenon of 'recovered memories' is that recovered memories reflect veridical traumatic events that were previously repressed. Other researchers argue that recovered memories are false memories, suggested by therapists. They emphasise that dubious assumptions about memory may contribute to the development of such false memories. The assumptions about memory were explored in a Dutch sample. Twenty-seven psychotherapists and 50 undergraduate students completed a questionnaire about memory and repression. A large proportion of the subjects held problematic assumptions about the workings of memory. Though most said that memory is not an accurate reflection of reality, metaphors provided by the subjects suggest that the reconstructive nature of memory was less well acknowledged. These findings may have implications for psychotherapy.

THE ACCURACY OF AUTOBIOGRAPHICAL MEMORY: A REPLICATION OF BARCLAY & WELLMAN (1986)

Harald Merckelbach, Ineke Wessel, and Robert Horselenberg

Limburg University, The Netherlands

Ten volunteers kept written records of self-selected, daily events for a one-week period. After 4 months, they were given a surprise recognition test. This test consisted of original memories and several types of foils. In line with the previous findings of Barclay and Wellman, it was found that acceptance of foils as one's own memories is a relatively common phenomenon. This suggests that pseudo memories may also occur in the absence of suggestions and repeated interviews and, more generally, that autobiographical memory is intrinsically unreliable.

INDIVIDUAL DIFFERENCES IN THE RECOLLECTION OF EMOTIONAL EXPERIENCES: THE CASE FOR ALEXITHYMIA

Marie-Pascale Noël and Bernard Rimé

Catholic University of Louvain, Belgium

Subjects scoring low vs. high on an alexithymia scale (i.e., measuring the ability to recognise and describe one's feelings) were compared in a situation of recollection of a strong emotional experience. Compared with the low alexithymic, the high alexithymic evaluated their emotion as less intense, they provided shorter descriptions of the factual and emotional aspects of the event, reported less often bodily sensations and feelings but yet judged their recollections as more painful. They also reported to have disclosed the event less often and with a longer delay elapsed between the event and the first disclosure.

VARICEAL HEMORRHAGE AND POST-TRAUMATIC STRESS DISORDER

Ronan E. O'Carroll, G. Masterton, R. Gooday, and P.C. Hayes

University of Sterling, Scotland, U.K.

It is claimed that PTSD may be common following traumatic medical events. We tested the hypothesis that PTSD would be prevalent in patients with liver disease who had experienced a major variceal haemorrhage. We recruited 24 patients with chronic liver disease who had survived variceal haemorrhage of more than 4 units of blood. All were fully conscious at the time and had full recall of the bleed, and were assessed on average 2 years following the bleed. None of the patients met DSM-III-R criteria for PTSD. The implications of the present findings are discussed.

ATTENTION, CONCENTRATION, MEMORY, AND EXECUTIVE FUNCTIONS AFTER PROLONGED TRAUMATIC EXPERIENCE

Oget Oktem-Tanör

University of Istanbul, Turkey

Research with people exposed to prolonged and extraordinary trauma have documented cognitive dysfunctions. A previous study presented 6 cases who showed deficits of attention and registration. I concluded that their memory problem lay in the initial phase of acquisition; that is, they failed to acquire the information due to their impaired attentional faculties; otherwise their memory processes such as retention and retrieval were intact. It is worthwhile to investigate whether this attentional failure is part of the executive functional system and accompanied by other executive dysfunctions or if it is simply an impairment of immediate memory. To investigate this point the following tests were used: WMS-R sub tests, Verbal Memory Processes test; Stroop test, Fluency tests, some Luria tests, and the WCST.

CHILDREN'S MEMORY FOR THE HURRICANE: A CONTENT ANALYSIS

Janat Parker, Lorraine Bahrick, Brenda Lundy, Robyn Fivush and Mary Levitt

Florida International University and Emory University, USA

One hundred 3- and 4-year-old children recalled events surrounding Hurricane Andrew. The stress experienced as a result of the storm was defined as low, moderate, or severe according to the severity of the child's storm exposure. The structured interview assessed memory for pre-hurricane preparations, the hurricane itself, and the post-hurricane recovery period. A detailed analysis was made of 1) spontaneous versus cued recall, 2) recall of actions, descriptions, and emotions, and 3) elaborations. Analyses of the total number of propositions showed that 4-year-olds recalled more than 3-year-olds and that a quadratic function related amount recalled and severity level. The curvilinear function of stress and recall was evident in the overall recall and in the spontaneous recall; it was not as robust for the cued recall. Older children showed more elaborated recall than young children but the number of elaborations recalled was not related to the severity level of the storm. These results highlight the curvilinear relationship between stress and amount of recall regardless of the particular content of memory.

HOW MUCH DO CHILDREN REMEMBER ABOUT TRAUMATIC PERSONAL INJURY?

Carole Peterson

Memorial University of Newfoundland, Canada

Children (2–13 years) who suffered trauma injuries necessitating hospital emergency room treatment served as subjects. They were interviewed a week and 6 months later about both injury and hospital treatment. Adult witnesses corroborated the children's information. All children provided considerable information, although increasingly with age, and made few errors. Details were classified into 3 categories: central, peripheral-inside the emotional events, or peripheral-outside those events. All categories were distinct, with recall differing depending upon detail category. The degree of distress experienced at injury or hospital had surprisingly little effect on the amount or accuracy of information recalled.

EFFECTS OF PARENTAL SUGGESTIONS, INTERVIEWING TECHNIQUES, AND AGE ON YOUNG CHILDREN'S EVENT REPORTS

Debra A. Poole & D. Stephen Lindsay

Central Michigan University, USA and University of Wales, Wales, U.K.

Immediately after participating in activities with "Mr. Science," 2–8-old (N=114) children answered non suggestive questions about their experiences. Parents later read them a story that contained accurate and inaccurate information about this visit. Subsequently, the children answered non leading, leading and source-monitoring questions on two occasions, approximately 1 day and 1 month after exposure to misinformation. The children made erroneous reports following misleading suggestions (e.g., 58 descriptions of suggested events in free recall during Interview 2). Age trends were influenced by the types of questions, the timing of the interviews, and whether the suggested events did or did not involve bodily touch.

WAS ANNA O.'S BLACK SNAKE HALLUCINATION A SLEEP PARALYSIS NIGHTMARE?

Russell A. Powell and Tore A. Nielsen

Grant MacEwan Community College and Sleep Disorder Centre Montreal, Canada

The final traumatic event recalled by Anna O. during her cathartic treatment with Joesef Breuer was a terrifying hallucination she once had of a black snake attacking her sick father. We argue that this episode -- during which Anna O.'s arm was reportedly "asleep" due to limb occlusion -- was actually a sleep paralysis nightmare (SPN). We further argue that, contrary to recent speculation, SPNs are probably not reliable indicators of a history of sexual abuse. Therapists should also be aware that some reports of sexual assault may be hypnagogic hallucinations associated with narcolepsy, a condition which usually goes undiagnosed.

COGNITIVE ENCODING AND COGNITIVE INTERVIEWING IN EYEWITNESS RECALL.

Jacques Py, Magali Ginet, and Natascha Rainis

Université Pierre Mendez, France

Participants viewed an emotion-arousing film following instructions to encode the film according to either standard memory procedures or to a "cognitive" method of encoding inspired by Fisher and Geiselman's cognitive interview technique (i.e., pay attention to context, to as many details as possible, and consider different observational perspectives). One week later, the two groups recalled the film events within their standard or cognitive interview procedures. Cognitive encoding and cognitive interviewing independently enhanced recall; however, the beneficial effects of cognitive encoding upon recall performance were considerably larger than those of the cognitive interview.

EFFECTS OF EXTERNAL (ENVIRONMENTAL) AND INTERNAL (EMOTIONAL) CONTEXTS ON RECOGNITION OF UNFAMILIAR FACES

Natascha Rainis

Université Pierre Mendez, France

Investigations of the effects of emotion upon eyewitness memory have generally suggested a negative relationship between the two, but results have been inconsistent. Our participants memorised photos of unfamiliar faces presented within either negative, positive, or neutral contexts. One week later, subjects discriminated old from new faces. On the recognition test, faces were presented with either an old context, a new semantically related context, a new unrelated context, or no context. As predicted, negative emotional contexts reduced correct face recognition performance (hits) compared to the positive and neutral conditions. However, presentation of a face in a semantically related context moderated the effects of negative emotion on eyewitness memory.

HOW QUESTION FORM AND BODY-PARTS DIAGRAMS CAN AFFECT THE CONTENT OF YOUNG CHILDREN'S DISCLOSURES

Jane Rawls

Private Practice, Hamilton, New Zealand

Thirty 5-year-old children individually interacted in a "dress-up" game with a male research assistant at their school and were sometimes asked to keep secret parts of that physical interaction. Each child was interviewed four times about those events 1 and 2 weeks later. Combined, these four interviews followed the format used in legal "evidential" interviews, and comprised either a) open-ended questions only; b) closed questions only; c) both open and closed questions. Analyses of the videotaped interviews included: the types of questions and props (body-part diagrams) used by the interviewer; and each child's percentage of accurate reporting on who did what to whom (how, where, when, and in what sequence), the amount and type of fantasy they described, and the number and types of "secrets" they disclosed. Videotaped interviews were viewed by a panel of six professionals (lawyers, psychologists or evidential interviewers, police). The professionals gave their opinion on the acceptability and legal admissibility of the interviews, and the believability of children's reports in relation to the law.

RETROSPECTIVE MEMORY OF TRAUMATIC EVENTS IN UNIVERSITY STUDENTS: PARAMETERS OF RECALL AND CURRENT SYMPTOMATOLOGY

Martha L. Rogers, Caleb Ho, Jody Ward, and Eric Nelson

Rosemead School of Psychology and Biola University, USA

This study investigated the relationship between the nature and extent of traumatic events and dissociative or PTSD symptomatology as well as parameters of recall. University students ($N = 217$) were surveyed regarding past personal history of traumatic events and current symptomatology utilising several standardised instruments. Subjects were classified into five groups based on their characterisation of their memory of their most traumatic event memory: (1) always remembered fully and had talked about it (45%), (2) always remembered fully and had not talked about it (26%), (3) always remembered the event, did not talk about it and lost memory of significant details (15%), (4) event always remembered, did talk about the event, but lost memory of significant details (7%), and (5) event not always remembered--forgotten entirely for a time (1.8%). Parameters of retrospective traumatic memory reports, past trauma histories, selective aspects of autobiographic memories, current PTSD and dissociative symptomatology of these four groups are compared quantitatively and qualitatively.

DEPRESSED MOOD, LEVEL OF PROCESSING AND IMPLICIT AND EXPLICIT MEMORY FOR EMOTIONAL WORDS

José A. Ruiz-Caballero

Universidad Nacional de Education a Distancia, Spain

A central theory of Bower's (1981) network theory of affect is that mood leads directly to mood-congruence effects. We assessed the presence of a bias for negative information in explicit memory (free-recall) and implicit memory (word-stem completion) tasks among sub clinically depressed Ss compared to non depressed Ss, using the typical levels of processing manipulation. The results showed a mood-congruent bias for both implicit and explicit memory. As expected, the depressed Ss recalled significantly more negative words than positive words. Similarly, for the depressed Ss, the priming effect was larger for mood-congruent words than for mood-incongruent words. Emotionally congruent information was more accessible and recoverable than emotionally incongruent information in both depressed and non depressed Ss. The theoretical implications of these findings for implicit and explicit memory biases associated with depressed mood are discussed.

REMEMBRANCE OF THINGS PAST: THE RECONSTRUCTION OF TRANSSEXUALS' MEMORIES IN AUTOBIOGRAPHICAL MEMORIES

Marilyn Safir

University of Haifa, Israel

Transsexuals' (TSs) retrospective clinical and autobiographical reports reveal they "knew" by age two/three that a terrible mistake had occurred. Their psychological gender mismatched their biological sex. These accounts are discordant with those of two or three-year olds. Tully (1992) suggests TSs learn of and employ gender dysphoric explanations to understand their developmental histories in late adolescence. They restructure childhood memories to fit this new framework. Grimm (1987) reported that many subjects, following reading and discussions with other TSs, fabricate a history to fit medical criteria for approval for Sex Reassignment Surgery. Similarities in TSs' and abuse survivors narratives of childhood memories are noted and contrasted with those of young children.

SHOULD I BELIEVE THIS? REALITY MONITORING OF INVENTED AND SELF-EXPERIENCED EVENTS FROM EARLY AND LATE TEENAGE YEARS

Siegfried Sporer and Susan C. Hamilton

University of Aberdeen, Scotland, U.K.

According to the reality monitoring approach, memories of internally imagined and externally experienced events differ systematically. Can these differences also be found in accounts of self-experienced vs. invented highly complex autobiographical events, and can these differences be reliably detected by judges? In a 2 x 2 factorial design truthfulness (invented vs. self-experienced) and life period (under 15 vs. over 15) were varied. 240 adults (160 females, 80 males wrote either an account about a self-experienced or an invented personally significant experience. Subsequently, they rated first their own account with the Self-rating Memory Characteristic Questionnaire and another randomly assigned account with the Judged Memory Characteristic Questionnaire. For all of the scales, self-ratings were much higher than ratings by an external judge, and the independent variables had much stronger effects on self-ratings than on ratings by external judges. For self-ratings, there were multivariate main effects for truth status and life period. For ratings by external judges only differences between invented and self-experienced events emerged.

DO CHILDREN RESPOND ACCURATELY TO FORCED CHOICE QUESTIONS: YES OR NO?

Nancy E. Walker, S. M. Lunnig, and J.L. Eilts

Creighton University, USA

One format employed by those who interview children following traumatic events is the forced choice question. Recently, researchers have questioned the utility and accuracy of that question form, and some have suggested that forced choice questions be eliminated from interviews of children. The purpose of this study was twofold: (a) To assess developmental trends in children's responses to forced choice questions, and (b) to assess the impact of training on children's use of "I don't know" responses to forced choice questions. Sixty-one kindergarten, second, and fifth grade children participated in this 2 (gender) x 2 (condition) x 3 (grade) study. We found a developmental trend in children's ability to respond accurately to forced choice questions about a brief videotaped incident, as well as a significant tendency for children to select the more recently heard forced choice option. "Don't know" training partially ameliorated this effect. Legal and practical implications of these findings are discussed.

WHAT MISINFORMATION FINDINGS CAN TELL US ABOUT THE RECOVERED MEMORY DEBATE

Daniel B. Wright

University of Bristol, U.K.

Over the past 20 years, psychologists have asked people to watch videos and slide sequences of various crimes and then misinformed them about some details. People often report the misinformation. The misinformation research was originally done in the context of eyewitness testimony, not recovered memories. The misinformation research, and particularly the recent laboratory findings where entire events are created, does provide a mechanism to help explain why some recovered memories are false, but does not address whether some recovered memories are accurate. Further, more research is necessary using events/situations that are better analogs for the recovered memory situations.

IMAGERY AND FALSE MEMORY CREATION

Maria S. Zaragoza, Karen J. Mitchell, and Sarah Drivdahl

Kent State University, USA

Recent studies from our laboratory (Zaragoza & Mitchell, 1996; Mitchell & Zaragoza, 1996) have established that repeated exposure to suggestion can increase false memory for suggested events. The present study tested the hypothesis that visual imagery, especially if repeated, promotes the development of false memory for suggested events. A second goal was to assess the relative roles of visual imagery versus other sorts of reflective processing in the development of false memories. The results showed that, although visual imagery facilitated false memory induction, repeatedly reflecting on the meaning and implication of suggested events was more conducive to false memory creation.

PARTICIPANTS

Dr. Gwen Adshead
Broadmoor Hospital
Crowthorne Berkshire
RG45 7EG UK

Dr. Bernice Andrews
Department of Psychology
Royal Holloway, University of London
Egham, Surrey
TW20 0EX UK
uhjt054@vms.rhbnc.ac.uk

Ms. Marla Arvay
c/o Arvay Finlay
4th Floor, 888 Fort Street
Victoria, BC V8W 1H8, CANADA
marvay@horizon.bc.ca

Dr.Cahide Aydin
Ege Universitesi
Tip Fakultesi
Piskiyatri Klinigi
35100 Bornova-Izmir, TURKEY
aydin@psikiyatri.ege.edu.tr

Dr. Benjamin Beit-Hallahmi
Department of Psychology
University of Haifa
Haifa 31905, ISRAEL
rsps707@uvm.haifa.ac.il

Dr. Miriam S. Bendiksen
Bendiksen & Bendiksen
Virikveien 17
3212 Sandefjord
NORWAY

Dr. Ellen Berah
Dept of Psychological Medicine
Monash University
Clayton, Victoria 3168
AUSTRALIA
ellen.berah@med.monash.edu.au

Dr. Oguz Berksun
Ankara University
Tip Fakultesi
Psykiatri Bolumu
Dikimevi, Ankara
TURKEY

Dr. Lucy Berliner
Harborview Sexual Assault Centre
325 9 Avenue
Seattle, WA 98104
USA
lucyb@u.washington.edu

Dr. Dorthe Berntsen
Institute of Psychology
University of Aarhus
Asylvej 4, 8240 Risskov
DENMARK
dorthe@psy.aau.dk

Dr. William Brewer
Department of Psychology
University of Illinois
603 E. Daniel St.
Champaign, IL 61820
USA
wbrewer@s.psych.uiuc.edu

Dr. Chris Brewin
Cognition, Emotion, and Trauma Unit
Department of Psychology
Royal Holloway, University of London
Egham, Surrey TW20 0EX, UK
c.brewin@rhbnc.ac.uk

Dr. John Briere
Psychiatry and Behavioral Sciences
USC School of Medicine
1937 Hospital Place
Los Angeles, CA 90003-1071, USA
jbriere@hsc.usc.edu

Dr. Juliet Broadmore
Wellington Family Planning Clinics
24 Reading St.
Karori, Wellington 5
NEW ZEALAND
julietb@netlink.co.nz

Dr. Denis Brouillet
Psychologie Cognitive
Universite Montpellier III
BP 5043
34032 Montpellier Cedex
FRANCE
brouille@bred.univ-montp3.fr

Dr. Kevin Browne
School of Psychology
University of Birmingham
Birmingham B15 2TT, UK
brownek@psychol.bham.ac.uk

Dr. Maggie Bruck
Department of Psychology
1205 Dr. Penfield
McGill University
Montreal, PQ H3A 1B1
CANADA
bruck@hebb.psych.mcgill.ca

Dr. Catherine Cameron
Organizational, Behavioral Sciences
Claremont Graduate School
123 E. Eighth Street
Claremont, CA 91711-3955
USA

Dr. Etzel Cardeña
Department of Psychiatry
USUHS
4301 Jones Bridge RD
Bethesda, MD 20814
USA
cardena@usuhsb.usuhs.mil

Dr. Eve B. Carlson
Department of Psychology
Beloit College
700 College Street
Beloit, WI 53511
USA
carlsone@idcnet.com

Dr. Ashley V. Conway
Bowden House Clinic
London Road
Harrow On The Hill
Middlesex, England HA1 3JL, UK

Dr. Christine Courtois
Three Washington Circle
Suite 206
Washington, DC 20037, USA
ccourtois@aol.com

Dr. Mark Creamer
National Centre for PTSD
Austin & Repatriation Medical Centre
Locked Bag 1, West Heidelberg
Victoria 3081
AUSTRALIA
m.creamer@psych.unimelb.edu.au

Dr. Hans Crombag
Faculty of Law
University of Limburg
P.O. Box 616, 6200 MD
Maastricht
THE NETHERLANDS
hans.crombag@metajur.rulimburg.nl

Dr. Peter Dale
NSPCC East Sussex
2, Sedlescombe Road South
St Leonards on Sea, East Sussex
England TN38 OTA, UK

Dr. Constance Dalenberg
CSPP-SD
6160 Cornerstone Ct. East
San Diego, CA 92121
USA
cdalenberg@mail.cspp.edu

Dr. Graham Davies
Department of Psychology
University of Leicester
Leicester LE1 7RH, UK
gmd@leicester.ac.uk

Dr. Joaquín de Paúl
Department of Psychology
University of the Basque Country
P.O. Box 1249
20080 San Sebastian
SPAIN
ptpdeock@sc.ehu.es

Dr. Sietske Dijkstra
Department of Women's Studies
University of Utrecht
THE NETHERLANDS
sdijkstr@fsw-extern.fsw.ruu.nl

Dr. Denis Donovan
The Children's Centre for Developmental
  Psychiatry
6675 -13 Ave N, Suite 2-A
St. Petersburg, FL 33710-5483
USA
dmdonvan@ix.netcom.com

Dr. Eric Eich
Department of Psychology
University of BC
2136 West Mall
Vancouver, BC V6T 1Y7
CANADA
ee@cortex.psych.ubc.ca

Dr. Diana M. Elliott
UCLA School of Medicine
Harbor–UCLA Medical Center
1000 West Carson Street
Torrance, CA 90509
USA

Dr. Spencer Eth
Department of Veterans Affairs
Medical Center, West Los Angeles
11301 Wilshire Boulevard
Los Angeles, CA 90073
USA
eth.spencer@forum.va.gov

Dr. Robyn Fivush
Department of Psychology
Emory University
Atlanta, GA 30322
USA
fivush@fs1.psy.emory.edu

Dr. Jette Fog
Institute of Psychology
Aarhus University
Asylvej 4, 8240 Risskov
DENMARK
jettef@psy.aau.dk

Dr. Ron Frisch
Psychology Department
University of Windsor
Windsor, ON N9B 3P4
CANADA
frisch@server.uwindsor.ca

Ms. Magalie Ginet, D.E.A.
Psychologie Sociale de Grenoble
Université Pierre Mendes France
47 38040 Grenoble CEDEX 9
FRANCE

Dr. Camilla Gobbo
Dipt. di Psicologia
Universita' Delgli Studi di Padova
via Venezia 8 - 35131
Padova
ITALY
gobbo@psico.unipd.it

Dr. Felicity Goodyear-Smith
Auckland Univ. Medical School
380 Wright Road RD2 Albany
Auckland
NEW ZEALAND
f.goodyear-smith@auckland.ac.nz

Dr. Luise Greuel
Institute Psychology & Cognition
Universitat Bremen
IPK, Postfach 33 04 40
28334 Bremen
GERMANY

Ms. Frances Grunberg
2028 West 36th Avenue
Vancouver, B.C., V6M 1K9
CANADA

Ms. Petra Haenert
Diplom-Psychologin
Homannstr. 17
24106 Kiel
GERMANY

Dr. Inge Fabricius Hansen
A.F. Beyers Vej 23 St. th.
2720 Vanlose
Copenhagen, DENMARK

Dr. Evan Harrington
Department of Psychology
Temple University
Weiss Hall
Philadelphia, PA 19103, USA
evan-h@vm.temple.edu

Dr. Daphne Hewson
Department of Psychology
Macquarie University
NSW 2109, AUSTRALIA
dhewson@bunyip.bhs.mq.edu.au

Dr. Phillip Higham
Department of Psychology
UNBC, 333 University Way
Prince George, BC V2N 4Z9
CANADA
highamp@unbc.edu

Ms. Elaine Hunter
Department of Psychology
University of London
Department of Psychology
Egham, Surrey TW20 0EX, UK
e.hunter@rhbnc.ac.uk

Dr. Ira E. Hyman, Jr.
Psychology Department
Western Washington University
Bellingham, Washington 98225, USA
hyman@henson.cc.wwu.edu

Dr. Michael Kenny
Sociology & Anthropology
Simon Fraser University
Burnaby, BC V5A 1S6
CANADA
michael_kenny@sfu.ca

Dr. Michael Kopelman
Division of Psychiatry and Psychology
United Medical and Dental Schools of
   Guy's and St Thomas's
St Thomas's Hospital
Lambeth Palace Road
London SE1 7EH, UK

Dr. Kerry Lee
Department of Psychology
Humanities and Social Sciences
Bond University
Gold Coast, QLD 4229
AUSTRALIA
klee@pcmail.bond.edu.au

Dr. Ingrid Lindegren
Legal Psychologist
Gronviksvagen 52
S-161 40 Stockholm
SWEDEN

Dr. D. Stephen Lindsay
Department of Psychology
University of Victoria
P.O. Box 3050
Victoria, B.C., V8W 3P5
lindsay@uvic.ca

Dr. Elizabeth F. Loftus
Department of Psychology
University of Washington
Box 351525
Seattle, WA 98195-1525
USA
eloftus@u.washington.edu

Dr. Steven J. Lynn
Department of Psychology
State University of New York at Binhamton
Binghamton, N.Y., 13902, USA
slynn@binghamton.edu

Ms. Peggy Mahoney
Child Abuse Prevention and Counseling
  Society of Greater Victoria
730 Quadra Street
Victoria, BC V8V 4Z5, CANADA

Dr. Giuliana Mazzoni
Dipartimento di Psicologia
Via S. Niccolo', 89/a
50125 Firenze
ITALY
gium@cesit1.unifi.it

Dr. Judith McDougall
Psychology Department
Victoria University of Wellington
P.O. Box 600 Wellington
NEW ZEALAND
judith.mcdougall@vuw.ac.nz

Dr. Amina Memon
Psychology Program
University of Texas at Dallas
P.O. Box 830688, GR41
Richard, TX 75083-0688
USA
amemon@utdallas.edu

Dr. Harald Merckelbach
Department of Experimental Abnormal
  Psychology
Limburg University
P.O. Box 616, 6200 MD
Maastricht
THE NETHERLANDS
h.merckelbach@dep.rulimburg.nl

Ms. Sherrill Mulhern, D.E.A.
Laboratoire de Rumeurs
92 rue Perronet
92200, Neuilly sur Seine
FRANCE
smulhern@pasteur.fr

Dr. Israel Nachson
Department of Criminology
Bar-Ilan University
Ramat Gan 52900
ISRAEL

Dr. Tara Ney
Island Psychological Services
Health Care Consultants
Ste. 214-2187 Oak Bay Ave.
Victoria, BC V8R 1G1
CANADA
gkblank@uvic.ca

Dr. Narina N. Nightingale
Department of Psychology
University of Wyoming
Laramie, WY 82071
USA
narina@uwyo.edu

Dr. Marie-Pascale Noël
NECO Faculte de Psychologie
10, place du Cardinal Mercier
1348 Louvain la Neuve
BELGIUM
noel@neco.ucl.ac.be

Dr. Ronan O'Carroll
Senior Research Fellow
Department of Psychology
University of Stirling
Stirling, Scotland FK9 4LA
UK
reo1@stir.ac.uk

Dr. Oget Oktem-Tanör
Istanbul Medical Faculty
Department of Neurology
34390 CAPA - Istanbul
TURKEY

Dr. Janat Parker
Department of Psychology
Florida International University
Miami, FL 33199
USA
parkerjf@servax.fiu.edu

Dr. Carole Peterson
Department of Psychology
Memorial University
St. John's, Newfoundland A1B 3X9
CANADA
carole@play.psych.mun.ca

Dr. Margaret-Ellen Pipe
Department of Psychology
University of Otago
Dunedin
NEW ZEALAND
mepipe@psy.otago.ac.nz

Dr. Debra Poole
Department of Psychology
Central Michigan University
Mt. Pleasant, MI 48859
USA
debra.a.poole@cmich.edu

Dr. Russell A. Powell
Department of Social Sciences
Grant MacEwan Community College
P.O. Box 1796
Edmonton, AB T5J 2P2
CANADA
powellr@admin.gmcc.ab.ca

Dr. Jacques Py
Psychologie Sociale de Grenoble
Université Pierre Mendez France
4738040 Grenoble CEDEX 9
FRANCE
py@ccomm.grenet.fr

Ms. Natasha Rainis, D.E.A.
Psychologie Sociale de Grenoble
Université Pierre Mendez France
4738040 Grenoble CEDEX 9
FRANCE
rainis@grenet.fr

Dr. Jane Rawls
Clinical and Child Psychologist
3 Te Aroha Street
Hamilton
NEW ZEALAND

Dr. J. Don Read
Department of Psychology
University of Lethbridge
4401 University Drive
Lethbridge, AB T1K 3M4
CANADA
read@hg.uleth.ca

Dr. Noelle Robertson
Psychology, Hadleigh House
Leicester General Hospital
Gwendolyn Road
Leicester LE5 4PW, UK

Dr. Martha Rogers
Clinical & Forensic Psychology
17662 Irvine Boulevard, Suite 12
Tustin, CA 92680, USA
rtandb@aol.com

Dr. Marilyn P.Safir
Department of Psychology
University of Haifa
Haifa 31905
ISRAEL
msafir@psy.haifa.ac.il

Dr. Jonathan Schooler
Department of Psychology
University of Pittsburgh
635 LRDC
Pittsburgh PA 15260
USA
jonathan@lrdc2.lrdc.pitt.edu

Dr. Art Shimamura
Department of Psychology
University of California - Berkeley
Berkeley, CA 94720
USA
aps@garnet.berkeley.edu

Dr. Daniel Shuman
School of Law
Southern Methodist University
P.O. Box 750116
Dallas, TX 75275-0116
USA
dshuman@mail.smu.edu

Dr. Marie-Christine Simon de Bergen
La Residence Sociale
3 Avenue de L'Europe
92300 Levallois Perret, FRANCE
scheps@ext.jussieu.fr

Dr. Eva Smith,
Professor of Law
Institute of Legal Science, A
University of Copenhagen
6, Studiestraede, DK-1455
Copenhagen K, DENMARK

Dr. Siegfried L. Sporer
Department of Psychology
University of Aberdeen
Old Aberdeen, Scotland AB9 2UB, UK
sporer@aberdeen.ac.uk

Dr. Max Steller
Institut fur Forensische Psychiatrie
Freie Universitaet Berlin
Limonenstr. 27
D -12203 Berlin, GERMANY
msteller@zedat.fu-berlin.de

Dr. Sherry H. Stewart
Department of Psychology
Dalhousie University
Halifax, Nova Scotia B3H 4J1
CANADA
sstewart@ac.dal.ca

Dr. Bettina von Lovenberg
Institut fur Forensische Psychiatrie
Freie Universitat Berlin
Limonenstr. 27
D-12203 Berlin
GERMANY
msteller@zedat.fu-berlin.de

Dr. Willem Wagenaar
Department of Experimental and
   Theoretical Psychology
Leiden University
P.O. Box 9555, (Wasenaarseweg 52)
2300 RB Leiden
THE NETHERLANDS
wagenaar@rulfsw.leidenuniv.nl

Dr. Nancy E. Walker
Department of Psychology
Creighton University
Omaha, NE 68178, USA
nwalker@creighton.edu

Dr. Cathy S. Widom
School of Criminal Justice
SUNY–Albany
135 Western Avenue
Albany, NY 12222, USA
cw887@albany.albany.edu

Dr. Linda Williams
Director of Research
Stone Center
Wellesley College
106 Central St.
Wellesley, MA 02181, USA
lwilliams@wellesley.edu

Dr. Daniel B. Wright
Department of Psychology
University of Bristol
8 Woodland Road BS8 1TN, UK
d.b.wright@bristol.ac.uk

Dr. Rachel Yehuda
Department of Psychology
The Mount Sinai School of Medicine
One Gustave L. Levy Place
New York, NY 10029-6574, USA
yehuda.rachel@bronx.va.gov

Dr. Maria S. Zaragoza
Department of Psychology
Kent State University
Kent, Ohio 44242, USA
mzaragoz@phoenix.kent.edu

INDEX

DATE DUE

MAY 0 4 1999			
MAY 2 7 1999			
FEB 0 8 2000			
RET'D OCT 3 1 2000			
RET'D JUL 1 8 2002			
APR 2 5 2004			
RET'D JUL 0 2 2004			